THE OXFORD HANDBOOK OF

THE COGNITIVE SCIENCE OF RELIGION

THE OXFORD HANDBOOK OF
THE COGNITIVE SCIENCE OF RELIGION

Edited by

JUSTIN L. BARRETT

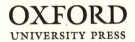

Oxford University Press is a department of the University of Oxford. It furthers
the University's objective of excellence in research, scholarship, and education
by publishing worldwide. Oxford is a registered trade mark of Oxford University
Press in the UK and certain other countries.

Published in the United States of America by Oxford University Press
198 Madison Avenue, New York, NY 10016, United States of America.

© Oxford University Press 2022

All rights reserved. No part of this publication may be reproduced, stored in
a retrieval system, or transmitted, in any form or by any means, without the
prior permission in writing of Oxford University Press, or as expressly permitted
by law, by license, or under terms agreed with the appropriate reproduction
rights organization. Inquiries concerning reproduction outside the scope of the
above should be sent to the Rights Department, Oxford University Press, at the
address above.

You must not circulate this work in any other form
and you must impose this same condition on any acquirer.

Library of Congress Cataloging-in-Publication Data
Names: Barrett, Justin L., 1971– editor.
Title: The Oxford handbook of the cognitive science of religion / [edited by Justin L Barrett].
Description: New York, NY : Oxford University Press, [2022] |
Includes bibliographical references and index.
Identifiers: LCCN 2021025253 (print) | LCCN 2021025254 (ebook) |
ISBN 9780190693350 (hardback) | ISBN 9780190693374 (epub)
Subjects: LCSH: Psychology and religion. | Psychology, Religious. | Cognitive science.
Classification: LCC BF51 .O94 2022 (print) | LCC BF51 (ebook) |
DDC 200.1/9—dc23
LC record available at https://lccn.loc.gov/2021025253
LC ebook record available at https://lccn.loc.gov/2021025254

DOI: 10.1093/oxfordhb/9780190693350.001.0001

3 5 7 9 8 6 4 2

Printed by Integrated Books International, United States of America

Contents

List of Contributors   ix

PART I: HISTORICAL, THEORETICAL, AND METHODOLOGICAL FOUNDATIONS OF CSR

1. Ghostly Relationships: Differentiating Cognitive Science of Religion and Psychology of Religion   3
   JUSTIN L. BARRETT

2. The Historical Genesis of Cognitive Science of Religion   13
   E. THOMAS LAWSON

3. Philosophical Foundations of Cognitive Science of Religion   27
   AKU VISALA

4. The Cognitive Study of Religious Activity: Beyond Religion and Belief   48
   PASCAL BOYER

PART II: RELIGIOUS CONCEPTS

5. Gods: Cognition, Culture, and Ecology   67
   BENJAMIN GRANT PURZYCKI

6. The Nature of Humans   90
   REBEKAH A. RICHERT AND KIRSTEN A. LESAGE

7. The Nature of the World   110
   JULIE B. SCOTT AND JUSTIN L. BARRETT

PART III: RELIGIOUS ACTIONS

8. Explaining and Solving Practical Problems Supernaturally   133
   RACHEL E. WATSON-JONES AND CRISTINE H. LEGARE

vi   CONTENTS

9. Mortuary Practices   145
   CLAIRE WHITE

PART IV: RELIGIOUS OBJECTS

10. Scripturalism: A Theory   167
    BRIAN MALLEY

11. Special Objects   191
    TYLER S. GREENWAY

PART V: RELIGIOUS EXPERIENCES

12. Conceiving Religious Dreams and Mystical Experiences:
    A Predictive Processing Investigation   215
    ROBERT E. SEARS

13. Extreme Rituals   237
    DIMITRIS XYGALATAS

PART VI: FORMING RELIGIOUS SYSTEMS

14. Key Ingredients for a World Religion: Insights from Cognitive
    and Evolutionary Science   257
    JAMES VAN SLYKE AND D. JASON SLONE

15. What Is the Role of Ritual in Binding Communities Together?   278
    HARVEY WHITEHOUSE AND CHRISTOPHER M. KAVANAGH

16. The Failure of Religious Systems   303
    HUGH TURPIN AND JONATHAN A. LANMAN

PART VII: CSR'S RELATIONS AND IMPLICATIONS

17. Neuroscience of Religion   327
    UFFE SCHJOEDT AND MICHIEL VAN ELK

18. Soul Mates? Conflicts and Complementarities in the
    Evolutionary and Cognitive Sciences of Religion   349
    RICHARD SOSIS, JOHN SHAVER, BENJAMIN GRANT PURZYCKI,
    AND JORDAN KIPER

19. CSR and Religious Belief: Epistemic Friends or Foes?	371
HANS VAN EYGHEN	
20. The Cultural and Developmental Niche of Religious Cognitions: Educational Implications of the Cognitive Science of Religion	389
REBEKAH A. RICHERT	
21. Lived Faith and Cognitive Intuitions: Some Theological Implications of Cognitive Science of Religion	411
LAIRD R. O. EDMAN AND MYRON A. PENNER	
Index	431

LIST OF CONTRIBUTORS

Justin L. Barrett is President of nonprofit Blueprint 1543, which does consultation for grant projects at the intersection of religion and the sciences. He has held positions at Fuller Graduate School as Professor of Psychology, and led the Office for Science, Theology, and Religion, as well as the Thrive Center for Human Development prior to that. Before Fuller, he held a post as senior researcher of the Centre for Anthropology and Mind and The Institute for Cognitive and Evolutionary Anthropology at Oxford University. He is one of the founders of the field of cognitive science of religion and is the author of numerous articles, chapters, and books concerning the topic.

Pascal Boyer studied philosophy and anthropology at University of Paris and Cambridge, where he did his graduate work with Professor Jack Goody, on memory and oral literature. He has done anthropological fieldwork in Cameroon on the transmission of the Fang oral epics and on Fang traditional religion. Since then he has worked mostly on the experimental study of cognitive capacities underlying cultural transmission, particularly in the domain of religious beliefs and behaviors. Pascal Boyer is the author of Religion explained (2001) and Minds Make Societies (2018). After teaching in Cambridge, San Diego, Lyon, and Santa Barbara, P. Boyer moved to his present position as Henry Luce Professor of Individual and Collective Memory at Washington University, St. Louis.

Laird R. O. Edman is a Professor of Psychology at Northwestern College in Orange City, Iowa. Much of his work centers on the implications of theory and research in the Cognitive Science of Religion for religious belief and practice. He has dozens of presentations and several book chapters and articles exploring these issues. Edman is currently writing a monograph with Myron A. Penner focusing on how CSR can inform our understanding of religious worship design. He has also published on critical thinking pedagogy and epistemology, and he is the recipient of four faculty of the year teaching awards from three different universities.

Michiel van Elk completed his PhD in Cognitive Neuroscience at the Donders Institute in Nijmegen (cum laude). He worked as a visiting researcher at the University of California Santa Barbara (2010), as a Marie Curie post-doctoral fellow at the École Polytechnique Fédérale de Lausanne in Switzerland (2010–2012), as a Fulbright Scholar at Stanford University (2017), as a Research Fellow at the Netherlands Institute for Advanced Studies (NIAS) in Amsterdam (2019-2010), and as Assistant Professor at the University of Amsterdam (2013-2020). Since 2020, Elk is affiliated as Associate Professor to the University of Leiden and as an affiliate researcher at VU University. Supported by grants from the John Templeton Foundation, NWO, and the BIAL Foundation, he supervises the PRSM Lab, which focuses on the study of psychedelic, religious, spiritual, and mystical (PRSM) experiences. By using a variety of different techniques, the aim of the lab is to understand how PRSM experiences come about, the effects they have on our behavior and well-being, and the philosophical implications of these experiences for our views on the self and reality.

Tyler S. Greenway is the Research Director at the Fuller Youth Institute and a Research Faculty member at Fuller Theological Seminary. He studies the psychology of religion, with a focus on application in religious contexts. He has published his work in a variety of scientific journals and edited volumes. He holds a Ph.D. and M.A. in Psychological Science from Fuller Theological Seminary and an MDiv from Calvin Theological Seminary.

Christopher Kavanagh is an Associate Professor at the College of Contemporary Psychology at Rikkyo University, Tokyo, and a Researcher at the Centre for the Study of Social Cohesion at the University of Oxford. His primary research interests are in the social and psychological dynamics of ritual events, East Asian religions, intergroup psychology, and research methodologies that combine field and lab-based experiments. He is also an enthusiastic advocate for Open Science practices, serves as assistant editor for the *Religion, Brain and Behavior* journal, and co-hosts the *Decoding the Gurus* podcast: examining online gurus, cult dynamics, and the psychology of conspiracy theories.

Jordan Kiper is Assistant Professor of Anthropology and Human Rights at the University of Alabama, Birmingham (UAB). Drawing from cognitive science, human rights, and philosophy, his research has examined the social conditions that induce commitments to peace or armed conflict, with particular interests in propaganda, nationalism, moral cognition, and the dynamics of religious systems. His work has also considered the influence of various types of propaganda and speech acts, including hate speech, on decision-making, intergroup perceptions, and support for violence. To explore these issues, he has conducted experimental studies and fieldwork in post-conflict regions of the Balkans, including Bosnia-Herzegovina, Croatia, and Serbia. Much of his current research is collaborative and cross-cultural.

Jonathan A. Lanman is Senior Lecturer in Cognitive Anthropology and Assistant Director of the Institute of Cognition and Culture at Queen's University Belfast. His work on atheism and secularization aims to provide an account of why some individuals become theists and others become non-theists, why some nations have higher proportions of non-theists than others, and why some non-theists engage in anti-religious social action. Alongside Lois Lee, Stephen Bullivant, and Miguel Farias, he co-led the international, interdisciplinary research program *Understanding Unbelief* from 2017-2021.

E. Thomas Lawson is Professor Emeritus of Comparative Religion at Western Michigan University, Kalamazoo, Michigan USA, and Honorary Professor of Cognition and

Culture at Queen's University, Belfast, Northern Ireland. He is the author of *Religions of Africa, Traditions in Transformation*, and coauthor with Robert N. McCauley of *Rethinking Religion: Connecting Cognition and Culture*, and *Bringing Ritual to Mind: Psychological Foundations of Cultural Forms*. He is the Executive Editor of the *Journal of Cognition and Culture* and the author of numerous articles in scholarly journals.

Cristine Legare is a professor of psychology and the director of the Center for Applied Cognitive Science at The University of Texas at Austin. Her research examines how the human mind enables us to learn, create, and transmit culture. She conducts comparisons across age, culture, and species to address fundamental questions about cognitive and cultural evolution.

Kirsten Lesage is a Developmental Psychologist. She received her Ph.D. in 2020 in Developmental Psychology from the University of California, Riverside and her B.A. in 2013 in Psychology and Spanish from Northwestern College. Her research interests focus on (1) the cultural evolution of how causal explanatory systems are transmitted (vertical and oblique), such as language, testimony, social learning, and rituals, (2) the emergence of explanatory worldviews in early childhood (folk, scientific, religious, supernatural), and (3) the role of the sociocultural context in the development of religious cognition and supernatural beliefs (e.g., concepts of God, prayer, supernatural causality). Some of her more recent work includes a set of cross-cultural studies examining Latinx parents' and children's causal explanations for biological illnesses (in the US and Colombia). Lesage is currently a Postdoctoral Research Associate for the Developing Belief Network – an international network of social scientists examining the development and diversity of religious cognition and behavior and studying variation in the acquisition and transmission of religious beliefs and practices.

Brian Malley is a lecturer in Psychology at the University of Michigan. His work addresses the interaction of individual cognition and cultural traditions, particularly in scripturalism and ritual. He is the author of *How the Bible works: An anthropological study of Evangelical Biblicism* (AltaMira, 2004).

Myron A. Penner is a professor of philosophy at Trinity Western University in Langley, British Columbia. His areas of research and specialization include epistemology, philosophy of science, philosophy of religion, and cognitive science of religion. His publications include journal articles in Faith and Philosophy, International Journal for Philosophy of Religion, Dialogue, and Toronto Journal of Theology. His current research focus is on scientific approaches to studying religion, which he is pursuing while a Visiting Professor in the Department of Psychology at the University of British Columbia. He is also involved in various collaborative projects with natural scientists exploring the intersection of science and religion.

Benjamin Grant Purzycki is an Associate Professor in Aarhus University's Department of the Study of Religion. He studies how and why religious traditions evolve to overcome problems associated with cooperation and coordination. In addition to managing

xii   LIST OF CONTRIBUTORS

large international teams, he has conducted fieldwork in the Tyva Republic in southern Siberia.

Rebekah A. Richert is a full professor of psychology, the director of the Childhood Cognition Lab at the University of California, Riverside, and a PI of the Developing Belief Network, an international, collaborative research network studying the acquisition and transmission of religious beliefs. Dr. Richert takes a cognitive developmental approach to study how children's developing social cognition influences their understanding of religion, fantasy, and media.

Uffe Schjoedt is an associate professor in psychology of religion at Aarhus University in Denmark. His neuroscientific research includes experimental work on the neural correlates of religious experience, as well as theoretical work on the relationship between religious experience and predictive processing. He is co-editor of the journal *Religion, Brain & Behavior*, and his research has been published in journals such as *Proceedings of the National Academy of Sciences, Social Cognitive and Affective Neuroscience,* and *Psychological Science*.

Julie B. Scott is a doctoral student in intercultural studies and holds a Crowell Ph.D. fellowship for the Center for Missiological Research at Fuller Theological Seminary in Pasadena, California. Her primary interests in research are the multidisciplinary and cross-cultural intersections of religion, cognitive psychology, cognitive science of religion, and missiology. She has authored and edited several scholarly books and articles in religion and mission studies, including editing for the *Oxford Handbook for Mission Studies* (forthcoming) and authoring and editing for the *Small Dictionary for the Study of Religion in English and Chinese* (forthcoming). She holds a B.A. in religion, M.A. in intercultural studies, MDiv, and is currently pursuing her Ph.D. studies in the intersection of intuitive cognition and intercultural missiology.

Robert E. Sears is a lecturer at TCA College in Singapore. His research and teaching interests span theology, philosophy, and various scientific disciplines, though his academic publications have largely dealt with the psychology of dreams and mystical experiences. He holds an MDiv and Ph.D. in Intercultural Studies from Fuller Theological Seminary in the United States.

John Shaver is an evolutionary anthropologist concerned mostly with understanding the relationships between social inequality, cooperation, and conflict. His recent research focuses on how religion impacts maternal fertility as well as maternal and child health. He has conducted demographic, ethnographic, and experimental research in the Czech Republic, Fiji, Mauritius, New Zealand, and the United States.

D. Jason Slone is a Professor in the Department of Philosophy and Religious Studies at Georgia Southern University. He holds a Ph.D. in Comparative Religion from Western Michigan University (2002), where he studied under CSR founder E. Thomas Lawson. He is the author of *Theological Incorrectness* (Oxford. 2004), the editor of *Religion and*

Cognition (Routledge. 2006), the co-editor of *The Attraction of Religion* (Bloomsbury. 2015), and the co-editor of *The Cognitive Science of Religion* (Bloomsbury. 2019).

Richard Sosis is James Barnett Professor of Humanistic Anthropology at the University of Connecticut. His work has focused on the evolution of religion and cooperation, with particular interests in ritual, magic, religious reproductive decision-making, and the dynamics of religious systems. To explore these issues, he has conducted field-work with remote cooperative fishers in the Federated States of Micronesia and with various communities throughout Israel. He is cofounder and co-editor of the journal *Religion, Brain & Behavior*, which publishes research on the bio-cultural study of religion.

Hugh Turpin is a postdoctoral research fellow at the University of Oxford. His research draws on cognitive, sociological, and socio-anthropological theories and methods to investigate processes of change in religious and moral worldviews. His particular specialization has been Irish secularization, and he is in the final stages of preparing his first book, *Unholy Catholic Ireland: Secular Morality, Religious Hypocrisy, and Irish ex-Catholicism*, for publication with Stanford University Press.

Hans Van Eyghen is assistant professor at Tilburg University. He previously worked at the Catholic University of Louvain and VU Amsterdam. His work focuses on the cognitive science of religion and religious epistemology. His recent book *Arguing from Cognitive Science of Religion: Is Religious Belief Debunked?* addresses the question of whether cognitive theories of religious belief undermine the epistemic status of religious belief.

James A. Van Slyke, PhD. is program director and associate professor of psychology at Fresno Pacific University. His first book was *The Cognitive Science of Religion* (Ashgate Press, 2011) and he also co-edited two books entitled *Theology and the Science of Moral Action: Virtue Ethics, Exemplarity and Cognitive Neuroscience* (Routledge Press, 2012) and *The Attraction of Religion: A New Evolutionary Psychology of Religion* (Bloomsbury Publishing, 2015). He has published articles in *Zygon, Religion, Brain & Behavior*, and *Evolutionary Psychological Science*.

Aku Visala is an Adjunct Professor in Philosophy of Religion and Research Fellow of the Finnish Academy at the University of Helsinki, Finland. He has held postdoctoral positions at the universities of Oxford (UK), Princeton (USA), and Notre Dame (USA). His work is located at the intersection of philosophy, theology, and the cognitive sciences. His publications include *Naturalism, Theism and the Cognitive Study of Religion* (Routledge 2011), *Conversations on Human Nature* (with Agustin Fuentes, Routledge 2015), and *Vapaan tahdon filosofia* ("A Philosophy of Free Will", Helsinki University Press 2018). He is currently working on a monograph on free will in science and theology. In addition to numerous research articles, he is the author of textbooks on philosophy of religion and the relationship between theology and science.

Rachel Watson-Jones is a Senior Principal Usability Engineer with Dell Technologies. In her current role, she leads both qualitative and quantitative research projects to optimize the user experience of commercial customers. Previously, she was a Postdoctoral Fellow within the Department of Psychology at the University of Texas at Austin. She has authored or coauthored numerous book chapters and scholarly articles in journals such as *Psychological Science, Evolution & Human Behavior*, and *Cognitive Science*. She holds an M.A. in Experimental Psychology and a Ph.D. in Cognitive and Evolutionary Anthropology from the University of Oxford.

Claire White is an Associate Professor in the department of religious studies at California State University, Northridge. She holds the first tenure-track appointment in the Cognitive Science of Religion in a religious studies department in the United States. Her work addresses the cognitive and evolutionary underpinnings of religion and grief. She is the author of *An Introduction to the Cognitive Science of Religion: Connecting Evolution, Brain, Cognition, and Culture*.

Harvey Whitehouse is Professor of Social Anthropology and Director of the Centre for the Study of Social Cohesion at the University of Oxford. His research focuses on the role of ritual in the evolution of social complexity, much of it conducted collaboratively with psychologists, historians, archaeologists, and evolutionary theorists. He is well known for his theory of "modes of religiosity" set out in a trilogy of books: *Inside the Cult* (1995), *Arguments and Icons* (2000), and *Modes of Religiosity* (2004). His latest book, *The Ritual Animal: Imitation and cohesion in the evolution of social complexity* (forthcoming with OUP), describes the results of many years of collaborative research on how different modes of ritual performance emerge, reproduce, and spread, and explores the implications of this for the future of human cooperation.

Dimitris Xygalatas is an Associate Professor of Anthropology and Psychological Sciences at the University of Connecticut. His research explores some of the things that unite and divide us, focusing on religion and ritual, sports, cooperation, and the interaction between cognition and culture. He has held positions at the universities of Princeton, Aarhus, and Masaryk, where he served as Director of the Laboratory for the Experimental Research of Religion. At UConn, he directs the Experimental Anthropology Lab, which develops methods and technologies for studying human interaction scientifically in real-life settings.

PART I

HISTORICAL, THEORETICAL, AND METHODOLOGICAL FOUNDATIONS OF CSR

CHAPTER 1

GHOSTLY RELATIONSHIPS

*Differentiating Cognitive Science of Religion
and Psychology of Religion*

JUSTIN L. BARRETT

SOMETIMES science is spooky. In April 2019, the University of Otago, in New Zealand, presented its annual ScienceTeller conference, this one called "Science and the Afterlife." Hosted by Jesse Bering, director of the Centre for Science Communication, and Jamin Halberstadt, professor of psychology, the conference was at once a science communication event and a psychological conference. The popular-science writers Mary Roach and Michael Shermer were keynote speakers, but leading psychologists in the study of concepts of death and the afterlife Virginia Slaughter and Natasha Tassell-Matamua also presented research from their own labs. The audience laughed heartily when writer-producer Paul Yates screened an episode of his comedy television series *Wellington Paranormal*; but things became a bit more sober when psychologist Quentin Atkinson shared research concerning the evolution of sacrifice, and Dr. Azim Shariff explained the social utility of hell. Such was the dual character of the conference.

A far less obvious duality also characterized the conference. Much of what was presented would have been perfectly at home at a meeting of division 36 of the American Psychological Association, the Society for the Psychology of Religion and Spirituality. Beliefs concerning what happens to a self, soul, spirit, or mind at the death of one's body surely relates to one's "religion" or "spirituality." Simultaneously, much of the ScienceTeller conference's content would have been familiar to those who identify with the scholarly area known as cognitive science of religion (CSR). Was it a CSR event or a psychology of religion event? It was both.

As sketched by E. Thomas Lawson (chap. 2, this volume), what has become known as CSR began as an initiative of anthropologists and religious studies scholars who were turning to psychology and the cognitive sciences to generate causal explanatory accounts for the recurrence and persistence of certain forms of cultural expression (Barrett, 2011, 2017b), such as the beliefs in the existence and action of superhuman beings (Boyer, 1994; Guthrie 1980, 1993), and religious rites and rituals (Lawson & McCauley, 1990; Whitehouse 2000). Psychologists came later, and so CSR developed largely independently of the much more established area in psychology known as psychology of religion (PoR). As the ScienceTeller conference made clear, however, it was, and is, no longer easy to distinguish between CSR and PoR. Both areas may turn to psychological research to account for the rise, persistence, and spread of beliefs, attitudes, practices, and identities concerning gods, spirits, souls, and afterlives. And yet, at least analytically, CSR and PoR have some differences in emphasis that are worth retaining.

This volume is a handbook for the cognitive science of religion. My intention in bringing together the chapters that I have is to create a foundation for the next twenty years of CSR scholarship. The present volume summarizes where CSR has been and where it is, and looks toward where it might go. To use a mountaineering metaphor, it establishes a base camp in preparation for the next climb toward CSR's summit. Yet we find that psychology of religion is sharing the same base camp even though its climbers are headed for a different summit. Without a clearer distinction among the directions to each of the summits, and some discrimination among provisions for making the next climb, scholarly mountaineers may find themselves on the wrong trek.

I therefore briefly synthesize the takeaways from the ScienceTeller conference with the aim of illustrating the often subtle differences between CSR and PoR. I then extend the lessons for CSR to the organization of this volume.

COMPARING PSYCHOLOGY OF RELIGION AND COGNITIVE SCIENCE OF RELIGION

A psychologist of religion attending the ScienceTeller conference may have discerned the following account joining up the various presentations.

> Some individuals have unusual dreams, near-death experiences, or other personal events that suggest that our conscious awareness is somehow distinguishable from our current physical bodies. These experiences may be caused by a pathology or of unknown origin. The development of children's understanding of death does not begin to stabilize around adult ideas of biological death until middle childhood, and so it may be that children are particularly susceptible to taking these usual experiences as strong evidence of the existence of spirits, ghosts, former lives, or afterlives. From childhood, we are also very susceptible to the power of cultural narratives involving these ideas that seek to explain the anomalous experiences. Once in place, such narratives may perform important social and psychological functions and need not be pathological.

One could construct such an account from Virginia Slaughter's explanation of how children's beliefs about death develop; from Deborah Kelemen's gripping anecdote concerning a late twentieth-century Louisiana boy's uncanny memories of being killed while a World War II pilot and her subsequent presentation of developmental research conducted with Natalie Emmons that demonstrates children's receptivity to ideas about pre-birth lives; from Natasha Tassell-Matamua's careful documentation of various near-death experiences and the people who have them; and from Jesse Bering's various experiments showing how easily children let suggestions about invisible beings shape their behavior.[1]

Such an account of afterlife experiences and beliefs captures many common features of PoR. In keeping with the spirit of William James's *Varieties of Religious Experiences* (1902), PoR gives a prominent role to personal, idiosyncratic experiences. These may be worship experiences, meditative states, or dreams and visions (Hood & Francis, 2013). Sometimes, but not always, psychologists of religion openly debate whether these experiences and the religious beliefs they seem to generate are pathological or not. Though Sigmund Freud leaned toward a negative assessment of all religious thought (Freud, 1989), subsequent psychologists have tended to be more discriminating between religious thought that is pathological versus that which is neutral or even beneficial. For instance, clinical psychologists of religion may distinguish between positive religious coping and negative religious coping (Gall & Guirguis-Younger, 2013). And though cultural settings are often regarded as important background conditions in a PoR account, the primary PoR unit of analysis is the individual. What does the individual believe, feel, and do religiously or spiritually? To what degree are these beliefs, feelings, identifications, and actions the result of personal history and socialization or enculturation? This primary focus on individuals leads PoR to have a strong sensitivity to the idea that being religious or spiritual isn't an all or nothing situation but comes in degrees. Individuals, then, can vary in religiosity or spirituality, and numerous instruments have been created to measure this variability (e.g., see Hood et al. 2018). Though PoR has concerned causes of religious experiences and beliefs, in recent decades it has stressed more greatly consequences of religious commitments on adherents (Barrett, 2010).

If one were to draw out a CSR explanation for afterlife beliefs from the ScienceTeller conference, the emphases would be slightly different, and the account might go this way:

> Because of maturationally common features of individual cognitive development, it is easy to think about selves as decoupled from ordinary human bodies. As Slaughter, Kelemen, and Bering all suggest, biological death is not easily conceived of as identical to psychological death. Perhaps the evolved psychological systems that handle mental states have different natural histories than those handling biological states. In any case, to the extent that mental states such as personal desires and memories are indicative of selves, the notion of selves existing before or after this biological life finds very "fertile ground" (as Kelemen notes) in individual human cognition.

---

[1] Videos from the ScienceTeller 2019 conference can be found at this YouTube channel: https://www.youtube.com/channel/UCbnpMDWkKipU7iBIfdDJn-A (accessed January 2020). The program of speakers for the event is available here: https://www.otago.ac.nz/scienceteller/programme/index.html.

Indeed, it may be harder to imagine not having existed at some point in the past or not existing at some point after death than it is to imagine having indefinite existence. Consequently, from childhood we are very receptive to cultural narratives that match with these cognitive predilections. For that reason, narratives that do not fit well (as in denials of prebirth existence, or prebirth existence being too embodied in an ordinary sense) may take more instruction and other cultural scaffolding for us to acquire. Furthermore, cultural narratives concerning disembodied ghosts and spirits who may be watching us and possibly morally interested (see Bering's and Halberstadt's studies), may make us less inclined to try to get away with cheating each other. Trustworthy people and groups with greater cooperation bred from trustworthiness, will often have a fitness advantage over less trustworthy individuals or fractious communities. Thus, individual and/or cultural evolution may have favored narratives of a certain sort. Some of these may be elaborated into practices concerning sacrifice (Atkinson) or beliefs about who will persist after death and who won't (see Joshua Jackson's presentation) and beliefs concerning afterlife punishment (Shariff). Individual human psychology, then, may at once be constrained by past evolutionary dynamics and also exercise constraint on contemporary cultural expression, expression that may further encourage or discourage certain modes of individual thought or action.

Such a CSR-style account has many points of overlap with the PoR account. Both appeal to various types of scientific data to postulate psychological dynamics that bear upon human propensities to think about and act upon certain ideas that are commonly regarded as "religious." Nevertheless, a CSR-style account possesses important differences of emphasis.

The most important difference between CSR and PoR is that CSR primarily concerns group-level expression as its focal unit of analysis, and not individual expression. CSR asks, "Why do people generally believe in the afterlife?"; PoR is more likely to ask, "Why does that person believe in the afterlife?" CSR may investigate why one group of people has a belief in former lives but another does not; whereas PoR may be more concerned with why two people from the same family deviate in their beliefs concerning former lives.

This difference in primary unit of analysis, in turn, impacts the role of "culture" in explanations. CSR takes cultural expression to be the thing that needs to be explained and turns to individual-level psychology and social-level interactions among individuals as primary mechanisms for explaining the type of cultural expression under consideration. This explanatory strategy is on display throughout this handbook and receives greater treatment by Lawson (chapter 2), Aku Visala (chapter 3), and Pascal Boyer (chapter 4). To oversimplify, for CSR, individual psychology has causal force on "culture"; for PoR, "culture" exercises causal force on individual psychology.

The unit-of-analysis difference in emphasis between CSR and PoR also helps explain why it is that CSR has often said little about "religious experiences" (but see Andresen, 2001, and Sears, this volume), particularly idiosyncratic experiences of individuals. Why individuals have the experiences they have is not what CSR typically sets out to explain.

Individual experiences become more interesting to CSR when they become shared or are interpreted in common cultural terms. At that point, they enter into the explanatory space that has been CSR's focus.

A further, but related, reason that personal experiences are not typically discussed in CSR is CSR's heavy use of selectionist models to account for recurrence of cultural forms. Because an individual's experience does not count as a group feature until it has been successfully reproduced or shared, much of the explanatory emphasis is on the mechanisms of successful transmission of the experience rather than the genesis of the experience. Analogously, evolutionary biologists often spend less time considering why this mutation rather than that mutation arose (they are often just labeled "random") and more time discussing the selection pressures that operated on a mutation to either preserve or eliminate it in a population. CSR scholars are typically more interested in the psychological, social, or other "selection pressures" on ideas or experiences than in the ideas or experiences themselves. For the same reason, CSR also rarely concerns itself with whether an idea had origin in pathology.

Because CSR does not focus on individual expression, one rarely sees mention of the standard PoR notions of religiosity or spirituality in its writings. Another reason questions of the degree of religiosity, religiousness, or spirituality in individuals are not the typical stuff of CSR is that CSR has taken a fractional (McKay & Whitehouse, 2015), building blocks (Taves, 2011), or piecemeal (Barrett, 2017a) approach to the topical space. That is, many working in the CSR area think we can make progress in the study of "religion" if we recognize that "religion" is, at best, a heuristic category rather than a causally coherent object of study (Barrett, 2017a). Because belief in an afterlife may have different causes and effects than belief in gods or ritual efficacy, for instance, we should not assume that these different forms of cultural expression cohere in all times and places. Consequently, being more-or-less "religious" may prove to be meaningful in only a carefully circumscribed context or defined in a very particular way.

For sake of comparison, consider another domain of cultural expression with very irregular boundaries: sport. Only if we have in mind a narrow domain of activities that we want to call "sports" will it be very useful to talk about one person being greater or lesser in "sportiness." Once we allow archery, baseball, bowling, boxing, distance running, downhill skiing, gymnastics, horseback riding, ice hockey, racecar driving, swimming, and weightlifting into the same category of "sport," the intercorrelation of competency among all of these is likely to be very low indeed. Sportiness becomes meaningless. Aside from specific cultural contexts (e.g., in which it is a proxy for degree of commitment to and participation in conventional Christianity), "religiosity" may have little explanatory utility.

On the other hand, breaking "religion" into constituent parts for study may be importantly incomplete if the parts are never put back together again so that we can better understand the whole of particular societies' religious traditions and how the various beliefs, commitments, experiences, ceremonies, rituals, and the rest play off of each other. How do beliefs in superhuman beings motivate ritualized behaviors that may contribute to the formation of social identities? Indeed, an important future direction for CSR will be to make more efforts to put the pieces together and attempt more comprehensive accounts of the traditions of particular groups.

I have not spent these few pages comparing PoR and CSR to argue for the superiority of one over the other or to try to discourage cross-fertilization and collaboration. Indeed, the ScienceTeller conference was a great example of allowing borders to blur. Many of the presenters have made noteworthy contributions to both CSR and PoR. I expect, however, that by drawing out the differences in emphasis between the two, we will better be able to see the relative strengths of each, and that unnecessary confusion between them can be avoided. PoR's tools for considering personal experiences may, for instance, importantly inform why some classes of religious thought are more prevalent in one society versus another because of, say, how different rituals help generate them. At times, it may be a mistake for a CSR scholar to treat personal experience as analogous to a random mutation. Such experiences may not be so random after all. Similarly, it may be that religious experts or leaders may be unusually high in degree of commitment and passion to certain beliefs and practices—approaching what PoR scholars have called "religiosity"—and so the PoR study of such individuals may help inform a CSR-style cultural-evolutionary account of the role of religious experts in spreading ideas that would be hard to spread otherwise. In this way, PoR may enrich CSR explanations.

On the cautionary side, attending to differences in emphasis and research strategies may prevent hasty claims of falsification or vindication. Stewart Guthrie (1980, 1993) has argued that humans have a natural tendency to anthropomorphize the natural world, which leads to the positing of humanlike beings such as spirits and gods. In an effort to add psychological precision to his argument, I drew upon research in the cognitive sciences concerning the detection of intentional agents, which, in the late 1990s seemed to show that our cognitive system(s) for detecting agents operated largely on low-level perceptual features of the environment and would readily treat even two-dimensional figures on computer screens as minded agents given the right cues of goal-directed movement (Scholl & Tremoulet, 2000). The idea, then, was that because humans readily see nonhumans as minded beings, they could easily entertain the idea that nonhuman beings were active in the world around them. Occasionally, they may even "detect" action that couldn't be attributed to a human or known animal and, thus, they might postulate a new kind of agent (Barrett, 2004). Though a key mechanism is postulated to be a piece of individual psychology, Guthrie's account, and my recasting of it, was meant to help explain why belief in gods, ghosts, and the like, are common in human groups, not why this belief appears in some individuals and not others. And yet, some psychologists have attempted to see whether differences in degree of sensitivity to detecting agents corresponds to differences in degree of religiosity or commitment to God's existence (Petrican & Burris, 2012; Riekki et al., 2014; van Elk et al., 2016). Notice that this is not the CSR claim, but it is an interesting PoR question inspired by the CSR account. Evidence bearing on one claim does not completely map onto the other, and so the evidence for and against such an association should not be too quickly taken to support or challenge the CSR claim. CSR and PoR will help each other best when explanatory precision is safeguarded.

The State of the Field

This handbook represents an attempt to snapshot the current state cognitive science of religion. The Part I, "Historical, Theoretical, and Methodological Foundations of CSR," broadly sets the stage. Its three chapters introduce readers to the historical, theoretical, and methodological foundations of CSR. Religious studies scholar E. Thomas Lawson offers a history of CSR and introduces some of the foundational theories. Philosopher Aku Visala then provides an overview of the philosophical foundations of CSR. Anthropologist-psychologist Pascal Boyer closes with an overview of the typical theoretical and methodological commitments of CSR. Together these chapters situate CSR and the rest of the volume in its intellectual space and help to remove some misunderstandings about the field that are occasionally voiced, such as that it was developed with Abrahamic religions as the primary subject matter, that it is intended to replace historical and ethnographic studies, and that it is committed to a nativist, modular model of the mind. None of these are fair characterizations of CSR, as Part I demonstrates.

Rather than tackle "religion" as a whole, as is typical in CSR, Parts II through VI address the subject matter by getting a bit more specific, dividing the topical space into religious concepts, actions, objects, and experiences. Part II, "Religious Concepts," begins with anthropologist Benjamin Purzycki discussing gods of various sorts. Psychologists Rebekah Richert and Kirsten Lesage then present a cognitive approach to how human beings are conceptualized, including the relationship of bodies, souls, and spirits. Next, theologian Julie Scott and I synthesize the cognitive and developmental research concerning how people tend to conceive of the natural world, such that they are drawn to see design, purpose, and even intentionality behind it.

Religious actions are discussed throughout the volume, but the two chapters in Part III are particularly illustrative. Chapter 8, by psychologists Rachel Watson-Jones and Cristine Legare, describes how people commonly use rituals, superstitions, and other cultural practices to solve practical problems. Then, in chapter 9, psychologist and religious studies scholar Claire White offers a cognitive appraisal of mortuary rituals.

Part IV, "Religious Objects." Anthropologist-psychologist Brian Malley provides a framework for thinking about sacred texts in chapter 10, "Scripturalism: A Theory," and psychologist Tyler Greenway offers a cognitive account of how mundane objects come to be regarded as special in chapter 11, "Sacred Objects."

Although CSR does not consider religious experiences as frequently as does PoR, it does not lack tools for considering experiences that come to be deemed religious or that might emerge out of religious practices. In Part V, two chapters give examples of how cognitive approaches might be applied to such phenomena. In chapter 12, anthropologist Robert Sears considers the mechanisms by which dreams may come to be regarded as religious. In chapter 13, Dimitris Xygalatas considers what happens when people undergo "extreme rituals" such as fire-walking or self-mutilation.

With the basic pieces in place, Part VI begins to put the pieces back together again. How do various components combine to form religious systems? Psychologist James Van Slyke and religious studies scholar D. Jason Slone address this question in chapter 14, "Key Ingredients for a World Religion." In chapter 15, anthropologists Harvey Whitehouse and Christopher Kavanagh focus on the role of certain types of religious practices to binding communities together around religious beliefs and identities. Part VI ends with chapter 16, "The Failure of Religious Systems," a discussion by cognitive anthropologists Hugh Turpin and Jonathan Lanman.

The final section of the book turns to the question of how CSR is related to two neighboring fields and to questions arising from philosophy and theology. As already noted, CSR and PoR often overlap. CSR is also sometimes conflated with two other scientific approaches to the study of religion: neuroscience of religion and evolutionary studies of religion. As with PoR, good fences, with well-maintained gates, make good neighbors, and so Part VII considers CSR's relationship to neuroscientific approaches (Uffe Schjoedt and Michiel van Elk, chapter 17) and to evolutionary studies of religion (Richard Sosis, John Shaver, Benjamin Purzycki, and Jordan Kiper, chapter 18). These chapters both sharpen the differences and highlight the most promising points of cooperation or complementarity among these scientific approaches. CSR shares many findings and tools with PoR, evolutionary studies, and (to a lesser extent) the neuroscience of religion. Although they aim at different summits in the same mountain range, these scientific approaches to religious phenomena may, at times, share the same base camp and supplies.

A volume of this sort would not be complete without some attention to the growing excitement about the philosophical, theological, and educational implications around CSR's findings and theories. Chapter 19, by philosopher Hans Van Eyghen, concerns whether CSR improves or threatens the epistemic status of some religious beliefs, including the existence of God. Rebekah Richert returns in chapter 20 with some reflections on how findings from CSR might bear on religious education. The handbook ends with psychologist Laird Edman and philosopher Myron Penner offering their reflections on how CSR might (or might not) be brought to bear on elements of Christian theology.

It has recently been observed that the dream that cognitive science would emerge as an integrated discipline in its own right has not come to pass (Núñez et al., 2019). The six parental disciplines (anthropology, artificial intelligence/computer science, linguistics, neuroscience, philosophy, and psychology) have largely retained practitioners' primary identity, and cognitive science has mostly become a subfield of psychology, with only very modest cross-fertilization from the other disciplines. As theologian Lluis Oviedo has observed (personal communication, July 2019), the situation seems more positive in CSR. Many CSR scholars move between disciplinary affiliations and draw on the findings of various disciplines, synthesizing them into treatments with certain distinctive features, including those enumerated above. As this handbook illustrates,

CSR cannot properly be regarded as a subfield of anthropology, psychology, or religious studies; it is something altogether new that draws upon the strengths of these disciplines and others.

In the twenty years since CSR was first named, considerable progress has been made. If CSR continues to draw on fresh insights from the various cognitive sciences and from its sister sciences of religion, its next twenty years promise to be even more exciting.

REFERENCES

Andresen, J. (Ed.). (2001). *Religion in mind: Cognitive perspectives on religious belief, ritual, and experience*. Cambridge, UK: Cambridge University Press.

Barrett, J. L. (2004). *Why would anyone believe in God?* Walnut Creek, CA: AltaMira Press.

Barrett, J. L. (Ed.). (2010). *Psychology of religion* (Vols. 1–4). Oxfordshire: Routledge.

Barrett, J. L. (2011). Cognitive science of religion: Looking back, looking forward. *Journal for the Scientific Study of Religion, 50*(2), 229–239. doi:10.1111/j.1468-5906.2011.01564.x

Barrett, J. L. (2017a). Could we advance the science of religion (better) without the concept "religion"? *Religion, Brain & Behavior, 7*(4), 282–284. http://dx.doi.org/10.1080/2153599X.2016.1249926

Barrett, J. L. (2017b). On keeping cognitive science of religion cognitive and cultural. In L. Martin & D. Wiebe (Eds.), *Religion explained? The cognitive science of religion after twenty-five years* (pp. 193–202). London: Bloomsbury.

Boyer, P. (1994). *The naturalness of religious ideas: A cognitive theory of religion*. Berkeley: University of California Press.

Freud, S. (1989). *The future of an illusion*. New York: W. W. Norton.

Gall, T. L., & Guirguis-Younger, M. (2013). Religious and spiritual coping: Current theory and research. In K. Pargament, J. Exline, & J. Jones (Eds.), *APA handbook of psychology, religion, and spirituality* (pp. 349–364). Washington, DC: American Psychological Association.

Guthrie, S. E. (1980). A cognitive theory of religion. *Current Anthropology, 21*, 181–194.

Guthrie, S. E. (1993). *Faces in the clouds: A new theory of religion*. New York: Oxford University Press.

Hood, R. W., & Francis, L. J. (2013). Mystical experience: Conceptualizations, measurement, and correlates. In K. Pargament, J. Exline, & J. Jones (Eds.), *APA handbook of psychology, religion, and spirituality* (pp. 391–405). Washington, DC: American Psychological Association.

Hood, R. W., Hill, P. C., & Spilka, B. (2018). *The Psychology of Religion: An Empirical Approach, Fifth Edition*. New York: The Guildford Press.

Lawson, E. T., & McCauley, R. N. (1990). *Rethinking religion: Connecting cognition and culture*. Cambridge, UK: Cambridge University Press.

McKay, R., & Whitehouse, H. (2015). Religion and morality. *Psychological Bulletin, 141*(2), 447–473. http://dx.doi.org/10.1037/a0038455

Núñez, R., Allen, M., Gao, R., Rigoli, C. M., Relaford-Doyle, J., & Semunuks, A. (2019). What happened to cognitive science? *Nature Human Behavior, 3*, 782–791. doi:10.1038/s41562-019-0626-2

Petrican, R., & Burris, C. T. (2012). Am I the stone? Overattribution of agency and religious orientation. *Psychology of Religion and Spirituality, 4*(4), 312–323. https://doi.org/10.1037/a0027942

Riekki, T., Lindeman, M., & Raij, T. T. (2014). Supernatural believers attribute more intentions to random movement than skeptics: An fMRI study. *Social Neuroscience, 9*(4), 400–411. https://doi.org/10.1080/17470919.2014.906366

Scholl, B. J., & Tremoulet, P. D. (2000). Perceptual causality and animacy. *Trends in Cognitive Sciences, 4*(8), 299–310.

Taves, A. (2011). *Religious experience reconsidered: A building block approach to the study of religion and other special things.* Princeton, NJ: Princeton University Press.

van Elk, M., Rutjens, B. T., van der Pligt, J., & van Harreveld, F. (2016). Priming of supernatural agent concepts and agency detection. *Religion, Brain & Behavior, 6*(1), 4–33. doi:10.1080/2153599X.2014.933444

Whitehouse, H. (2000). *Arguments and icons: Divergent modes of religiosity.* Oxford: Oxford University Press.

CHAPTER 2

THE HISTORICAL GENESIS OF COGNITIVE SCIENCE OF RELIGION

E. THOMAS LAWSON

INTRODUCTION

THE scholarly and eventually scientific study of religion comes with complicated origins and includes intricate multi- and interdisciplinary features. Historians, philosophers, theologians, psychologists, sociologists, and anthropologists have all found "religion" to be a subject worthy of interpretation and explanation. The discipline of comparative religion developed within the context of theological schools, but in the twentieth century it broadened to include departments of religion within secular academic institutions. This chapter will focus primarily on the relationship between comparative religion and the newly, but rapidly, developing cognitive science of religion (CSR), which was initially suggested in a context of secular comparative religion but soon attracted the attention of scholars in a number of disciplines, including cognitive anthropology and cognitive psychology and, eventually, evolutionary psychology. Recently, neuroscientists have also joined the discussion. This chapter will focus on the emergence of CSR by examining a series of questions, the first of these being . . .

WHAT PROBLEM WAS THE DISCIPLINE OF COMPARATIVE RELIGION TRYING TO SOLVE?

Every inquiry, whether scientific or not, begins with a puzzlement. In the case of the scientific study of religion from cognitive and evolutionary perspectives, the puzzlement was recognized long before scientifically minded scholars developed the means to solve it. The initial form of the problem emerged as soon as people, eons ago, recognized that certain forms of their own thought and behavior, which they took for granted, differed in both form and content from that of their neighbors, often in strikingly different ways. The emergence much later of the discipline of comparative religion consisted of an escalation, development, and adumbration of ways to face this puzzlement of differences by searching for ways that might lead to an understanding of the nature of those differences. Explicitly thinking about them sometimes suggested that they were in conflict, or that they might be variations on a common theme, or even that they were not as different as they seemed. Comparative religion, then, featured systematic thought that emerged out of common-sense perceptions of subtle and even glaring differences in the encounter with the thought and behavior of strangers. This kind of thinking was present in the minds of theologians, too, but also, eventually, in the thought of psychologists and anthropologists as well.

At its best, comparative religion, despite its earlier theological context, intended to develop an appreciative awareness of the great variety of religious ideas and practices, by whatever means were available within the humanities. The initial focus of comparative religion consisted of the treatment of ritual practices, mythic narratives, doctrinal statements, and even the philosophical status of truth claims, all oriented from within the confines of a specific religious tradition and its academic and priestly institutions. As Sam Preus (1987) has shown, by the sixteenth century, not only was which form of *Christianity* is true (namely, its Catholic and Protestant versions) a pressing question, but also, given the increasing exploration of the rest of the globe, which *religion* is true?! Particularly important for these earlier scholars was the gathering of the sacred texts of the "other" religious traditions (e.g., the sacred books of the East) and translating them into European languages, on the assumption that, once so translated, their very strangeness would diminish or even evaporate, and their underlying meanings would be revealed.

Added to this developing corpus of texts by comparative religionists (also referred to as "historians of religion") was a whole set of ethnographic descriptions, by anthropologists as well as by travelers and missionaries in distant countries, of people who transmitted their cultural knowledge and practice orally. Much of this information was gathered in the context of colonialism and has been subjected to rigorous critique (Said, 1979), and the theological context has not gone unscathed (Wiebe, 1990).

By the early twentieth century, everything necessary was in place for a genuine comparative religion in universities and in theological schools. With this big influx of information came a large problem set, and a quest for a method (or group of methods) for dealing with the issues that inevitably arose with the realization that all knowledge is "comparative." It became primary to recognize the importance of giving accurate accounts of the thought and practices of the various religions in their cultural contexts. One of the goals of comparative religion was to be descriptively adequate to the information available and to make sense of this fascinating new information by postulating its possible meanings.

The goal of the method of description of comparative religion was to be historically correct, culturally accurate, resolutely interpretive, and logically taxonomic. The historical aspect of comparative religion focused on the origins and development of a specific religious tradition, including whether or not it had a founder. The interpretive element attempted to find and disclose the meaning of the thought and behavior in practice. The cultural aspect focused on linguistic matters such as accurate translation. The taxonomic analysis engaged in the act of naming the different traditions, often regarded as systems of thought and practice with greater or lesser modes of theological discourse. Issues about the truth or falsity of religious claims were typically assigned to philosophy.

Within this general framework, the major question comparative religion paid attention to was to what extent (given a basic assumption that the similarities among religious ideas and practices were relatively superficial) concepts about superhuman agents, ritual officials, ritual scenarios, mythic narratives, theological systems, and doctrinal formulae differed from each other, and to what extent systematic thought about these beings, practices, narratives, doctrines, and so forth, provided sufficient grounds for clarifying the meaning of the religious elements. Inevitably, specific issues, such as whether the practices and the concepts associated with these elements were literal or symbolic, emerged as matters of great significance. Did the texts—uncovered by scholars of oral traditions and acquired by ethnographic research—really mean what they appeared to mean, or were these statements very indirect ways of conveying special information requiring special methods to comprehend them?

Scholars interested in religious thought and behavior discussed not only questions of meaning but also utility or function. Émile Durkheim (1965) and other scholars had an important influence on comparative religion by arguing that it was more important to focus on the usefulness or "function" of the ideas and practices of religions than on their truth content. Durkheim also insisted on the autonomy of this kind of inquiry. It was what religion *does* that mattered, and there was only one proper level on which to understand it: the social. In fact, the idea of the autonomy of the social level took hold, not only in the humanities, but also in the social sciences, to the detriment of psychological and biological modes of inquiry.

In sum, the general approach of comparative religion (and ethnographic study, for that matter) was hermeneutic; that is to say, the goal was the faithful interpretation of religious thought and behavior. The search was interpretive rather than explanatory, if by "explanatory" we mean a search for causal explanations that might lead to an account of why and how people produced, transmitted, and acquired such ideas, and why and how they felt the urge to practice them. Although the comparativists were aware that sociological, psychological, and even biological issues were at stake, they were willing to leave any such speculation to the social and cultural sciences. They had problems enough in finding the best descriptions and the most adequate meanings of religious thoughts and practices. In the long run, what they made available to a scientific mode of inquiry were notions such as gods, revelations, sacrifice, purity, danger, evil, moral codes, priests, hierophanies, initiation, and afterlife, along with important ideas about the historical development of religious institutions. At some point it became obvious that a scientific inquiry of some sort into the factors required to understand such thought and its attendant behavior was called for, and the cognitive revolution, which went beyond the strictures of behaviorism to focus on mental processes, provided a promising opportunity to do so.

What Problems in Comparative Religion Was Cognitive Science of Religion Trying to Solve, and Why?

By the second half of the twentieth century, a few scholars in comparative religion had begun to be well versed in the abundance of new information about religions that was available. They were also inspired by anthropologists engaged in ethnographic study in small-scale societies and by psychologists who recognized the importance of cross-cultural studies. Practitioners of comparative religion began to do fieldwork themselves in Asia and Africa, encountering the actual practices in situ that had only been read about but not observed in an earlier period. They also began to ask questions about the cognitive processes at work when people made theological statements or participated in religious rituals. Previously, this information had mainly been viewed from the proverbial armchair. Inevitably, this gave rise to the realization that it was necessary to begin to develop hypotheses about the data and even to devise experiments to test the emerging hypotheses.

Take, for example, the many narratives that had been transmitted both orally and textually in the data set. Did religious people take those accounts literally or symbolically? If they were symbolic, what was it about their content that required such special treatment? If they were literal, how did the concepts square with standard, common-sense knowledge about the world? Such questions gained in significance as the linguistic and cognitive revolution began to make an intellectual impact across disciplines, especially in the social and behavioral sciences. Even the disciplines emerging in the humanities, such as generative linguistics, argued that despite the apparent differences among human languages, they all had a common underlying structure (Chomsky, 1965). The search for a "universal grammar," a tacit cognitive mechanism that facilitated language acquisition and stability, attracted considerable energy and attention. Given that language differences were clearly cultural, it was not surprising that religious differences were seen as cultural as well. And if languages, at least at the syntactic level of analysis, proved to be governed by universal principles, why not religions as well? That is, a suitable causal explanation would need to account for both the variability and recurrence of religious expression across cultures. Mere appeal to "cultural" factors or historical peculiarities would not do the job.

Inspired by the work of Noam Chomsky and others, E. Thomas Lawson (1976) suggested that religious ritual was amenable to a similar kind of analysis; whereas anthropologists, such as Dan Sperber (1975), argued for a specifically cognitive approach to symbolic thought in general, by emphasizing the deep-seated mental equipment that makes experience possible. Anthropologists Pascal Boyer (1994), Stewart Guthrie (1993), and Harvey Whitehouse (1995); philosopher of science Robert McCauley and comparative religionist Thomas Lawson (Lawson & McCauley, 1990); and psychologist Justin Barrett (Barrett & Keil, 1996) began to explore ideas that would ultimately lead to the development of a cognitive science of religion. This convergence of thought is striking. Breakthroughs were occurring in both the humanities and the social and psychological sciences. For example, in cognitive developmental psychology, the idea that infant minds are best characterized as domain-general, generic information processors was set aside because experimental evidence showed otherwise: different schedules for the acquisition of information depend on the type of information involved (e.g., information about agents, capacity to imitate, false beliefs, and so on). New methodological advances were crucial, such as looking-time and habituation and dishabituation techniques. Boyer, Sperber, Lawson, Barrett, McCauley, and Whitehouse were having conversations, not only with each other, but also with the cognitive psychologists Ulric Neisser and Frank Keil, and others. In comparative religion, there was dissatisfaction with the explicit and implicit theological assumptions that were guiding the research, and discussions Luther H. Martin, Donald Wiebe, and Tom Lawson were having led to the formation of the North American Association for the Study of Religion (NAASR). This organization explicitly focused on secular and naturalistic approaches to the study of religious thought and behavior, and it began to invite cognitive anthropologists, as well as cognitive and evolutionary psychologists, to present papers at its meetings.

The first systematic treatment of religious thought and its associated practices to have special focus on religious ritual was a work by Lawson and McCauley ([1990]; see also Martin & Wiebe, 2017). They discussed the relationship between interpretation and explanation; analyzed intellectualist, symbolist, and structuralist approaches; showed the special role that language played in the quest for knowledge about religion; introduced a specifically cognitive approach to symbolic-cultural systems; outlined a formal and highly specified theory of religious ritual systems; and examined the semantic issues that emerged from such analysis. In addition to all of this, the book made many predictions that awaited testing in empirical and experimental studies.

The period from 1990 to 2000 was a very fertile period of scientific inquiry into religion from a cognitive and, eventually, evolutionary perspective and included much discussion about the importance of theoretical development and the envisioning at some stage of empirical and experimental studies that the theories suggested were both necessary and practicable. Very important, therefore, was the original work of Justin Barrett and Frank Keil (1996), who did the first experimental study in cognitive science of religion, one explicitly informed by notions emerging in cognitive science. This study made the crucial distinction between "theologically correct" thought and the quite different intuitive religious thought. The former was the consequence of deep reflection, whereas the latter was intuitive, rapid, and spontaneous. For example, when the people in this study were told stories about the gods, they systematically misremembered key aspects of the story. So, even though they had reflectively developed highly abstract notions of the gods, their cognitive biases about the limitations of all beings became apparent even in their judgments that the gods were bound by temporal and spatial categories. This early work was, in fact, a development of very important studies in cognitive science about heuristics and biases by Amos Tversky and Daniel Kahneman (1974) and also schema theory (Piaget, 1928, Bartlett, 1932), which now clearly became relevant for the study of religious thought and practice.

Cognitive science is an interdisciplinary endeavor that attempts to develop experimentally based theories that explain how minds work and why they work the way they do rather than some other way. Religious reasoning and theological reasoning (and the differences between them) are obviously relevant domains of thought in this endeavor (Lawson, 2012). That being so, the data provided by both ethnography and comparative religion provide all kinds of interesting but puzzling phenomena that are worthy of both a cognitive analysis and an evolutionary explanation. For example, in various religious traditions, the notion of gods, superhuman, or supernatural beings plays a significant role in human affairs. How do such notions arise? Why are they transmitted so successfully? Comparative religion accepts these notions as interesting, and can even trace their trajectories historically, but it does not offer or even attempt to offer a causal account of their emergence, transmission, and persistence through time. The power of CSR comes from its capacity to provide compelling, novel, and often experimentally based accounts for the emergence, transmission, and persistence of what appear to be similar sets of ideas and practices that are historically and geographically isolated and have been subject to philosophical critique and competing worldviews.

In the effort to answer these questions that ensued, two lines of theoretical development have emerged. The first involves a study of the human capacity for agency detection in the context of the important notion of "theory of mind." The second involves an inquiry into the tendency of this capacity to become hyperactive under special conditions. Theory of mind is the capacity to attribute mental states to others, which is to say, conceive of them as agents capable of acting intentionally. A host of experiments began to show the very early development of the human capacity to detect agents and to distinguish them from everything else in the world (Rochat, 2001). The tendency to attribute agency to an object even when it is not an agent (e.g., geometric figures) is also endemic in cognitive activity, not only in adults but also very young children (Biro & Leslie, 2007; Carey & Spelke, 1994; Gergely & Cisbra, 2003). Since thinking about ancestors, gods, and spirits frequently concerns speculations about those beings' thoughts and motives and occasionally concerns detection of their actions, perhaps the characteristics of these cognitive processes will provide clues for understanding the emergence, transmission, and persistence of god concepts, and the like.

Illustrative Specific Topics of Consideration

CSR focused on topics such as ritualized behavior, theological correctness, and successful narrative themes and began to provide important new insights about recalcitrant problems that arise from such human practices and concepts.

Ritualized Behaviors

Ritualized behaviors are not the only cognitive processes that cognitive scientists began to explore, however. Take, for example, a notion that is present in many religious traditions—namely, the compulsion to avoid contamination and impurity. In religious contexts people frequently engage in elaborate ritual activities to remove contamination, even if it is invisible. Hands that are clean are repeatedly washed; garments that are spotless are purified; buildings that are safe are protected, and so on. One avenue of investigation is the exploration of the significance of this kind of ritual activity from a cognitive evolutionary perspective. Boyer and Liénard (2006) suggest that humans implicitly understand, and are prepared to act on, the difference between signals of imminent danger versus potential danger. The built-in evolutionary response to imminent danger is freezing, fleeing, or fighting. The enemy is visible, and the threat obvious. The predator turning its gaze to you, or obviously stalking you, is an immediate threat and triggers action. But many dangers are hidden. People become ill without an obvious or visible cause, or they behave in self-destructive ways for no apparent reason. This means that there are unseen dangers around that call for protection. Special kinds of action are required to perform such a protective role, whereas when the danger is immediate and obvious, the required action is immediate and obvious as well. The stimuli such as eye-gaze, stalking, and charging behavior are easily decodable signals. The stimuli for *potential* danger, however, do not consist of a clear set of warnings: these threats could be anything, anywhere. In fact, they are invisible. One moment you are well, and suddenly you are at death's door. What happened? You need protection against these invisible forces, and "ritualized" behavior often works. Of course, this realization suggests that a kind of explicit reasoning is taking place, but ethnographic work shows that this is not the case. Typical responses to a "why" question about ritual performance include "I don't know why we do it," "We have always done it that way," "Ask her! She might know because I don't, but we had better do it because it feels right." Performing ritual behavior is much more like acting on an instinct than explicitly following a set of instructions. Where does this "instinct" come from, and how do cultural conditions trigger it? To answer this question, a turn to cognitive and evolutionary psychology may be fruitful.

Religious Rituals

Another question that has arisen has to do with why some rituals are performed frequently and others rarely. Whitehouse (2004) and McCauley and Lawson (2002) have explored this problem both theoretically and empirically. The focus in both lines of investigation is on mnemonic issues. Both projects examined the question of what makes religious ideas memorable. McCauley and Lawson argued that the principle of superhuman agency distinguishes between two kinds of ritual profiles—*special agent rituals* and *special patient rituals*. In special agent rituals, the most direct connection to the gods is through the current ritual's agent. In special patient rituals, the most direct connection is either through the patient or recipient of the ritual action or through the act itself by way of the use of a special ritual instrument.

Unlike special patient rituals, special agent rituals are typically associated with sensory pageantry, unusual sights, sounds, and smells, which clearly makes them more memorable.

Why are some rituals reserved for an exclusive set of participants, while others are open to anybody who cares to participate? That is because some rituals are more central and therefore more important to the ritual participants, and their benefits, more consequential.

> Those rituals where superhuman agents function as the agent in the ritual . . . will always prove more central to a religious system than those where superhuman agents serve some other function (as, for example, when they serve as the passive recipient of a sacrifice. (Lawson & McCauley, 1990, p. 125)

When the god is more directly present in the action, the ritual matters most. Again,

> the theory predicts that the relative centrality of a religious ritual to the broader religious system . . . is a function (1) of the relative *proximity* of a culturally postulated superhuman agent to the manifest local agent within that ritual's structural description . . . and (2) of the *role* of that most proximal culturally postulated superhuman agent in the structural description. (Lawson & McCauley, 1990, p. 176; original emphasis)

Thus, rituals that have ritually closer *proximity* to the presence of a god (in terms of the number of previous rituals that enable the current one) and whether that proximity is manifest in the *role* of the agent versus that of the patient bear upon intuitions governing centrality and just who can participate in the ritual.

Theological Correctness

Why do people's judgments about the characteristics of the gods typically differ from theologically orthodox views? Theologically orthodox beliefs, or, as we sometimes refer to them, "theologically correct" statements, are the result of a great deal of reflection and often the consequence of vigorous and persistent debates about theological contents. They have a history in a specific religious tradition. But judgments about the gods that are based on religious intuitions, which come quite naturally, tend to be influenced by quite ordinary cognitive processes that are focused on the standard properties of agents. They often have a decidedly anthropomorphic flavor (Barrett & Keil, 1996; Guthrie, 1993).

Successful Narrative Themes

Ethnographers have often noticed the similarities in narratives from different cultural contexts. Is this just an accident, or do strong factors shape certain kinds of ideas no matter what the context? Scholars interested in the epidemiology of ideas (such as Dan Sperber, 1996) have suggested the notion of *attractors*. If we ask why narratives from different cultural contexts have such similar forms, the simple answer is that they are the kinds of narrative that are more successfully transmitted. They are successfully transmitted because, even given variation among a set of similar ideas, interesting microprocesses are at work. Sperber (2012) argues that when we study those processes, we see two things happening: both a preservation of what is being transmitted and the construction of a version of it that "suits the capacities and interests of the transmitter." But instead of compromising the stability of cultural items that are successfully transmitted, the items transmitted remain remarkably stable. Why? "Well, bits of culture remain self-similar not because they are replicated again and again but because variations that occur at almost every turn in their repeated transmission, rather than resulting in 'random walks' drifting away in all directions from an initial model, tend to gravitate around cultural attractors" (Sperber, 2012 p.180, Sperber, 1994). For example, any of Grimm's fairy tales, such as Red Riding Hood, survive the process of oral transmission because of their powerful and memorable themes: the threatening wolf, the innocent young maiden, and the happy ending. There may well be versions in which the wolf does eat the maiden, but the happy ending in which he does not is the more powerful narrative and, therefore, more likely to be transmitted.

WHY DID THE STANDARD MODEL OF CSR EMERGE?

Once evolutionary theory entered the picture and the dialogue among disciplines began to take shape, alternate modes of inquiry began to develop. At a certain point during this process, sufficient theoretical discussion and even experimental work had taken place to establish the framework for a standard model of cognitive science of religion. There were more agreements than disagreements, for example, about the role superhuman agents play or the importance of theory of mind. It became obvious that the early researchers had identified a number of areas of agreement about the cognitive dimensions of religious notions (Boyer, 2018). The first of these is a focus on minimally counterintuitive concepts (sometimes referred to as "modestly counterintuitive concepts"; see, e.g., McCauley, 2011). Religious concepts do not require any special mental equipment to account for their emergence. At most, they employ quite ordinary intuitive concepts, such as "intentional agent," with only one additional aspect seeming to be necessary for this particular mode of thought to do its job—namely, a counterintuitive aspect, such as *being invisible* or *superknowing*. Counterintuitive intentional agents, in particular, easily generate useful intuitions. These agents are not only regarded as being approachable but can also intentionally establish actions required to make one's social life work. Intentional agents of this sort are implicated and involved in ritual behavior. They either play a major role in the ritual action or provide backup for agents who are acting in their stead, whose job it is to bring about, for example, changes in status. This kind of ritual behavior is widespread, as any survey of data presented in comparative religion texts and ethnographic reports will show. The study of such accounts demonstrates a deep concern for such notions as contagion and contamination along with ritual practices emphasizing purification. And though they are not universal, ideas of the afterlife are certainly widespread and prominent in many religious traditions, as are notions of moral obligation. Intense discussions and analyses of these notions have taken place and significant experimental work has been published.

As so often happens in science, once a robust standard model is in place, there is much that the next generation can now take for granted (because the project has established relatively firm foundations), and thus they can see beyond the initial parameters. Theories are refined; new ideas can be explored, new techniques acquired, new dimensions examined, and new lines of research undertaken. As I have argued elsewhere (Lawson, 2017), a progressive rather than a degenerative research program is underway.

Although evolutionary concerns had never been ignored, they were not initially in the forefront in the cognitive approach to religion, for the simple reason that, before you can speculate about what role natural selection played in the emergence of the kinds of cognitive processes involved in religious thought and behavior, you had better have a reasonably clear idea about what religious thought and behavior are like, and what makes them susceptible to a cognitive analysis in the first place. You had better be sure that giving an evolutionary account of cognitive processes makes sense. Fortunately, a great deal of work, both about the notion of instincts and cognitive capacities, was already being developed (Barkow et al., 1992; Hirschfeld & Gelman, 1994).

Once the notion of human cognitive capacities had been developed, the theoretical and experimental work on religion became more specific, by showing, for example, that religion was an aggregate phenomenon that could be analyzed in terms of domain-specific capacities (Boyer, 2001). This meant that we could talk about individual systems, such as the *action representation system* (Lawson & McCauley, 1990), the *hazard precaution system* (Boyer & Liénard, 2006), the *hypersensitive agency detection system* (Barrett, 2004), which could all be calibrated by cultural input and understood as capable of maturation in a developmental context (McCauley, 2011).

WHAT ARE NEW DIRECTIONS FOR CSR?

Cognitive science of religion (CSR) is a progressive research program (Lawson, 2017), interdisciplinary in nature, that is maturing theoretically and developing experimentally. It should be no surprise that its initial interests have been broadened. For example, the study of religious behavior has been broadened to include extreme rituals (Xygalatas, 2012), religious experience (Taves, 2016), and the basis of institutions (Boyer, 2018), and new methodologies such as modeling and simulation (Lane, 2013). I will focus briefly on the latter.

McCauley and Lawson (1993) had already proposed the notion of employing artificial minds as methodological devices for explaining symbolic-cultural systems such as religious thought and behavior. They suggested the use of competence theorizing as the key for penetrating the intricacies of ritual representations. Initially, this approach to religious thought and behavior made little impression on scholars who were interested in the scientific study of religion. Instead, these scholars, after acknowledging the benefit of analyzing cognitive systems and processes, turned their attention to evolutionary considerations, which were thought to be more fruitful areas of inquiry. Much of subsequent inquiry focused on showing that religion was an aggregate notion of many different modular processes, each of which required its own explication, and all of which were viewed as a consequence of evolution. This move resulted in many insights about such notions as the role played by theory of mind, agency detection, and so on, in the formation of cultural structures. Furthermore, this work led to lower levels of analysis at the neurological level of investigation and inspired some investigators to become expert in the use of such techniques as functional magnetic resonance imaging and brain stimulation (Schjoedt & Andersen, 2017). But this did not mean that modeling and simulation had no role to play in the development of the scientific study of religion. Good ideas eventually get their day.

Glimpses of this new direction can be seen in the work of Lane (2013) and Lane et al. (forthcoming), who bring computational modeling and simulation to bear on cognitive theories, such as Lawson and McCauley's competence theory and Whitehouse's divergent modes of religiosity. In his 2013 article, Lane laid out the rationale for taking CSR in a modeling direction; whereas, in his forthcoming paper (with Shults and McCauley), he subjects the Lawson and McCauley's competence theory to a rigorous analysis. Lane shows that these theories are empirically grounded and sufficiently specific to withstand computational modeling and testing. Lane argues that all of them (a) offer empirical testable hypotheses; (b) are theoretically compatible with lower levels of scientific analysis; (c) are broad enough to represent the diversity of religious concepts and behaviors; (d) are specific enough to generate data that can be tested against historical and future datasets; and (e) are multilevel in character.

What Are the Merits of CSR in Solving Problems the Methods of Comparative Religion Could Not?

The merits of CSR lie in the recognition of the importance of the explanatory function of science, instead of settling for interpretive strategies. This was a problem incidentally, not only in comparative religion, but also in the social sciences, where human exceptionalism often plays a major role in social scientific discourse.

CSR has also helped us recognize the importance of identifying the different functions that intuitive and reflective judgments play in religious thought and behavior.

This identification has clarified the tension between idealized religion, as it is frequently pictured in comparative religion texts (which are heavily focused on the great thinkers of the various religious traditions), and actual religious practice, which, though it includes reflective thought, is far more widespread in people's intuitive responses to superhuman agencies. Comparative religion textbooks are remarkably similar in that they label the major religions; include so-called primitive religions; and focus on beliefs, practices, founders, and doctrinal development.

CSR has also called attention to the role our cognitive capacities play in undergirding ritual practices, even when the standard modes of reflection in different cultural traditions suggest their irrelevance and even disharmony with the ideal cultural norms. Historians of religion often spend more time emphasizing the history of theological modes of thought than the history of the religious practices of ordinary folk, for example, the crucifix on the wall, the altar on the mantle shelf, the caution at crossroads, the string of beads on the wrist, and the silent prayer.

CSR encourages us to acknowledge the deep relationship between religious cognition and adaptive modes of behavior disclosed in evolutionary theorizing. In particular, CSR is helping us develop an understanding of how many religious representations are byproducts of quite standard and ordinary mental representations, and are not only born of esoteric and rare moments in cultural transmission. Their power arises from their association with evolutionary adaptations, not necessarily from their adaptiveness.

Finally, CSR helps us recognize the real reasons for the persistence of forms of religious thought and behavior despite standard cultural knowledge that would seem to provide obstacles to their persistence. Religious thought and behavior is much harder to eliminate than the cultured despisers of religion ever imagined. Part of the reason for this persistence of religion lies in its attention-grabbing qualities, a fact which has been demonstrated experimentally a number of times (Boyer & Ramble, 2001).

What Are the Limitations of CSR?

Even if we achieve an accurate and compelling causal explanation of religion capable of leading to an understanding of why religious thought persists, many forms of human knowledge that are relevant to the study of religion remain to be captured by the scientific net. For example, how consciousness emerges from the systematic firing of neurons continues to be a puzzlement. Serious investigation into the origin of consciousness might provide important clues about so-called altered states of consciousness. We certainly need to learn much more about the varieties of religious experience. William James made a good start in 1902, but there remains a great deal of work to do.

It is important to keep emphasizing that scientific explanations are never complete. Even though scientific knowledge is dependable for many purposes, it is provisional in nature. The next set of experiments might reveal unexpected anomalies or, occasionally, even overturn entire theoretical frameworks.

Although CSR has finally highlighted the commonalities, and even the universal recurring features of religion, the fact of the matter is that not all religious ideas are the same. There are important differences among individual religious representations, religious ritual practices, and, on the wider level, religious systems. Why are there differences and how important are they? While anthropologists tend to overemphasize the differences, sometimes to the extent of denying that there is a human nature, and succumb to cultural relativism, focusing on differences in specific situations can bring to light important features, for example by focusing on the differences between imagistic and doctrinal religions (Whitehouse, 2004).

We should always ask, what has been left out?

References

Biro, S., & Leslie, A. M. (2007). Infants' perception of goal-directed actions: Development through cue-based bootstrapping. *Developmental Science*, *10*, 379–398.

Barkow, J., Tooby, J., & Cosmides, L. (1992). *The adapted mind*. Oxford: Oxford University Press.

Barrett, J., & Keil, F. (1996). Anthropomorphism and God concepts: Conceptualizing a non-natural entity. *Cognitive Psychology*, *31*, 219–247.

Barrett, J. L. (2004). Counterfactuality in counterintuitive religious concepts. *Behavioral and Brain Sciences*, *27*(6), 731–732.

Bartlett, F. C. (1932). *Remembering: A study in experimental and social psychology*. Cambridge, UK: Cambridge University Press.

Boyer, P. (1994). *The naturalness of religious ideas*. Los Angeles: University of California Press.

Boyer P. (2001). *Religion explained*. New York: Basic Books.

Boyer, P. (2018). *Minds make societies: How cognition explains the world humans create*. New Haven, CT: Yale University Press.

Boyer P., & Liénard, P. (2006). Why ritualized behavior? Precaution systems and action parsing in developmental, pathological and cultural rituals, *Behavioral and Brain Sciences*, *29*(6), 595–650.

Boyer P., & Ramble, C. (2001). Cognitive templates for religious concepts: Cross-cultural evidence for recall of counter-intuitive representations. *Cognitive Science*, *25*, 535–564.

Carey, S., & Spelke, E. (1994). Domain-specific knowledge and conceptual change. In L. A. Hirschfeld & S. A. Gelman (Eds.), *Mapping the mind: Domain specificity in cognition and culture* (pp. 169–200). New York: Cambridge University Press.

Chomsky, N. (1965). *Aspects of the theory of syntax*. Cambridge, UK: MIT Press.

Durkheim, É. (1965). *The elementary forms of religious life*. New York: Free Press. (Original published in 1915).

Gergely, G., & Cisbra, G. (2003). Teleological reasoning in infancy: The naïve theory of rational action. *Trends in Cognitive Sciences*, *7*, 287–282.

Guthrie, S. E. (1993). *Faces in the clouds: A new theory of religion*. New York: Oxford University Press.

Hirschfeld, L. A., & Gelman, S. A. (Eds.). (1994). *Mapping the mind: Domain specificity in cognition and culture*. Cambridge, UK: Cambridge University Press.

James, W. (2004). *The varieties of religious experience: a study in human nature*. New York: Barnes & Noble Classics. (Originally published in 1902.)

Lane, J. (2013). Method, theory and multi-agent artificial intelligence: Creating computer models of complex social interaction. *Journal for Cognitive Science of Religion*, *1*(2), 161–180.

Lane, J., Shults, F. L., & McCauley, R. N. (Forthcoming). Modeling and simulation as pedagogical and heuristic tool for developing theories in cognitive science: An example from competence theory.

Lawson, E. T. (1976). Ritual as language. *Religion, 6*, 123–139.

Lawson, E. T. (2012). Religious thought and behavior. *WIREs Cognitive Science*. doi:10.1002/wcs.1189.

Lawson, E. T. (2017). Cognitive science and the growth of knowledge. In L. H. Martin & D. Wiebe (Eds.), *Religion explained? Cognitive science of religion after twenty-five years* (pp. 7–16). London: Bloomsbury.

Lawson, E. T., & McCauley, R. N. (1990). *Rethinking religion: Connecting cognition and culture.* Cambridge, UK: Cambridge University Press.

Martin, L., & Wiebe, D. (Eds.). (2017). *Religion explained? Cognitive science of religion after twenty-five years.* London: Bloomsbury Press.

McCauley, R. N., & Lawson, E. T. (1993). Connecting the cognitive and the cultural: Artificial minds as methodological devices in the study of the sociocultural. In R. G. Burton (Eds.), *Natural and artificial minds* (pp. 102–121). Albany: State University of New York Press.

McCauley, R. N., & Lawson, E. T. (2002). *Bringing ritual to mind: Psychological foundations of cultural forms.* Cambridge, UK: Cambridge University Press.

Piaget, J. (1928). *Judgment and reasoning in the child.* Routledge & Kegan Paul.

Preus, S. (1987). *Explaining religion: Criticism and theory from Bodin to Freud.* Oxford: Oxford University Press.

McCauley, R. N. (2011). *Why religion is Natural and Science is Not.* Oxford: Oxford University Press.

Rochat, P. R. (2001). Social contingency detection and infant development. *Bulletin of the Menninger Clinic, 65*(3: Special issue), 347–360.

Said, E. (1979). *Orientalism.* New York: Barnes and Noble.

Schjoedt, U. & Andersen, M. (2017). How does religious experience work in predictive minds?. *Religion, Brain & Behavior. 7.* 1–4.

Sperber, D. (1975). *Rethinking symbolism.* Cambridge, UK: Cambridge University Press.

Sperber, D. (1994). The modularity of thought and the epidemiology of representations. In L. A. Hirschfeld & S. A. Gelman (Eds.), *Mapping the mind: Domain specificity in cognition and culture* (pp. 39–67). Cambridge, UK: Cambridge University Press.

Sperber, D. (1996/1975). Why are perfect animals, hybrids, and monsters food for symbolic thought? *Method & Theory in the Study of Religion, 8*(2), 143–169.

Sperber, D. (2012.). Cultural attractors. In J. Brockman (Ed.), *This will make you smarter*, New York: Harper Perennial. 180-183.

Taves, A. (2016). *Revelatory events: novel experiences and the emergence.* Princeton, NJ: Princeton University Press.

Tversky, A., & Kahneman, D. (1974, September 27). Judgment under uncertainty: Heuristics and biases. *Science*, [n.s.] *185*(4157), 1124–1131.

Whitehouse, H. (1995). *Inside the cult: Religious innovation and transmission in Papua New Guinea.* Oxford: Oxford University Press.

Whitehouse, H. (2004). *Modes of religiosity: A cognitive theory of religious transmission.* Walnut Creek, CA: Altamira Press.

Wiebe, D. (1990). *The irony of theology and the nature of religious thought.* Montreal: McGill-Queen's University Press.

Xygalatas, D. (2013). Effects of religious setting on cooperative behavior: a case study from Mauritius, *Religion, Brain & Behavior, 3*:2, 91–102, DOI: 10.1080/2153599X.2012.724547.

CHAPTER 3

PHILOSOPHICAL FOUNDATIONS OF COGNITIVE SCIENCE OF RELIGION

AKU VISALA

INTRODUCTION

TALK about the philosophical foundations of cognitive science of religion (CSR) can be easily misunderstood. One may be tempted to think of CSR as a single discipline, theory, or approach, which could (or should) have a unified foundation. However, this is not the case. Instead, it is more accurate to consider CSR an umbrella term for more-or-less loosely connected hypotheses, theories, and approaches for explaining religious-type phenomena that spans different fields, from religious studies to anthropology and from cognitive science to evolutionary biology and neuroscience. Because of this diversity, many different philosophical assumptions are at play in the field.

There are recurring themes or questions in CSR that are labeled "methodological" or "philosophical." The philosopher and cognitive scientist Robert McCauley is undoubtedly a pioneer in the field. A brief glance into his collected volume *Philosophical Foundations of the Cognitive Science of Religion* (2017) reveals the following questions:

1. What is the relationship of interpretative methods and causally explanatory methods in the study of religion?
2. The related question of the disciplinary identity of the study of religion, for example, does it consider itself a science or a humanistic discipline?
3. What culture is and how it is related to the workings of human cognition?
4. How should we understand reductionism and pluralism in interdisciplinary relationships?

Researchers working in the field of CSR have various answers to these questions, but there is clear convergence around certain kinds of responses. In what follows, I will examine these questions, especially numbers 1 to 3, and suggest that a pattern emerges. (I leave number 4 mostly aside, since other chapters in this handbook deal with CSR's relationship to other fields in more detail.) CSR sees itself as a scientific research program that emphasizes causal explanation and experimentation, pushes for a close dialogue between religious studies and cognitive science, and, finally, insists that certain aspects of cultures and religions are best explained by invoking the workings of human cognitive mechanisms.

In the preface to his volume, McCauley states that getting CSR going required as much philosophizing as theorizing. When arguing for a new approach to the study of religion in the late 1980s and early 1990s, McCauley and his close colleague E. Thomas Lawson focused on demonstrating how theories from the cognitive sciences could be used to provide explanations of the kinds of phenomena religious scholars were interested in, such as rituals (Lawson & McCauley, 1990). They wanted to make room for an approach to religion that would consider the results of the scientific study of the mind and provide scientific-style causal explanations. Such an approach, they suggested, would only enrich the traditional approaches, not replace them or explain them away. A defense of this approach is still needed today, according to McCauley and his colleagues, as much as it was twenty or thirty years ago.

What follows is an outline of the recurring themes and core commitments of CSR that could be labeled philosophical. As I have already suggested, people in CSR seem to adopt commitments and make assumptions along certain lines, not by random. These commitments and assumptions hardly form "foundations" of CSR (though as a field of research striving toward a naturalistic analysis of its subject matter, it does not require a foundation supplied by philosophy), but they are used to structure how the field is presented and how it is defended against its critics.

The Byproduct Thesis and Five Core Commitments

To better understand the issues discussed under the philosophical foundations banner, it is instructive to look more carefully at the early (ca. 1990–2010) defenders and architects of CSR, especially McCauley and the anthropologist Pascal Boyer. The central motivation of these "early fathers" of the field was to formulate and defend an approach to the study of religion that would provide causal explanations for cultural phenomena (as opposed to interpretations, simple comparisons, or some such). Religious ideas, practices, and behaviors, they believed, could be, at least to some extent, explained. Furthermore, the explanations would not be based on other social- or cultural-level phenomena but on the cognitive and psychological phenomena studied by the cognitive sciences.

This is one of the field's central claims: unlike traditional social science approaches in which group-level phenomena are explained by other group-level phenomena, the main idea in CSR is that some aspects of group-level phenomena can be explained as the expressions or effects of individual-level phenomena. Moreover, the individual-level phenomena in question are not interpretation-type descriptions of folk-psychological mental content, but cognitive processing.

These basic assumptions (that is, some group-level phenomena can be explained by individual cognitive processes) can be applied to any cultural phenomena, not just religion. The third central assumption, however, was specifically about religion. This was the claim that there is no specifically religious cognition. This *byproduct thesis* can be clearly observed in McCauley's (2017) description of the central commitments of the early representatives of the field, including himself, Lawson, Boyer, Stewart Guthrie, and Harvey Whitehouse, just to name a few. The byproduct thesis can be further broken down into three commitments:

1. Employing the theories, methods, and findings of the cognitive sciences to the study of religion would yield significant new findings.
2. The mind has no special department for religion; that is, there is no specifically religious cognition.
3. Many forms of religious cognition are byproducts of mechanisms that have not emerged to process religious ideas but to solve other problems in the social and physical environment.

Unlike in some approaches in religious studies, the early cognitive scientists assumed that "the religious mind" is not a collection of cognitive systems specialized to process religious thinking and behavior. Instead, religious information is processed by cognitive systems whose main function is to process nonreligious, everyday information. This deceptively simple assumption allows the cognitive scientist of religion to apply and extend theories of everyday cognitive processing to include religious thinking and behavior.

As McCauley's third point suggests, the byproduct thesis is sometimes taken to be a thesis about the evolutionary history of religion. According to this interpretation, religious thoughts and behaviors were not selected for some specific benefit—that is, they are not adaptations. Instead, they are byproducts of ordinary cognitive systems, which are adaptations for nonreligious purposes. I will return to this issue later. Regardless of the adaptation versus byproduct issue, I want to suggest that the core of the byproduct thesis is a methodological commitment to the usefulness of the cognitive sciences. If a specifically religious cognition, separate from other areas of cognition, existed, it could be studied by religious studies alone. But this is exactly what CSR is against: religious studies theorizing about cognitive functions by itself. As we will soon see, a consequence of the byproduct thesis is that it takes religion to be a collection of various ideas, behaviors, and practices, not necessarily connected by some underlying essence or core.

In his book *Cognitive Aspects of Religious Symbolism*, Pascal Boyer (1993, p. 7) outlines his view of what a cognitive science of religion should look like. His formulation is still one of the most informative, and it summarizes the core commitments of early CSR very well:

1. The study of religion should be explanatory in nature, rather than interpretative.
2. Culture is not, as Boyer puts it, "an independent level of reality," but a collection of shared and widely distributed ideas, practices, and artifacts that are in people's minds.
3. The information-processing capacities of the human mind are relevant in explaining cultural and social phenomena, including ideas, practices, and behaviors. This is because the basic information-processing capacities of the mind are more-or-less resistant to cultural differences.
4. Theories and hypotheses regarding the information-processing capacities of human minds should be derived from cognitive and behavioral sciences, not from disciplines that operate on the cultural and social level of analysis.
5. The study of religion should not be reduced simply to either cognitive anthropology or history or some other discipline.

I will expand on these commitments in the following sections.

Naturalizing Religion and Culture: From Interpretation to Explanation

The byproduct thesis and the overall resistance to interpretative approaches go together. Some have argued that religion has a certain "essence" or core, such as the *sacred* or the sense of the *holy*. Against this, CSR maintains that the science of religion does not allow for this; religious ideas and behaviors are byproducts of ordinary, nonreligious cognition. It follows from this commitment that CSR pursues the causal explanations of the sciences, not the hermeneutical approach of the humanities. Many have, nevertheless, viewed the study of religion as a humanistic, interpretative discipline, committed, not to explaining religious ideas and actions, but to interpreting their meaning for those who are committed to them. From this point of view, explanation looks very much to be "reductionistic" (meant pejoratively). Contrariwise, the early CSR theorizers maintained that the science of religion should also seek to provide causal explanations.

Lawson and McCauley (1990) have done pioneering work in mapping out the differences and similarities between the interpretative and explanatory approaches in anthropology and the study of religion. They do not claim that the explanatory approach CSR champions will overcome or replace other approaches; instead, they "maintain that both interpretation and explanation are possible and that they can fruitfully interact to increase our knowledge. They are complementary not competitive" (Lawson & McCauley, p. 2). Along the lines of this *explanatory pluralism*, McCauley has consistently maintained that cognitive explanations of religious phenomena are always partial ones and do not provide an overall "theory of religion." Others in the field have not always displayed such humility. In his popular book *Religion Explained*, Boyer (2001, pp. 48–49) argues that CSR can and will explain many of the central features of religion, better and more scientifically than its competitors, including how it emerged, why it is so widespread, why it is so persistent even in our scientific age, and why people take religious beliefs to be plausible.

The core of interpretative approaches to human action is the claim that cultural phenomena in general, and religious phenomena in particular, are special kinds of phenomena, and as such they cannot be subjected to the type of causal explanations that the natural sciences successfully endorse. Boyer (1993) writes:

> The hermeneutic stance is based on the fundamental premise that phenomena of meaning cannot be the object of explanation because they cannot be causally related to other, notably physical phenomena. Against this framework, the "naturalised" view of cultural phenomena is based, precisely, on the assumption that "meanings," or in less metaphysical terms, thought events and processes, are the consequence and manifestation of physical phenomena. (p. 8)

The reason the hermeneutical approaches reject causal explanation is, in Boyer's view, the claim that cultural and religious phenomena cannot be understood in terms of physical phenomena; rather, they inhabit a world of their own—the world of meaning. However, as plausible this premise might seem, it is a mistake.

Let us take one representative of the interpretative approach as an example. According to the American anthropologist Clifford Geertz, human action cannot be causally explained because human action occurs in a meaningful context of ideas and reasons. In his classic article "Thick Description: Toward an Interpretive Theory of Culture," Geertz (1973) points out that his concept of culture is a semiotic one and explains:

> Believing, with Max Weber, that man is an animal suspended in webs of significance he himself has spun, I take culture to be those webs, and the analysis of it to be therefore not an experimental science in search of a law but an interpretive one in search of meaning. (p. 5)

Because culture consists of "webs of meaning and significance," it cannot be described as simple behavior; rather, it requires *thick description* to be properly understood. Geertz's example involves two boys who both contract their eyelids rapidly: in one, this is an involuntary twitch; in the other, it is a conspiratorial signal to his friend. As movements they are identical, but the difference in terms of meaning is enormous: one is a communication with a special message, and the other is meaningless. If the idea of thick description—namely, that describing actions includes describing the reasons and intentions of the actors—is taken seriously, then, Geertz argues, we should see actions as interconnected in a web of cultural meaning. As such, they cannot be explained by invoking general laws. Notice that Geertz explicitly associates explanations with the term "law"; explanation is subsumption under a general law. Instead of explanation, actions should be understood in reference to the meaningful context in which they occur. There can be no causal explanation of action because intentions and reasons do not exhibit law-like regularities.

Boyer and other representatives of CSR react strongly against views like Geertz's. They maintain not only that causal explanations of actions are possible but also that human actions can be, at least to some extent, predicted and put in a larger context of scientific knowledge. Human action is not as completely context dependent as it appears to be. Cognitive science, according to Boyer (1993),

> makes at the least the *principle* of the connection [of cognition and meaning] intelligible, by observing that the rule-directed manipulation of tokens of abstract symbols by machines of whatever nature (mechanical, electronic or biological) can simulate some regularities in thought processes. In other words, the shift to "physicalist" or materialist interpretation of cognition is made possible, because cognitive science has at least a minimal "causal story" to explain how thought processes can be actualised in material processes, as well as some practical implementations of that story. (p. 9)

There are two central claims here: (a) reasons, beliefs, inferences, and other mental processes do indeed exhibit some kinds of law-like patterns, and (b) these patterns have their source in underlying cognitive mechanisms implemented by human brains. Notice again that these two claims do not entail the complete rejection of interpretation as a useful method. Indeed, there surely is human action that only makes sense in a certain cultural context. CSR is committed only to the claim that there might be similar patterns across cultures and religions, and that these patterns can be explained by invoking the features of human cognition that are resistant to cultural differences.

Here CSR contrasts not only with the interpretative or hermeneutical study of culture, but also with the standard sociological approaches. Positions according to which cultures, religions, and societies exist relatively independently of individual minds are said to be *methodologically holistic*. One classical example is Émile Durkheim's sociological program. Durkheim claimed that the social world consists of "social facts" that are external to the individual. Whereas a natural scientist studies the facts of nature, a sociologist studies the facts of social life, which are as stable as natural facts. So societies (norms, roles, institutions, etc.) have priority over individuals. Further, Durkheim's program proposes that these social facts can be explained by describing their function and beneficial effects in the society. In other words, the explanatory strategy is *functionalistic*. The existence of an institution, norm, or a practice (e.g., religious practice) is explained by its beneficial consequences for society in general. The holist explains group-level events (cultures, societies) with other group-level events. Cultures and societies are parts of nature even though biological or psychological causes do not explain many features of social world.[1]

Many of the early CSR theorizers were critical of such views. Inspired by the evolutionary psychologists who were criticizing the *standard social science model* (Cosmides & Tooby, 1992, pp. 24–30), the CSR theorizers directed attack to the psychological assumptions that are inherent in sociology. Standard social science often ignores the ways in which the human mind shapes the social world. Instead, it seems to presuppose that collective representations, emotions, and tendencies are not caused by individual cognition, but by the conditions in which the social group, in its totality, is placed. Social systems are abstract wholes that supersede individual psychology. The central psychological assumption underlying this idea is that because complex and diverse behavior and thinking is absent in infants, it follows that adult mental capacity and organization originates from the social world. The mind is a "blank slate" until culture and society make their mark on it.

I will return to the nature of human cognition (see the section "Cognition, Culture, and Modularity"). Here, it will suffice to highlight the central point: for CSR, cultures and religions are not, as Geertz and Durkheim would have it, "symbolic systems or belief systems." Instead, they are collections of various kinds of mental and public representations whose nature and pervasiveness can be explained by invoking material causes (brains, environment, etc.). The cognitive anthropologist Scott Atran (2002) argues:

> Cultures and religions do not exist apart from the individual minds that constitute them and the environments that constrain them, any more than biological species and varieties exist independently of the individual organisms that compose them and the environments that conform them. They are not well-bounded systems of definite clusters of beliefs, practices, and artifacts, but more or less regular distributions of causally connected thoughts, behaviors, material products, and environmental objects. To naturalistically understand what "cultures" are is to describe and explain the material causes responsible for reliable differences in these distributions. (p. 10)

Since cultures and religions are ultimately not "entities" or "systems" outside the mind and the environment in which it is situated, the factors that explain culture and religion must exist in human minds (and their environments), and not in other "social entities," "social systems," or similar forces.

Boyer and Atran seem to be committed to a strong claim that all social facts are nothing more than an accumulation of cognitive processes and should be explained as such. Others, such as McCauley, seem to adopt a weaker line, according to which patterns in the operation of cognition might explain the prevalence of some aspects of some shared ideas and practices. Whether one takes the claim in its strong or weak form, the core commitment rejects the idea that social and cultural facts are *completely*

---

[1] For defenses of this type of social science, see, for example, Kincaid (1997).

independent from cognitive and psychological processes. In other words, when we want to explain an aspect of culture or society, we should not do it by simply invoking some other cultural or social event or tendency. We should, instead, "look downstairs" and invoke an underlying cognitive mechanism.

It is not difficult to see why these claims produce a distinctive approach to the category "religion." Perhaps the most central problem in the study of religion is whether there is a set of phenomena, ideas, or experiences that are distinctively religious and thereby escape psychological social-scientific explanations or analysis. The *religionists* or "anti-reductionists" answer this question affirmatively and maintain that there is a generative underlying principle in religion, such as the aforementioned sacred or holy. According to this view, religious ideas and behaviors are spiritual and imaginative creations that are highly resistant to explanations based on nonreligious, psychological, social, and biological factors.[2]

In opposition to religionism and "anti-reductionism," CSR takes a naturalistic stance and argues that "religion" is simply a vague collection of ideas, practices, and artefacts that does not necessarily have a core or essence at all. This claim has significant consequences. First, it attempts to circumnavigate the definitional quagmire into which one inevitably sinks when attempting to define religion. Instead of providing a refutable definition of what counts as religion, CSR seeks to study the phenomena that are sometimes categorized under the term but cannot necessarily be clearly demarcated from other, nonreligious phenomena. Therefore, CSR is not interested in drawing a clear boundary between religious and nonreligious rituals, religious or nonreligious ways of thinking about agents, or religious and nonreligious unusual experiences. Second, by rejecting the idea that religion forms its own, irreducible domain, one also rejects the assumption that religious beliefs, ideas, concepts, and practices have functionally specialized cognitive mechanisms. The denial of a specifically religious cognition is simply the byproduct thesis, as mentioned earlier.

The CSR approach to the category "religion" has one extremely important consequence. Boyer (2001) suggests that by assuming even a somewhat unified category of religion or a religious essence, one is liable to think that all aspects of religion, including representations about gods, spirits, ancestors, various rituals, beliefs about an afterlife and misfortune, as well as spiritual practices, can be explained in the same way. In other words, all religious phenomena have the same explanation. Boyer calls this thinking a "magic bullet" because it attempts to use one principle to explain all diverse religious phenomena. If we take the diversity of religious phenomena seriously, we should conclude that there cannot be a single theory of religion; instead, each phenomenon under the category religion might have a different explanation (Boyer, p. 298). This "piecemeal" approach to religion is widely endorsed by representatives of CSR.[3]

---

[2] For an overview of the debate, see McCutcheon (1999).
[3] Barrett (2011, p. 231) refers to it as "the piecemeal approach."

Cognition, Culture, and Modularity

If we adopt the piecemeal approach and reject the autonomy of the social realm, we can now ask how one should go about explaining cultures and religions. This brings us to Boyer's third and fourth commitments. Barrett (2007, p. 59) elaborates these as follows:

1. Basic functions of the human mind do not vary across cultures because human minds emerge from similar biological foundations (brains) in basically uniform natural environments.
2. Human minds are not "general purpose learning machines," but rather house a great number of cognitive systems that perform highly specialized tasks.
3. Specialized cognitive systems shape our perceptions and inferences, and sometimes even distort them instead of just faithfully recording "what is out there."
4. Specialized cognitive systems produce recurrent patterns in human thinking and behavior by constraining and informing possible ways of thinking and acting. Thus, recurrent patterns in, say, religious thinking and acting, can be explained by evoking these systems.

At least some mechanisms of the human mind are resistant to cultural variation. No one denies the obvious fact that individual minds are significantly shaped by their cultural and social context, everything from language to cultural practices. However, some information-processing tendencies can be observed across cultures. These can be utilized to explain pan-human cultural tendencies, such as religious ideas and practices. These universal, or near-universal, operations include various folk theories, such as folk psychology, folk biology, and folk physics, as well as basic inference, perceptual, and memory systems.

CSR maintains that anthropologists, religious scholars, sociologists, and others necessarily make psychological assumptions about, for instance, learning and the validity of folk-psychological belief-desire explanations (as Geertz seems to do), as well as about the transmission of ideas and practices. Often, the assumption is that "people who grow up in a certain group just 'absorb' whatever cultural models are held valid in that culture, and that this process of absorption is both simple and passive" (Boyer, 1993, p. 14). There is, however, plenty of evidence that human minds are not such general-purpose learning machines. This is the basis of the cognitive revolution: the human mind is not just a receptacle for whatever information happens to be in its environment; it actively selects, shapes, and even distorts information. Some pieces of information are easier to learn than other pieces of information. Some pieces of information tend to be distorted or amplified in a specific way. Thus the information-processing capacities of the human mind constrain the set of ideas and practices that could become widely shared in human communities.

The results of the cognitive sciences can also be used to launch a critique of the folk-psychological model of action explanation implicit in the hermeneutical and interpretative approach. We humans intuitively explain our actions by invoking simple belief-desire explanations: Why did Henry go to the pub? He went to the pub because he wanted a beer and believed that the pub had beer. However, we now know from cognitive psychology and related fields that folk psychology is at least partly mistaken. Belief-desire explanations of behavior often break down on both the individual and group levels. Sometimes, they even turn out to be post hoc rationalizations—that is, invented after the fact to make sense of actions driven by entirely different, subpersonal causes. Folk psychology also seems mistaken in its assumption that cognitive processes are transparent for those who have them. Geertz, for instance, seems to assume the existence of *first-person authority* in judging what is going on in an individual's mind. Against this, the cognitive perspective insists that some of the cognitive processes of the mind are invisible to the individuals themselves. For these reasons, CSR maintains that we should not derive our hypotheses and theories about the human mind entirely from social and cultural studies. This basic claim is endorsed widely in the field, including by Boyer, as well as by Lawson and McCauley (1990, p. 2).

The fact that the mind is not a general-purpose learning machine but a collection of specialized systems is crucial for CSR. It is crucial because it allows CSR to explain different aspects of religious thinking and behavior by invoking separate and functionally distinct cognitive mechanisms. The two concepts used in this context are "modularity" and "domain specificity."

The *modularity hypothesis* views the human mind as a collection of modules (units or individual systems) that are relatively independent and have specialized functions. The extent and the nature of modularity is hotly debated.[4] Fodor (1983) suggested that the mind consists of central processes that are not modular, such as judgment and decision-making, and peripheral systems that are modular, such as perceptual systems. Other versions of the modularity hypotheses have also been put forward. According to the *massive modularity hypothesis*, not only are the peripheral processes of the mind modular, but so are the central processes. The massive modularity hypothesis, defended, for instance, by Peter Carruthers (2006) and Dan Sperber (2005), extends the idea of modular structure to all cognitive processes, including judgment and decision-making.

Although many proponents of CSR have endorsed the massive modularity hypothesis,[5] it does not seem to me to be a necessary part of CSR's foundations. Most CSR researchers accept the following theses: (a) there are specialized systems that have

[4] See Barrett and Kurzban (2006). See also the debate between Peter Carruthers (defending massive modularity), Jesse Prinz (arguing against all modular architecture) and Richard Samuels (defending restricted modularity) in Stainton (2006, p. 1–56).

[5] Sperber (1996, pp. 119–134) follows evolutionary psychologists when he claims that there is no reason to presume that higher-level thought processes could not be modular. Both Atran and Boyer talk about inference systems and conceptual modules and connect them with massively modular architecture (e.g., Atran, 2002, pp. 57–58). Barrett only talks about "mental tools" and "specialized systems." McCauley remains agnostic about massive modularity.

cognitive effects ranging from perceptual to conceptual processes; (b) some operations of specialized systems are inaccessible to introspection; and (c) most specialized systems operate automatically. These do not, by themselves, entail massive modularity.

The modularity thesis should be kept separate from the claim that mental processes are *domain specific*. Domain specificity is not a claim about cognitive architecture but a claim about patterns in information processing: instead of having a set of general reasoning abilities that they apply to all tasks, humans have a number of different sets of cognitive abilities that are specialized to process only certain types of information in certain ways. The term *domain* is defined as "a body of knowledge that identifies and interprets a class of phenomena assumed to share certain properties and to be of a distinct and general type" (Hirschfeld & Gelman, 1994, p. 21). This definition would allow for the existence of domains such as physical entities and processes, substances, living kinds, numbers, artifacts, mental states, social types, and the like. According to this understanding, domains partition our world (classification of things, concept formation), operate as functional and widely distributed devices (cognitive competencies arising to solve particular adaptive problems), and have dedicated mechanisms (modules operating outside conscious awareness).[6] Domains and modules rarely coincide, however: although all modules have their own domain-specific input conditions, domains are usually considered to be more general and broader than the domain of a single module.

Given these distinctions, it seems that a commitment to domain specificity is enough for CSR. It appears that CSR is indeed committed to the claim that human cognition (at least in adults) houses a number of distinct domains of intuitive knowledge, such as folk physics, folk biology, and folk psychology. Boyer calls these domains *intuitive ontologies* that constrain and channel the adoption and transmission of new information. Although Boyer himself seems to be committed to massive modularity, CSR derives its explanatory power mainly from the existence of the domains of intuitive knowledge, not from the massive modularity thesis.

Cognitive and Evolutionary Explanations and the Naturalness of Religion

Moving on to Boyer's (1993) third and fourth commitments (see the section, "The Byproduct Thesis and Five Core Commitments"), we can now examine more carefully how domain-specific cognition explains cultural and social phenomena. As we have already seen, CSR seeks to explain ideas and behaviors rather than interpret them. One benefit of explanations based on cognitive accounts is that they produce testable

---

[6] See, e.g., Atran 1994.

hypotheses. A commitment to a scientific study of religion is a commitment to test and to evaluate theories and hypotheses based on empirical evidence. Here we see a criticism directed at other forms of religious studies, especially those oriented toward producing interpretations. The criticism is simply that interpretations and thick descriptions, such as ethnographic reports, cannot be directly tested and shown to be true or false. Against this, CSR should seek to formulate hypotheses that can, at least in principle, be subjected to empirical testing, in either the laboratory or real-life contexts.

Traditionally, philosophers of science have suggested that science explains its targets by invoking general laws. An individual event is explained when it is subsumed under a law as an individual instance of a more general pattern. The ultimate model for such a process is, of course, physics, which supposedly will provide the ultimate and most general laws of nature. This *covering law model*, however, fell out of favor toward the end of the twentieth century, for a number of reasons. For our purposes, the most important reason is this: philosophers of science have acknowledged that special sciences, especially the life sciences and behavioral sciences, only seldom explain anything via general laws. Instead, they invoke mechanisms and structures, thereby producing causal models.

Philosopher Robert Cummins (2000) gives us a useful model of psychological explanation. According to Cummins, psychology does not even aim at covering law explanations. Instead, when a law-like tendency in psychology is identified, it is seen as the target of an explanation, not as the explainer. The targets of psychological explanations are not individual psychological events or singular actions, but patterns, tendencies, and dispositions. These are often referred to as *effects*. After an effect has been identified (a bias in information processing, for instance), an explanation for it is sought in the stable activity of an underlying cognitive mechanism (a capacity). What explains psychological effects are the workings of cognitive and neural mechanisms. In this sense, laws explain nothing in psychology, they simply describe what needs to be explained. The explanation is provided by the model of how the mechanisms work.

Along these lines, CSR can be seen as an attempt to explain group-level tendencies and patterns by invoking the workings of individual-level—and interindividual-level—mechanisms. The target of the explanation is the set of widespread religious ideas and practices across human cultures (which may include explaining why particular types of these are differentially emphasized in a particular group). There seems to be a general human disposition to prefer religious concepts and behaviors. What explains the widespread nature of these ideas and practices are the universal cognitive mechanisms underpinning all transmission of cultural information. Because of their relatively invariant operations across different cultures, they drive cultural and religious information toward certain forms; they are the factors that drive the selection process of cultural evolution.

CSR explanations differ, to some extent, from basic psychological explanations, because they seek to explain the social-level effect, not individual-level effects. Ultimately, CSR aims at being a social and cultural science, not psychological and behavioral science. The link between the social and individual levels is *cultural selection*. Although there are a number of differences, the cultural selection of ideas and behaviors is analogous to biological selection. Features of biological organisms can be explained as adaptations to certain selective pressures. Similarly, patterns of ideas can be explained as outcomes of selection pressures created by the social environment and the cognitive mechanisms that process those ideas.

Sperber systematically developed the idea of selective explanation, and it was subsequently taken up by Barrett, Boyer, and other early CSR researchers. As Sperber (1996) suggests in *Explaining Culture*, to explain culture is to explain why certain ideas are more contagious than others. This explanation is partly provided by the constraints of human cognitive processing: some ideas are easier to learn, memorize, and transmit than others. The argument of CSR is that the operations of functionally specialized cognitive systems in different domains cumulatively make some representations "easy" to transmit, and that many of those called "religious" are in this group.

To illustrate the notion of selective explanation, Visala and Barrett (2019) have suggested the following analogy: Imagine that every day you bait and set a live animal trap in your garden and consistently catch rabbits more than any other type of animal. You want to explain why you are catching more rabbits than, say, squirrels or foxes. It may be that something about the trap or the bait is especially good for catching rabbits (as opposed to squirrels or foxes) or simply that far more rabbits around to be caught than any other kind of animal. In the case of culture and religion, our minds are traps for cultural ideas. No one denies that human minds universally produce and entertain huge numbers of catchy ideas, such as spirits, gods, souls, afterlives, and so on. What CSR suggests is that individual minds do not catch such ideas simply because there are so many around. Instead, there are so many around because the human mind catches these kinds of ideas more easily than it does, for instance, complex mathematical, scientific, or even just really weird ideas (McCauley, 2011). If the byproduct thesis is the central methodological assumption of CSR, this notion of the *cognitive naturalness* of religion is the central hypothesis: our belief-forming mechanisms are biased in such a way as to create a tendency or a disposition to acquire, think, and transmit some ideas we call "religious" instead of some other kinds of ideas.

As the chapters in this handbook reveal, there are many hypotheses on the table about why ideas about gods, spirits, souls, and afterlife are among those that are particularly catchy. I will not treat or even list those hypotheses here, since readers can find this information in other chapters of this handbook. Instead, I will address the issue of CSR and evolutionary explanations because it is relevant for the discussion of cultural selection (see also Sosis et al., Chapter 18, this volume). It is important to note that CSR uses evolutionary theorizing for different functions:

1. Cultural evolution is considered analogous to biological evolution and it is invoked in explaining the selection of religious ideas and practices.
2. In accounting for the emergence of human cognitive architecture by invoking evolutionary scenarios.

3. In sometimes locating and accounting for the role of religious thought or practices in human evolution itself.

The first function is widely accepted: CSR is indeed in the business of explaining the cultural selection of religious ideas. Furthermore, some CSR researchers spend many pages trying to account for the emergence of the mind in evolutionary terms (Boyer, 2001; Tremlin, 2006). Some have even suggested that Darwinian evolution should form a metatheory for all study of culture and sociality (Slingerland, 2008a). From 2010 onward, interest in the role of religion in human evolution also increased. Ara Norenzayan (2013) and Dominic Johnson (2015), to mention just a few scholars, have put forward hypotheses about the adaptive role of some aspects of religious belief and behavior.

The exact relationship of CSR and evolutionary explanation, however, remains unclear. Should CSR be committed to evolutionary explanations or even to the adoption of Darwinism as a metatheory for the whole field? It seems that two interpretations of CSR are available. On the first view, CSR does not need evolutionary biology and therefore does not need to take the evolutionary background of the human mind and human culture into its focus. CSR's closest scientific partners would be found in cognitive psychology and developmental psychology (Barrett 2012). According to the second interpretation, evolutionary considerations, and especially evolutionary psychology, are crucial for CSR; that is, CSR has a story to tell about the evolution of religion and the evolution of the human mind.

Interestingly, evolutionary considerations are almost completely missing from the work done in CSR in the 1990s. The index of Lawson and McCauley's (1990) book *Rethinking Religion*, for instance, does not even contain the word "evolution." Even in Boyer's early works, such as *The Naturalness of Religious Ideas* (Boyer, 1994), for example, evolution comes up only in connection to discussions about selectionist models of explanation; the evolution of cognitive systems or religion is not discussed at all. In the 2000s, Boyer went on to connect his work more closely with evolutionary psychology, but the divide between evolutionary and nonevolutionary preferences remained. Atran and Boyer clearly find such considerations important, whereas Barrett, Lawson, and McCauley do not. Barrett (2007, p. 59) even briefly notes that "evolutionary theoretical foundation is not strictly necessary" for CSR.

It is nevertheless useful to distinguish evolutionary explanations from cognitive explanations. Much ink has been spilled over the question of whether religion is an evolutionary byproduct or an adaptation. These should not be seen as mutually exclusive alternatives, mainly because of the complexity of the notion of "adaptation" itself. As biologist Jeffrey Schloss (2009) points out, the claim that religion is an adaptation is vague. It might very well be that some religious beliefs and practices are adaptations, and others not. Furthermore, it might turn out that some religious behaviors were originally adaptations to a specific set of circumstances but are no longer adaptive. Finally, it may be that some religious behaviors began as byproducts but then turned out to be favored by natural selection in some environments (*exaptations*). These are all live hypotheses. Moreover, cognitive and evolutionary explanations seem to exist on distinct levels of explanation. Sometimes this distinction is made in terms of *proximate* and *ultimate* explanations. Cognitive systems could be taken as proximate explanations of cultural selection, while the ultimate explanation of human cognition is provided by evolutionary biology and psychology. Perhaps CSR theories could be subsumed under a larger Darwinian explanation. Religion could be a byproduct on the psychological level, but that does not give us any clues as to how it might be understood at the biological level.

VARIETIES OF NATURALISM IN CSR

Finally, we still have one set of issues that is mostly left untouched—namely, the question of reduction, interdisciplinary relationships, and the identity of religious studies. These issues are pertinent because of CSR's defense of a properly *naturalistic* "science of religion." The "sciencing up" of religious studies consists of a process of naturalization; religious phenomena and their possible explanations are conceptualized in terms friendly to naturalism. In the process of formulating this position, McCauley and other pioneers of CSR had to deal with accusations of "reductionism."

Naturalism is notoriously slippery term. *Methodological naturalism* can be taken as one of the key commitments of the field. Methodological naturalism means simply that when explaining religious phenomena, one should invoke only natural processes and mechanisms, as opposed to supernatural or nonnatural ones. The naturalist, understood in this sense, does not invoke supernatural entities like gods and spirits in scientific explanations. It is relatively easy to put gods, spirits, and souls on the supernatural side; it is much more difficult to say exactly what qualifies as "natural." According to philosopher Steve Clarke (2009), naturalists often disagree on what kinds of entities can feature in naturalist ontology (whether mental states, intentions, social facts, or abstract entities like numbers, for instance, can be included), but they do agree on the core epistemological thesis of naturalism: naturalism is first and foremost a methodological thesis about the primacy of scientific methodology.

One should carefully distinguish methodological naturalism, which is a pragmatic commitment to scientific methods and background assumptions, from *ontological naturalism*, which is the full-blown commitment to a broadly naturalistic metaphysics, whatever that would entail. We can further distinguish hard and soft versions of ontological naturalism. *Strict, hard,* or *reductive naturalism* is often taken to entail a belief that the world is a physically closed system, and therefore everything in the world (including religion) can be sufficiently explained in terms reducible to physics. The natural sciences provide us with knowledge of these physical causes and effects. All other forms of inquiry are either reducible to the sciences or suffer elimination. With respect to religion and the study of religion, this program requires that religion must have an explanation in terms of natural sciences (or an explanation that is reducible to natural sciences). It also includes the idea that the academic disciplines dealing with human culture, societies, behaviors, and religions must be unified with the natural sciences with respect to methods and ontological assumptions.[7]

In contrast to strict naturalism, there are many versions of *broad, nonreductionist, emergent,* or *soft naturalism.* Nonreductive physicalism holds that the natural world is physically constituted but includes complex entities and processes that cannot be explained by the physical sciences or by explanations that are reducible to physical explanation. This entails rejecting the claim of the explanatory completeness of physics. Given this view, mental states, for instance, can be seen as relatively independent of the physical states that realize them in the sense that they can have explanatory relevance of their own. A similar analysis can be extended to cultural and social phenomena, which do indeed consist of physical parts, but cannot be explained in terms of their parts (Fodor, 1974).

As I have argued elsewhere at length (Visala, 2011), CSR need not be committed to hard naturalism but can make do with something like soft, nonreductive naturalism. If the core naturalistic commitment to scientific methodology is preserved, there is no need for strict a priori rejection of "ontologically vague" entities or social facts. Soft naturalism already has a clear foothold in CSR. Robert McCauley's account of intertheoretic relationships and explanatory pluralism is one such foothold. According to McCauley (2007), we should not a priori reject explanatory factors; instead, we should focus on the practical and contextual success or usefulness of different kinds of explanations in answering specific problems. "For the explanatory pluralist," he writes, "all explanations are partial explanations; all explanations are from some perspective, and all explanations are motivated by and respond to specific problems" (McCauley, p. 150). Such pluralism would reject any simple reduction or unification of cultural and social sciences to biology or psychology. This is because the reduction or elimination of established scientific theories or disciplines is highly unlikely, because these established disciplines have usually uncovered relatively stable causal relationships. Instead of reduction or unification, these disciplines should seek to build bridges between their theories and those of neighboring disciplines by discovering *interlevel identities*—that is, by identifying phenomena that are the subject of different disciplines.

Although McCauley's pluralism is developed in the context of the psychology and neuroscience interface, its morals are quite easily applicable to the relationship of cognitive science and the study of religion. Given the explanatory pluralist view, CSR should not be seen as an attempt to reduce religious studies to cognitive science or to unify its assumptions with cognitive science and biology but, instead, as an attempt to create explanatorily relevant links between ultimately autonomous disciplines. We can understand CSR theorizing as an attempt to create interlevel connections and to inform theorizing both in the behavioral sciences, by pointing out how the study of religious phenomena might provide new material for psychological theories, and in the study of religion, by providing psychologically plausible assumptions about the human mind.

[7] See, for example, Slingerland (2008a, 2008b).

The explanatory pluralist would not, however, insist on complete intertheoretic mapping. If the theories of religious studies make assumptions that do not map onto the assumptions of the cognitive sciences, this is not necessarily fatal to religious studies. Even if theorizing about religion were strongly informed by cognitive science, the study of religion itself would retain its autonomy in the sense that its theories need not necessarily map onto those of neighboring disciplines. Inquiry into religious phenomena can proceed in a piecemeal fashion, more "locally" than "globally," and it can be based on the usefulness of different kinds of explanations rather than a priori commitment to a set of naturalistically acceptable causes. Although CSR is compatible with the autonomy of religious studies as a discipline, it is important to realize that CSR does not, strictly speaking, entail it. This is because of its commitment to the byproduct thesis outlined here. If "religion" is a collection of different kinds of ideas and practices spanning different levels (social, cultural, cognitive, neural), perhaps they do not form a coherent subject after all. This, however, is an open question.

Mechanical Philosophy and CSR

One of the most recent developments in the philosophical foundations of CSR has been the turn toward the mechanistic analysis of explanations. In philosophy of life sciences, a new perspective has emerged. The *new mechanical philosophy of science* (e.g., Glennan 2017; Craver 2007; Craver & Darden 2013; Craver & Tabery 2016; Woodward 2003) promises to plot a course between the obsolete covering law model and the simple reductionism of hard naturalism. It does this by shifting the focus from laws and theories to models and mechanisms, which (so proponents argue) better reflect the everyday practices of biology, neuroscience, and psychology, for instance. A handful of scholars associated with CSR have adopted the mechanical approach and applied it to the foundations of CSR (Asprem & Taves, 2018; Visala 2011, 2018; Pyysiäinen 2009a, 2009b). The basic idea behind the new mechanical philosophy is in line with Cummins's view of psychological explanation (see the section, "Cognitive and Evolutionary Explanations and the Naturalness of Religion") but this time applied to all life sciences: these sciences do not explain by placing individual events under a general law; instead, they explain regularities in the actions of complex wholes (organisms, psychological systems, etc.) by invoking the operations of their constituent parts—namely, mechanisms (Bechtel & Wright 2007).

Adopting the mechanist approach would provide a number of benefits for CSR. First, it would retain CSR's commitment to "looking downstairs" for explanations without the commitment to strong forms of naturalism and theory reduction. Recall the discussion about naturalism earlier: the core of naturalism is a commitment to scientific methodology. By adopting the mechanist approach, CSR could maintain its commitment to scientific methodology without making strong assumptions about the "physicality" of cognitive mechanisms and the "vagueness" of social and cultural phenomena. In other words, there would be no need to draw strict a priori boundaries as to what counts as a properly naturalist and scientific approach, which would avoid, at least to some extent, the opposition between a "science-like approach" and the humanities. This is made possible by the notion of "mechanism" itself: mechanisms are not just the micromechanisms of brains, for instance; they can be partly social and cultural (Ylikoski, 2017). CSR could work with other social and cultural studies to try to identify various mechanisms across the disciplinary board.

Another benefit of mechanical philosophy of science for CSR is that it casts the explanation-interpretation divide in a new light. As we have seen, the defenders of interpretation and their opponents, including Boyer, take causal explanations as involving laws or law-like tendencies. For the hermeneuticians, culture cannot be explained because intentions and other mental states are context sensitive and do not follow laws. For their opponents, laws and regularities exist because mental states are products of physical systems like brains. Mechanical philosophy would reject the underlying assumption that both groups seem to share, that scientific explanation requires general laws or even law-like tendencies. This denial would go a long way in breaking down the distinction between interpretation and explanations altogether. Egil Asprem and Ann Taves (2018) suggest that interpretations might very well be incorporated into the mechanistic scheme: the subject's mental content (her intentions, beliefs, etc.) could be parts of the mechanisms that produce her actions. So, individual actions—for example, Geertz's conspiratorial wink—may very well have mechanistic explanations without being "reduced" to robotic responses or universal human tendencies. Indeed, interpretation might just turn out to be one specific case of mechanistic explanation.

CONCLUSION

I have now briefly identified and outlined some of the philosophical and foundational issues related to CSR. I began by discussing the byproduct thesis and the interpretation-explanation divide. I suggested that early CSR provided a distinctive way around this divide and argued for a specific approach to explaining religion and culture. According to this view, certain aspects of cultural evolution (the "stickiness" of gods, spirits, and religious behaviors) can be explained by invoking the underlying cognitive mechanisms. In other words, CSR aims to be a science of group-level culture and religion rather than a science of individual cognition. I concluded by examining naturalism, interdisciplinary relationships, and the ways in which CSR might benefit from adopting a pluralist and mechanistic philosophy of science. Hopefully, mechanistic thinking might also inspire future research in the area and help to identify more carefully the targets of CSR explanations. I hope that what I have said here will highlight the fact that even a naturalistic field of research like CSR cannot avoid deep philosophical waters.

Questions for Future Research

1. How would the practice of CSR be affected if its rather traditional view of cognition (computationalist, functionalist) were to be severely challenged?
2. What is the role of evolutionary explanation in CSR?
3. How could we apply the new mechanistic philosophy of science to CSR?
4. How could work in the philosophical foundation of CSR inspire new experimental work?

References

Asprem, E., & Taves, A. (2018). Explanation and the study of religion. In B. Stoddard (Ed.), *Method today: Redescribing approaches to the study of religion* (pp. 133–157). London: Equinox.

Atran, S. (1994). Core domains versus scientific theories: Evidence from systematics and Itza-Maya folk biology. In L. Hirschfeld & S. Gelman (Eds.), *Mapping the mind: Domain specificity in cognition and culture* (pp. 316–340). Cambridge: Cambridge University Press.

Atran, S. (2002). *In gods we trust: The evolutionary landscape of religion*. Oxford: Oxford University Press.

Barrett, H. C., & Kurzban, R. (2006). Modularity in cognition: Framing the debate. *Psychological Review, 213*(3), 628–647.

Barrett, J. (2007). Is the spell really broken? Bio-psychological explanations of religion and theistic belief. *Theology and Science, 5,* 57–72.

Barrett, J. (2011). Cognitive science of religion: Looking back, looking forward. *Journal for the Scientific Study of Religion, 50*(2), 229–239.

Barrett, J. (2012). *Born believers: The science of children's religious belief*. New York: Free Press.

Bechtel, W., & Wright, C. (2007). Mechanisms and psychological explanation. In P. Thagard (Ed.), *Philosophy of psychology and cognitive science* (pp. 31–79). Amsterdam: North-Holland.

Boyer, P. (1993). Cognitive aspects on religious symbolism. In P. Boyer (Ed.), *Cognitive aspects of religious symbolism* (pp. 4–47). Cambridge, UK: Cambridge University Press.

Boyer, P. (1994). *The naturalness of religious ideas: A cognitive theory of religion*. Berkeley: University of California Press.

Boyer, P. (2001). *Religion explained: The evolutionary origins of religious thought*. New York: Basic Books.

Carruthers, P. (2006). *The architecture of the mind: Massive modularity and the flexibility of thought*. Oxford: Clarendon Press.

Clarke, S. (2009). Naturalism, science, and the supernatural. *Sophia, 48,* 127–142.

Cosmides, L., & Tooby, J. (1992). The psychological foundation of culture. In L. Cosmides, J. Tooby, & J. Barkow (Eds.), *The adapted mind* (pp. 19–136). Oxford: Oxford University Press.

Craver, C. (2007). *Explaining the brain: Mechanisms and the mosaic unity of neuroscience*. New York: Oxford University Press.

Craver, C., & Darden, L. (2013). *In search of mechanisms: Discoveries across the life sciences*. Chicago: University of Chicago Press.

Craver, C., & Tabery, J. (2016). Mechanisms in science. In E. N. Zalta (Ed.), *The Stanford encyclopedia of philosophy* (Spring edition). http://plato.stanford.edu/archives/spr2016/entries/science-mechanisms/

Cummins, R. (2000). "How does it work" versus "what are the laws"? Two conceptions of psychological explanation. In F. Keil & R. Wilson (Eds.), *Explanation and cognition*, (pp. 117–144). Cambridge, MA: MIT Press.

Fodor, J. (1974). Special sciences (or: the disunity of science as a working hypothesis). *Synthese*, *28*, 97–115.

Fodor, J. (1983). *The modularity of mind*. Cambridge, MA: MIT Press.

Geertz, C. (1973). *The interpretation of cultures: Selected essays*. New York: Basic Books.

Glennan, S. (2017). *The new mechanical philosophy*. Oxford: Oxford University Press.

Hirschfeld L., & Gelman, S. (Eds.). (1994). *Mapping the mind: Domain specificity in cognition and culture*. Cambridge, UK: Cambridge University Press.

Johnson, D. (2015). *God is watching you: How fear of God made us human*. Oxford: Oxford University Press.

Kincaid, H. (1996). *Philosophical foundations of the social sciences*. Cambridge, UK: Cambridge University Press.

Lawson, E. T., & McCauley, R. N. (1990). *Rethinking religion: Connecting cognition and culture*. Cambridge, UK: Cambridge University Press.

McCauley, R. N. (2007). Reduction: Models of cross-scientific relations and their implications for the psychology-neuroscience interface. In P. Thagard (Ed.), *Philosophy of psychology and cognitive science* (pp. 105–158). Amsterdam: North-Holland.

McCauley, R. N. (2011). *Why religion is natural, and science is not*. Oxford: Oxford University Press.

McCauley, R. N. (2017). *Philosophical foundations of the cognitive science of religion: A head start*. London: Bloomsbury.

McCutcheon, R. T. (Ed.). (1999). *The insider/outsider problem in the study of religion*. London: Cassell.

Norenzayan, A. (2013). *Big Gods: How religion transformed cooperation and conflict*. Princeton, NJ: Princeton University Press.

Pyysiäinen, I. (2009a). Reduction and explanatory pluralism in the cognitive science of religion. In I. Czachesz & T. Bíró (Eds.), *Changing minds: Religion and cognition through the ages* (pp. 15–29). Leuven: Peeters.

Pyysiäinen, I. (2009b). *Supernatural agents*. Oxford: Oxford University Press.

Schloss, J. & Murray, M. (2009). Introduction: Evolutionary theories of religion—science unfettered or naturalism run wild? In *The believing primate: Scientific, philosophical, and theological reflections on the origin of religion* (pp. 1–25). New York: Oxford University Press.

Slingerland, E. (2008a). *What science offers to the humanities*. Cambridge, UK: Cambridge University Press.

Slingerland, E. (2008b). Who is afraid of reductionism? The study of religion in the age of cognitive science. *Journal of the American Academy of Religion, 76*(2), 375–411.

Sperber, D. (1996). *Explaining culture: A naturalistic approach*. Oxford: Blackwell.

Sperber, D. (2005). Modularity and relevance: How can a massively modular mind be flexible and context-sensitive? In P. Carruthers, S. Laurence, & S. Stich (Eds.), *The innate mind: Structure and contents* (pp. 53–68). New York: Oxford University Press.

Stainton, R. J. (Ed.). (2006). *Contemporary debates in cognitive science*. Malden, MA: Blackwell.

Tremlin, T. (2006). *Minds and gods: The cognitive foundations of religion*. New York: Oxford University Press.

Visala, A. (2011). *Naturalism, theism, and the cognitive study of religion: Religion explained?* Farnham: Ashgate.

Visala, A. (2018). Pro-science rhetoric or a research program? Naturalism(s) in the cognitive-evolutionary study of religion. In H. Van Eyghen, R. Peels, & G. van den Brink (Eds.), *New developments in the cognitive science of religion* (pp. 51–70). Cham: Springer.

Visala, A., & Barrett, J. (2019). In what senses might religion be natural? In P. Copan & C. Taliaferro (Eds.), *The naturalness of belief: New essays on theism's rationality* (pp. 67–84). Lanham, MD: Lexington Books.

Woodward, J. (2003). *Making things happen: A theory of causal explanation*. New York: Oxford University Press.

Ylikoski, P. (2017). Social mechanisms. In S. Glennan & P. Illari (Eds.), *The Routledge handbook of mechanisms and mechanical philosophy* (pp. 401–412). Abingdon, UK: Routledge.

CHAPTER 4

THE COGNITIVE STUDY OF RELIGIOUS ACTIVITY

Beyond Religion and Belief

PASCAL BOYER

INTRODUCTION

COGNITIVE studies have renewed our understanding of religious thought and behavior in domains as diverse as the organization of religious concepts like "ancestors" or "gods" (J. L. Barrett, 2000), their connection to human memory (Boyer & Ramble, 2001), the notions of an afterlife or reincarnation (White, 2016), the cognitive effects of rituals (Liénard & Boyer, 2006; Whitehouse, 2000), the tacit assumptions that govern prayer (J. L. Barrett, 2001) or those involved in funeral ceremonies (McCorkle, 2010; White et al., 2017), the connections between religious doctrines and social organization (Shariff et al., 2010), and many more.

Besides enriching our picture of how minds acquire and transmit religious concepts, the accumulation of empirical data and models leads to some counterintuitive conclusions concerning some of the central notions in the traditional study of religions. Psychological evidence and the historical record suggest that we should probably dispense with the notions of "religion" and "belief." As I explain below, both create considerable confusion and probably hinder the proper understanding of important findings in the cognitive study of religious activity.

WHY "RELIGION" IS A HINDRANCE

Students of religion frequently point out that the domain of religious thought and behavior is intrinsically diverse, with considerable historical and cultural variation in practices and ideas. This is certainly true, but this observation is usually combined with the assumption that there must be some features that are common to the various cultural products we call "religious," and to only those products. This, however, is very misleading. If anything, one achievement of the cognitive science of religion (CSR) over the last decades has been to show that no cognitive or behavioral processes are unique to religion. For instance, the concepts of gods and spirits that are usually central to religious activity are also found in legends, superstitions, fiction, dreams, and other kinds of fantasy (Boyer, 2003). The ways they are transmitted from one individual to another follow memory and relevance routes that apply to many other kinds of mental representations (J. L. Barrett & Nyhof, 2001). The tacit principles that organize religious ceremonies are found in many other areas of stereotyped or ritualized behavior (Eilam et al., 2006; Liénard & Boyer, 2006). Religious prohibitions are generally based on a disgust psychology geared to protection against pathogens (Schnall et al., 2008; Tybur et al., 2012). The experiences considered central to people's religious conviction or conversion are similar to experiences that occur in many nonreligious contexts (Taves, 2009). In sum, there is nothing sui generis about any aspect of religious thought and behavior.

The term "religion" is also misleading in another way, because it leads us to ignore important distinctions between types of "religious" activities. It has often led scholars to extend to all religious activities some features that were in fact true only of highly specific religious phenomena, which just happened to be more familiar to scholars. Most scholars of religion were (and still are) acquainted with some of the traditions of the "organized religion" of their time and place, such as Hinduism, Buddhism, Islam, or Christianity, as a direct result of growing up in places where those traditions were central to social life.

But religious activities in many human groups, indeed for most of human prehistory and history, took place away from such traditions. They occurred in the social interaction within small groups, with no literary traditions, doctrines, or scholarship. These activities, as I will describe, are so different from what the religions scholars are familiar with that using the same term, "religion," to describe them, almost inevitably leads to a serious distortion of both kinds of tradition.

This is not to say that the various kinds of activities we call religious share no similar features. The problem is that these are not features that matter in explaining thought and behavior. To reprise a classical illustration, there is no single biological category of "trees." Trees belong to various clades, such as Magnoliophyta (most flowering trees), Pinophyta (most conifers), ginkgoes, ferns, and others. Whether the term "tree" is useful is a matter of practical goals. For landscape designers, architects, or firefighters and for all animals that need shade or shelter, it makes sense to consider all trees as one kind of thing. But for biologists, who are trying to understand the evolution, ecology, or reproduction of plants, a birch tree has more in common with buttercups than with a spruce tree, so that the category "tree" is useless.

This is precisely the problem with the notion of religion, which confuses two main types of religious activity and makes it difficult to understand how either appeared in human cultures or survived cultural transmission. Despite the prudence of many religious scholars, the use of a single term has hampered our understanding of the cognitive and social processes involved.

INFORMAL RELIGIOUS ACTIVITY: BEFORE AND BESIDES RELIGIONS

Most of the features that we think are generally true of "religions" and that apply, for instance, to Buddhism, Christianity, Islam, Hinduism, and other familiar faiths, are very recent inventions. They almost certainly never occurred before historical times, and before the existence of large-scale societies with religious organizations. So, considering these "world religions" may be a bad starting point for an evolutionary model of religious thought and behavior. What are those misleading features?

- The existence of a doctrine in the sense of a stable set of common, coherent beliefs.
- The notion of faith.
- The pursuit by religious organizations of a common goal in terms of religious activity.
- The presence of priests or other specialists (ulema, rabbis, etc.) who are trained in the doctrine.
- The notion of religious communities or affiliations.
- Concern with the end of the world (eschatology) or the origins of evil (theodicy).

All these features are characteristic of religions in the modern world, but it would be very misleading to see them as relevant to the emergence and transmission of religious ideas in general, since they only appeared under very special social conditions.

There were religious representations and activities before there were religions, and there are many types of religious thought and behavior that are not associated with such organizations. I will use the term *informal religious activity or "wild" religious traditions*, to denote (a) all the apparently religious behaviors that occurred in human societies before the emergence of religious organizations—prehistoric religion; (b) all religious activities that currently take place in human societies that have no such religious organizations; and (c) all peripheral, often nonnormative or officially disapproved religious activities in places that do have religious organizations. In short, wild traditions are religious activity before, besides, and beyond religions.

The term *wild religious traditions* would be of no use if they had no distinctive features. What does this kind of religious activity look like?

1. It is pragmatic, in the sense that people mostly engage in it to achieve a particular goal or change actual states of affairs in the world, and they expect these religious activities to produce the desired change.

2. It is about misfortune and ways to palliate or remedy it, illness of course, but also accidents, failures in one's endeavors, etc.

3. It has special (superhuman) agents, since people construe both misfortune and protection from potential danger in terms of the causal powers of spirits, ancestors, ghosts, souls.

4. Its activities are often directed by specialists who are thought to have special qualities or competence in dealing with ancestors, souls, or spirits. These specialists undergo no systematic training, and there are no "schools" or particular traditions. They generally begin to practice after a period of apprenticeship with an established specialist. There is no organization of such specialists. There usually is some competition among practitioners, and reputations can fluctuate.

In brief, people's wild religious traditions are based on the notion that spirits or other such agents can cause misfortune, and that certain specific individuals are better equipped than most to counter that influence, although the way this is effected is inscrutable. This core may, of course, be accompanied by many other kinds of religious activities, such as divination, magic, or ancestor cult practices. I focus on spirits and misfortune because they are found everywhere and have important common features. By contrast, ancestor cults are more typical of sedentary, agrarian societies than nomadic ones or foragers in general.

This description may seem very close to what is usually called shamanism, and that, of course, is no accident; shamanism was and is one of the most widespread forms of religious activity before and outside organized religions. In anthropology, the term *shamanism* is usually taken, in a rather restrictive sense, to denote the specific belief systems and religious activities of Amerindian and Siberian populations. In a broader sense, it could be used to encompass all systems in which a specialist enters a trance or possession state that allows him or her to deal with spirits and restore their clients' well-being (Singh, 2018).

Briefly, that kind of religious activity focuses on pragmatic goals, especially on handling cases of misfortune, and centers on notions of spirits, souls, ancestors, and small-scale deities. This is true of most shamanism-like religious behavior in small-scale societies that are without religious organizations. But informal activity of this kind is also found in virtually all societies that do have established religions, usually in peripheral "cults."

WILD TRADITIONS ARE UBIQUITOUS: WHY RELIGIONS WIN BATTLES AND LOSE THE WAR

To present-day, Western-based scholars of religion, informal religious activity may appear marginal or unimportant, which would explain why it is not central to models of religious thought and cognition. But the fact remains that some form of what I call wild traditions was, for most of human prehistory and history, the most prevalent form of religious activity. This is also the case for contemporary cultures—that is, before conquest and colonization imposed organized religions on small-scale societies. Using the cross-cultural samples from the Human Relations Area Files, Michael J. Winkelman measured the probability of associations between particular features of "magic-religious practitioners." For instance, some of these practitioners are seen as special by virtue of their training; others are said to have inner qualities that make them different from typical individuals. Some use trance or possession, while others base their diagnoses on divination or tradition. Winkelman's systematic study shows that these traits are not randomly distributed but form three major clusters (Winkelman, 1990, p. 27ff.). One of the clusters is the *priest* complex, which includes religious officers who are full-time specialists and have high social status and political influence, whose functions often combine performing religious rituals with wielding judicial or legislative power. A second cluster is the *shaman and healer* complex, where specialists typically use trance or other altered states of consciousness to address problems such as illness or misfortune, or address such issues through divination and various forms of treatment. Finally, a *medium* complex combines those historical situations where individuals claim direct inspiration from ancestors or deities (Winkelman, 1990, p. 27ff.).

These different clusters of features do not appear randomly. If a society only has one type of "magic-religious" specialist, it is always a healer or shaman (understood as the types defined here). If it has two types of specialists, the second type is generally closer to the priest cluster. Finally, mediums seem to appear in places that already have shaman-healers and priests. There is also an obvious connection between socioeconomic complexity and the appearance of these different types. In foraging economies, which were typical of human existence for most of our evolution, only shaman-healers are present. Priests usually appear in agrarian economies, starting with lineage elders in charge of ancestor cults and culminating in the priestly castes of city-states and kingdoms. Mediums seem to emerge, largely as a form of resistance, in the context of large-scale societies with priests (Winkelman, 1986, 1990).

The cross-cultural evidence, then, shows that the one form of religious activity that is constant across human cultures and certainly predates priest-based religions, is what Winkelman calls the "shaman-healer complex," which is roughly identical to what I call informal religious activity here to avoid the connotations of traditional terms like "shaman." But the cross-cultural evidence marshaled by Winkelman also points to the crucial fact that priestly (organized) religions are invariably combined with either shamans or mediums—in other words, they never really supplant those forms of religious activity.

It might be tempting to think of religions as replacing earlier, primitive cults. That is indeed how religions themselves describe their historical emergence—as the appearance of a system of ideas and practices that makes all other religious activities redundant, as well as misguided or nefarious. In reality, the emergence of religious organizations did not and does not result in the elimination of ancestor worship, mediumship, or shamanistic practices, for several reasons. First, not all human groups turned into large-scale, unified polities characterized by extensive social stratification and division of labor. Second, religious organizations in most places, for most of human history, had to contend with the constant presence of shamans and mediums, and other similar, informal religious-service providers. Indeed, a good deal of the history of doctrinal religions is the history of their fight against these competitors. In all places with doctrinal religions also exists a variety of alternative providers—personally identified specialists such as shamans, healers, diviners, and mediums. So religious organizations can win many battles, mostly because of their political influence, but they seem to lose the war, because the resurgence of an alternative provision of religious services is inevitable.

This raises the question, Why do people resort to informal providers to supplement the services of official religions? The demand must be there, and it seems to be quite compelling since people resort to these services even though they often are frowned upon, marginalized, or even prohibited by established churches or castes of priests. It seems that informal shamans, mediums, and healers respond better than religious organizations to a very specific demand that religious organizations do not meet.

One possible explanation, proposed by Harvey Whitehouse, lies in the contrast between doctrinal and imagistic practices. The doctrinal practice of religions is a form of intellectual training, the accumulation of a great number of relevant and explicitly connected propositions, and it is characteristic of doctrinal religions. By contrast, the imagistic mode of transmission that is more characteristic of mediums and shamans consists of rare but exceptionally salient experience, so striking that its details remain engraved in memory. Doctrinal practices constantly run the risk of generating as much tedium as conceptual clarity, while imagistic ones can become so incoherent that most conceptual content is lost (Whitehouse, 2000, 2004).

This contrast between doctrinal practice and imagistic practice, however, may apply only to some situations of competition between institutional and informal religious activities. In many places, people who consult shamans and diviners do not seek or receive imagistic revelations from them. What they want and get are solutions to particular problems, such as illness, infertility, an accident, bad crops, and diseased herds. In other words, the main benefit conferred by religious specialists may lie in their addressing specific cases of misfortune.

Misfortune as a Challenge to Religions

A universal concern in human individuals is to explain the specifics of misfortune, as opposed to the general laws that bring about untoward, as well as happy, circumstances. The great anthropologist E. E. Evans-Pritchard famously illustrated the point in his ethnography of the Zande (1937), using the example of a hut that collapsed while people were sitting under its roof. Most Zande people accept the general principle that explains the collapse—they know that termites gnaw away at wooden pillars, which at a certain point are bound to cave in. But they also wanted to explain why that particular structure collapsed at that particular moment and injured those particular people. These are the questions a diviner is supposed to address, and the explanation is usually couched in terms of witchcraft, describing the accident as a deliberate attack on the part of specific individuals, who wanted it to happen and made sure it hit the intended victims.

This quest for specific, personal, practical answers may be one reason religions generally fail to eradicate their informal competition. Priests and their doctrines promote the notion of large-scale superhuman agents, gods whose jurisdiction extends to an entire city-state, kingdom, or empire, affecting all and sundry in the same manner. Gods are described in terms of doctrinal principles that operate in very generic terms. Sumerian and Egyptian gods are said to demand temples, offerings, and ceremonies. According to the doctrines, the gods will respond to human action by protecting the city or empire when they are placated, or by flooding entire kingdoms or sending devastating plagues when they are not.

All this is about the society in its entirety, not particular individuals. The ceremonies organized by official priests are supposed to guarantee the survival of the city-state or the empire's victory over its enemies, but they do not palliate the disaster of a particular farmer's bad crops. By contrast, the local superhuman agents that shamans and mediums claim to interact with are specifically involved in social interactions with particular people. These souls, spirits, and ancestors are described as individuals having local connections, so to speak. The ancestors, clearly, are construed as concerned with what happens in their lineage. The souls and spirits of shamanistic ceremonies are said, for instance, to have stolen the soul of a particular person. Naturally, this distinction is something of an oversimplification. In many cases, the representatives of religions end up performing ceremonies for particular situations, and there is more overlap between the functions of priests and shamans than this model would suggest. Still, the divergence is real and may explain why there is always sustained demand for services besides those provided by established religions.

There is a clear asymmetry in the interaction of religions with wild traditions. Religious organizations arise in the context of state societies and, in most cases, prosper only to the extent that they are closely associated with state bureaucracies. In traditional palace societies or city-states, priests are part of the political hierarchy. The connection may be looser, as in the case of Hinduism and Islam. But the connection is a general one.

Religions as Hegemonic Discourse

Religious organizations do not generally emerge and prosper as independent entities in a free market of religious providers. On the contrary, their close association with political power makes it impossible for many religious organizations to reach a hegemonic or monopolistic position, because the state does not allow dissenter groups to constitute themselves as alternatives to the official religion.

Informal religious activities are almost universally described by the official organization's priests and scholars as inferior and nefarious in comparison to the services provided by the organization. That is the case in many different traditions. The history of Christianity, for instance, illustrates this in its incessant Sisyphean struggle against, not just heretical or schismatic sects, but also a variety of shamans, magicians, possessed mediums, and other competitors. This is also true of other traditions. Muslim ulema deplore the persistence of magic and divination, for example, and Buddhist monks have to compromise with various cults and magical practices that are far from orthodoxy or orthopraxy. To some extent, this conflict corresponds to the contrast between "great" and "little" traditions (Redfield, 1989) that is familiar to anthropologists (see Tambiah, 1970, for more detailed discussion).

This distinction poses a difficult problem for religious scholarship. Inevitably, the historical record is extremely skewed toward religious organizations, which leave deeds, contracts, rulings, chronicles, and all manner of records that constitute the raw materials historians can work from. By contrast, wild tradition practices can be documented based only on fragmentary evidence, private records, and so on. That is why we know very little about actual religious activities in the Roman Empire, of either the domestic cults or the ecstatic cults such as that of Cybele, and have vastly more documentation of the official state religious rituals, which were probably of very little importance to most people.

Worse, the record is not just asymmetrical but also distorted; in many cases, our knowledge of non-organized religions stems principally if not exclusively from the descriptions of priests and other scholars of the religious organizations, whose perceptions of their competitors are, of course, far from impartial. For instance, some information about the Cybele cults in the late empire comes from such tainted sources. Some of these priests and scholars are elite intellectuals who ridicule the cults; others are Christian apologists who resent the attractiveness of a cult that shares many superficial features with Christianity. It takes special forensic skills for historians to build a plausible model of what the cult really was like, on the basis of such sources. This creates a contrast between underreported informal activity and overdocumented activity by religious organizations that is detrimental to our understanding of actual religious thought and behavior. In most historical situations, the ideas of religious organizations are clearly hegemonic.

This distorted base of evidence becomes a problem when religious organizations benefit from the same hegemony in our models of religion. For instance, some anthropologists and psychologists of religion have argued that religious organizations were crucial to the development of large-scale societies (Norenzayan & Shariff, 2008; Shariff et al., 2010). This argument is based on the difference, familiar from religious historiography and anthropology, between the superhuman agents posited by religious organizations—typically powerful gods whose jurisdiction extends to an entire polity or even the cosmos—and those centred on local spirits, deities associated with specific locations, or the ancestors of particular lineages. A further assumption is that, because the gods of religious organizations, especially in archaic religions, are construed as punishing gods who closely monitor people's behavior, the people who adhere to this belief are more likely to refrain from antisocial behavior, which, in turn, will make large-scale societies more viable (Shariff & Norenzayan, 2011). Some critics of the model have argued that the link between belief in gods and prosocial behavior may be very weak (Gomes & McCullough, 2015), and that the ancestors and spirits of more traditional religious systems are also said to monitor people's behaviors and punish deviations from social norms (Boyer & Baumard, 2016).

Leaving aside these difficulties, a crucial problem lies in the assumption that the "Big Gods" described by the scholars or scribes of religious organizations are actually central to most people's beliefs and motivations. The model assumes, for example, that for most people most of the time, religious thought and behavior will be associated with those cosmic gods concepts. But the anthropological record seems to suggest the opposite. In communities that have been studied by anthropologists, there seems to be an overwhelming supply of small-scale deities, local spirits, and ancestors' souls, in addition to the large-scale gods. And these small-scale deities seem to matter more, in the sense that they are involved in the explaining or preventing illness and misfortune, as well as in punishing wrongdoers.

This is only one example of the way in which the hegemony that is characteristic of religious organizations in many historical societies seems to be reflected in their influence on cognitive theories of religion. Another such influence concerns the very nature of religious representations, in particular the notion of "belief" that underpins many descriptions and models in the study of religion, including in the cognitive models.

THE PROBLEM WITH "BELIEF"

Beliefs are not necessarily central to religious thought and behavior. That is to say, it is certainly naive (and probably ethnocentric) to think that the motivations of religious practitioners, and the explanation for their behavior, are couched in terms of *beliefs*, especially if we take the meaning of term in its usual sense of information that is declarative, accessible to conscious inspection, and explicitly held to be true.

One of the most important findings in the early years of the cognitive science of religion was that the notion of belief commonly used in religious studies was highly misleading. As Justin Barrett and others have described based on experimental studies in Hindu, Christian, Buddhist, and other traditions (J. L. Barrett, 1999; J. L. Barrett & Keil, 1996; Slone, 2004), "theological correctness" refers to the phenomenon whereby people maintain an explicit representation of their own beliefs that is largely in agreement with official doctrine; meanwhile, implicit tasks show that their spontaneous judgments are based, not on the doctrine, but on intuitive expectations, which are often diametrical to the official beliefs (Malley 2004). Christians or Hindus may maintain that their gods are everywhere in our world and attend to the whole cosmos at the same time—their overt beliefs. Yet their performance on implicit tasks reveals that they expect the gods to be in some places (e.g., above and in front of them) rather than others, or that they expect gods to attend to each problem in turn (J. L. Barrett, 1998; J. L. Barrett & Keil, 1996). In a similar way, Calvinists may state their belief in predestination and accept that virtuous works will not affect their god's judgment, yet at the same time, in everyday conversations, imply that good deeds will indeed have a positive effect (Slone, 2004).

So, what is the cognitive status of explicit religious beliefs? As Dan Sperber and others have argued, typical religious statements of belief are not beliefs in the strong sense inherited from the philosophy of mind (Mercier & Sperber, 2009; Sperber, 1997). Understanding their cognitive effects requires making a distinction between intuitive and reflective beliefs. Intuitive beliefs are representations of our world, produced more or less automatically by our cognitive systems, for example, the belief that the object placed behind a screen is still present even though it is not visible, or the belief that an animate agent is moved by internal states rather than external forces, or the belief that a particular facial expression indicates anger or fear. As should be obvious from these examples, intuitive beliefs can be conscious, but the processes that led to their production generally are not. In contrast, other beliefs consist in comments on, inferences from, or comparisons of intuitive beliefs and, more generally, come in a metarepresentational format—for example, "the proper interpretation of 'mc^2 = e' is true," or "it is true that 'three persons are one being'" (Sperber, 1997).

This description of beliefs as metarepresentational helps us to understand why there is nothing irrational in attaching credence to statements whose contents are not precisely or entirely represented. But this framework does not by itself account for the fact that individuals may be committed to the truth of their metarepresented beliefs, and that such beliefs may in some contexts drive people's motivation.

Perhaps this is clearer in the context of less important "beliefs," where there is no direct connection between a motivation to act ("I must do x because of p") and a subjective sense of certainty ("there is some truth in the statement that p"). This is the case with the so-called magical beliefs elicited in the course of experimental studies, in particular, those conducted by Paul Rozin and his colleagues (1986), suggesting that *magic* is an ever-present propensity of human minds. In Rozin's experiments, people are, for instance, reluctant to drink from a glass labeled "poison," even when they wrote the label and poured water into it themselves. There is a great variety of such effects, which are, of course, all the more fascinating for being demonstrated in people who, outside the particular contexts, are adamant that they do not "believe" in magic. The lesson seems to be that, regardless of our self-image as rational thinkers, we are all, in some sense, vulnerable to occasional lapses into magical thinking. That, at least, is the way these experimental studies are usually interpreted.

But the interpretation may be misleading. Our intuitive psychology generally assumes that

1. the mind includes a central belief box, where the organism's current beliefs are stored and combined to produce new inferences;
2. decision-making is the outcome of stored representations in that belief box combined with a hierarchy of the organism's goals, presumably stored in some "current preference box" buffer.

Both assumptions are fraught with difficulties, however, as many psychologists and philosophers have pointed out (Apperly & Butterfill, 2009; H. C. Barrett & Kurzban, 2006; Dennett, 1986; Gendler, 2008; Stich, 1983).

In an alternative, more plausible description of cognitive architecture, the mind is best construed as a collection of relatively autonomous inference systems, each of which is specialized to process specific kinds of input, particularly different aspects or domains of reality (Ermer et al., 2007; Sperber & Hirschfeld, 2004). This implies a different description of belief-fixation and decision-making:

1. The mind does not include a central belief box but a (probably rather large) number of belief-adjudicating modules that are automatically activated by the similarities in content and scope among any *n*-tuplet of beliefs produced by different domain-specific modules.
2. Decision-making is the outcome of current goal competitions, informed by competition between those belief-adjudicating systems.

Under these assumptions, what happens when people see a glass labeled "poison" is that some threat-detection systems are automatically activated, because the label matches one of their input conditions—a cue indicating that a substance dangerous to ingest. Other pieces of conceptual information, for example, "the label truly represents the contents" or, on the contrary, "I wrote and stuck this label on the glass myself," "this is all a game suggested by the experimenter," and so forth, do not enter in the threat-detection module's processing because they simply do not match its input format. So these experiments are indeed revealing—but not of magical thinking. They show that any change of preferences induced by some modular processes, somewhere in the mind, is sufficient to sway decision-making when all else (i.e., the preferences induced by other modules) is neutral with regard to that decision. This is interesting, and should be studied, but it does not require magical beliefs in the strong sense of the term.

The same reasoning applies to other cases of magical beliefs. Anthropologists tend to describe people as committed to a prior belief—for example, that sticking pins in a doll may harm people or reciting a particular incantation will get people to fall in love with them. But that is a rather impoverished version of the cognitive processes involved. It seems more plausible in cognitive terms, and more consistent with the anthropological evidence, to think of such actions as involving a variety of cognitive systems, some of which provide no specific information to the effect that sticking pins in a doll can have any external effects, while at least some cognitive modules can effect the conceptual mapping between the doll's body-like shape and a particular person's body (Sørensen, 2007).

In some communities, there is a large amount of explicit discourse to the effect that magic really works. But the cognitive description proposed here would suggest that this discourse about magic, with which people are familiar, is not what triggers their intuitions or behaviors but is an interpretation of their own behaviors. That is, once we make choices that seem "magical" (as a result of the processes described here), we may have to justify them to others and ourselves. So in some cultural contexts, like those of Rozin's subjects, people can say, "It's silly but I can't help it." In other contexts, we can draw on a culturally salient model of magic to say, "It does make sense and I, like others, know that it often happens." Given that there must be many occasions when our modular systems yield choices we cannot really justify, there is ample ecological space for discourse about magic to become culturally stable.

THE DARK MATTER OF RELIGIOUS REPRESENTATIONS

Standard models in the cognitive science of religion account for religious concepts and activities in the CSR program in terms of relevance-driven cultural transmission. Such models emphasize the connection between the cognitive effects of particular representations, on the one hand, and their spread, on the other (Boyd & Richerson, 1985; Sperber, 1985). Specifically, CSR models imply that religious representations are more likely to be acquired, stored, and represented because they produce specific cognitive effects that can be experimentally studied in individuals (even modern individuals, since the properties of the relevant cognitive systems are assumed to be pan-specific; J. L. Barrett, 2000; Boyer, 1994; Lawson & McCauley, 1990). For instance, one crucial component of both wild and organized religions, according to CSR models, is the notion that superhuman agents are characterized by a combination of (a) some explicitly specified counterintuitive properties, such as physical or biological properties; and (b) some tacitly assumed regular properties of agents, in particular, mental properties, as expected by our intuitive psychology (J. L. Barrett, 2000). Such agents are the focus of religious systems in both wild and historical religions. Also, the description of the agent and its "special" features is central to the formal description of ceremonies (Lawson & McCauley, 1990).

However, we cannot understand the spread of religious representations unless we have a precise description of the cognitive processes involved. This is where common notions such as "religion" or "belief" get in the way of a proper understanding of cultural dynamics. The notion of "religion" is misleading in two different ways. First, as mentioned in the chapter introduction, it suggests that there are common and unique features to the representations commonly called "religious," which goes against the empirical evidence. Second, as discussed in more detail here, the term *religion* glosses over crucial differences, in particular between wild traditions, on the one hand, and religious organizations, on the other.

The incoherent concept of religion leads scholars to ignore what could be called the "dark matter" of religious representations. Astronomers identify a large amount of matter in the universe that did not register on previous measures and was not described in previous models. In a similar way, the religious representations activated in the minds of most people at most times and in most human societies belong to the domain of what I describe here as wild religious traditions. This is also true for the minds of people living in societies with religious organizations. The anthropological and historical record demonstrates that there are virtually no human societies in which people actually think exclusively in the ways their religious organizations prescribe. In this sense, it is highly misleading to describe fifteenth-century Italians as Catholic or their North African contemporaries as Muslim, for example. Obviously, these descriptions capture the nature of the religious organizations, doctrines, and practices those people were exposed to. But the labels also suggest, in a more problematic way, that these people's representations and behaviors can be predicted based on these religious affiliations. When models of cultural evolution are based on such simplifying but also misleading assumptions, they strive to explain a phenomenon that simply did not occur.

The cognitive approaches to religious representations started with the realization that explaining these domains of culture would require a tight integration of religious studies, from history and anthropology, with the findings and models of biology and psychology (J. L. Barrett, 2000; Lawson & McCauley, 1990). Conversely, we should strive to make our cognitive models compatible with the actual anthropological and historical record. Following these two imperatives should lead us to abandon notions that we imported from common folk theories that have little place in scientific theorization. The folk-psychological notion of "belief" is partly incoherent—it serves our practical purposes as a rough and ready description of our, and others', minds (Dennett, 1987), but it cannot be part of a scientific account of cognition (Stich, 1983). The notion of "religion" glosses over social differences, such that explanatory models of one kind of "religion" certainly cannot apply to the other. A more advanced cognitive science of religious representations will create a greater consilience between historical, anthropological, biological, and psychological findings and models.

QUESTIONS FOR FUTURE RESEARCH

1. What are the different forms of interaction (avoidance, complementarity, conflict, suppression) between informal religious activity and doctrinal traditions?
2. What are the effects of either informal religious activity or religious doctrines on moral intuitions?

3. Can we have a good understanding of religious history if we only focus on the explicit, conscious part of religious representations?

4. What experimental or observational methods could reveal the implicit, nonconscious aspects of religious thoughts?

REFERENCES

Apperly, I. A., & Butterfill, S. A. (2009). Do humans have two systems to track beliefs and belief-like states? *Psychological Review*, 116(4), 953–970. doi:10.1037/a0016923

Barrett, H. C., & Kurzban, R. (2006). Modularity in cognition: Framing the debate. *Psychological Review*, 113(3), 628–647.

Barrett, J. L. (1998). Cognitive constraints on Hindu concepts of the divine. *Journal for the Scientific Study of Religion*, 37, 608–619.

Barrett, J. L. (1999). Theological correctness: Cognitive constraint and the study of religion. *Method & Theory in the Study of Religion*, 11, 325–339.

Barrett, J. L. (2000). Exploring the natural foundations of religion. *Trends in Cognitive Sciences*, 4(1), 29–34.

Barrett, J. L. (2001). How ordinary cognition informs petitionary prayer. *Journal of Cognition and Culture*, 1(3), 259–269.

Barrett, J. L., & Keil, F. C. (1996). Conceptualizing a nonnatural entity: Anthropomorphism in God concepts. *Cognitive Psychology*, 31(3), 219–247.

Barrett, J. L., & Nyhof, M. (2001). Spreading non-natural concepts: The role of intuitive conceptual structures in memory and transmission of cultural materials. *Journal of Cognition and Culture* 1(1), 69–100.

Boyd, R., & Richerson, P. J. (1985). *Culture and the evolutionary process*. Chicago: University of Chicago Press.

Boyer, P. (1994). *The naturalness of religious ideas: A cognitive theory of religion*. Berkeley: University of California Press.

Boyer, P. (2003). Religious thought and behaviour as by-products of brain function. *Trends in Cognitive Sciences*, 7(3), 119–124.

Boyer, P., & Baumard, N. (2016). Projecting WEIRD features on ancient religions. *Behavioral and Brain Sciences*, 39. doi:10.1017/S0140525X15000369

Boyer, P., & Ramble, C. (2001). Cognitive templates for religious concepts: Cross-cultural evidence for recall of counter-intuitive representations. *Cognitive Science*, 25, 535–564.

Dennett, D. C. (1986). *Content and consciousness*. London: Routledge & Kegan Paul.

Dennett, D. C. (1987). *The intentional stance*. Cambridge, MA: MIT Press.

Eilam, D., Zor, R., Szechtman, H., & Hermesh, H. (2006). Rituals, stereotypy and compulsive behavior in animals and humans. *Neuroscience & Biobehavioral Reviews*, 30(4), 456–471.

Ermer, E., Cosmides, L., & Tooby, J. (Eds.). (2007). *Functional specialization and the adaptationist program*. New York: Guilford Press.

Evans Pritchard, E.E. (1937). *Witchcraft, oracles and magic among the Azande*, Oxford: Clarendon Press.

Gendler, T. S. (2008). Alief in action (and reaction). *Mind & Language*, 23(5), 552–585. doi:10.1111/j.1468-0017.2008.00352.x

Gomes, C. M., & McCullough, M. E. (2015). The effects of implicit religious primes on dictator game allocations: A preregistered replication experiment. *Journal of Experimental Psychology: General*, 144(6), e94.

Lawson, E. T., & McCauley, R. N. (1990). *Rethinking religion: Connecting cognition and culture.* Cambridge, UK: Cambridge University Press.

Liénard, P., & Boyer, P. (2006). Whence collective rituals? A cultural selection model of ritualized behavior. *American Anthropologist, 108*(4), 814–827.

Malley, B. (2004). *How the Bible works: An anthropological study of evangelical Biblicism.* Walnut Creek, CA: AltaMira Press.

McCorkle, W. W. (2010). *Ritualizing the disposal of the deceased: From corpse to concept.* New York: Peter Lang.

Norenzayan, A., & Shariff, A. F. (2008). The origin and evolution of religious prosociality. *Science, 322,* 58–61.

Redfield, R. (1989). *The little community and peasant society and culture.* Chicago: University of Chicago Press.

Rozin, P., Millman, L., & Nemeroff, C. (1986). Operation of the laws of sympathetic magic in disgust and other domains. *Journal of personality and social psychology, 50*(4), 703.

Schnall, S., Haidt, J., Clore, G. L., & Jordan, A. H. (2008). Disgust as embodied moral judgment. *Personality and Social Psychology Bulletin, 34*(8), 1096–1109.

Shariff, A. F., & Norenzayan, A. (2011). Mean gods make good people: Different views of god predict cheating behavior. *International Journal for the Psychology of Religion, 21*(2), 85–96. doi:10.1080/10508619.2011.556990

Shariff, A. F., Norenzayan, A., & Henrich, J. (2010). The birth of high gods: How the cultural evolution of supernatural policing influenced the emergence of complex, cooperative human societies, paving the way for civilization. In M. Schaller, A. Norenzayan, S. J. Heine, T. Yamagishi, & T. Kameda (Eds.), *Evolution, culture, and the human mind* (pp. 119–136). New York: Psychology Press.

Singh, M. (2018). The cultural evolution of shamanism. *Behavioral and Brain Sciences, 41,* E66. doi:10.1017/S0140525X17001893.

Slone, D. J. (2004). *Theological incorrectness: Why religious people believe what they shouldn't.* Oxford: Oxford University Press.

Sørensen, J. (2007). *A cognitive theory of magic.* Lanham, MD: AltaMira Press.

Sperber, D. (1985). Anthropology and psychology: Towards an epidemiology of representations. *Man, 20*(1), 73–89.

Sperber, D. (1997). Intuitive and reflective beliefs. *Mind & Language, 12*(1), 17.

Sperber, D., & Hirschfeld, L. A. (2004). The cognitive foundations of cultural stability and diversity. *Trends in Cognitive Sciences, 8*(1), 40–46.

Stich, S. P. (1983). *From folk psychology to cognitive science: The case against belief.* Cambridge, MA: MIT Press.

Tambiah, S. J. (1970). *Buddhism and the spirit cults in North-East Thailand.* Cambridge, UK: Cambridge University Press.

Taves, A. (2009). *Religious experience reconsidered: A building-block approach to the study of religion and other special things.* Princeton, NJ: Princeton University Press.

Tybur, J. M., Lieberman, D., Kurzban, R., & DeScioli, P. (2012). Disgust: Evolved function and structure. *Psychological Review.* doi:10.1037/a0030778

White, C. (2016). The cognitive foundations of reincarnation. *Method & Theory in the Study of Religion, 28*(3), 264–286.

White, C., Marin, M., & Fessler, D. M. T. (2017). Not just dead meat: An evolutionary account of corpse treatment in mortuary rituals. *Journal of Cognition and Culture, 17*(1–2), 146–168.

Whitehouse, H. (2000). *Arguments and icons: Divergent modes of religiosity*. Oxford: Oxford University Press.

Whitehouse, H. (2004). *Modes of religiosity*. Walnut Creek, CA: AltaMira Press.

Winkelman, M. J. (1986). Magico-religious practitioner types and socioeconomic conditions. *Behavior Science Research, 20*(1–4), 17–46.

Winkelman, M. J. (1990). Shamans and other "magico-religious" healers: A cross-cultural study of their origins, nature, and social transformations. *Ethos, 18*(3), 308–352.

PART II

RELIGIOUS CONCEPTS

CHAPTER 5

GODS: COGNITION, CULTURE, AND ECOLOGY

BENJAMIN GRANT PURZYCKI

INTRODUCTION

AROUND the world, people talk of all manner of spiritual beings, such as souls, wraiths, gods, and devils. These "unseen or spiritual agencies," as Charles Darwin (2004) described them, reside in the minds of individuals in every human society (Brown, 1991). Let us call these agents "gods." Some gods are relegated to the realm of myth and do little in the way of influencing human relationships. Others are thought to be active in human affairs, and people have, correspondingly, devised culturally postulated forms of behaviors that can alter their temperaments (e.g., ritual, etiquette, and moral conduct). In unique ways, current cognitive approaches in the science of religious beliefs are coming to terms with both the universality and the cultural particularities of gods, both mythical and active.

Although it is rarely explicitly recognized by researchers in the cognitive science of religion (CSR), the late Roy D'Andrade (1981) presaged CSR's primary modus operandi when he expressed the goal of cognitive anthropology, which is to make sense of how "cultural content 'interfaces' with psychological processes." One of the main assumptions of the approach is that through "repeated social transmission," cultural information eventually takes "forms which have a good fit to the natural capacities and constraints of the human brain." It follows then that "when similar cultural forms are found in most societies around the world, there is reason to search for psychological factors which could account for these similarities" (p. 182).[1]

---

[1] Because this vantage point offers a view of change in "cultural forms," the field is also inherently evolutionary. I restrict the bulk of the current discussion to proximate cognitive mechanisms underlying religious cognition, not evolutionary processes (see Sosis et al., this volume) and the many routes of social learning (Kendal et al., 2018).

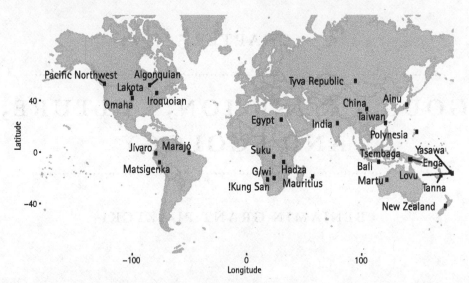

FIGURE 5.1 Peoples and places referenced herein. Some points are roughly centered on general associated geographical regions.

At its inception, CSR followed this line of inquiry (Atran 2002; Boyer, 1994; Guthrie, 1980; McCauley & Lawson, 2002). Despite the abundant knowledge we have of religious traditions being "good fits" for the social (Reynolds & Tanner, 1995) and natural (Berkes, 2012) environments in which people live, there remains one consequence of focusing on "natural capacities and constraints." Specifically, the field has largely ignored (cf. Atran et al., 2002) important factors in human social ecologies that also play a role in the genesis and persistence of religious beliefs and practices.[2] Indeed, because religious systems conform to, mediate, and/or exacerbate the kinds of dilemmas humans face, CSR is in a good position to pinpoint the "natural capacities and constraints" contributing to these particular kinds of fits as well.

This chapter seeks to motivate this line of inquiry by first taking a close look at the complicated relationship between culture and cognition. It then focuses on the cognitive processes purported to underlie how people process the gods and treats such processes as distinct from our explicit cultural models of gods' specific qualities. Using this model of cognition and considering a wide array of ethnographic examples from around the world (see Figure 5.1), it then points to social and natural environments as important inputs to cognitive and social systems. It concludes with a brief sketch of the horizon ahead.

---

[2] This "eco-blindness" may be in part an artifact of the reluctance of the field's progenitors to examine the possibility that religious culture might have payoffs that would be called "adaptive" (see Sosis, 2009; Sosis et al., this volume). This is a curious position to maintain, considering that the idea that there are beliefs that are more "fit" than others is an inherently ecological proposition inasmuch as "fit" means "intuitive" or "less taxing" to understand (see below).

Culture as Information

Let us assume that "culture" is socially transmitted representational information stored in the minds of individuals (Boyd & Richerson, 1985; D'Andrade, 1981; Sperber, 1996; Strauss & Quinn, 1997). In this view, culture is an aggregate or distributed property of individual-level ideas, beliefs, and concepts, and the "culturalness" of such information is measured by its ubiquity in a specific population.[3] As difficult as it can be, sticking with this definition has a few benefits, particularly in trying to make sense of the gods at the level of human cognition.

One benefit of maintaining this conception is that we can avoid making the all too frequently committed logical error of explaining away beliefs—or any other shared, socially transmitted trait—with culture (D'Andrade, 1999; Hirschfeld, 2018). Although one *can* make sensible predictions about whether or not an individual will share a particular belief with their group via social learning and seek to explain why some information is ubiquitous in a population, one cannot adequately explain *culture* by appealing to itself (*petitio principia*).[4] It is reasonable, then, to look for other factors at varying analytical levels and timescales that are exogenous to social learning, thus accounting for the presence of certain cultural traits (e.g., individual decisions, psychological processes, learning biases, cultural evolutionary forces, and the environment).[5] By avoiding these basic but common errors, isolating and sticking to this sense of "culture" fosters more precision in making sense of other *non*cultural analytical levels.[6]

---

[3] In this view, then, "culturalness" is not necessarily indicated by how sustained information is through time (Morin, 2015; Strauss & Quinn, 1997) or whether or not it is beneficial (cf. Richerson & Boyd, 2005). Culture is not any other nontransmitted byproduct of entertaining a belief (e.g., the inference that Santa Claus has an infinite but compromised gastrointestinal system or any other variety of Meno's Problem), and it is not populations of bodies cohabiting an area that share some information (Watts, Sheehan, et al., 2015).

[4] The central debates in the evolutionary social sciences are contemporary iterations of some very old problems. Here, the gods are our *explanandum*. In a superficially repackaged iteration of the eternal nature-nurture debate, many arguments continue over the better *explanans*: the external (e.g., social learning and environment) or the internal environment (e.g., noncultural cognition; Barrett, 2008; Gervais & Henrich, 2010; Purzycki & Willard, 2016). In my view, this debate can only be interesting to the extent that the terms are clearly specified and what counts as satisfactory "explanation" is agreed upon. They rarely are.

[5] Similarly, culture remains an inadequate explanation for beliefs when compared to a control group that doesn't have them (or simply varies on a given trait). This logical error—denying the antecedent— takes the following form: (1) If P, then Q. (2) Not P, therefore not Q. With relevant content, one argument is (1) if people are taught to, then they will believe in that god; (2) these folks are not taught to, therefore they don't believe in that god. Compare this to (1) if he's a psychologist, then he thinks that culture matters; (2) he's not a psychologist, therefore he doesn't think culture matters. These arguments are equally fallacious on logical grounds, yet many presume—and often defend—the former. In the present view, culture can only be said to have an effect on individuals to the degree that it is held by both them and their communities and that these factors somehow motivate or correspond to motivations for behavior (see Purzycki, Pisor, et al., 2018).

[6] We need to be careful, however. Considering that humans have exceptionally long periods of development when we develop a variety of habits that aren't readily articulated, "culture" often acts

Cognition as Information Processing and Production

Consider cultural information to be a relatively *shallow* part of human cognition. It is socially transmitted data that we can reflectively and purposefully recruit (see Purzycki & Willard, 2016, for elaboration; cf. McCauley, 2011; Sperber, 1997). As such, it is fairly effortless to ethnographically elicit from others, given that its prevalence is high. Take the following statement: "Oh, say can you, by the early light." Filling in these blanks is a cognitive process that includes retrieving cultural information to complete a statement that is consistent with a cultural model—that is, the aggregate sense of the "correct" answer (Romney et al., 1986). Features of gods, such as their forms, particulars of what they know and care about, and their roles in the cosmos, vary considerably, and it is at this level of cognition that such details reside.

However, a considerable amount of human cognition and expression is not obviously "cultural" in the sense used here. Retrieving "see" and "dawn's" in the foregoing example is not a conscious process for cultural insiders; we don't have to consciously rifle through our mental libraries, and retrieving information is not a learned process. Moreover, we infer a considerable amount of information about our world without any explicit instruction or transmission. On the *deeper* end of cognition, then, are these difficult-to-articulate processes that constrain, restructure, process, and utilize cultural information (among other things). These processes are much more difficult to elicit from people, and tightly controlled experiments are often required to determine their influence (e.g., emotions). One of the more maddening riddles in trying to understanding humans is coming to terms with the fact that our shallow cognition can provide messages that are (in)consistent with the outputs of our deeper cognitive processes (Barrett & Keil, 1996; Purzycki & Willard, 2016); that is, we can both express and mask our intuitions.

Cultural information interacts with nonexplicit cognitive processes all the time, and environmental inputs trigger deep and, ultimately, shallow cognition. Indeed, the closer we look, the more challenging it is to isolate the links between cognition, culture, and environment. To illustrate: let's say we asked 20 people in a community to list foods sold at the grocery store and found some consistency in the items listed and the order in which they were listed. We do not necessarily need to appeal to culture to explain this, since we are not actively teaching our children and peers to organize their mental models of foods in this fashion. Rather, it may have something to do with cultural information (e.g., names and types of foods) interacting with internally generated representations of structured features of the environment. We might list fruits and vegetables first, not

like instinct, and oftentimes, cultural information can indirectly lead people to think or behave in similar ways. For example, the fact that many university students will sit in the same unassigned seat in a classroom day after day without explicit instruction to do so seems remarkable only if we ignore the long-lasting habituation effects of the very explicitly instructed rules (equally without reason) learned in primary school. Similar facets of religion are likely to be the case. As such, ruling out one explanation or the other—or, better still, accounting for which bears more explanatory weight—requires a better understanding of how religious traits develop throughout the life history of individuals.

because we have been taught to do so or value produce more than condiments, but because we see them first when we enter the store. Perhaps shop planners have a cultural model of the way to organize grocery stores, but consumers' internally stored structures of foods are probably generated by the extraction of information from our environments, compiled into a model, and shared by virtue of retrieval processes. Calling this process "cultural" is convenient, but it is entirely contingent on what we mean by "socially" or "culturally transmitted." In the strict sense used here, individuals have independently convergent models that *look* cultural and consist of cultural data, but they are not explicitly transmitted across minds.

Compare this to the case of the Müller-Lyer illusion, where two lines appear to be different lengths by virtue of the direction of their forked ends. As it turns out, susceptibility to this illusion is not universal; !Kung San adults and Suku children are not fooled by it (Segall et al., 1963). This might be the result of perceptual systems habituating themselves to the angles in our "carpentered worlds" (Stewart, 1974). As far as we know, people who fall for the illusion are not socially transmitting their susceptibility to it. As such, "culture" remains an inadequate explanation here as well. To say that this variation is caused by culture overstates culture's significance by conveniently relaxing social transmission as an essential component of its definition (cf. McCauley & Henrich, 2006). Instead, growing up in rooms with walls that are perpendicular to the floor and ceiling alters and stabilizes certain perceptual expectations that lead one to perceive an illusion in a particular way. These examples illustrate how difficult it is to tease apart cognition, culture, and the environment, let alone measure them as analytically isolated phenomena. Empirically, the causal arrows among them are arguably even more elusive. They also illustrate how (in)consistent the content of our deeper and shallow faculties can be with each other, and how (in)consistent they can be with features of the social and natural environments. Bearing this discussion in mind, we now turn to the deeper cognitive components that handle the gods in order to delineate them from the explicit, shallow set of beliefs that people share.

UNIVERSALS AND WHAT GODS ARE

In one sense, gods are a specific subclass of cultural concepts that individuals learn from their parents and peers. A variety of factors from revelation, personality, and experience can account for individual variation in beliefs. Yet gods around the world exhibit many recurring features that correspond to deeper cognitive processes. As noted, the strategy cognitive scientists of religion employ is to identify a psychological process that corresponds with some feature of gods and then appeal to that process to explain those features. Many such accounts exist; gods have been variously characterized as corresponding to psychological systems dedicated to (a) attachment and bonds (Granqvist et al., 2010), (b) dominance hierarchies (Garcia, 2015), (c) death anxiety (Becker, 1973; Jackson et al., 2018), (d) the need to understand the world (see Evans-Pritchard, 1965), and (e) fulfillment of basic emotional needs (Turner et al., 2017). Rather than discuss these possibilities, I wish to provide a more basic staple of CSR—namely, that gods are powerful humanlike agent concepts that know and care about human affairs.

Gods Are Minds

Gods are simultaneously humanlike (i.e., anthropomorphic) and unhumanlike (Guthrie, 1980, 1995; Nyhof & Johnson, 2017; Shaman et al. 2018). Even when gods are conceived as having an animal form or have animal parts, they remain essentially humanlike. Anubis, the Egyptian god who ushered people into the afterlife, had the head of a jackal but a human body. During hallucinogenic interactions with spirits, the Ecuadorian Jívaro interact with spirit animals who appear in dreams as ancestor spirits (Harner, 1973, pp. 134–138). Here, despite shapeshifting, the soul is ultimately associated with a human form and communicates with the seeker. In most communities, gods are not abstractions, weird mindless bodies, sacred vibrations, or transdimensional ideas—they are appreciated *as* minds with interests and concerns.

As humanlike minds, they tend to understand our symbolic communication. Even when the ultimate sacred entity is believed to be a vast, flowing force, we see such anthropomorphism at work. From the Siouan *wakan tanka*, Algonquian *manitou*, and Chinese *dao* to the Iroquoian *orenda*, the Polynesian *mana*, and the Indian *karma*, such sacred forces are often translated as "Great Spirit," "Power," or "Force" and individuals readily think of them as agentic entities when talking about them or associated as instruments of gods. For example, some studies suggest that people claim that *karma* "punishes" people for certain behaviors (White et al., 2018) or that the Buddha uses *karma* to punish people (Purzycki & Holland, 2019). According to George Sword, a Lakota (Sioux) elder, "*Wakan Tanka* [literally, "sacred vastness"] was everywhere all the time and observed everything that each one of mankind did and even knew what anyone thought, that he might be pleased or displeased because of something that one did" (Walker, 1991). One such devotional practice that was performed before a bison hunt consisted of burning incense of buffalo chips to release the spirit of a bison, which "goes to *Wakan Tanka*, and pleases him so that he will help in the chase" (p. 77). In these examples, it appears effortless to describe a cosmic force as an instrument of punishment or an undulating, creative force as a mind with perceptions, goals, and a sense of smell.

What accounts for this effortlessness? We have cognitive systems designed to infer and interpret our world in terms of mental states: one general suite of deeper cognitive mechanisms purported to be critical for beliefs in the gods is our ability to infer that other things and beings have minds. This set of mechanisms is variously called "mindreading," "theory of mind," or the "intentionality system" (Baron-Cohen, 1995; Barrett, 1998; Guthrie, 1980; Johnson & Bering, 2006; Premack & Woodruff, 1978; Van Leeuwen & van Elk, 2019). Humans are also natural dualists; because we systematically separate mind from body, the idea of a mind *without* an obvious body is not a far-fetched possibility (Chudek et al., 2017).

Gods Are Knowledgeable

Explicitly, not all gods are held to know everything (i.e., omniscient) and even those that are, are not consistently thought of as such. Some gods are downright oblivious; others can be fooled and manipulated into serving human ends. In the Tyva Republic of southern Siberia, spirits are not generally thought of as knowledgeable about everything on earth, and they are tied to local regions and resources. In reply to the question of whether or not spirits knew what transpired in other regions, one herder said that they didn't, but that *those* resident spirits knew (Purzycki, 2010). One Tyvan musician mused, "Believing that there are many spirits makes more sense than believing in one god. There are a lot of rivers and mountains. How can one god watch over everything?" (Levin, 2006, p. 29).

These views are not necessarily representative of all Tyvans' thinking on these matters (Purzycki, 2016), but they do suggest that, at least explicitly, whether a god is omniscient is psychologically irrelevant if *many* gods are always watching everywhere anyway. In some cases, even nonresident deities can obtain knowledge of people. The banished creator god of the Matsigenka of Peru, for example, dwells on the distant horizon and cannot directly interact with people. But because he gets his information about local goings-on from armadillos who run between him and the villages, he is nevertheless informed (Caissa Revilla Minaya, personal communication, 2018).

Though good quantitative data are scarce, gods do seem to be generally more knowledgeable than people are; they seem to have access to information that is otherwise immediately inaccessible. Figure 5.2 shows a series of density plots depicting responses to a set of questions about deities' breadth of knowledge (typically two in each site) across eight samples (Purzycki et al., 2016b). The two deities were selected on the basis of one knowing, punishing, and being more interested in human morality (referred to as the "moralistic god"), whereas the other was also a locally important deity but relatively less knowledgeable, punitive, and moralistic (referred to as the "local god"). One question was about whether or not these gods can see inside people's minds, and the other was whether they know about things that happened in some place that was distant from where participants lived. Most people within and across societies answered affirmatively for both types of gods.

Exceptions are the local deities in Yasawa (McNamara & Henrich, 2018) and Mauritius (Xygalatas et al., 2018), who answered bimodally (i.e., with two peaks). In both places—unlike at the other field sites—it is taboo or illegal to worship the selected local spirits. This may have influenced the responses if individuals tried to make the gods appear less powerful than they are believed or inferred to be (thus overriding deeper intuitions about deities), but this is just one possibility. Some gods, like the Hadza's Haine and Ishoko, are often represented as the sun and the moon (Apicella, 2018; Power, 2015). As celestial bodies, they may be thought of as able to see everything by virtue of their positions relative to the earth, and not because of any specifically articulated cultural belief about the breadth of their knowledge. There are many possible explanations, but

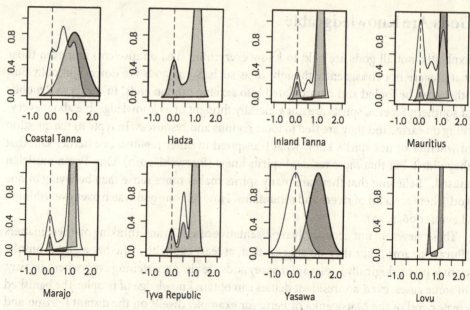

FIGURE 5.2 Density plot of 15 deities' knowledge breadth across eight field sites. Data are means from two binary scale items (yes = 1, no = 0) measuring gods' knowledge of people's thoughts and feelings and the behaviors of people from a geographically distant location for moralistic (*dark*) and locally salient (*white*) deities. Dotted lines indicate values of zero for both questions. Moralistic deities for Coastal Tanna, Marajó, and Yasawa are the Christian God. Note that Lovu lacks local deity data and that the Hadza distributions completely overlap.

speculation and debate are no match for good data, rigorous analysis, and theory that would make addressing this question an interesting enterprise.

Our ability to mentalize likely makes it easier to reflect on the thoughts and knowledge of the gods. And while there appears to be cross-population variation in how mentalizing systems develop (Shahaeian et al., 2011), it remains unclear how the development of general mentalizing corresponds to religiosity and religious cognition. Some research suggests that our *defaults* about other minds are generally closer to omniscience than ignorance. A variety of experimental studies suggest that, though the youngest children typically assume that all agents (including people) approach having full knowledge, only older children can infer that gods (including imaginary friends) have full knowledge while their mothers and other agents do not (Barrett et al., 2001; Heiphetz et al., 2016; Knight et al., 2004; Wigger, 2016; Wigger, Paxson, & Ryan, 2013). In other words, experience prunes this over-attribution of knowledge away from actual minds, but retains the inference for gods. However, *explicitly* reasoning through the implications of omniscience is quite taxing for children (Lane et al., 2012, 2014) and adults (Barrett, 1998; Purzycki et al., 2012; Purzycki, 2013) alike.

Herein lies a curious set of insights the field is currently disentangling: *People tend to naturally infer that agents know more than they should. As we grow, we appear to retain this inference with respect to the gods, yet reason differently about flesh-and-blood agents.*

Full-blown omniscience is not easy to consistently reason about, but it is nevertheless consistent with our defaults about gods knowing more. This problem is easier to think about if we appreciate the distinction between shallow and deep levels of cognition described earlier. As a belief, omniscience is quite easy to learn and express: *God knows everything.* Millions of believers might say this yet systematically fail to *reason* consistently about it. In other words, "God knows everything" is a shallow belief, and the idea that a god knows *anything* is made possible by virtue of mentalizing systems. Yet using deeper processes to *reason* consistently about this shallow information is not as easy. Moreover, gods might tend to know more than normal people not because people learned to say it, but because this is a cognitive default that was never eliminated through socialization processes. Can the same be said of gods' moral interests?

Gods Are Interested

The gods might know more than humans. So what? One domain of information that gods may be *especially* inclined to know (i.e., that we are especially inclined to associate them with) is called "socially strategic information" (Boyer, 2000). This information is whatever "activates the mental systems that regulate social interaction" (Boyer, 2001, p. 152), which in the right context can be just about anything. It is important to know who is an insufferable kleptomaniac. It is advantageous to know whom you can rely on with your deepest, darkest secrets. It is also important to know who is wealthy, who is in charge, and who talks to outsiders. In Boyer's view, gods don't have to be *explicitly* (i.e., culturally and shallowly) associated with such information. Instead, this is the work of a deeper cognitive process. In general, then, gods may be primed to have what has been called "perfect access" to important information whether or not they are explicitly thought of as omniscient. This might make them especially salient in individual minds.

How deep is the association between gods and socially strategic knowledge? Some research suggests a strong link between the perception of minds in general and moral cognition[7] (Gray et al., 2012), and some researchers have suggested that the relationship between religion and morality is quite robust (McKay & Whitehouse, 2015). When it comes to processing information about gods' knowledge, a response-time study (Purzycki et al., 2012) found that across four different omniscient agents (God, Santa, a surveillance government, and an alien species that observed the earth), people were quicker to respond to questions about socially strategic information (e.g., "Does X know that Y robs banks?") than to more mundane information (e.g., "Does X know that Y has blue shoes?"). In another study (Purzycki, 2013), American Christians who claimed that God knew everything, answered more affirmatively when asked socially strategic questions than mundane questions (i.e., God might know everything, but he *really* knows moral behavior).

---

[7] "Morality" here refers to norms of interpersonal behaviors with a cost or benefit to others. Consider the behavioral implications of a so-called moralization bias of gods' minds.

How shallow and widespread is the association between gods and moral interest? Some debate this point on theoretical grounds (Johnson, 2015; Norenzayan, 2013), but others have examined the question empirically. Boehm (2008) surveyed ethnographies of foraging populations (i.e., hunter-gatherer-fisher) and found that while all of the sampled deities were reported to care about some moral behaviors (e.g., cheating, murder, theft, etc.), they largely cared about—and punished—violations of what he called "nonmoral" taboos (e.g., issues surrounding ritual, sex, birth, etc.). Tyvans explicitly hold that local spirits are concerned with ritual and resource maintenance; and there is little conceptual overlap between these beliefs and what they think characterizes "good" and "bad" people (Purzycki, 2016). Nevertheless, when asked directly, Tyvans were more likely to claim that deities knew about moral behaviors that occurred in their territory (Purzycki, 2013). Here then, is a conundrum: even though spirits aren't *explicitly* thought of as morally concerned (i.e., shallow cognition), they nevertheless might be *deeply* associated with morality, conditional on external factors such as location.

Using the same data set used in the previous section, Figure 5.3 suggests that this association might be quite general (see, too, Purzycki, et al. in press). We asked participants to rate how important it is for deities to punish lying, murder, and theft (three questions about two deities). Recall that one deity was specifically selected based on the breadth of its moral concern, punishment, and knowledge (the dark distributions in the figure). Indeed, these explicitly "moralistic" deities are often more "moralistic" than important

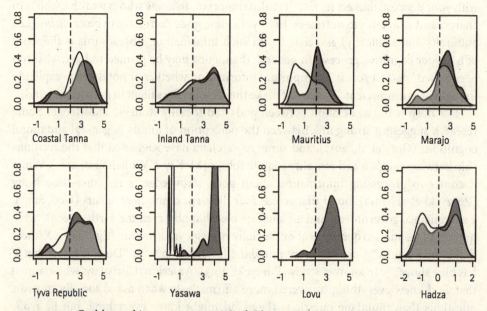

FIGURE 5.3 Gods' moral interests across eight field sites. Data are means (scale 0 to 4) of three scale items measuring moral interests of moralistic (*dark*) and locally salient (*white*) deities. Dotted lines are at midpoint of scale. Moralistic deities for Coastal Tanna, Marajó, and Yasawa are the Christian god. Note that Lovu site lacks local deity data and the Hadza distributions are on a different scale (−1, 0, and 1).

local deities are. However, local deities are also largely conceived of being as morally concerned as well, though to a lesser degree. Even when they may be explicitly thought of as concerned with other things, again, with the exception of Mauritius and Yasawa, the bulk of responses are above the halfway mark (2 for most sites) on the scale.

These data are consistent with the idea that underneath the shallow cultural surface, people are more inclined to reason about gods' interests as moralistic when asked about them. In other words, people might not talk about local deities as being morally concerned, but when they are directly asked specific questions, the responses can converge because of the deeper association with agency and moral cognition.[8] Perhaps individuals are projecting their own disgust with immoral behavior onto the gods. If so, we should see similar patterns for other things that people value beyond the moral domain (e.g., are jazz percussion enthusiasts more likely to infer that God likes Max Roach?) However, as we discuss in the final section, explicit cultural models of gods' concerns are not obviously individual projections. Rather, they correspond to collective concerns.

Gods Are Powerful

Gods certainly come in handy when we are rationalizing our own behavior, but they also appear to motivate and prevent our actions through a combination of their watchful gaze (Krátký et al., 2016; Yilmaz & Bahçekapili, 2016; cf. Northover et al., 2017), the threat of punishment or not keeping us safe from harm (Johnson, 2005; Purzycki et al., 2016b), and the promise of rewards. Gods also have special roles and powers, which makes them both cognitively salient and worth worrying about.

Gods' relative strength and mysteriousness led Darwin (2004) to suspect that our obligations to them and "reverence or fear" of them (p. 140) are deeply connected with our social instincts of shame and remorse. Not all gods are obviously or actively feared, but they all appear to have powers that humans do not and are likely implicated as beings one shouldn't mess with if given the chance. Because of this relative power, we may also see their desires, when expressed, as especially worth fulfilling, if only to maintain our reputation in their eyes. According to one account, the G/wi of the Kalahari apparently lack devotional practices to their supreme creator deity N!adima. They nevertheless do offer rites to thunderstorms and celestial phenomena (e.g., the new moon and the sun) "in order to show man's lack of arrogance and thereby to avoid [N!adima's] displeasure (Silberbauer, 1972, p. 319). As in the aforementioned case of the Matsigenka, even deities

---

[8] Of course, this bias may be somehow influenced by the more explicitly moralistic tradition present in these communities. Purzycki, et al. (in press) show the bias remains even after holding constant the correlation with moralistic gods. From a cognitive perspective—one I wish to maintain here—the question of why exposure to a moralistic deity would somehow inform models of local gods still requires some deeper account (e.g., assuming that people aren't telling each other that because god X cares about morality, god Y should as well, what process is responsible for this inference?).

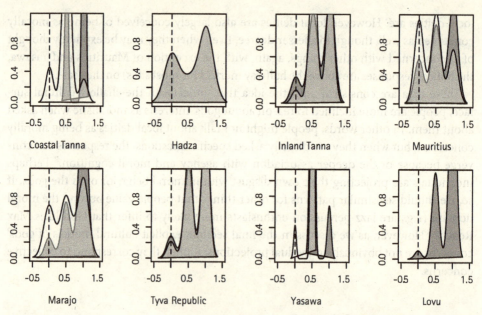

FIGURE 5.4 Gods' punishment across eight field sites. Data are means of two dichotomous scale items measuring punishment of moralistic (*dark*) and locally salient (*white*) deities. Dotted lines are at the minimum of scale. Moralistic deities for Coastal Tanna, Marajó, and Yasawa are the Christian god. Note that Lovu site lacks local deity data and the Hadza data completely overlap. Note, too, that there is more overlap in the Mauritius and Yasawa distributions than in the previous figures.

not thought to be directly involved in or knowledgeable about human affairs can still "inspire" certain behaviors.

Because gods are powerful and interested, people may be more inclined to conceive of them as capable of having a negative impact on human destinies, however indirectly (e.g., through karma or luck). Figure 5.4 indicates just how universal gods' "punishments" might be. These questions were about whether gods punished people for their behavior or had a hand in what happens to people after they die. Across these field sites and 15 deities, aggregate responses to questions concerning gods' punishments are more frequently affirmative than not. This finding might be partly due to the fact that we selected locally important deities based on ratings of freely listed gods in each field site. If, for instance, many spirits and gods "existed" in a specific field site, but people listed only a handful of the salient gods, these increased scores may be indicative of a bias in recollection (i.e., gods that punish are easier to recall), but it may also reflect a general ignorance of religious pantheons; individuals wouldn't recall them because they're rarely exposed to them (see Box 5.1).

This section discussed some of the cognitive foundations of beliefs in gods. Gods, spirits, ghosts, and other spiritual agents are represented as minds with the capacity to know and care about human behavior. Gods also tend to be represented as more powerful than normal humans, and at least among those discussed herein, more prone to

Box 5.1

Cognition, expertise, and theological inconsistency. Spiro (1987) lamented the folly of "confus[ing] the teachings of a philosophical school with the beliefs and behavior of a religious community" (p. 194). Indeed, if we want to understand a religious system, the last thing we should do is rely too heavily on a sage, priest, theologian, shaman, or sacred text. The reasons for this are manifold. First, the view you would get from one of these authoritative sources would have little resemblance to how the average person thinks or behaves. Bodies of specialized knowledge are articulated, developed, and transmitted under conditions that can sustain such investment. Second, there are enough inconsistencies between authoritative sources that it would be difficult to reliably establish—without appropriate analyses— what the "authoritative" view would actually be. Indeed, scholars and theologians have had a difficult time coming to terms with omniscience (Abbruzzese, 1997; Kapitan, 1991). Third, authorities can be inconsistent with themselves. In addition to the practical variation in expenditure to make sense of one's tradition and the kinds of inconsistencies borne out by competing experts, some of the inconsistencies between authoritative views of religious belief and behavior are due to how our minds work (Barrett 1998, 1999; Slone, 2004). On the one hand, we might say that God knows everything and is everywhere because that's what some preachers said, and the Bible (sometimes) suggests this is the case. However, it's fairly easy for us to think about God "hearing our prayers" (as though he couldn't just anticipate our thoughts without anyone else having to hear them) or "coming down from Heaven" (as though he were physically limited to some realm). These inconsistencies suggest that we use our default modes of reasoning about actual agents—specifically *human* beings—to talk about gods' perceptual abilities.

punish people (cf. Barrett et al., 2019). The source of these universals is easily chalked up to the interaction between social environments and deep cognitive faculties but explaining the details of these interactions remains a peripheral activity in the field. Nevertheless, this foundational set of cognitive processes can also help guide us through some of the dizzying variation that exists in religious beliefs by asking the question of when, where, and why this suite of cognitive systems becomes engaged in the "wild" (Hutchins, 1995).

LOOKING AHEAD: COGNITION, VARIATION, AND ECOLOGY

The study of ecology involves the investigation of how energy is distributed in a given system. Studying the ecology of religion, then, attends to how religious concepts and behaviors contribute to the direction of energy flows (i.e., the costs and benefits) in a given community (Reynolds & Tanner, 1995; Sosis & Bulbulia, 2011). As should be clear by now, much of the cognitive science of religion is implicitly couched ecologically.

Indeed, D'Andrade's view, cited in the introduction to the chapter, was ecological inasmuch as psychological processes will anchor cultural representations and therefore reduce variation by virtue of their shared similarity (i.e., they're cheaper to learn). Cognitive processes and behaviors act as valves for the flow of information. In many ways, gods and religious behaviors function the way valves do in energetic systems (McCullough & Willoughby, 2009; Morgan et al., 2016; cf. Schjoedt et al., 2013).

Gods are also associated with behaviors that directly mediate the distribution of energy in the form of consumable resources. Why associate such mediations with gods, and how are cognitive processes responsible for the genesis of such associations? How do deeper cognitive processes produce mutant shallow beliefs that go on to become widespread, and what kind of cognitive states make us more receptive to adopting them? How does the mental act of representing gods redirect resources? These questions are explored in the remainder of the chapter.

Imagine a technology that (a) quickly motivates action by making users think they are being watched, with a risk of repercussions; (b) partly consists of intuitive, and difficult-to-disprove, notions; and (c) taps into moral cognition and our sense of obligation. Imagine being able to trigger this system whenever a problems rears its head and can only be resolved through collective action and/or restraint. As I hope is more obvious at this point, this "system" is the gods. Gods and the practices done in their name(s) often conform to the very real problems that people face. Moreover, variation in gods suggests that they flexibly attend to novel perturbations of the social order. As discussed above (see the section "Gods are Minds"), some aspects of gods "fit" with the deeper cognitive processes responsible for mentalizing. Gods also "fit"—both trivially and importantly—to factors in the social and natural environments in which people live. Indeed, many religious beliefs and practices converge independently of shared social histories (Botero et al., 2014; Watts, Greenhill, et al., 2015). How does cognition help us account for such phenomena? This area remains poorly understood.[9] Of course, gods' environmental "fits" are just as mental as their correspondences to deeper faculties, but carefully attending to local, individual-level cognitive processes that contribute to global patterns currently remains beyond our grasp (and, in some cases, our purview). A sensible first step forward, then, is to examine how beliefs correspond to inputs from the social and natural environments.

From elephant-headed Ganesha of India to the giant beaver Wishpoosh of the American Pacific Northwest, gods are portrayed in innumerable ways that are clearly inspired by features of the natural environment. Of course, people in places without elephants or beavers aren't likely to incorporate them into religious pantheons without some external influence, corresponding internal processing, and subsequent social transmission. To illustrate, take the spider, an important figure in the stories of various Siouan-speaking groups of the American Great Plains. Like all tricksters, this character

---

[9] While some view gods and religious behaviors as actually minimizing these problems' effects (Purzycki et al., 2014; Shariff et al., 2014; Sosis & Alcorta, 2005; Wilson, 2002), my focus here to point to the cognitive processes behind gods' conformity to such problems.

GODS: COGNITION, CULTURE, AND ECOLOGY   81

(variously called Iktomi, Unktomni, Inktomni, etc.) is simultaneously funny and troublesome, clever and foolish, and downright irresponsible but also brings humans some of the most important facets of their culture. Tricksters are portrayed as excessively human and prone to thievery because of their insatiable appetites (Erdoes & Ortiz, 1999; Hyde, 1998). Among the Omaha of Nebraska, Ictinike is often portrayed as a monkey, even though monkeys are not indigenous to North America (Welsch, 1981). A partial explanation for this is that the Omaha incorporated the monkey after seeing monkeys in the circuses that traveled throughout the Great Plains (Mark Awakuni-Swetland, personal communication, 2005). Moreover, monkeys' similarity to humans and playful craftiness might have been a better psychological-conceptual fit for the trickster figure than spiders, which might provide another piece of the explanatory puzzle.[10]

Some fits with the external environment are not so trivial. For example, some research shows an association between child-rearing practices (benevolent vs. malevolent) and the temperaments attributed to deities (Lambert et al., 1959; cf. Spiro & D'Andrade, 1958). The distribution of decision-making power in societies (e.g., from top-down tyranny to direct, distributed democracy) appears to correspond to religious beliefs and the distribution of sacred power (Peregrine, 1996; Swanson, 1960; Wallace, 1966). Some examine the role material wealth plays on the genesis and an increased receptivity to adopting beliefs in moralistic gods (Baumard et al., 2015; Mullins et al., 2018; Purzycki, Ross, et al., 2018). One long-standing line of inquiry examines the association between belief in morally concerned gods and social complexity (Johnson, 2005; Norenzayan et al., 2016; Peoples & Marlowe, 2012; Purzycki et al., 2016b; Watts, Greenhill, et al., 2015).

Around the world, gods' explicit concerns largely revolve around a few major themes of human behavior (Purzycki & McNamara, 2016): how we treat ourselves and each other (e.g., based on our sense of morality, virtue, and etiquette), how we treat the gods (e.g., by virtue of ritual and belief), and how we treat the natural world (e.g., through resource maintenance and ecological practices). These behaviors show striking patterns, and like other aspects of religious commitment, they appear to be synchronic and diachronic *responses* to particular problems (Bendixen & Purzycki, 2020). Examples are abundant.

The Enga of Papua New Guinea always performed rites devoted to the ancestors when threats to their well-being were especially acute (Wiessner & Papu, 1998, p. 182). In New Zealand, religious commitment spiked after a major earthquake (Sibley & Bulbulia, 2012). Taiwanese activists transformed Mazu, traditionally the goddess of the sea, into a goddess of antinuclear power (Shih, 2012). Pope Francis's encyclical *Laudato si'* (*Praise Be to You*) rebrands the Catholic god as an environmentalist (see Chaplin,

---

[10] In Chinese literature, Sun Wukong, the monkey, is the puckish trickster. It may be chance that these two disparate traditions converged, but if monkeys actually are puckish and thieving and universally appreciated as a little too humanlike, it shouldn't be surprising that they fit this role so well. While this "conceptual fit" might partly account for how rapidly the association with the monkey spread (as opposed to some other animal), the account remains rather stark without some transmission component.

2016). Deities and religious practices have been directly linked to the regulation of resources around the world (Hartberg et al., 2016; Reynolds & Tanner, 1995); specific case studies include—but aren't limited to—the Martu in Australia (Bliege Bird et al., 2013), the Tsembaga of Papua New Guinea (Rappaport, 2000), the Balinese (Lansing, 2012), the Ainu of Japan (Watanabe, 1972), and groups throughout Inner Asia (Jordan, 2003; Purzycki, 2010). Instead of reflecting individual whims or the deeper cognitive structures that have been detailed here, gods and the sacred are not only systematically associated with practical, shared problems—a fact that scholars of the field have long recognized (Durkheim, 2001; Wilson, 2002); they also co-evolve in their association with such problems.

How these complicated processes operate remains conjectural, but CSR is well positioned to contribute to the discussion by detailing the internal mechanics that generate and help maintain such a system, particularly with respect to the gods. By way of a rough sketch of the process (for more sophisticated treatments, see Berkes, 2012, pp. 217–238; Hinde, 2010; Turner & Berkes, 2006; Wood, 2017), people first have to address threats when they occur and become especially taxing. If these are problems of collective action or coordination, people are likely to use relatively cost-effective (i.e., intuitive, salient, and widespread) means to rally people together. Because gods are intuitive, powerful, and interested, they may inspire and expedite action in the absence of cheaper, more-effective secular means. Myths and appeals to gods' concerns convey values (Matthews, 1992) that feed back to group commitments and—provided corollary behaviors are effective—back to the severity of the problem. This crude sketch is one of many possible accounts for why gods and behaviors done under their "influence" are "distributed" spatially, temporally, and across particular social dilemmas; the contours of salient problems correspond to this "distribution" of gods and the shallow information of which they are composed. This prospect—coupled with the abundant ethnographic evidence—only bolsters the promise in making sense of the internal mechanics of the human mind as critical factors in accounting for the presence of gods and the roles they play in human affairs.

Questions for Future Research

1. What do gods care about cross-culturally?
2. Do the behaviors that gods care about cross-culturally correspond to locally salient threats to social cohesion?
3. Are gods optimal solutions for problems associated with the distribution of resources?
4. What are the differences between the social problems gods addressed by gods and the problems resolved by secular means?
5. Do gods' explicitly held concerns actually motivate behavior?

Acknowledgments

Many thanks go to Justin Barrett for the invitation to write this chapter and to Sarey Martin for management of the present volume. I was supported by the Max Planck Institute for Evolutionary Anthropology while writing this chapter. I also gratefully acknowledge the many individuals who participated in and executed the Evolution of Religion and Morality Project (Purzycki Henrich, et al., 2018), without whom presenting the data herein would not have been possible. Readers may access the data at https://github.com/bgpurzycki/Evolution-of-Religion-and-Morality and the code at https://gist.github.com/bgpurzycki/490e9d0ee8c7c3446e1f5df231e41a07.

References

Apicella, C. L. (2018). High levels of rule-bending in a minimally religious and largely egalitarian forager population. *Religion, Brain & Behavior, 8*(2), 133–148. doi:10.1080/2153599X.2016.1267034

Atran, S. (2002). *In gods we trust: The evolutionary landscape of religion.* Oxford: Oxford University Press.

Atran, S., Medin, D., Ross, N., Lynch, E., Vapnarsky, V., Ek', E. U., Coley, J., Timua, C., & Baran, M. (2002). Folkecology, cultural epidemiology, and the spirit of the commons: A garden experiment in the Maya lowlands, 1991–2001. *Current Anthropology, 43*(3), 421–450. doi:10.1086/339528

Baron-Cohen, S. (1995). *Mindblindness: An essay on autism and theory of mind.* Cambridge, MA: MIT Press.

Barrett, J. L. (1998). Cognitive constraints on Hindu concepts of the divine. *Journal for the Scientific Study of Religion, 37*(4), 608–619.

Barrett, J. L. (2008). Why Santa Claus is not a god. *Journal of Cognition and Culture, 8,* 149–161. doi:10.1163/156770908X289251

Barrett, J. L., & Keil, F. C. (1996). Conceptualizing a nonnatural entity: Anthropomorphism in god concepts. *Cognitive Psychology, 31*(3), 219–247.

Barrett, J. L., Richert, R. A., & Driesenga, A. (2001). God's beliefs versus mother's: The development of nonhuman agent concepts. *Child Development, 72*(1), 50–65. doi:10.1111/1467-8624.00265

Barrett, J. L., Shaw, R. D., Pfeiffer, J., Grimes, J., & Foley, G. (2019). Good gods almighty: A report concerning divine attributes from a global sample. *Journal of Cognition and Culture, 19*(3-4), 273–290.

Baumard, N., Hyafil, A., Morris, I., & Boyer, P. (2015). Increased affluence explains the emergence of ascetic wisdoms and moralizing religions. *Current Biology, 25*(1), 10–15. doi:10.1016/j.cub.2014.10.063

Becker, E. (1973). *The denial of death.* New York: Simon and Schuster.

Bendixen, T., & Purzycki, B. G. (2020). Peering into the minds of gods: What cross-cultural variation in gods' concerns can tell us about the evolution of religion. *Journal for the Cognitive Science of Religion, 5*(2), 142–165.

Berkes, F. (2012). *Sacred ecology* (3rd ed.). New York: Routledge.

Bliege Bird, R., Tayor, N., Codding, B. F., & Bird, D. W. (2013). Niche construction and dreaming logic: Aboriginal patch mosaic burning and varanid lizards (*Varanus gouldii*) in Australia. *Proceedings of the Royal Society B: Biological Sciences*, 280(1772), 20132297. doi:10.1098/rspb.2013.2297

Boehm, C. (2008). A biocultural evolutionary exploration of supernatural sanctioning. In J. Bulbulia, R. Sosis, E. Harris, , R. Genet, & K. Wyman (Eds.), *Evolution of religion: Studies, theories, and critiques* (pp. 143–152). Santa Margarita, CA: Collins Foundation Press.

Botero, C. A., Gardner, B., Kirby, K. R., Bulbulia, J., Gavin, M. C., & Gray, R. D. (2014). The ecology of religious beliefs. *Proceedings of the National Academy of Sciences*, 111(47), 16784–16789. doi:10.1073/pnas.1408701111

Boyd, R., & Richerson, P. J. (1985). *Culture and the evolutionary process*. Chicago: University of Chicago Press.

Boyer, P. (1994). *The naturalness of religious ideas: A cognitive theory of religion*. Berkeley: University of California Press.

Boyer, P. (2000). Functional origins of religious concepts: Ontological and strategic selection in evolved minds. *Journal of the Royal Anthropological Institute*, 6(2), 195–214. doi:10.1111/1467-9655.00012

Boyer, P. (2001). *Religion explained: The evolutionary origins of religious thought*. New York: Basic Books.

Brown, D. (1991). *Human universals*. Boston: McGraw-Hill.

Chaplin, J. (2016). The global greening of religion. *Palgrave Communications*, 2, Article 16047. doi:10.1057/palcomms.2016.47

Chudek, M., McNamara, R. A., Birch, S., Bloom, P., & Henrich, J. (2017). Do minds switch bodies? Dualist interpretations across ages and societies. *Religion, Brain & Behavior*, 8(4), 354–368. doi:10.1080/2153599X.2017.1377757

D'Andrade, R. G. (1981). The cultural part of cognition. *Cognitive Science*, 5(3), 179–195. doi:10.1016/S0364-0213(81)80012-2

D'Andrade, R. G. (1999). Culture is not everything. In E. L. Cerroni-Long (Ed.), *Anthropological theory in North America* (pp. 85–103). Westport, CT: Bergin and Garvey.

Darwin, C. (2004). *The descent of man*. New York: Penguin Classics. (Original work published in 1871).

Durkheim, É. (2001). *The elementary forms of religious life*. New York: Oxford University Press. (Original work published in 1915).

Erdoes, R., & Ortiz, A. (Eds.). (1999). *American Indian trickster tales*. New York: Penguin Books.

Evans-Pritchard, E. E. (1965). *Theories of primitive religion*. Oxford: Clarendon Press.

Garcia, H. A. (2015). *Alpha God: The psychology of religious violence and oppression*. New York: Prometheus.

Gervais, W. M., & Henrich, J. (2010). The Zeus problem: Why representational content biases cannot explain faith in gods. *Journal of Cognition and Culture*, 10(3), 383–389. doi:10.1163/156853710X531249

Granqvist, P., Mikulincer, M., & Shaver, P. R. (2010). Religion as attachment: Normative processes and individual differences. *Personality and Social Psychology Review*, 14(1), 49–59. doi:10.1177/1088868309348618

Gray, K., Young, L., & Waytz, A. (2012). Mind perception is the essence of morality. *Psychological Inquiry*, 23(2), 101–124. doi:10.1080/1047840X.2012.651387

Guthrie, S. E. (1980). A cognitive theory of religion. *Current Anthropology*, 21(2), 181–203. doi:10.1086/202429

Guthrie, S. E. (1995). *Faces in the clouds: A new theory of religion.* New York: Oxford University Press.

Harner, M. J. (1973). *The Jivaro: People of the sacred waterfalls.* New York: Anchor Books.

Hartberg, Y., Cox, M., & Villamayor-Tomas, S. (2016). Supernatural monitoring and sanctioning in community-based resource management. *Religion, Brain & Behavior*, 6(2), 95–11. doi:10.1080/2153599X.2014.959547

Heiphetz, L., Lane, J. D., Waytz, A., & Young, L. L. (2016). How children and adults represent God's mind. *Cognitive Science*, 40(1), 121–144. doi:10.1111/cogs.12232

Hinde, R. A. (2010). *Why gods persist: A scientific approach to religion.* London: Routledge.

Hirschfeld, L. A. (2018). The Rutherford atom of culture. *Journal of Cognition and Culture*, 18(3–4), 231–261. doi:10.1163/15685373-12340029

Hutchins, E. (1995). *Cognition in the wild.* Cambridge, MA: MIT Press.

Hyde, L. (1998). *Trickster makes this world: Mischief, myth and art.* New York: North Point Press.

Jackson, J. C., Jong, J., Bluemke, M., Poulter, P., Morgenroth, L., & Halberstadt, J. (2018). Testing the causal relationship between religious belief and death anxiety. *Religion, Brain & Behavior*, 8(1), 57–68. doi:10.1080/2153599X.2016.1238842

Johnson, D. (2015). *God is watching you: How the fear of God makes us human.* New York: Oxford University Press.

Johnson, D. D. P. (2005). God's punishment and public goods: A test of the supernatural punishment hypothesis in 186 world cultures. *Human Nature*, 16(4), 410–46. doi:10.1007/s12110-005-1017-0

Johnson, D., & Bering, J. (2006). Hand of God, mind of man: Punishment and cognition in the evolution of cooperation. *Evolutionary Psychology*, 4(1), 14747049060040013O. doi:10.1177/147470490600400119

Jordan, P. (2003). *Material culture and sacred landscape: The anthropology of the Siberian Khanty.* Walnut Creek, CA: AltaMira Press.

Kendal, R. L., Boogert, N. J., Rendell, L., Laland, K. N., Webster, M., & Jones, P. L. (2018). Social learning strategies: Bridge-building between fields. *Trends in Cognitive Sciences*, 22(7), 651–665. doi:10.1016/j.tics.2018.04.003

Knight, N., Sousa, P., Barrett, J. L., & Atran, S. (2004). Children's attributions of beliefs to humans and God: Cross-cultural evidence. *Cognitive Science*, 28(1), 117–126. doi:10.1207/s15516709cog2801_6

Krátký, J., McGraw, J. J., Xygalatas, D., Mitkidis, P., & Reddish, P. (2016). It depends who is watching you: 3-D agent cues increase fairness. *PloS One*, 11(2), Article e0148845. doi:10.1371/journal.pone.0148845

Lambert, W. W., Triandis, L. M., & Wolf, M. (1959). Some correlates of beliefs in the malevolence and benevolence of supernatural beings: A cross-societal study. *Journal of Abnormal and Social Psychology*, 58(2), 162–169. doi:10.1037/h0041462

Lane, J. D., Wellman, H. M., & Evans, E. M. (2012). Sociocultural input facilitates children's developing understanding of extraordinary minds. *Child Development*, 83(3), 1007–1021. doi:10.1111/j.1467-8624.2012.01741.x

Lane, J. D., Wellman, H. M., & Evans, E. M. (2014). Approaching an understanding of omniscience from the preschool years to early adulthood. *Developmental Psychology*, 50(10), 2380–2392. doi:10.1037/a0037715

Lansing, J. S. (2012). *Perfect order: Recognizing complexity in Bali*. Princeton, NJ: Princeton University Press.

Levin, T. (2006). *Where rivers and mountains sing: Sound, music, and nomadism in Tuva and beyond*. Bloomington: Indiana University Press.

Matthews, H. F. (1992). The directive force of morality tales in a Mexican community. In R. D'Andrade and C. Strauss (Eds.), *Human motives and cultural models* (pp. 127–162). Cambridge, UK: Cambridge University Press.

McCauley, R. N. (2011). *Why religion is natural, and science is not*. Oxford: Oxford University Press.

McCauley, R. N., & Henrich, J. (2006). Susceptibility to the Müller-Lyer illusion, theory-neutral observation, and the diachronic penetrability of the visual input system. *Philosophical Psychology, 19*(1), 79–101. doi:10.1080/09515080500462347

McCauley, R. N., & Lawson, E. T. (2002). *Bringing ritual to mind: Psychological foundations of cultural forms*. Cambridge, UK: Cambridge University Press.

McCullough, M. E., & Willoughby, B. L. B. (2009). Religion, self-regulation, and self-control: Associations, explanations, and implications. *Psychological Bulletin, 135*(1), 69–93. doi:10.1037/a0014213

McKay, R., & Whitehouse, H. (2015). Religion and morality. *Psychological Bulletin, 141*(2), 447–473. doi:10.1037/a0038455

McNamara, R. A., & Henrich, J. (2018). Jesus vs. the ancestors: How specific religious beliefs shape prosociality on Yasawa Island, Fiji. *Religion, Brain & Behavior, 8*(2), 185–204. doi:10.1080/2153599X.2016.1267030

Morgan, J., Clark, D., Tripodis, Y., Halloran, C. S., Minsky, A., Wildman, W. J., Durso, R. & McNamara, P. (2016). Impacts of religious semantic priming on an intertemporal discounting task: Response time effects and neural correlates. *Neuropsychologia, 89*, 403–413.

Morin, O. (2015). *How traditions live and die*. Oxford: Oxford University Press.

Mullins, D. A., Hoyer, D., Collins, C., Currie, T., Feeney, K., François, P. (2018). A systematic assessment of "Axial Age" proposals using global comparative historical evidence. *American Sociological Review, 83*(3), 596–626. doi:10.1177/0003122418772567

Norenzayan, A. (2013). *Big Gods: How religion transformed cooperation and conflict*. Princeton, NJ: Princeton University Press.

Norenzayan, A., Shariff, A. F., Gervais, W. M., Willard, A. K., McNamara, R. A., Slingerland, E., & Henrich, J. (2016). The cultural evolution of prosocial religions. *Behavioral and Brain Sciences, 39*, doi:10.1017/S0140525X14001356

Northover, S. B., Pedersen, W. C., Cohen, A. B., & Andrews, P. W. (2017). Artificial surveillance cues do not increase generosity: Two meta-analyses. *Evolution and Human Behavior, 38*(1), 144–153. doi:10.1016/j.evolhumbehav.2016.07.001

Nyhof, M. A., & Johnson, C. N. (2017). Is God just a big person? Children's conceptions of God across cultures and religious traditions. *British Journal of Developmental Psychology, 35*(1), 60–75. doi:10.1111/bjdp.12173

Peoples, H. C., & Marlowe, F. W. (2012). Subsistence and the evolution of religion. *Human Nature, 23*(3), 253–269. doi:10.1007/s12110-012-9148-6

Peregrine, P. (1996). The birth of the gods revisited: A partial replication of Guy Swanson's (1960) cross-cultural study of religion. *Cross-Cultural Research, 30*(1), 84–112. doi:10.1177/106939719603000104

Power, C. (2015). Hadza gender rituals—epeme and maitoko—considered as counterparts. *Hunter Gatherer Research, 1*(3), 333–358. doi:10.3828/hgr.2015.18

Premack, D., & Woodruff, G. (1978). Does the chimpanzee have a theory of mind? *Behavioral and Brain Sciences, 1*(04), 515–526. doi:10.1017/S0140525X00076512

Purzycki, B. G. (2010). Spirit masters, ritual cairns, and the adaptive religious system in Tyva. *Sibirica, 9*(2), 21–47. doi:10.3167/sib.2010.090202

Purzycki, B. G. (2013). The minds of gods: A comparative study of supernatural agency. *Cognition, 129*(1), 163–179. doi:10.1016/j.cognition.2013.06.010

Purzycki, B. G. (2016). The evolution of Gods' minds in the Tyva Republic. *Current Anthropology, 57*(S13), S88–104. doi:10.1086/685729

Purzycki, B. G., & McNamara, R. A. (2016). An ecological theory of gods' minds. In H. De Cruz & R. Nichols (Eds.), *Cognitive science of religion and its philosophical implications* (pp. 143–167). New York: Continuum.

Purzycki, B. G., & Holland, E. C. (2019). Buddha as a god: An empirical assessment. *Method & Theory in the Study of Religion, 31*(4–5), 347–375.

Purzycki, B. G., Finkel, D. N., Shaver, J., Wales, N., Cohen, A. B., & Sosis, R. (2012). What does God know? Supernatural agents' access to socially strategic and non-strategic information. *Cognitive Science, 36*(5), 846–869. doi:10.1111/j.1551-6709.2012.01242.x

Purzycki, B. G., Haque, O. S., & Sosis, R. (2014). Extending evolutionary accounts of religion beyond the mind: Religions as adaptive systems. In F. Watts & L. P. Turner (Eds.), *Evolution, religion, and cognitive science*: Critical and constructive essays (pp. 74–91). Oxford: Oxford University Press.

Purzycki, B. G., Apicella, C., Atkinson, Q. D., Cohen, E., McNamara, R. A., Willard, A. K., Xygalatas, D., Norenzayan, A., & Henrich, J. (2016a). Cross-cultural dataset for the evolution of religion and morality project. *Scientific Data, 3*, Article 160099. doi:10.1038/sdata.2016.99

Purzycki, B. G. Apicella, C., Atkinson, Q. D., Cohen, E., McNamara, R. A., Willard, A. K., Xygalatas, D., Norenzayan, A., & Henrich, J. (2016b). Moralistic gods, supernatural punishment and the expansion of human sociality. *Nature, 530*(7590), 327–330. doi:10.1038/nature16980

Purzycki, B. G., Henrich, J., Apicella, C., Atkinson, Q. D., Baimel, A., Cohen, E., McNamara, R. A., Willard, A. K., Xygalatas, D., & Norenzayan, A. (2018). The evolution of religion and morality: A synthesis of ethnographic and experimental evidence from eight societies. *Religion, Brain & Behavior, 8*(2), 101–132. doi:10.1080/2153599X.2016.1267027

Purzycki, B., Willard, A., Kundtová Klocová, E., Apicella, C., Atkinson, Q., Bolyanatz, A., Cohen, E., Handley, C., Henrich, J., Lang, M., Lesorogol, C., Mathew, S., McNamara, R., Moya, C., Norenzayan, A., Placek, C., Soler, M., Weigel, J., Xygalatas, D., Ross, C., & Vardy, T. in press. The Moralization Bias of Gods' Minds: A Cross-Cultural Test. *Religion, Brain & Behavior*.

Purzycki, B. G., Pisor, A. C., Apicella, C., Atkinson, Q., Cohen, E., Henrich, J., McElreath, R., McNamara, R. A., Norenzayan, A., Willard, A. K., & Xygalatas, D. (2018). The cognitive and cultural foundations of moral behavior. *Evolution and Human Behavior, 39*(5), 490–501. doi:10.1016/j.evolhumbehav.2018.04.004

Purzycki, B. G., Ross, C. T., Apicella, C., Atkinson, Q. D., Cohen, E., McNamara, R. A., Willard, A. K., Xygalatas, D., Norenzayan, A., & Henrich, J. (2018). Material security, life history, and moralistic religions: A cross-cultural examination. *PLoS One, 13*(3), Article e0193856. doi:10.1371/journal.pone.0193856

Rappaport, R. A. (2000). *Pigs for the ancestors: Ritual in the ecology of a New Guinea people* (2nd ed.). Long Grove, IL: Waveland Press.

Reynolds, V., & Tanner, R. (1995). *The social ecology of religion* (2nd ed.). New York: Oxford University Press.

Richerson, P. J., & Boyd, R. (2005). *Not by genes alone: How culture transformed human evolution*. Chicago: University of Chicago Press.

Romney, A. K., Weller, S. C., & Batchelder, W. H. (1986). Culture as consensus: A theory of culture and informant accuracy. *American Anthropologist, 88*(2), 313–338.

Schjoedt, U., Sørensen, J., Nielbo, K. L., Xygalatas, D., Mitkidis, P., & Bulbulia, J. (2013). Cognitive resource depletion in religious interactions. *Religion, Brain & Behavior, 3*(1), 39–55. doi:10.1080/2153599X.2012.736714

Segall, M. H., Campbell, D. T., & Herskovits, M. J. (1963). Cultural differences in the perception of geometric illusions. *Science, 139*(3556), 769–771. doi:10.1126/science.139.3556.769

Shahaeian, A., Peterson, C. C., Slaughter, V., & Wellman, H. M. (2011). Culture and the sequence of steps in theory of mind development. *Developmental Psychology, 47*(5), 1239–1247. doi:10.1037/a0023899

Shaman, N. J., Saide, A. R., & Richert, R. A. (2018). Dimensional structure of and variation in anthropomorphic concepts of God. *Frontiers in Psychology, 9.* doi:10.3389/fpsyg.2018.01425

Shariff, A. F., Purzycki, B. G., & Sosis, R. (2014). Religions as cultural solutions to social living. In A. Cohen (Ed.), *Culture reexamined: Broadening our understanding of social and evolutionary influences* (pp. 217–238). Washington, DC: American Psychological Association.

Shih, F.-L. (2012). Generating power in Taiwan: Nuclear, political and religious power. *Culture and Religion, 13*(3), 295–313. doi:10.1080/14755610.2012.706229

Sibley, C. G., & Bulbulia, J. (2012). Faith after an earthquake: A longitudinal study of religion and perceived health before and after the 2011 Christchurch New Zealand earthquake. *PLoS One, 7*(12), e49648. doi:10.1371/journal.pone.0049648

Silberbauer, G. B. (1972). The G/wi Bushmen. In M. G. Bicchieri (Ed.), *Hunters and gatherers today* (pp. 271–326). Prospect Heights, IL: Waveland Press.

Sosis, R. (2009). The adaptationist-byproduct debate on the evolution of religion: Five misunderstandings of the adaptationist program. *Journal of Cognition and Culture, 9*(3), 315–332. doi:10.1163/156770909X12518536414411

Sosis, R., & Alcorta, C. (2005). Is religion adaptive? *Behavioral and Brain Sciences, 27*(06), 749–750.

Sosis, R., & Bulbulia, J. (2011). The behavioral ecology of religion: The benefits and costs of one evolutionary approach. *Religion, 41*(3), 341–362. doi:10.1080/0048721X.2011.604514

Sperber, D. (1996). *Explaining culture: A naturalistic approach*. Malden: Wiley-Blackwell.

Sperber, D. (1997). Intuitive and reflective beliefs. *Mind & Language.*. Retrieved February 4, 2014, from http://cogprints.org/402/

Spiro, M. E., & D'Andrade, R. G. (1958). A cross-cultural study of some supernatural beliefs. *American Anthropologist, 60*(3), 456–466.

Stewart, V. M. (1974). A cross-cultural test of the "carpentered world" hypothesis using the Ames distorted room illusion. *International Journal of Psychology, 9*(2), 79–89. doi:10.1080/00207597408247094

Strauss, C., & Quinn, N. (1997). *A cognitive theory of cultural meaning*. Cambridge, UK: Cambridge University Press.

Swanson, G. E. (1960). *The birth of the gods: The origin of primitive beliefs*. Ann Arbor: University of Michigan Press.

Turner, J. H., Maryanski, A., Petersen, A. K., & Geertz, A. W. (2017). *The emergence and evolution of religion: By means of natural selection*. New York: Routledge.

Turner, N. J., & Berkes, F. (2006). Coming to understanding: Developing conservation through incremental learning in the Pacific Northwest. *Human Ecology, 34*(4), 495–513. doi:10.1007/s10745-006-9042-0

Van Leeuwen, N., & van Elk, M. (2019). Seeking the supernatural: The interactive religious experience model. *Religion, Brain & Behavior, 9*(3), 221–251. doi:10.1080/2153599X.2018.1453529.

Walker, J. R. (1991). *Lakota belief and ritual*. Lincoln, NE: Bison Books.

Wallace, A. F. C. (1966). *Religion: An anthropological view*. New York: McGraw-Hill.

Watanabe, H. (1972). The Ainu. In M. G. Bicchieri (Ed.), *Hunters and gatherers today* (pp. 448–484). Prospect Heights, IL: Waveland Press.

Watts, J., Greenhill, S. J., Atkinson, Q. D., Currie, T. E., Bulbulia, J., & Gray, R. D. (2015). Broad supernatural punishment but not moralizing high gods precede the evolution of political complexity in Austronesia. *Proceedings of the Royal Society of London B: Biological Sciences, 282*(1804), 20142556. doi:10.1098/rspb.2014.2556

Watts, J., Sheehan, O., Greenhill, S. J., Gomes-Ng, S., Atkinson, Q. D., Bulbulia, J., & Gray, R. D. (2015). Pulotu: Database of Austronesian supernatural beliefs and practices. *PLoS One, 10*(9), Article e0136783. doi:10.1371/journal.pone.0136783

Welsch, R. L. (1981). *Omaha tribal myths and trickster tales*. Lincoln, NE: J & L Lee.

White, C., Kelly, J. M., Shariff, A., & Norenzayan, A. (2018). Thinking about karma and God reduces believers' selfishness in anonymous dictator games. [Preprint]. PsyArXiv. doi:10.31234/osf.io/w4dfp

Wiessner, P. W., & Papu, N. (1998). *Historical vines: Enga networks of exchange, ritual, and warfare in Papua New Guinea*. Washington, DC: Smithsonian Institution Press.

Wigger, J. B. (2016). Children's theory of God's mind: Theory-of-mind studies and why they matter to religious education. *Religious Education, 111*(3), 325–339. doi:10.1080/00344087.2016.1169879

Wigger, J. B., Paxson, K., & Ryan, L. (2013). What do invisible friends know? Imaginary companions, God, and theory of mind. *International Journal for the Psychology of Religion, 23*(1), 2–14. doi:10.1080/10508619.2013.739059

Wilson, D. S. (2002). *Darwin's cathedral: Evolution, religion, and the nature of society*. Chicago: University of Chicago Press.

Wood, C. (2017). Ritual well-being: Toward a social signaling model of religion and mental health. *Religion, Brain & Behavior, 7*(3), 223–243. doi:10.1080/2153599X.2016.1156556

Xygalatas, D., Kotherová, S., Maňo, P., Kundt, R., Cigán, J., Klocová, E. K., & Lang, M. (2018). Big Gods in small places: The random allocation game in Mauritius. *Religion, Brain & Behavior, 8*(2), 243–261. doi:10.1080/2153599X.2016.1267033

Yilmaz, O., & Bahçekapili, H. G. (2016). Supernatural and secular monitors promote human cooperation only if they remind of punishment. *Evolution and Human Behavior, 37*(1), 79–84. doi:10.1016/j.evolhumbehav.2015.09.005

CHAPTER 6

THE NATURE OF HUMANS

REBEKAH A. RICHERT AND KIRSTEN A. LESAGE

INTRODUCTION

IN this chapter, we consider how humans conceive of other humans, and the interacting roles of cognitive biases and cultural processes in the development of these conceptions. Data collected from young children and adults suggest that humans conceptualize themselves and other humans as consisting of "an essential something" beyond a body and mind. We argue that a cognitive bias that leads to essentialist reasoning, combined with cultural practices directed at altering that essence (i.e., rituals), provide a uniquely human cognitive foundation for concepts of a human quintessence. In particular, we propose that humans utilize a *folk anthropology* that attributes an intrinsic and central constituent of human character (what makes humans human), and is the product of conceptual predilections to categorize objects into discrete groups with an unseen essence and cultural practices that build upon these cognitive foundations.

INTUITIVE THEORIES AND COGNITIVE DEVELOPMENT

Forming a useful conception of what it means to be human is a fundamental accomplishment for children. This conception includes understanding that humans have physical bodies that conform to fundamental laws of nature and depend on life-giving biological processes. Children must also come to understand that humans have mental processes that function as causes and motivators of human action. To grasp these aspects of humans, children rely on and refine intuitive theories about the nature of humans (Gelman & Legare, 2011). Intuitive theories differ from scientific theories in that they are implicit as opposed to explicit and imprecise as opposed to precise; however, intuitive

THE NATURE OF HUMANS   91

theories function similarly to scientific theories in their cognitive functioning, which includes "organiz[ing] experience, generat[ing] inferences, guid[ing] learning, and influenc[ing] behavior and social interactions" (Gelman & Legare, 2011, p. 379). A large body of research has outlined the development of three core intuitive theories that support and constrain children's learning about the world in general, and their perceptions of humans, in particular: folk physics, folk biology, and folk psychology. In developing an intuitive sense of the nature of humans, children coordinate inferences derived from these three theories. We first describe these three foundational theories (Wellman & Gelman, 1992), and then we propose an additional folk theory (folk anthropology) that becomes coordinated in an understanding of the nature of humans.

Folk Physics

Folk physics involves reasoning about the physical laws that constrain objects (Baillargeon, 2008). Core foundations of folk physics are demonstrated early in infancy; infants as young as 2.5 to 4 months old expect physical events to conform to principles of continuity (that objects move in continuous paths), cohesion (that bounded objects remain whole unless acted upon), and persistence (objects do not phase in and out of existence or pass through other objects; Baillargeon, 2008). For example, the attention of 2.5- to 4-month-olds was greater for a display in which an object seemed to pass through a solid barrier or through an impossibly small opening than it was for possible normal physical events (Spelke et al., 1992). That is, babies appear to be surprised by objects that appear to be violating some elements of basic physics. Young infants also are surprised if an object breaks apart as it moves through space (Needham, 1999) and do not expect an object to spontaneously change location (Newcombe et al., 1992). Throughout early childhood, the continued development of the folk-physics system involves developing spatial cognition and applying an understanding of the physical world to the use of tools to overcome physical obstacles (see Bjorklund & Causey, 2018).

Folk Biology

Folk biology involves reasoning about living kinds (Gelman & Legare, 2011). Even newborns demonstrate preferential looking toward lights that move as humans would move (Bardi et al., 2011), and young infants differentiate animate from inanimate objects based on their ability to move themselves (Schlottman & Ray, 2010). By age 4, children's folk theories of biology include an understanding of the properties of living things (Inagaki & Hatano, 2002; Wellman & Gelman, 1998). These properties include growth (Hatano & Inagaki, 1994; Inagaki & Hatano, 1996; Hickling & Gelman, 1995; Rosengren et al., 1991), movement (Gelman & Gottfried, 1996), nourishment (Inagaki & Hatano, 2002), reproduction (Keil, 1995), and inheritability (Keil, 1989; Sousa et al., 2002). For example, in a study by Inagaki and Hatano (1996), 5-year-old children accurately differentiated that plants (e.g., flowers) and animals (e.g., chickens) grow, but that man-made artifacts (e.g., a tea cup) do not. Moreover, 4-year-olds are able to order pictures of a plant in its correct growth sequence (e.g., seed–plant–flower) and readily recognize an incorrect growth sequence (e.g., flower–plant–seed; Hickling & Gelman, 1995).

Folk Psychology

Folk psychology is thinking about human actions in terms of beliefs, desires, intentions, and goals (Gelman & Legare, 2011). Some studies have suggested that an intuition that agents have unobservable intentions, thoughts, and beliefs begins to emerge by the age of 1 year (Sommerville & Woodward, 2005; Wellman et al., 2001; Woodward & Guajardo, 2002). Additionally, infants appear to expect human action to conform to principles of efficiency (i.e., minimal effort with maximal reward) and consistency (i.e., coherence between cognition and behavior; Baillargeon et al., 2016). For example, Woodward and Guajardo (2002) found that infants between the ages of 9 and 12 months understand the goal of reaching for an object or pointing to an object as a deliberate, object-directed action. The understanding that human mental states and emotions con-tribute to human behaviors continues to develop through the early childhood years (Wellman & Liu, 2004).

Coordination of Intuitive Theories in the Developing Concept of Humans

Because humans have physical bodies that (a) exist in time and space, (b) require sus-tenance and conform to a life cycle, and (c) embody emotional and cognitive states that cause behavior, intuitions about "what makes humans human" require the coordination of inferences derived from these folk systems of thought. For example, during certain phases of development, children conflate some aspects of folk biology with folk psy-chology, associating "being alive" with having intentional agency (Shtulman, 2017). Thus children might claim that a cloud is alive because it appears to move through space on its own, but that a tree is not alive because it does not move through space.

Humans are sensitive to cues that indicate which system of inference should be used to process different kinds of information. In particular, very young infants are sensi-tive to cues of agency (e.g., self-propelled motion) and will develop different predictions about the movements of animate agents and inanimate objects (Kuhlmeier et al., 2004). Importantly, the human body itself is a cue to intentional agency. Chudek et al. (2018) tested Fijian and Canadian participants' intuition that a "mind" could move from one shape (a pentagon) to another (a smaller pentagon) to help the original shape achieve a goal (to get some cake). Approximately 70% of children in both samples, and approxi-mately 60% of Fijian adults (the Canadian adults were not tested), inferred that a mind had transferred from the original shape to another shape if the original shape had eyes. This inference was less common (though not completely absent) in both children and adults if the shape did not have eyes as a cue to agency (Chudek et al., 2018).

The coordination of these systems of thinking could lead to three potential intuitions about the nature of humans and how human bodies and mental states contribute to what makes humans human. A *materialist intuition* would be an intuition that humans are strictly and solely composed of bodies and brains—a form of materialism (see Churchland, 1981). Forstmann and Burgmer (2018) described this stance as a reductive physicalism, which they defined as the view that mental states are either actually physical states or only descriptions of physical states, but do not exist independently of physical states. Similarly, Hodge (2008) has argued that there is minimal evidence for an intuitive separation of mental and bodily processes, especially when exploring funerary cultural practices that focus heavily on respect for the human body upon death.

A *dualist intuition* is the intuition that minds are separate from bodies (Bloom, 2004; Bering, 2006). Forstmann and Burgmer (2018) described this as substance dualism, which they defined as the stance that mental states exist entirely separately from physical bodies and can exist in the absence of a physical body. Much of the research supporting claims of an intuitive Cartesian substance dualism are based on research suggesting that young children form separate representations of the mind and the body early in childhood, and that even infants successfully make animate-inanimate distinctions (Bloom, 2004). For example, infants tend to look longer at objects on a screen that appear to be following each other in a game of tag (i.e., animated, or having a mental state) than at objects that appear to be moving randomly on the screen (i.e., inanimate, or not having specific goals or desires).

A *tripartite intuition* is the intuition that in addition to the body and mind, humans have an essential something" (from here on referred to as a "quintessence") that confers individual identity beyond that conferred by the body or the mind alone. In other words, humans may conceive of other humans as consisting of an identity-granting essence that is separate from the body and also separate from mental processes (Richert & Harris, 2006).

The largest body of research on intuitions about the nature of humans has focused on the (presumed) presence of a mind-body substance dualism in children and adults. Much of this research is based on the hypothesis that a developing theory of mind (i.e., the attribution of unseen goals, intentions, desires, and motivations to others' actions) can account for this intuitive dualism. We first summarize this body of research and then articulate the limitations of this approach for explaining data suggesting a primary role for essentialist reasoning in conceptualizations of the nature of humans.

Folk Psychology and Dualism

The presence of mind-body dualism has been documented early in development (Bloom, 2004), as well as across human cultures and human history (Roazzi et al., 2013;

Slingerland & Chudek, 2011; Slingerland, 2018). The developmental research on dualism has focused on children's developing understanding of the functions of the mind and brain and their beliefs about whether a person's identity is contained in the mind or the body.

In one of the earliest studies of the developing understanding of the mind-brain distinction, Johnson and Wellman (1982) found that by the age of 4, children understand that the brain is internal to a person and is responsible for mental functions. Johnson and Wellman (1982) argued that children younger than age 9 do not differentiate the functions of the brain from the functions of the mind; however, subsequent research has documented the development of this distinction in early childhood. To understand how children come to differentiate the mind from the brain, Corriveau et al., (2005) examined the natural language in which children hear the words *mind* and *brain* between the ages of 2 and 5 by looking through a database of children's language environment (CHILDES, the CHIld Language Data Exchange System). Parents were much more likely to use the word *mind* than *brain*, and when the word *mind* was used, it was more likely to be used to refer to mental functioning. Furthermore, Gottfried and Jow (2003) noted that in children's storybooks written in English, the word *brain* was used far less often than the word *heart*, and that the word *heart* was often used in metaphorical contexts that denoted emotional states.

To test how children coordinate intuitions about the mind and the body in conferring identity, Johnson (1990) asked participants which abilities, preferences, or identity characteristics would transfer with a person (i.e., the donor) if their mind were transferred into another body (i.e., the recipient). Children between the ages of 5 and 7 indicated that their own cognitive (e.g., knowing words), behavioral (e.g., being kind), and identity (e.g., name) aspects would transfer along with their brain into the body of a pig or a baby. Children also claimed that these aspects would transfer if their brain were transplanted into another child, but they were less likely to claim that the reverse was true (i.e., that the transplant of another child's brain into their own body would bring along those characteristics of the other child). Thus, children seem to view their own identity as being tied to both their own brain and their own body, but others' identity as tied to their brain but not their body.

Using a similar hypothetical transplant method, Gottfried et al., (1999) questioned children between the ages of 3 and 5 about the brain of a donor animal being transplanted into the brain of a recipient animal. The children were asked if the thoughts, memories, vocalizations (e.g., mooing), and appearance would travel with the donor's brain into the recipient animal's body. Gottfried et al. found that children ages 3 to 5 did not indicate that the identity characteristics of the donor animal would transfer with that animal's brain into another animal's body. They documented that the association of these functions with a traveling brain emerges around age 8 or 9. The combined findings from Johnson (1990) and Gottfried et al. (1999) suggest that children younger than age 9 or 10 will agree that the identity characteristics of a person will travel with that person's brain into the body of an animal, but they are less prone to claim that identity travels with a brain in animal-to-animal transfer.

These two studies focused on children's concepts of the brain; however, children associate the mind with identity before they associate the brain with identity. Corriveau et al. (2005) used Gottfried et al.'s (1999) transformation method to examine the beliefs of 5- to 7-year-old children (as well as a sample of adults) about what properties would change about a child if a wizard magically changed the child's mind or brain into that of a horse. Corriveau et al.'s study focused on whether the child would maintain her or his name, memories, preferences, and knowledge. Younger children were more likely to indicate that the child's identity would change if the mind were transformed than if the brain were transformed. Older children and adults also indicated that the identity would change if the brain were transformed. These findings suggest that although children associate the physical brain with mental functions, an early emerging intuition is that the mind is more important than the brain in conferring identity by virtue of being the repository for one's name, memories, preferences, and knowledge. This view of the mind is supported by a cultural context that supports privileging the mind as the "container" of identity (e.g., Corriveau et al., 2005).

Cohen and Barrett (2008) further unpacked how individuals conceptualize what happens when a mind is transplanted into a new body. Young adults indicated what kinds of abilities and preferences transfer if a person's mind is transferred into the body of another person. The participants' responses were scored as indicating whether the donor's mind would displace or fuse with the mind of the recipient. The majority of participants indicated that the donor's mind would completely displace the mind of the recipient.

Using a slightly different method, Hood et al. (2012) asked participants about an animal that had been cloned. British 6-year-olds indicated what properties a hamster would retain if its body were duplicated by a magic machine. In this method (in which the body rather than the mind is duplicated), children were more likely to indicate that physical states (e.g., having a blue heart) rather than mental states (e.g., memory) would duplicate into the new hamster. The participants were also less likely to say that memory states would transfer into a duplicated body if the original hamster had been given a name. Thus, in the case of a duplicated body, children privilege the duplication of physical states over that of mental states, suggesting a view that the mind is associated with a particular physical form (or a unique person's body). These findings suggest that although children appear to view the human mind as more identity-granting than the human body, they also view the unique connection between a given individual's mind and her or his body as critical for conferring that person's identity, especially if that person has a name.

Forstmann and Burgmer (2014) conducted a series of similar studies using adults, asking them what kinds of properties would carry over from an animal or a human into a duplication (i.e., clone) of that animal or human. As with the children in Hood et al.'s (2012) study, participants were more likely to indicate that physical rather than mental characteristics would be shared between the original animal/human and its duplicate.

Conducting research with adults in the United Kingdom and in a community in Brazil that has cultural beliefs in spirit possession, soul flight, and the afterlife, Cohen et al., (2011) asked participants to imagine they had (a) left their bodies, (b) left their bodies and entered a rock, or (c) left their bodies and entered a plant. They were then asked whether physical and psychological processes would cease or continue. In their questions, Cohen et al. diverged from prior research that had delineated processes as belonging to one of two categories: (a) a category that includes psychobiological (e.g., feel queasy), perceptual (e.g., taste)/emotional (e.g., feel scared), and epistemic (e.g., believe; Bering & Bjorklund, 2004) states, or (b) a category that includes psychobiological (e.g., hear) and mental (e.g., know; Astuti & Harris, 2008) states..

Cohen et al. (2011) instead distinguished two categories of processes as being either *body dependent* or *body independent* based on participants' responses to the first set of questions asking them to imagine they had left their bodies. Although there was much cross-cultural agreement on which processes were body dependent (e.g., feeling the wind, smelling things, tasting things) and which were body independent (e.g., hoping, learning, knowing), there were informative cultural differences in some processes. Specifically, the participants from Brazil were more likely than the participants from the United Kingdom to indicate that the following processes were body dependent: "feel sexual desire, feel angry, feel excited, feel scared, hate things, feel upset, feel disgust, feel sad" (Cohen et al., p. 1292).

In their general responses, participants were more likely to associate the continuation of both body-dependent and body-independent processes when they were asked to imagine going into an object (plant or rock) than when they were asked to simply imagine leaving their body (Cohen et al., 2011). Furthermore, the participants from Brazil were more likely than the UK participants to associate continued body-dependent processes with transition into a rock. And the Brazilian participants were equally likely to claim that body-independent processes would continue in a general disembodiment and in transfer into a plant or rock. In contrast, the UK participants were less likely to endorse the continuation of body-independent processes if the person has left their body and entered into a rock or plant (Cohen et al., 2011).

Research with adults in the United States and India indicates variation in how the body and the mind are viewed in conferring identity (Mahalingam & Rodriguez, 2006). Both the American and Indian participants believed the social identity (ethnicity/caste) of an individual would not change if their brain were transplanted into a new body. In contrast, the American adults believed the brain-transplant recipient would act in ways consistent with the ethnicity of the donor brain; whereas, the Indian participants believed that actions would travel with a low-status brain into a high-status body, but not vice versa. In other words, a person's actions may change if they receive a new brain, but a person's ethnicity or caste is defined by their body, not their brain.

Folk Theories Summary

Previous research has indicated that by the age of 7 or 8, children associate the mind with a person's preferences, actions, and desires. Studies that ask children and adults to think about the mind in novel ways (e.g., a mind going from one body into another) also seem to suggest that people view the mind as housing an individual's identity. However, studies that prompt children and adults to think about the body (e.g., cloning studies) or about whether changes to the brain result in changes to one's social category indicate that children not only conceive of identity as being connected to the mind, but also indicate that there is something unique about the *connection* between a given individual's mind and body that confers a unique identity to each individual (Hood et al., 2012). Therefore, to fully capture intuitions about the nature of humans, researchers should consider the role of essentialist reasoning about individuals and categories.

Folk Anthropology

The body of research summarized so far suggests that cognitive biases toward substance dualism and the folk theory of mind cannot fully account for how humans conceptualize other humans. As Hirschfeld (2013) has argued, the human capacity for mentalizing is insufficient to explain patterns in how we interpret and predict the actions of others. In fact, most people rely on heuristics related to others' nonmental properties, such as age, gender, occupation, race, and rank, when interpreting and predicting others' actions (e.g., Hirschfeld et al., 2007). Associating an individual with a social category employs essentialist reasoning to explain or predict human behavior (Rhodes et al., 2012).

We propose that as children are developing folk theories of physics, biology, and psychology, they are simultaneously developing a folk system of inference about the quintessence of individual persons and the cultural practices that engage or alter that essence. We call this foundational theory a *folk anthropology*, and we propose it incorporates three main components not included or accounted for in other folk theories: (a) the attribution of a quintessence to each individual person (e.g., a soul), (b) intuitions that the quintessence exists outside the life cycle (e.g., in prelife and afterlife beliefs), and (c) a belief that the quintessence can be altered by cultural, supernatural, and/or religious activities that change the fundamental nature of humans (e.g., rituals).

Essentialism

For the purposes of this chapter, three descriptions of essentialism are especially productive for delineating how humans view other humans. First, "psychological essentialism is a pervasive cognitive bias that leads people to view members of a category as sharing a deep, underlying, inherent nature (a category 'essence'), which causes them to be fundamentally similar to one another in both obvious and nonobvious ways" (Rhodes et al., 2012, p. 1). Second, according to Medin (1989), "People act as if things (e.g., objects) have essences or underlying natures that make them the thing that they are" (p. 1476). Third, and as Gelman (2009) noted, "Despite outward changes in appearances over the lifetime of an individual (e.g., from infant to adult) and despite outward variation in appearance across members of a category (e.g., from typical to atypical instances), people believe that category members share an immutable feature or substance (essence) that causes category members to be what they are and have the properties that they do" (p. 124).

Thus, as conceptualized in the field of cognitive development, essentialism supports the development of category learning by scaffolding children's transfer of learning about an individual member of a category (e.g., Fido grows) to other members of that category (e.g., all dogs grow; Gelman et al., 1994). Essentialist reasoning is found across cultures and ages, though the way it manifests varies by culture (Gelman, 2009). Gelman and Diesendruck (1999) have argued that psychological essentialism is skeletal in nature, such that the cognitive bias toward essentialism provides a placeholder into which children put information about the nature of an individual or category. The role of essentialist reasoning is most commonly highlighted in research on children's language learning and categorization (Gelman, 2009). However, essentialist reasoning can also be applied to thinking about social categories and what makes groups of people unique (e.g., race, religion, gender) (Rhodes et al., 2012).

In a classic study, Jane Elliott demonstrated how easy it is to prime social essentialism in children (cited in Stewart et al., 2003). She told her classroom of third graders that brown-eyed children are better than blue-eyed children. By the time lunch was over, the classroom had developed a caste-like system in which the brown-eyed children ostracized the blue-eyed children. As Mahalingam (2007) outlined, the bias toward attributing essences to humans and to social categories reflects both a cognitive bias that supports category learning and inferences, and social biases that maintain the sociological power structures that serve individuals in power.

Individuals may also judge the inheritance of personal characteristics (e.g., identity, beliefs, behaviors, skills, genetics) in essentialist terms (Moya et al., 2015). For instance, in a set of cross-cultural studies in Peru, Fiji, and the United States examining differences in folk theories of the influence of parenting, participants were presented with vignettes in which the protagonist had either (a) been adopted by a nonbiologically related family at birth (adoption condition) or (b) had migrated with her biological family to a different culture after birth (migration condition; Moya et al., 2015). The participants were then asked a series of questions about whether the protagonist would be more likely to share a particular trait with her birth parents or her adoptive parents (e.g., music preference, intelligence, ear shape). Results showed high cultural variation in how similar the protagonist would be compared to the birth parents across the different personal characteristics, with only the US sample embracing the strong "nurture" view that parents shape children's beliefs and behaviors (Moya et al., 2015).

Gelman and Diesendruck (1999) additionally argued that because the bias toward essentializing provides a placeholder, the motivation to identify what fits into that placeholder can account for conceptual change. This cognitive "placeholder" can provide a fertile cognitive space both for the cultural influence of beliefs about what makes a person a person (e.g., concepts of the soul) and for cultural and ritual practices that imply individuals have an essence that makes them who they are. A pervasive implicit assumption that the brain functions as a container or repository for our mental capacities echoes this characterization (see Gottfried et al., 1999).

However, newer studies have suggested that individuals do not dichotomously or orthogonally categorize human functions as either mental or bodily. For example, a priming study with adults presented participants with a biological prime (video on the brain), an emotional prime (video about the Rwanda genocide), or no prime (control condition), followed by a gender-matched vignette about a student named Sam who was heading home for the summer at the end of the academic year when she or he was killed in an accident at the train station (Bek & Lock, 2011). The adult participants then reported their views on whether Sam continued to hold various states: biological (e.g., does Sam still suffer from hay fever?), psychobiological (e.g., is Sam still thirsty), perceptual (e.g., can Sam still see the sky?), emotional (e.g., can Sam still love his or her mum?), desire (e.g., does Sam still want to go to the party?), epistemic (e.g., does Sam still know how to do math?), and death-awareness (e.g., does Sam know that she or he is dead?). The emotional priming condition did not appear to have an effect on participants' judgments (as compared to the control condition), but the biological prime reduced some attribution of postdeath states continuing, such as emotional states (Bek & Lock, 2011).

Results also indicated that adults might categorize mental and physical states on three dimensions: the *physiological body* (biological, psychobiological, some perceptual), the *nonphysiological body* (epistemic, some perceptual), and *nonembodied* (emotions, desires; Bek & Lock, 2011). These findings indicate three, not two, dimensions in how children and adults conceptualize other humans. As we will see, a growing body of research suggests that in addition to conceptualization of humans as comprising minds and bodies, children have an intuition that humans also have an individualized essence that is complementary to, but still distinct from, a person's body and mind.

The Quintessence of a Person and the Soul

Evidence that human cognition incorporates a tripartite intuition about the nature of humans comes from studies in which participants were specifically asked to consider the functions of the body, mind, and soul and the role of each in conferring identity. Richert and Harris (2006) asked 6- to 12-year-old Catholic children whether a newborn baby had a brain, mind, and soul. The children were also asked whether the brain, mind, and soul stayed the same or changed over a person's lifetime and whether the baby would be the same person if the brain, mind, and soul were taken away. The children indicated that the mind and brain would change over time but that the soul was more likely to stay the same. Overall, they claimed that a baby would be a different person if the mind, brain, and soul were taken away; but the children younger than age 9 were less likely than older children to indicate that the baby would be a different person if the soul were taken away (Richert & Harris, 2006).

Then, utilizing the Johnson and Wellman (1982) method, the children indicated whether the baby could still perform behavioral (suck the thumb, close the eyes), cognitive (dream, think), and noncognitive (see, want) tasks if the baby's brain, mind, and soul were taken away (Richert & Harris, 2006). Across ages, children claimed that all functioning could likely continue without a soul but would likely not continue without a brain or mind. Finally, in response to open-ended questions about how the brain, mind, and soul function, children spontaneously attributed spiritual functions to the soul (e.g., it helps you tell right from wrong, is a life-giving force, afterlife) but not to the mind or the brain (Richert & Harris, 2006).

Using the Johnson (1990) method, Roazzi et al. (2013) expanded this research to determine whether people make further distinctions between the soul and the spirit of a person. They interviewed young adults from the United States, Brazil, and Indonesia. The participants were presented with a series of scenarios in which an individual's mind, soul, or spirit transferred into the body of another individual. The young adults then indicated whether the cognitive, physical, moral, and social abilities and the passion for those abilities transferred with a person's mind, soul, or spirit into a new body. In the United States, participants were more likely to associate the spirit with passion but the soul and mind with both passion and ability. In addition, social and moral attributes were more strongly associated with the soul and spirit than with the mind.

Studies have further unpacked the influence of individual differences in explicit concepts of the soul. Richert and Harris (2008) interviewed US undergraduates, asking participants questions about the ontological status of the mind and soul (does it exist, when does it begin, does it change over development, does it continue after death?) and the functions of the mind and soul (cognitive, spiritual). The participants also answered questions about whether scientists and doctors should be able to use stem cells in research, disconnect people from life support, and clone humans. The participants were more likely to indicate that the mind existed within the life cycle and changed with development but that the soul existed outside of the life cycle and remained the same. In addition, they attributed cognitive functions (i.e., the ability to solve problems, think, tell right from wrong, remember) to the mind and spiritual functions (i.e., the life force, afterlife, connection to higher power, spiritual essence) to the soul. In this study, participants considered emotion and reason to be both cognitive and spiritual functions. Regarding participants' ethical reasoning, participants who had a more spiritual concept of the soul were more likely to claim that stem cell research, human cloning, and euthanasia are not appropriate. In contrast, there was no relation between reasoning on the ethical questions and concepts of the mind (Richert & Harris, 2008).

Following up on this research, Richert and Smith (2012) found that young adults' beliefs about the nature of the soul were related to their stance on beginning-of-life ethical dilemmas (e.g., abortion, stem cell research) but not end-of-life ethical dilemmas (i.e., removal of life support, euthanasia). In particular, beyond the predictive power of religious affiliation, the participants were more likely to disapprove of abortion and stem cell research if they believed that the soul exists before conception and remains constant over the life span.

Further studies have indicated the importance of considering individual differences in whether individuals take a materialist, dualist, or tripartite stance in their understanding of what makes humans human. Lindeman et al., (2015) characterized different ways in which Finnish adults conceptualize the relation between the soul, the mind, and the body. Based on the six categories developed by Bering and Bjorklund (2004), participants indicated if the mind, soul, and body were necessary for various functions. Lindeman et al. (2015) found that three clusters of participants emerged, which they labeled *monists*, *emergentists*, and *spiritualists*. The monists indicated that only the brain was necessary for all functions; the emergentists reported the view that both the brain and the mind were necessary for all functions; and the spiritualists considered the brain, mind, and soul all to be necessary for functions. Regardless of their cluster, the participants were least likely to claim that the soul was necessary for biological, psychobiological, and perceptual processes. Individuals who were in the spiritualist cluster also were more likely to hold paranormal beliefs and to believe that the soul was immortal. Even spiritualists, however, associated the soul with fewer of the listed properties than the mind or brain.

Prelife and Afterlife Beliefs

The existence of a tripartite concept of humans, *mind-body-quintessence*, is also apparent in research asking children and adults about their prelife and afterlife beliefs. In one of the first developmental studies of afterlife beliefs, Bering and Bjorklund (2004) interviewed 4- to 12-year-old US children (religious affiliation not reported) about what kinds of processes a mouse would still be able to perform after being eaten by an alligator. Adults were also interviewed. About 70% of kindergartners claimed that both cognitive (e.g., see, want) and psychobiological (e.g., thirsty, sleepy) processes continued after death; in contrast, close to 100% of later elementary school children claimed that psychobiological process would cease at death, in comparison with 70% who claimed cognitive processes would cease at death. Both adults and children were more likely to claim that epistemic, desire, and emotional states continue after death than biological, psychobiological, and perceptual states. In other words, in this US sample, belief in the continuity of both biological and psychological processes was present in kindergarten children but decreased by adulthood, with near universal agreement that biological processes cease and less certainty about whether psychological processes cease or continue.

In Spain, this pattern is stronger in children in Catholic schools than in secular schools (Bering et al., 2005), suggesting that the contexts in which children learn about the afterlife influence their judgments about what aspects of a person continue on after death. Harris and Giménez (2005) told 7- to 11-year-old Spanish children about the death of an elderly person in two narrative contexts: religious, which included references to a priest and being with God, and secular, which included references to a doctor and illness. The children were more likely to indicate that mental processes than bodily processes would continue after death, and were more likely to do so after hearing the religious narrative about death. This distinction was particularly pronounced in children older than age 10, who on average attributed the continuation of almost all mental functions after death (Harris & Giménez, 2005). Similarly, Astuti and Harris (2008) interviewed 5- to 17-year-old Vezo children and adults in rural Madagascar communities in which even young children are exposed to both biological death (mostly of animals) and afterlife beliefs (primarily through observing ritual communication with ancestors). Participants indicated which processes (bodily and mental) they believed continued to function after a person died. They were presented with two different narratives: a religious narrative in which the focus was on the construction of the ancestral tomb, and a nonreligious narrative in which the focus was on the bodily illness and death. In contrast to the studies by Bering and colleagues (Bering & Bjorklund, 2004; Bering et al., 2005), children were less likely than adults to claim that both bodily and mental functions continue after death, claiming instead these functions would cease at death. However, both children and adults were more likely to claim that mental functions would continue if they were responding in the context of the religious (tomb) narrative than in the context of the nonreligious (corpse) narrative. Additionally, the participants were asked if the body, mind, and spirit would cease to work at death. Participants were more likely to say the spirit continued to work after death, when compared with the body and mind; and adults were more likely to make this claim than children (Harris & Giménez, 2005).

Despite this evidence of cultural differences, the mechanisms through which these differences emerge remain unclear. For example, some studies have found that parents' beliefs and testimony are not related to children's afterlife beliefs (Misailidi & Kornilaki, 2015). Using a similar vignette to that of Bering and Bjorklund (2004)—but with a human protagonist—Misailidi and Kornilaki (2015) asked 5-, 7-, and 10-year-old Greek children if biological, perceptual, mental activity, epistemic-volitional, and emotional states would continue after death. As in other similar studies (e.g., Bering & Bjorklund, 2004), the 7- and 10-year-olds judged the biological and perceptual states as ceasing, whereas the 5-year-olds judged the biological, but not the perceptual, states as ceasing. However, across all three age groups, between 40% and 65% of children claimed that epistemic and emotional states would stop (Misailidi & Kornilaki, 2015).

Surprisingly, parents' own beliefs in the afterlife and their reports of how they talk to their children about death and the afterlife (e.g., "I use the terms 'soul' and/or 'spirit' when I discuss death with my child") were not correlated with children's own afterlife beliefs. Yet parents' reports indicated that how frequently they attended religious services was strongly related to their own afterlife beliefs. Although Misailidi and Kornilaki (2015) argued that this finding indicates that parental beliefs in an afterlife do not directly influence their children's beliefs, these findings may be conflated by how frequently children are exposed to death on a regular basis, as well as by parents' testimony in real-time (opposed to parental report).

Emmons and Kelemen (2014) extended the research on children's attributions of mental states in the afterlife to a study of the development of prelife belief—namely, the belief that individuals exist in some kind of spiritual state prior to birth. Participants were 5- to 12-year-old children from two Ecuadorian communities: an urban, primarily Catholic community and a rural community incorporating traditional beliefs and practices about spirits and witchcraft. Importantly, neither community had explicit doctrines supporting prelife existence, thus children's assumptions about prelife reflected their inferences about the nature of human existence. As with their responses to questions about the afterlife, children were more likely to associate mental states (specifically, emotions and desires) to prelife existence than physical and biological states (Emmons & Kelemen, 2014).

Even though the Ecuadorian children were more likely to attribute mental states than physical states to prelife existence, by the age of 11 to 12, at most, 34% of children endorsed the existence of mental states in prelife (Emmons & Kelemen, 2014), raising questions about whether this is indeed evidence of a cognitive bias toward mentalistic attributions or alternatively reflects the role of essentialism in conceptual change (see Gelman & Diesendruck, 1999). Indeed, developmental shifts in children's attribution of prelife experience to humans were related to their developing understanding of human biology and the nature of human conception. Therefore, one explanation for this pattern is that contexts (such as learning about human biology) promote the revision of the content of the quintessence placeholder to remove both physical and mental states as the primary features of individual essence and that other characteristics of a person assume prominence in that placeholder.

The Human Quintessence and Ritual Change

The choice of the term *folk anthropology* reflects the expectation that humans conceptualize other humans as being fundamentally changed by the religious and cultural practices that typically fall under the domain of anthropological research. The research on how children view the influence of cultural practices on a person's identity is minimal, but what little there is has been conducted on children's understanding of how ritual affects a person's identity and membership in the social group. For the purpose of this chapter, rituals are defined as culturally specific action sequences for which the intended outcomes and the causal mechanisms that produce those outcomes are causally opaque (Legare & Souza, 2012). Rituals serve social functions that are evolutionarily adaptive, such as identifying group members and maintaining group cohesion (Watson-Jones & Legare, 2016).

Emerging research on children's understanding of ritual suggests that children view rituals as altering the essence or soul of a person, more so than their body, brain, or mind. Children who have participated in ritual-type actions with a group have a stronger ingroup affiliation than children who participated in a nonritual group activity (Wen et al., 2016). Additionally, children will perform ritualized actions to help others achieve their goals (Nielsen et al., 2015) and are more likely to perform ritual-like actions if they have been previously ostracized by a group (Watson-Jones et al., 2014; Watson-Jones et al., 2016). Finally, Richert and Harris (2006) found that 4- to 12-year-old Catholic children were more likely to say the soul would be changed by a ritual (baptism) than the mind or the brain. Indeed, Slingerland (2018) has suggested that one interpretation of mortuary rituals is that they serve to break the connection between the individual and her or his body. Thus, emerging evidence paints a compelling picture of the role of a folk anthropology of persons in processing how rituals function in social groups and affect the individual members of social groups.

FUTURE RESEARCH

The hypothesized folk anthropology, building upon the attribution of a quintessence to individual humans, suggests the need for several programs of research. First, within theories of cognitive science of religion, theorists and researchers should more proactively examine the role that essentialism has played in the evolution and transmission of religious concepts, beliefs, and practices. Much CSR theorizing has been devoted to the important role of theory of mind and social cognition in the evolution and persistence of religious beliefs, actions, and concepts. However, the findings outlined here indicate the critical need for CSR theories to incorporate the developmental research highlighting the importance of essentialism in cognitive development.

Second, the developmental function of attributing to humans an individual quintessence needs to be delineated. On the one hand, developmental psychologists should consider how and when in cognitive development a quintessence becomes differentiated from the psychological, biological, and physical aspects of humans. On the other hand, belief in an individual quintessence may be the "glue" that holds an individual's psychological, biological, and physical characteristics together to make each individual the person they are. Developmental studies could be particularly useful for uncovering the role of essentialism in coordinating or differentiating these other foundational theory systems.

Third, future research should examine the extent to which individuals view cultural and religious rituals as changing the essence of an individual. For example, studies could examine whether certain rituals change the ontological category membership of an individual human (e.g., through spirit possession or mortuary rituals). Additionally, studies could examine whether there are similarities in the elements or structure of rituals that are expected to lead to essential changes in humans. Furthermore, studies should consider how rituals that change individual quintessence also support or leverage cognitions that lead to in-group and out-group categories, stereotypes, prejudice, and discrimination.

CONCLUSION

We propose that to fully characterize how human cognition processes the nature of humans, theorists and researchers should consider the existence of a folk system of inference akin to a *folk anthropology*, a folk system that incorporates intuitions that individuals have a quintessence that confers a unique identity, and that the social and environmental context of an individual, as well as the cultural practices, become part of that individual's quintessence. The hypothesized existence of this system of inference builds on other theorized systems in concepts of humans (psychology, biology, and physics), and we argue that the existence of this system more parsimoniously accounts for findings suggesting that humans view other humans as having a tripartite nature (body-mind-quintessence), and that the quintessence of a human can be altered by cultural practices that change the very nature of that person (e.g., christening or bris rituals, rituals of conversion, rites of passage, etc.).

QUESTIONS FOR FUTURE RESEARCH

1. What role has essentialism played in the evolution and transmission of religious concepts, beliefs, and practices?
2. What is the developmental function of attributing to humans an individual quintessence?
3. To what extent do individuals view cultural and religious rituals as changing the essence of an individual, and what are the associated developmental trajectories and influences on these intuitions?

ACKNOWLEDGMENTS

The writing of this chapter was supported by a grant to Rebekah A. Richert from the John Templeton Foundation (#JTF61062).

REFERENCES

Astuti, R., & Harris, P. L. (2008). Understanding mortality and the life of the ancestors in rural Madagascar. *Cognitive Science, 32*(2008), 713–740. doi:10.1080/03640210802066907

Baillargeon, R. (2008). Innate ideas revisited: For a principle of persistence in infants' physical reasoning. *Perspectives on Psychological Science, 3*(1), 2–13. doi:10.1111/j.1745-6916.2008.00056.x

Baillargeon, R., Scott, R. M., & Bian, L. (2016). Psychological reasoning in infancy. *Annual Review of Psychology, 67*, 159–186. doi:10.1146/annurev-psych-010213-115033

Bardi, L., Regolin, L., & Simion, F. (2011). Biological motion preference in humans at birth: Role of dynamic and configural properties. *Developmental Science, 14*(2), 353–359. doi:10.1111/j.1467-7687.2010.00985.x

Bek, J., & Lock, S. (2011). Afterlife beliefs: Category specificity and sensitivity to biological priming. *Religion, Brain & Behavior, 1*, 5–17. doi:10.1080/2153599X.2010.550724

Bering, J. M. (2002). Intuitive conceptions of dead agents' minds: The natural foundations of afterlife beliefs as phenomenological boundary. *Journal of Cognition and Culture, 2*, 263–308. doi:10.1163/15685370260441008

Bering, J. M. (2006). The folk psychology of souls. *Behavioral and Brain Sciences, 29*, 453–462. doi:10.1017/S0140525X06009101

Bering, J. M., & Bjorklund, D. F. (2004). The natural emergence of reasoning about the afterlife as a developmental regularity. *Developmental Psychology, 40*(2), 217–233. doi:10.1037/0012-1649.40.2.217

Bering, J. M., Blasi, C. H., & Bjorklund, D. F. (2005). The development of "afterlife" beliefs in religiously and secularly schooled children. *British Journal of Developmental Psychology, 23*(2005), 587–607. doi:10.1348/026151005X36498

Bjorklund, D. F., & Causey, K. B. (2018). *Children's thinking: Cognitive development and individual differences* (6th edition). Thousand Oaks, CA: Sage Publishing.

Bloom, P. (2004). *Descartes' baby: How child development explains what makes us human.* London: Arrow Books.

Chudek, M., McNamara, R. A., Birch, S., Bloom, P., & Heinrich, J. (2018). Do minds switch bodies? Dualist interpretations across ages and societies. *Religion, Brain & Behavior, 8*(4), 354–368. doi:10.1080/2153599X.2017.1377757

Churchland, P. M. (1981). Eliminative materialism and the propositional attitudes. *Journal of Philosophy, 78*, 67–90. doi:10.2307/2025900

Cohen, E., & Barrett, J. (2008). When minds migrate: Conceptualizing spirit possession. *Journal of Cognition and Culture, 8*(2008), 23–48. doi:10.1163/156770908X289198

Cohen, E., Burdett, E., Knight, N., & Barrett, J. (2011). Cross-cultural similarities in person-body reasoning: Experimental evidence from the United Kingdom and Brazilian Amazon. *Cognitive Science, 35*(2011), 1282–1304. doi:10.1111/j.1551-6709.2011.01172.x

Corriveau, K. H., Pasquini, E. S., & Harris, P. L. (2005). "If it's in your mind it's in your knowledge": Children's developing anatomy of identity. *Cognitive Development, 20*(2005), 321–340. doi:10.1016/j.cogdev.2005.04.005

Emmons, N. A., & Kelemen, D. (2014). The development of children's prelife reasoning: Evidence from two cultures. *Child Development, 85*(4), 1617–1633. doi:10.1111/cdev.12220

Forstmann, M., & Burgmer, P. (2014). Adults are intuitive mind-body dualists. *Journal of Experimental Psychology: General, 144*(1), 222–235. doi:10.1037/xge0000004

Forstmann, M., & Burgmer, P. (2018). A free will needs a free mind: Belief in substance dualism and reductive physicalism differentially predict free will and determinism. *Consciousness and Cognition, 63*(2018), 280–293. doi:10.1016/j.concog.2018.07.003

Gelman, S. A. (2009). Learning from others: Children's construction of concepts. *Annual Review of Psychology, 60*, 115–140. doi:10.1146/annurev.psych.59.103006.093659

Gelman, S. A., Coley, J. D., & Gottfried, G. M. (1994). Essentialist beliefs in children: The acquisition of concepts and theories. In L. A. Hirschfeld & S. A. Gelman (Eds.), *Mapping the mind: Domain specificity in cognition and culture* (pp. 341–366). Cambridge, UK: Cambridge University Press.

Gelman, S. A., & Diesendruck, G. (1999). What's in a concept? Context, variability, and psychological essentialism. In I. E. Sigel (Ed.), *Development of mental representation: Theories and applications* (pp. 87–111). Mahwah, NJ: Lawrence Erlbaum.

Gelman, S. A., & Gottfried, G. M. (1996). Children's causal explanations of animate and inanimate motion. *Child Development, 67*, 1970–1987. doi:10.1111/j.1467-8624.1996.tb01838.x

Gelman, S. A., & Legare, C. H. (2011). Concepts and folk theories. *Annual Review of Anthropology, 1*(40), 379–398. doi:10.1146/annurev-anthro-081309-145822

Gottfried, G. M., Gelman, S. A., & Schultz, J. (1999). Children's understanding of the brain from early essentialism to biological theory. *Cognitive Development, 14*(1), 147–174. doi:10.1016/S0885-2014(99)80022-7

Gottfried, G. M., & Jow, E. E. (2003). "I just talk with my heart": The mind–body problem, linguistic input, and the acquisition of folk psychological beliefs. *Cognitive Development*, *18*(1), 79–90. doi:10.1016/S0885-2014(02)00164-8

Harris, P. L., & Giménez, M. (2005). Children's acceptance of conflicting testimony: the case of death. *Journal of Cognition and Culture*, *5*(1–2), 143–164. doi:10.1163/1568537054068606

Hatano, G., & Inagaki, K. (1994). Young children's naïve theory of biology. *Cognition*, *50*, 171–188. doi:10.1016/0010-0277(94)90027-2

Hickling, A. K., & Gelman, S. A. (1995). How does your garden grow? Early conceptualization of seeds and their place in plant growth cycle. *Child Development*, *66*(3), 856-876. doi:10.1111/j.1467-8624.1995.tb00910.x

Hirschfeld, L. A. (2013). The myth of mentalizing and the primacy of folk sociology. In M. R. Banaji & S. A. Gelman (Eds.), *Navigating the social world: What infants, children, and other species can teach us* (pp. 101–106). Oxford Scholarship Online. doi:10.1093/acprof:oso/9780199890712.003.0019

Hirschfeld, L. A., Bartmess, E., White, S., & Frith, U. (2007). Can autistic children predict behavior by social stereotypes? *Current Biology*, *17*(12), R451–R452. doi:10.1016/j.cub.2007.04.051

Hodge, K. M. (2008). Descartes' mistake: How afterlife beliefs challenge the assumption that humans are intuitive Cartesian substance dualists. *Journal of Cognition and Culture*, *8*(2008), 387–415. doi:10.1163/156853708X358236

Hood, B., Gjersoe, N. L., & Bloom, P. (2012). Do children think that duplicating the body also duplicates the mind? *Cognition*, *125*(2012), 466–474. doi:10.1016/j.cognition.2012.07.005

Inagaki, K., & Hatano, G. (1996). Young children's recognition of commonalities between animals and plants. *Child Development*, *67*, 2823–2840. doi:10.2307/1131754

Inagaki, K., & Hatano, G. (2002). *Young children's naïve thinking about the biological world.* New York: Psychology Press.

Johnson, C. N. (1990). If you had my brain, where would I be? Children's understanding of the brain and identity. *Child Development*, *61*(4), 962–972. doi:10.1111/j.1467-8624.1990.tb02834.x

Johnson, C. N., & Wellman, H. M. (1982). Children's developing conceptions of the mind and brain. *Child Development*, *53*(1), 222–234. doi:10.2307/1129656

Keil, F. C. (1989). On the development of biologically specific beliefs: The case of inheritance. *Child Development*, *60*, 637–648. doi:10.2307/1130729

Keil, F. C. (1995). The growth of causal understandings of natural kinds: Modes of construal and the emergence of biological thought. In. D. Sperber, D. Premack, & A. Premack (Eds.), *Causal cognition: A multidisciplinary debate* (pp. 234–267). Oxford: Oxford University Press.

Kuhlmeier, V. A., Bloom, P. B., & Wynn, K. (2004). Do 5-month-old infants see humans as material objects? *Cognition*, *94*(2004), 95–103. doi:10.1016/j.cognition.2004.02.007

Legare, C. H., & Souza, A. L. (2012). Evaluating ritual efficacy: Evidence from the supernatural. *Cognition*, *124*(1), 1–15. doi:10.1016/j.cognition.2012.03.004

Lindeman, M., Riekki, T., & Svedholm-Hakkinen, A. M. (2015). Individual differences in conceptions of soul, mind, and brain. *Journal of Individual Differences*, *36*(3), 157–162. doi:10.1027/1614-0001/a000167

Mahalingam, R. (2007). Essentialism, power, and the representation of social categories: A folk sociology perspective. *Human Development*, *50*, 300–319. doi:10.1159/000109832

Mahalingam, R., & Rodriguez, J. (2006). Culture, brain transplants, and implicit theories of identity. *Journal of Cognition and Culture*, *6*(3–4), 453–462. doi:10.1163/156853706778554968

Medin, D. L. (1989). Concepts and conceptual structure. *American Psychologist*, *44*(12), 1469–1481. doi:10.1037/0003-066X.44.12.1469

Misailidi, P., & Kornilaki, E. N. (2015). Development of afterlife beliefs in childhood: Relationship to parent beliefs and testimony. *Journal of Developmental Psychology*, 61(2), 290–318. doi:10.13110/merrpalmquar1982.61.2.0290

Moya, C., Boyd, R., & Henrich, J. (2015). Reasoning about cultural and genetic transmission: Developmental and cross-cultural evidence from Peru, Fiji, and the United States on how people make inferences about trait transmission. *Topics in Cognitive Science*, 7(4), 595–610. doi:10.1111/tops.12163

Needham, A. (1999). The role of shape in 4-month-old infants' segregation of adjacent objects. *Infant Behavior and Development*, 22(2), 161–178. doi:10.1016/S0163-6383(99)00008-9

Nielsen, M., Kapitány, R., & Elkins, R. (2015). The perpetuation of ritualistic actions as revealed by young children's transmission of normative behavior. *Evolution and Human Behavior*, 36(3), 191–198. doi:10.1016/j.evolhumbehav.2014.11.002

Newcombe, N., Huttenlocher, J., & Learmonth, A. (1992). Infants' coding of location in continuous space. *Infant Behavior and Development*, 22(4), 483–510. doi:10.1016/S0163-6383(00)00011-4

Rhodes, M., Leslie, S.-J., & Tworek, C. M. (2012). Cultural transmission of social essentialism. *PNAS*, 109(34), 13526–13531. doi:10.1073/pnas.1208951109

Richert, R. A., & Harris, P. L. (2006). The ghost in my body: Children's developing concept of the soul. *Journal of Cognition and Culture*, 6, 409–427. doi:10.1163/156853706778554913

Richert, R. A., & Harris, P. L. (2008). Dualism revisited: Body vs. mind vs. soul. *Journal of Cognition & Culture*, 8, 99–115. doi:10.1163/156770908X289224

Richert, R. A., & Smith, E. I. (2012). The essence of soul concepts: How soul concepts influence ethical reasoning across religious affiliation. *Religion, Brain & Behavior*, 2(2), 161–176. doi:10.1080/2153599X.2012.683702

Roazzi, M., Nyhof, M., & Johnson, C. (2013). Mind, soul, and spirit: Conceptions of immaterial identity in different cultures. *International Journal for the Psychology of Religion*, 23(1), 75–86. doi:10.1080/10508619.2013.735504

Rosengren, K. S., Gelman, S. A., Kalish, C. W., & McCormick, M. (1991). As time goes by: Children's early understanding of growth in animals. *Child Development*, 62, 1302–1320. doi:10.1111/j.1467-8624.1991.tb01607.x

Schlottman, A., & Ray, E. (2010). Goal attribution to schematic animals: Do 6-month-olds perceive biological motion as animate? *Developmental Science*, 13(1), 1–10. doi:10.1111/j.1467-7687.2009.00854.x

Shtulman, A. (2017). *Scienceblind: Why our intuitive theories about the world are so often wrong.* New York: Basic Books.

Slingerland, E. (2018). *Mind and body in early China: Beyond orientalism and the myth of holism.* Oxford: Oxford University Press.

Slingerland, E., & Chudek, M. (2011). The prevalence of mind-body dualism in early China. *Cognitive Science*, 32(2011), 997–1007. doi:10.1111/j.1551-6709.2011.01186.x

Sommerville, J. A., & Woodward, A. L. (2005). Action experience alters 3-month-old infants' perception of others' actions. *Cognition*, 96, 1–11. doi:10.1016/j.cognition.2004.07.004

Sousa, P., Altran, S., & Medin, D. (2002). Essentialism and folkbiology: Further evidence from Brazil. *Journal of Cognition and Culture*, 2, 195–223. doi:10.1163/15685370260225099

Spelke, E. S., Breinlinger, K., Macomber, J., & Jacobson, K. (1992). Origins of knowledge. *Psychological Review*, 99(4), 605–632. doi:10.1037/0033-295X.99.4.605

Stewart, T. L., Laduke, J. R., Bracht, C., Sweet, B. A. M., & Gamarel, K. E. (2003). Do the "eyes" have it? A program evaluation of Jane Elliott's "blue-eyes/brown-eyes" diversity training exercise. *Journal of Applied Social Psychology*, 33(9), 1898–1921. doi:10.1111/j.1559-1816.2003. tb02086.x

Watson-Jones, R. E., & Legare, C. H. (2016). The social functions of group rituals. *Current Directions in Psychological Science*, 25(1), 42–46. doi:10.1177/0963721415618486

Watson-Jones, R. E., Legare, C. H., Whitehouse, H., & Clegg, J. M. (2014). Task-specific effects of ostracism on imitative fidelity in early childhood. *Evolution and Human Behavior*, 35(3), 204–210. doi:10.1016/j.evolhumbehav.2014.01.004

Watson-Jones, R. E., Whitehouse, H., & Legare, C. H. (2016). In-group ostracism increases high fidelity imitation in early childhood. *Psychological Science*, 27(1), 34–42. doi:10.1177/0956797615607205

Wellman, H. M., Cross, D., & Watson, J. (2001). Meta-analysis of theory-of-mind development: The truth about false beliefs. *Child Development*, 72, 655–684. doi:10.1111/j.1750-8606.2010.00154.x

Wellman, H. M., & Gelman, S. A. (1992). Cognitive development: Foundational theories of core domains. *Annual Review of Psychology*, 43, 337–375. https://doi.org/10.1146/annurev.ps.43.020192.002005

Wellman, H. M., & Gelman, S. A. (1998). Knowledge acquisition in foundational domains. In W. Damon (Ed.), *Handbook of child psychology* (Vol. 2). New York: Wiley.

Wellman, H. M., & Liu, D. (2004). Scaling of theory-of-mind tasks. *Child Development*, 75, 523–541. doi:10.1111/j.1467-8624.2004.00691.x

Wen, N. J., Herrmann, P. A., & Legare, C. H. (2016). Ritual increases children's affiliation with in-group members. *Evolution and Human Behavior*, 37(1), 54–60. doi:10.1016/j.evolhumbehav.2015.08.002

Woodward, A. L., & Guajardo, J. J. (2002). Infants' understanding of the point gesture as an object-directed action. *Cognitive Development*, 17, 1061–1084. doi:10.1016/S0885-2014(02)00074-6

CHAPTER 7

··

THE NATURE OF THE WORLD

··

JULIE B. SCOTT AND JUSTIN L. BARRETT

INTRODUCTION

> Goddess Mai Deer came down to the world for inspection on a snow-white
> sacred horse that shone brightly all over, to found on the blue waters only
> the top of Mount Sumeru, the highest mountain on earth leading to heaven.
> Then, suddenly she caught sight of a group of people living in a cave near the
> top of the mountain. Being only one chi (one-third meters) in height, they
> were riding horses as small as rabbits . . . Out of compassion for those little
> people Mai Deer sent two deities, one male and the other female, to bring
> them light. The male deity, named Sun, is on duty during daytime. He gives
> off both heat and red light. The female deity, called Moon, works during the
> night, giving off white light. They circle Mount Sumeru once a day in the
> track designed by Mai Deer.
> —a Mongolian origin myth (Hubin et al., 2011, pp. 293–294)

THIS Mongolian creation myth describes the origins of the sun and the moon. The
sun and moon were created for a purpose: to help bring light to the little people living
on Mt. Sumeru. The goddess Mai Deer is seen as the intentional creator of the sun
and moon.

Creation myths similar to this one are shared all over the world. Supernatural
agents created the world and everything in it, and designed them for a purpose. Are
there cognitive causes for this cross-cultural phenomenon? Do humans intuitively see
things in the natural world as purposeful and created by agents? In this chapter, we
will begin by describing how people conceive of the natural world, its properties, and
its origins. We will explore why supernatural agents are so frequently seen as the cause
of natural phenomena, and the research that has been done in the cognitive sciences
to help explain them. We will conclude this chapter with suggestions for further research in the cognitive science of religion (CSR) on how humans conceive of the natural world.

Natural Kinds and Ontological Categories

In the late twentieth century, development psychologist Frank Keil (1992) theorized that humans naturally think about different kinds of things in the world in terms of categories. Humans intuitively divide the world up into three basic kinds: natural kinds, nominal kinds, and artifacts. Humans hold distinctive expectations for the different kinds.[1] In this context, *natural kinds* are those things in nature which have not been created or constructed by humans. Mountains, rivers, plants, animals, and chemical elements and compounds are natural kinds. They follow a common set of laws, commonly called the "laws of nature." Pure *nominal kinds* are those concepts, which Putnam (1975) defined as "one-criterion concepts," such as triangles, circles, or odd and even numbers (Keil, 1992). They have just one simple definition, and can be accurately described by "only one if-and-only-if statements" (Keil, 1992, p. 38). For example, a triangle is a triangle if-and-only-if it has three edges which meet at three points (vertices). An *artifact* is something created by human beings for a purpose. Artifacts can be further divided into simple artifacts, such as chairs or hammers, and complex artifacts, such as cars or computers, which undertake multiple tasks (Keil, 1992).

The three categories of kinds are always conceived of in relation to objects of the same kind and to objects of other kinds (Erickson et al., 2010; Keil, 1992). The distinctions between each kind are not always clear-cut, but instead, can be thought of as falling along a continuum. For example, a simple artifact like a saw is more similar to a nominal kind than a natural kind, in that it is intended to have one and only one use (i.e., sawing wood).[2] A complex artifact such as a computer, however, can be thought of behaving more like a natural kind than a nominal kind, since it has complex uses (Keil, 1992).

Expectation Sets

The automatic tendency to categorize objects into ontological categories serves an important conceptual role. From the time they are infants, people make common inferences about objects depending on their kind (Erickson et al., 2010; Keil, 1992; Spelke, 1994). Drawing upon numerous lines of cognitive developmental research,

---

[1] By "intuitively," we mean that these thoughts and expectations are intuitive, and "do[] not require or do[] not allow for conscious inspection of the principles involved" (Barrett, 2008, p. 310). Cognitive developmental psychologists assume much of intuitive knowledge is, for the most part, unchanged across different cultural contexts, and they arise through people's normal development and interaction of their physical bodies with their natural and social contexts (Barrett, 2008).

[2] Whereas simple artifacts are usually made for only one use, they may be used for different purposes other than their original purpose. For example, a saw may be used as a mirror to see one's own reflection or even as a musical instrument, even though it is meant for sawing wood.

including Keil (1992), Boyer (1994, 2001) and Atran (2002), Barrett (2008, 2011) has proposed that people categorize objects using one or more of the following ontological categories: spatial entities, solid objects, living things, animates, and persons. These categories generate what he has called "expectation sets": sets of intuitions concerning the properties that an object is likely to have. These expectations are assumed and need not be directly and explicitly communicated. These expectation sets include: "Spatiality, Physicality, Biology, Animacy, and Mentality" (Barrett, 2008, p. 317).

The spatiality expectation set includes the notion that all physical objects exist only in one place in space and time (Barrett, 2008, 2011). The physicality expectation set (sometimes called naïve physics or folk mechanics) includes such expectations as physical objects, under normal circumstances, holding visible, tangible, solid, and cohesive characteristics (i.e., do not disintegrate upon movement of one part), and they move or stop moving only when some other object comes into contact with it (Baillargeon, 2004; Spelke, 1994; Spelke & Kinzler, 2007). The biology expectation set (often referred to as folk biology) includes the intuitive notions that living things grow and develop over time (Erickson et al., 2010; Hatano & Inagaki, 1994; Rosengren, et al., 1991), will eventually die (Hatano & Inagaki, 1994; Slaughter, 2005), give birth to like organisms (e.g., cats give birth to kittens and not lizards; Hatano & Inagaki, 1994), sustain life (vitalism; Erickson et al., 2010; Inagaki & Hatano, 2006, 2002; Keil, 1992, 2003), and are made of natural materials (vs. artificial metals or plastic; Simons & Keil, 1995). Animacy adds to the biological expectation set that animals and humans can act upon their environments and move themselves by their own volition (i.e., self-propelledness; Biro & Leslie, 2007; Friedman & Leslie, 2004; Premack, 1990). Finally, mentality is the expectation set which informs humans that a conscious mind and the properties of that mind are at work; humans assume that the mind has beliefs, memories, emotions, and desires which motivate its body's actions (often called, theory of mind [ToM] or folk psychology; Barrett, 2011; Friedman & Leslie, 2004; Wellman et al., 2001; Wellman & Liu, 2004).

These expectation sets are automatically activated in humans when they perceive a member of a relevant kind. For instance, when thinking about natural objects, such as rocks and shells, we intuitively assume expectations from the physicality and spatiality sets (i.e., visibility and being physically present in only one place and time) (Barrett, 2011; Purzycki & Willard, 2016). Animals and humans trigger the physicality and spatiality expectation sets, but also the animacy and, at least for humans and some animals, mentality expectations. As these expectation sets develop naturally in all human minds, we can expect to find the same intuitive expectations among every human population worldwide (Barrett, 2008, 2011; Purzycki & Willard, 2016).

Counterintuitive Religious Concepts

Religious ideas and entities do not occupy a separate intuitive ontological category, nor do they obey a unique set of expectations. Instead, they are shaped by the intuitive expectation sets mentioned above. However, Pascal Boyer (1994, 2001) has observed that religious concepts (among others) often differ from intuitive thoughts, in that they "violate" one or more properties of an expectation set, and thus, are *counter*intuitive (McCauley, 2011). For example, a ghost or human that walks through walls violates the physicality expectation set. This type of violation is called a *breach*, since it "breaches" the physicality expectation that physical, solid objects cannot pass through one another (Boyer, 2001). Another example of a breach would be a cat born to a cow. This property breaches the biology expectation set for animals. A breach of the mentality expectation set would be a person who "reads" others' thoughts. Religious ideas are full of these types of breaches (e.g., ancestral spirits or omniscient gods; McCauley, 2011).

Another type of violation against expectation sets is a *transfer* (Boyer, 2001). Transfers are when the principles of one ontological kind (e.g., solid objects or persons) are transferred to objects of another ontological type, which do not normally correspond to those expectations. For example, a talking tree is a transfer of our mentality expectations to a plant. Another example would be a "living" mountain. This transfers the biology expectation of vitality to a nonliving thing. Religious ideas and folklore are also full of transfers such as these (e.g., talking animals in Aesop's Fables or the talking snake in the Garden of Eden or Balaam's donkey in the Bible).

Minimally Counterintuitive Concepts and CI Agents

When the number of transfers or breaches of a counterintuitive concept is limited (one or two transfers, perhaps), cognitive scientists call these concepts "modestly counterintuitive" (McCauley, 2011), or, what Barrett has termed, "Minimally Counterintuitive" (MCI). MCI concepts are relatively easy and attractive for human brains to entertain, because they do not have too many counterintuitive elements, and, yet, are usually attention grabbing (Boyer, 1994, 2001).[3]

Boyer and others have shown through cross-cultural experiments that MCI concepts are often more memorable and likely to be communicated faithfully than regular, intuitive concepts, such as those of normal objects or even bizarre concepts (objects which meet all the expectation sets, but are just unusual, such as a 200 kilogram dog) (Barrett & Nyhof, 2001; Boyer & Ramble, 2001; Gregory & Greenway, 2017b), perhaps especially (or exclusively) by young people (Barrett, 2016, 2017b; Gregory & Greenway, 2017a; Hornbeck & Barrett, 2013). Not all MCI concepts become religious concepts, however, and common religious concepts are most often those MCI concepts that engage the ToM (i.e., have mental properties) (Gregory et al., 2019). Whereas some MCI concepts may be merely interesting (e.g., invisible trees or vanishing rocks), without being *minded* agents, they lack much inferential potential to factor into the common daily concerns of people

---

[3] Some MCI concepts have less inferential potential than others, since they do not relate to relevant matters for people (Barrett, 2008; Boyer, 2001). For example, the idea of an invisible rock may be MCI (an invisible physical object), but it is not likely to be personally relevant for most people. Therefore, the idea will most likely not be discussed and be forgotten (Barrett, 2008).

(Boyer, 2001) and are, thus, unlikely to become cultural concepts. On the other hand, MCI concepts which engage the ToM can hold personal relevance for people and help explain events (Barrett, 2004; Boyer, 2001). MCI concepts with ToM can appropriately be called *agents*, as they can affect their surrounding environments by their inner, mental states. Therefore, they are sometimes known as "counterintuitive agents," or CI agents.

INFERENTIAL POTENTIAL AND AGENTS

CI agents, in addition to the properties of regular agents, can provide "a vast source of explanatory capital," since they possess counterintuitive properties and are not held back by one or more laws of nature (McCauley, 2011, p. 183). Following Boyer (1996), Barrett calls this source of explanatory capital, "*inferential potential*," which he defines as "the ability for a concept or idea to readily generate explanations, predictions, and other inferences in a broad range of personally relevant contexts" (Barrett, 2011; see also Boyer, 2001). If an idea is relevant for a person in multiple situations, provides explanations for various events, and helps predict future events, it has good inferential potential.

CI agents hold the greatest inferential potential of all objects, as they can activate all five of the expectation sets: spatial, physical, biological, animacy, and mentality (Barrett, 2004; Boyer, 2001). It is important to remember that, for the most part, religious beliefs, like nonreligious ones, are *not* the result of well-thought-out, reflectively created belief statements (Boyer, 2001). Rather, they are the result of multiple mental systems providing intuitions that support and make relevant beliefs in a variety of situations. The counterintuitive properties of religious agents allow them to provide many possible meanings and intentions behind personally relevant events (Barrett, 2008; Boyer, 1994, 2001; McCauley, 2011).

It is not necessary for people to consciously reflect on explicit beliefs about CI agents, or to judge whether such intuitions are true or false, in order for the intuitions to seem appropriate in their particular mental systems (e.g., social, psychological, or moral; Barrett, 2008; Boyer, 2001). Rather, these intuitions seem plausible because they seem to provide the most helpful way of making sense of situations, and they satisfy the intuitions in a variety of mental systems. Ideas are more likely to be believed when a human has many experiences that seem to confirm the intuition, and the intuition is seemingly "backed up" by several mental systems (Boyer, 2001).

Philosopher Robert McCauley (2011) surmises that, because of the relative importance of other humans as causal forces in the human world, "agents are the mind's *natural* candidates for making things happen in the natural world as well" (McCauley, 2011, p. 183).[4]

---

[4] Jesse Bering (2011) makes similar observations about the hyper-sociality of humans, leading to a strong tendency to invoke agency very broadly. This insight underwrites Stewart Guthrie's (1993) treatment of anthropomorphism and has been recognized by other theorists as well (e.g., Pyysiäinen, 2003).

When an unexpected event happens, our mind, accustomed to seeing agents as the cause of events, automatically assumes that *someone* must have caused it, and thus, our "agency detection device," or ADD, as Barrett calls it, is activated (Barrett, 2017a; formerly HADD, Barrett, 2004). And if the action seems meaningful, then our ToM attributes the cause to something with a *mind*, goals, and desires. If we discover a normal agent (e.g., a human or a cat) is behind the event, then our ADD's identification of agency is reinforced as correct. However, if an agent cannot be discovered, then a person's mind may assume that he or she just cannot see the agent. If an agent *should* be visible under the conditions in question, but is not, ADD may still register the presence of an agent or agency. Thus, if there is a concept of a CI agent (e.g., an angel or ghost) readily present in the person's culture, even if the person had not previously believed in such things, it is easy for them to entertain the idea that a CI agent must be responsible for the event, even if this attribution is only held tentatively or rejected in the absence of validating social support (Barrett, 2004).

Because it is so intuitive for normal human beings to occasionally have their ADD detect agency when humans or animal agents are not suitable candidates, groups will likely have periodic experiences of agency more in conformity with postulated CI agents: angels or demons, ancestor spirits, ghosts or ghouls, gods or golems (McCauley, 2011). These are easy explanations for unexplained natural phenomena, especially those which seem meaningful or intentional. Events which are impossible for humans to affect, but could be possible for a CI agent to affect, are likely to be concluded as caused by a CI agent (Barrett, 2004).

TELEO-FUNCTIONING REASONING

When it comes to nature and the origin of natural kinds, likewise, humans intuitively seem to think that nature was intentionally made, and for a purpose. Pioneering developmental psychologist Jean Piaget (1997) argued that children naturally regard the natural world as created (he called this phenomenon "artificialism"). Even before children are old enough to receive any religious teaching (at the age of two or three), Piaget noticed that children spontaneously ask questions like, "Who made the sun?" "Why is there a moon?" or "Who is it [who] puts the stars in the sky at night?" (p. 256). Children seem to naturally have this sense that someone must have made the natural world, and for a reason.

Piaget (1997), however, also claimed that children think natural kinds are created by *humans*.[5] According to Piaget, any talk children have of God causing the natural world,

---

[5] Piaget (1997) explains, "When the child is invited to be precise," the child invents a myth that humans have created the natural kinds (p. 262).

before age 7 or 8, is a hollow echo of their parents' religious teaching—not reflecting any real understanding. Psychologist Olivera Petrovich (1997, p. 154) explains:

> Any reference to God made by the child Piaget attributes to parroting, i.e., unassimilated religious teaching, rather than to a sui generis concept. Only when children begin to distinguish psychological (viz., intentional) from physical causality, or . . . mental activity from mechanistic action, at age 7 or 8 years, does Piaget allows for a distinction between "human and divine or theological artificialism" in children's explanations of the natural world ([Piaget] 1977, p. 425).

According to Piaget, change occurs around the age of 7 or 8, when children are first able to distinguish between an agent's intentional causality and the result of physical, mechanistic action. With this change, children are able to distinguish between what humans create and what only God, Nature, or some other supernatural agent creates (Petrovich, 1997).

Origins of Natural Objects and Artifacts

More recent studies have revealed that Piaget underestimated younger children's abilities to distinguish between the creative properties of God and humans (Kelemen, 2004; Petrovich, 1997, 1999). In an experiment conducted by Petrovich (1999), a pair of photographs depicting natural objects (either living, e.g., dogs, daffodils, or non-living objects, e.g., pebbles and soil), regular artifacts (e.g., cup and ball) and artifacts representing living things (e.g., stuffed animals and plastic tomatoes), were shown to British preschool children. The children were asked to "look carefully" and tell whether the two things could be made by people or not (Petrovich, p. 10). The children were asked to justify their answers. The children mostly answered correctly: a natural object could not be made by humans, whereas an artifact could be made by humans (Petrovich, 1999).

In a similar experiment, conducted by Petrovich (1997), British preschoolers, mostly from Christian families, ages 4 to 5, were asked directly about the origins of plants, animals, and other natural things (e.g., the earth, rocks, and sky). The children were asked "to *think* how a selected natural item came into being first . . . before there were any such objects around" (Petrovich, p. 156). The children had three answer choices: people made them, God made them, or no one knew who made them. The results showed that children rarely answered that people were the origins of the natural kinds, and they instead chose "God" or "nobody knows" as the origin of the natural kinds (p. 157). Petrovich concluded that 4- to 5-year-old children may indeed understand God as having different creative abilities from humans (Petrovich, 1997).

E. Margaret Evans (2001) tested whether children preferred creationist accounts, evolutionary accounts, or emergentist accounts (natural things "just appeared" [p. 227]) for the origin of natural objects. She conducted an experiment involving American parents and their children, from grades K–2nd, 3rd–4th, and 5th–7th, who were from both fundamentalist Christian communities and various nonfundamentalist communities. In the experiment, the children and parents were asked "how the very first things got here on earth" (Evans, p. 227). The children were then shown seven pictures of animate objects (e.g., a bear, tuatara, lizard, and human), inanimate objects (e.g., a rock or crystal), and simple artifacts (e.g., a toy, chair, or doll). For each picture, the children were asked how strongly they agreed or disagreed with five statements about the item's origins. The five statements were categorized as: "Creationist ('God made it and put it on earth'), Artificialist ('A person made it and put it on earth'), Evolutionist ('It changed from a different kind of animal that used to live on earth'), [or] two spontaneous-generationist explanations ('It just appeared; It came out of the ground')" (Evans, p. 227).

The study found that all the children, regardless of their religious background, favored creationist explanations for the origins of animals and humans (Evans, 2001; Kelemen & DiYanni, 2005). Only the oldest age group of nonfundamentalist children showed a significant tendency to diverge from the creationist stance, and instead articulated the most common beliefs of their community, which, in this case, were a mix of creationist and evolutionist accounts (Kelemen & DiYanni, 2005; p. 5; Evans, 2001). Evans concluded that young children tend to intuitively believe that natural kinds are created intentionally; whereas older kids and adults start to reflect scientific learning in their answers about natural kinds' origins, if they were culturally conditioned to do so.

Children's Teleological Reasoning for Natural Objects

Children not only seem to prefer creationist accounts for the origins of natural things, but also understand natural things as teleological, or purposefully made. Recent research seems to suggest that children as young as preschoolers favor purpose-based explanations (i.e., teleological) over mechanistic, physical explanations (e.g., erosion) for natural phenomena (DiYanni & Kelemen, 2005; Kelemen, 1999a, 1999b, 2003; 2013). Children will generate their own purpose-based explanations for natural occurrences, even when they have not heard these explanations before.

Developmental psychologist Deborah Kelemen (1999a) has conducted many experiments testing the thesis that children will tend to choose or create teleological explanations for natural objects. In one experiment, American children, ages 4 to 5, and adults were given pictures of a wide variety of "living things, artifacts, and non-living natural objects" (Kelemen, p. 246). They were then asked what they believed the objects (e.g., a clock) and their physical parts (e.g., a clock hand) "were *for*." The children were allowed to say that the object was *not* made for anything. The results showed that children were more likely to give functional answers (e.g., "What is the clock for? Telling time") compared to adults, especially for natural objects and their constitutive parts (Kelemen, p. 249).

Kelemen (1999a) wanted to make sure that the children were not just giving functional answers because they did not understand the question or "were just randomly generating activities associated with the items" (Kelemen, p. 253). So, in a second study, Kelemen asked close-ended questions to investigate children's teleological tendencies. This time, a picture of a man, Ben, and one of a woman, Jane, were introduced, and a pair of photographs of natural things was put between them. The children were told that Ben and Jane "never ever agree with each other" over the cause of the natural things in the photographs (Kelemen, p. 255), and that one of them said that the objects in the pictures were "'made for something'" and the other person said that they were "'not made for anything.'" The children were asked which person they agreed with. The study was then conducted with adults.

The results showed that the children were more than twice as likely as the adults to agree with the person who said that the inanimate natural objects (e.g., icebergs and clouds) were "made for something." Furthermore, three-quarters of the children's answers endorsed the purpose-based (teleological) argument for all the items. Living objects were just as likely as artifacts to be purpose-based, the children said.[6] This series of experiments demonstrated that the American children tended to hold a function-based view of all natural kinds and their parts (Kelemen, 1999a).

In a further experiment, Kelemen (1999b) tested whether children also tend toward teleological reasoning when explaining the properties of living and nonliving natural kinds, whether biological, behavioral, or functional. For example, children were told to choose between a physical-reductionist explanation for why some "rocks were so pointy" and a teleological explanation (e.g., "They were pointy so that the animals wouldn't sit on them and smash them"; Kelemen, p. 1443). Kelemen's experiment demonstrated that children of all grades preferred teleological explanations over physical ones. Kelemen concluded that American children tend to see the properties of all kinds of natural objects as "made for something" (Kelemen, p. 1445) and that this is a natural tendency, since children are most often not explicitly taught teleological (purpose-based) explanations for the objects presented in her experiments (Kundert & Edman, 2017; Barrett, 2012; Kelemen, 1999b).

Are Children "Intuitive Theists"?

For children to be "intuitive theists," Kelemen observed that they would have to be able to distinguish the mental states of superhuman agents from those of more usual agents, such as humans, and also to "attribute design intentions to agents and understand an object's purpose as deriving from such intentions" (Kelemen, 2004, pp. 296–297). Barrett et al. (2001) provided one evidential step in that direction.

---

[6] Interestingly, in the closed-ended questions, the adults were just as likely as the children to say that *living things* were created for a purpose. Kelemen theorized that this may have been because the adults did not want to deny the value of living things or because for the adults, the closed-ended questions may have "tapped into religious convictions in ways the open-ended questioning . . . had not" (Kelemen, 1999a, p. 259).

They demonstrated that 3- to-5-year-old children of Protestant Christian parents were able to reason that God was superknowing and could even know things that humans could not, such as correctly identifying a hidden object in a closed container. Similarly, Yukatec Mayan children reasoned that various supernatural agents could be superknowing, whereas humans could not (Knight et al., 2004). These initial studies have been replicated, extended, and nuanced (e.g., Burdett et al., 2021, 2020). Nevertheless, it seems that one of Kelemen's prerequisites for "intuitive theism" stands supported: children can attribute different mental states to a supernatural agent from those they attribute to humans.

Regarding Kelemen's second prerequisite for "intuitive theism," Kelemen and DiYanni (2005) found evidence suggesting that children's thoughts about the purpose of natural kinds were, indeed, connected to their thoughts concerning an intentional designer. They conducted an experiment showing that, when British children aged 6 to 7 endorsed and/or generated their own purpose-based explanation of an artifact or natural kind, they also endorsed the idea that someone likely accounted for that purpose.[7] This close conceptual connection between seeing design, purpose, or order in the world, and assuming that these are the result of intentional agents, has received some indirect support from studies showing that children—perhaps as young as twelve-months-old—know that "agents are capable of creating order, whereas inanimate objects are not" (Newman et al., 2010, p. 17144).

Children's Essentialist and Teleological Beliefs Compared with Their Beliefs of Creationism of Natural Kinds

To sum up so far, recent experiments have suggested that

- children have natural creationist tendencies and think teleologically about natural kinds' origins;
- can distinguish between some CI agents' and humans' mental states; and
- understand that an object's purpose is the result of a creator's goal.

On a related note, past research has indicated that children's concepts of animals (Diesendruck et al., 1998; Gelman, 2003; Gelman & Wellman, 1991; Kalish, 1998) and even some human kinds (Astuti et al., 2004; Diesendruck & HaLevi, 2006; Hirschfeld, 1996) are largely essentialist, and therefore, children believe that animals and human kinds remain of the same type, despite superficial transformations (Diesendruck & Haber, 2009; Keil, 1992. Consequently, Diesendruck and Haber (2009) wanted to

---

[7] Kelemen notes that, of course, cultural teachings about religion strongly influence how children will understand supernatural concepts, and these may be full of counterintuitive theological concepts (e.g., Gods' omnipresence or omnipotence; Kelemen, 2004; Atran, 2002; Boyer, 2001).

find out whether children's essentialist and teleological explanations for natural kinds were related to their beliefs in God as the creator of the natural world.[8] The researchers reasoned that the belief "every creature has a God-given essence" and the belief in the teleological origin of natural things, at least superficially, correlate well with a religious belief in creationism (living things were created in their current form; Diesendruck and Haber, p. 100). In contrast, they argued, evolution assumes that species can and do change over time into other species, an idea that runs counter to essentialism.[9] They conducted an experiment with Jewish Israeli children and secular Israeli children, almost identical to Kelemen and DiYanni's (2005) origins experiment and Kelemen's (1999a) teleological experiments. The experimenters asked the children a set of questions designed to identify their essentialist beliefs in natural kinds, including the distinctive properties of those kinds (Diesendruck & Haber, 2009). The results did not show that children's essentialist beliefs about animals and teleological beliefs about artifacts predicted their beliefs in creationism. However, children's essentialist beliefs concerning people's membership in social categories and their teleological beliefs about both social and animal categories seemed to be related to cultural learning and creationism. Thus, cultural learning may impact children's developmental conceptions of kinds' domains.

Adult's Intuitive Teleological and Intentional Reasoning Concerning Nature

Children tend toward teleological and essentialist reasoning, correlate order with agents, and may even be "intuitive theists," believing in the purposeful creation of nature by an agent, but do these lines of intuitive thinking continue into adulthood? In one set of experiments, Romanian Romani adults with little schooling and no time constraints also tended to choose teleological explanations for natural phenomena (Casler & Kelemen, 2008). Likewise, Alzheimer patients chose teleological explanations over mechanistic explanations for natural phenomena (Lombrozo et al., 2007). In these studies, adults showed signs of teleological intuitions concerning the natural world, but do these findings also extend to educated, cognitively healthy adults when placed under cognitive load conditions?

Arguably, if adults have persisting teleological intuitions about the natural world that are overridden by formal education and cognitive effort, then increasing the cognitive

---

[8] Diesendruck and Haber defined essentialism as "the belief that members of certain categories have inherent and stable properties . . . which make members of one category fundamentally distinct from members of other categories (Medin & Ortony, 1989)" (Diesendruck & Haber, 2009, p. 100).

[9] (Diesendruck & Haber, 2009, p. 101) recognized that "the extent to which children apply essentialism and teleology" may differ among different domains (e.g., animals, human artifacts, and social categories) and that this might affect their potential relationship to beliefs in creationism.

load will reveal those intuitions. This basic rationale is used in many kinds of cognitive experiments, and speeded response is a common method for increasing cognitive load. In one speeded-response study, participants were forced to either affirm or deny a teleological explanation or a nonteleological explanation for a natural state of affairs, such as "earthworms tunnel underground to aerate the soil" or "polar bears are white because the sun bleaches them" (Kelemen et al., 2013). Some statements appropriately applied purpose, such as "women and men put on perfume/cologne in order to smell pleasant," and some applied incorrect purpose, such as "people chew food in order to strengthen their jaw muscles." Nonteleological items also included both "bad" and "good" causes, such as "polar bears are white because the sun bleaches them" (false) and "soda fizzes because carbon dioxide gas is released" (true). Participants were assigned to either a controlled condition, in which they could respond at their own pace, or a speeded condition, when they had to answer quickly. When they were forced to answer quickly, adults showed a greater tendency to endorse teleological explanations, which were rejected in the unspeeded conditions; this difference was not merely the result of increased errors across all item types. These findings applied to both physical scientists with advanced education (Kelemen et al., 2013) and Chinese university students (Rottman et al., 2017). Results suggest that formal education in particular cultural environments can tamp down or override natural inclinations to think teleologically about the natural world, but they do not entirely erase these predilections.

Additional cross-cultural evidence suggests that this persisting teleological reasoning may also support *intentional reasoning* about the origins of natural things. Using speeded responses, Järnefelt et al. (2015) discovered evidence that adults do indeed hold teleological, and even intentional, intuitions concerning natural phenomena. Even when adults explicitly said that they believed in a scientific framework for natural phenomena (e.g., evolution), they often mixed "agentive" understandings into their explanations for nature. For example, adults often expressed "evolution" as nature's way of helping animals meet their wants or needs, as if nature was itself an agent with mind-like intents and purposes. The results showed that adults are more likely to mix semireligious beliefs (such as nature's agentive characteristics) with scientific ideas than to completely abandon beliefs in the teleological development of nature.

In the first of these experiments, a mix of North American adults, some believers in a higher power, God, or gods and some nonbelievers, were shown forty pictures of living and nonliving natural objects (Järnefelt et al., 2015). The adults were asked to decide whether "any being purposefully made the thing in the picture." One group was tested with no time constraints, whereas the other had a time constraint of 865 milliseconds for each item. The results showed a marked rise in endorsements for a purposeful creation of natural phenomena in the speeded test, for both religious believers and nonreligious believers. This suggests that many people default to belief in the intentional design of natural phenomena by some nonhuman agent when they are not allowed the time to censor their thinking (whether they confessed to being religious or not). These experiments also revealed that adults who explicitly endorsed beliefs in God, or "the intrinsic agency of nature and the Earth" (labeled "Gaia" beliefs), tend to hold stronger beliefs in the purposeful design of nature than those without such explicit beliefs (Järnefelt et al., p. 75). Nevertheless, even confessing atheists seemed to hold implicit teleological beliefs about nature, and some who label themselves as atheists showed evidence of Gaia beliefs.

The test was repeated with explicitly atheist and nonreligious North American adults (Järnefelt et al., 2015). The results showed that these nonreligious adults were better able to inhibit their tendency to endorse natural phenomena as created, but nevertheless, under time constraints, atheist adults increasingly defaulted to a teleological explanation of both living and nonliving nature. Finally, the experiment was repeated a third time in Finland, where religious belief is far less normative in society, and there is less "God-talk" (Järnefelt et al., 2015, p. 81). Only explicitly nonreligious individuals (those who said that they do not believe in any higher power) were tested in order to compare with the North American atheists. As before, the results showed that under time constraints, adults increasingly defaulted to the view that nature was intentionally designed by "some being." In fact, the Finnish adults were, overall, somewhat *more* likely to endorse this teleological reasoning than were the North American atheists.

Some have argued that this persistent belief in nature's intentional design and agentive-like nature owes to the overwhelming presence of the creationist teachings and discourse of religions in society, especially in the United States (Järnefelt et al., 2015). These experiments, however, seem to support the interpretation that people's natural and intuitive cognitive predispositions, which develop early in childhood, endure into adulthood on "a more implicit and automatic level of processing" (Järnefelt et al., 2015, p. 73), a view consistent with a dual-process theory of cognition.[10] People's teleological reasoning may be inhibited by systematic concepts, scientific or otherwise, but their initial predisposition to teleological reasoning never fully disappears (Kundert & Edman, 2017).

These cognitive tendencies do not deny the importance of religious and cultural discourse in spreading religious and creationist beliefs about nature, but it seems that such cultural elaborations are built on intuitive foundations. Humans appear to be naturally inclined to see purpose behind nature and to readily attach this purpose to the intentions of intentional agents (Barrett, 2012). The idea of a divine creator, nature spirits that influence features of the world, or a personified Nature are readily accommodated by ordinary cognitive structures and their operating predilections. These experiments seem to show that even when people explicitly disavow a belief in supernatural agents on a reflective level, on an intuitive and nonreflective cognitive level, people remain believers in nature's intentional design by some sort of agent, whether it be Nature, Mother Earth, a god or gods, or some other supernatural agent (Järnefelt et al., 2015).

---

[10] For more discussion on dual-process theories of cognition, particularly as applied to religious thought, see Barrett (2011).

Open Questions

Numerous research questions about the cognitive foundations of beliefs about the natural world remain open for inquiry. Some concern the character of the foundations themselves, others bear on how these foundations might speak to cultural expression.

With regard to the first class of questions, it is not clear why humans have natural tendencies toward teleological thought. Does teleological reasoning make it easier to identify the potential utility of natural objects, and is this why it evolved? Or perhaps, teleological reasoning about the natural world is a byproduct of the artifact-rich environments humans grow up in. In fact, many of the plants and animals people interact with on a regular basis are where they are, or have some of the features they have, because of the purposeful activities of humans. Humans may not create dogs or cows in a literal sense, but contemporary dogs and cattle do have the features they have because of selective breeding for specific human purposes. What might the causal relationship between domestication practices and teleological thinking in humans be?

It may also be useful to CSR scholars if we knew more about specific or general intuitive teleological thought about the natural world. Does this thought apply equally to all classes of plants, animals, and natural nonliving kinds (such as rocks and rivers) or do some of these seem more purposeful than others? What about natural events such as thunderstorms, blizzards, or tsunamis? The research to date has concerned features of our world; less attention has been given to the question of how humans intuitively reason about the world or the cosmos as a whole.

This last point brings us to the second class of open questions, those concerning application to cultural expression. If teleological reasoning underwrites the generation and preservation of creation accounts, why do creation accounts commonly begin with some kind of primordial world? Is it because intuitive teleological thought most readily applies only to elements of the world but not the world as a whole? Likewise, many creation accounts involve the activities of multiple deities. Perhaps the apparently natural tendency to connect perceived purpose in the world to intentional agency favors attributions to collections of gods or natural spirits. That is, we may ask whether the dynamics identified by Kelemen and her colleagues sit more easily with the idea of a single creator deity or with pantheons, nature spirits, Gaia-type beliefs, or pantheism. Furthermore, this line of research could suggest whether some properties of deities fit better with the underlying natural cognition. Preschoolers seem to know that humans cannot account for the purpose preschoolers perceive in the natural world, but what kind of agency do they think is required? Is it merely more powerful agency than that of humans, or must an agent (or agents) also be more knowledgeable? Could it be that some dimensions of purpose—such as apparently purposeful beauty in the natural world—suggest that the intentional being that brought about that purpose is not just powerful but also good?

Finally, though we find it plausible that the intuitive cognition that Kelemen and others have identified facilitates the generation, transmission, and stabilization of many cultural forms that we might commonly call "religious," the case for this would be fortified by additional empirical demonstrations. Could it be shown, for instance, that mythological narratives that more closely approximate our natural intuitions in these areas are more readily remembered and more faithfully transmitted? Or could it be shown that narratives that deviate from the purported intuitive foundations gradually gravitate to more optimal (e.g., minimally counterintuitive) forms over time?

CONCLUSION

In summary, cognitive scientists have demonstrated that humans' minds intuitively make sense of the world by thinking about objects according to their kinds: natural, nominal, and artifacts. Humans intuitively hold different expectation sets (e.g., spatiality, physicality, mentality, etc.) about different kinds according to their ontological categories (e.g., solid objects, living things, etc.) This conceptual organization helps humans spend their mental energy efficiently, allowing them to make basic assumptions about the world based on kinds. When an idea fits most of our intuitive assumptions about the world, is it easier to think, express, and communicate relatively accurately; thus, it is more likely to spread and become a cultural idea (Sperber, 1996; Sperber & Hirschfeld, 2004). When an idea is minimally counterintuitive, by either transferring a principle or breaching an expectation of one ontological kind to another, it remains easy to think, but may also be especially memorable and likely to be communicated. CI agents have relatively good inferential potential, leading them to be used as explanations for many events that are relevant to people and communicated frequently. CI agents are often seen as the cause and origin of the world.

Many scientific experiments have shown that children seem to intuitively think that the natural world and its kinds are created and purposeful. Children distinguish between the creation of artifacts and of natural kinds. They also seem to naturally attribute the creation of natural kinds to a god or other CI agent. This childhood intuition never seems to completely go away, even in adulthood, and adults intuitively tend to revert to teleological explanations for the natural world and even intentional reasoning for it by an agent or agents. Gods, nature spirits, Gaia-type beliefs, and so forth, seem to fit well with our teleological intuitions about the world, and CI agents are rich in inferential potential. These cognitive tendencies help account for why such beliefs are so cross-culturally ubiquitous.

Further research questions revolve around the issues of why humans have the natural tendency toward teleological thought, the content of specific or general intuitive theological thoughts about the natural world, and cultural expressions of teleological thought. Finally, further research needs to provide empirical evidence to prove that intuitive cognition facilitates the creation, transference, and stabilization of many "religious" cultural forms.

Questions for Future Research

1. Why do humans have natural tendencies toward teleological thought?
2. Does teleological thought apply to all types of natural kinds and natural phenomena equally, or do some seem more purposeful than others?
3. Does intuitive teleological thought most readily apply only to elements of the world but not to the world as a whole?
4. Does the seeming natural tendency to connect perceived purpose in the world to intentional agency favor attributions to a single creator deity, or to pantheons, nature spirits, Gaia-type beliefs, or pantheism?
5. Does humans' intuitive, teleological reasoning of the natural world also assume characteristics of knowledge or goodness on account of creative agent(s)?
6. Are mythological narratives that are more closely aligned with humans' intuitions about the natural world more easily remembered and faithfully transmitted?

References

Astuti, R., Solomon, G. E. A., & Carey, S. (2004). Constraints on conceptual development. *Monographs of the Society for Research in Child Development, 69*(3), i–161.

Atran, S. (2002). *In gods we trust: The evolutionary landscape of religion.* Oxford: Oxford University Press.

Baillargeon, R. (2004). Infants' reasoning about hidden objects: Evidence for event-general and event-specific expectations. *Developmental Science, 7*(4), 391–424.

Barrett, J. L. (2004). *Why would anyone believe in God?* Walnut Creek, CA: AltaMira Press.

Barrett, J. L. (2008). Coding and quantifying counterintuitiveness in religious concepts: Theoretical and methodological reflections. *Method & Theory in the Study of Religion, 20*(4), 308–338. https://doi.org/10.1163/157006808X371806

Barrett, J. L. (2011). *Cognitive science, religion, and theology.* West Conshohocken, PA: Templeton Press.

Barrett, J. L. (2012). *Born believers: The science of children's religious belief.* New York: Free Press.

Barrett, J. L. (2016). The (modest) utility of MCI theory. *Religion, Brain & Behavior, 6*(3), 249–251. https://doi.org/10.1080/2153599X.2015.1015049

Barrett, J. L. (2017a). On keeping cognitive science of religion cognitive and cultural. In L. Martin & D. Wiebe (Eds.), *Religion explained? The cognitive science of religion after twenty-five years* (pp. 193–202). New York: Bloomsbury.

Barrett, J. L. (2017b). Religion is kid's stuff: Minimally counterintuitive concepts are better remembered by young people. In R. Hornbeck, J. Barrett, & M. Kang (Eds.), *Religious cognition in China: "Homo religiosus" and the dragon* (pp. 125–137). Cham, Switzerland: Springer International.

Barrett, J. L., & Nyhof, M. (2001). Spreading non-natural concepts: The role of intuitive conceptual structures in memory and transmission of cultural materials. *Journal of Cognition & Culture, 1*(1), 69–100. https://doi.org/10.1163/156853701300063589

Barrett, J. L., Richert, R., & Driesenga, A. (2001). God's beliefs versus mother's: The development of non-human agent concepts. *Child Development, 72*(1), 50–65. https://doi.org/10.1111/1467-8624.00265

Biro, S., & Leslie, A. M. (2007). Infants' perception of goal-directed actions: development through cue-based bootstrapping. *Developmental Science, 10*(3), 379–398. https://doi.org/10.1111/j.1467-7687.2006.00544.x

Boyer, P. (1994). *The naturalness of religious ideas: A cognitive theory of religion*. Berkeley: University of California Press.

Boyer, P. (1996). What makes anthropomorphism natural: Intuitive ontology and cultural representations. *Journal of the Royal Anthropological Institute, 2*(1), 83–97. https://jstor.org/stable/3034634

Boyer, P. (2001). *Religion explained: The evolutionary origins of religious thought*. New York: Basic Books.

Boyer, P., & Ramble, C. (2001). Cognitive templates for religious concepts: Cross-cultural evidence for recall of counter-intuitive representations. *Cognitive Science, 25*(4), 535–564. https://doi.org/10.1207/s15516709cog2504_2

Burdett, E. R. R., Barrett, J. L., & Greenway, T. S. (2020). Children's developing understanding of the cognitive abilities of supernatural and natural minds: Evidence from three cultures. *Journal for the Study of Religion, Nature and Culture, 14*(1), 124–151. http://doi.org/10.1558/jsrnc.39186

Burdett, E. R. R., Wigger, J. B., & Barrett, J. L. (2021). The minds of God, mortals, and in-betweens: Children's developing understanding of extraordinary and ordinary minds across four countries. *Psychology of Religion and Spirituality, 13*(2), 212–221. https://doi.org/10.1037/rel0000285

Casler, K., & Kelemen, D. (2008). Developmental continuity in teleo-functional explanation: Reasoning about nature among Romanian Romani adults. *Journal of Cognition and Development, 9*(3), 340–362. https://doi.org/10.1080/15248370802248556

Diesendruck, G., Gelman, S. A., & Lebowitz, K. (1998). Conceptual and linguistic biases in children's word learning. *Developmental Psychology, 34*(5), 823–839. https://doi.org/10.1037/0012-1649.34.5.823

Diesendruck, G., & Haber, L. (2009). God's categories: The effect of religiosity on children's teleological and essentialist beliefs about categories. *Cognition, 110*(1), 100–114. https://doi.org/10.1016/j.cognition.2008.11.001

Diesendruck, G., & HaLevi, H. (2006). The role of language, appearance, and culture in children's social category–based induction. *Child Development, 77*(3), 539–553. https://doi.org/10.1111/j.1467-8624.2006.00889.x

DiYanni, C., & Kelemen, D. (2005). Time to get a new mountain? The role of function in children's conceptions of natural kinds. *Cognition, 97*(3), 327–335. https://doi.org/10.1016/j.cognition.2004.10.002

Erickson, J. E., Keil, F. C., & Lockhart, K. L. (2010). Sensing the coherence of biology in contrast to psychology: Young children's use of causal relations to distinguish two foundational domains. *Child Development, 81*(1), 390–409. https://doi.org/10.1111/j.1467-8624.2009.01402.x

Evans, E. M. (2001). Cognitive and contextual factors in the emergence of diverse belief systems: Creation versus evolution. *Cognitive Psychology, 42*(3), 217–266. https://doi.org/10.1006/cogp.2001.0749

Friedman, O., & Leslie, A. M. (2004). Mechanisms of belief-desire reasoning. *Psychological Science, 15*(8), 547–552. https://doi.org/10.1111/j.0956-7976.2004.00717.x

Gelman, S. A. (2003). *The essential child: Origins of essentialism in everyday thought*. New York: Oxford University Press.

Gelman, S. A., & Wellman, H. M. (1991). Insides and essence: Early understandings of the nonobvious. *Cognition, 38*(3), 213–244. https://doi.org/10.1016/0010-0277(91)90007-Q

Gregory, J. P., & Greenway, T. S. (2017a). Is there a window of opportunity for religiosity? Children and adolescents preferentially recall religious-type cultural representations, but older adults do not. *Religion, Brain & Behavior, 7*(2), 98–116. https://doi.org/10.1080/2153599X.2016.1196234

Gregory, J. P., & Greenway, T. S. (2017b). The mnemonic of intuitive ontology violation is not the distinctiveness effect: Evidence from a broad age spectrum of persons in the UK and China during a free-recall task. *Journal of Cognitive and Culture, 17*(1–2), 169–197. https://doi.org/10.1163/15685373-12342197

Gregory, J. P., Greenway, T. S., & Keys, C. (2019). Gods and talking animals: The pan-cultural recall advantage of supernatural agent concepts. *Journal of Cognition and Culture, 19*(1–2), 97–130. https://doi.org/10.1163/15685373-12340050

Hatano, G., & Inagaki, K. (1994). Young children's naïve theory of biology. *Cognition, 50*(1–3), 171–188. https://doi.org/10.1016/0010-0277(94)90027-2

Hirschfeld, L. A. (1996). *Race in the making: Cognition, culture, and the child's construction of humankind*. Cambridge, MA: MIT Press.

Hornbeck, R., & Barrett, J. L. (2013). Refining and testing "counterintuitiveness" in virtual reality: Cross-cultural evidence for recall of counterintuitive representations. *International Journal for the Psychology of Religion, 23*(1), 15–28. https://doi.org/10.1080/10508619.2013.735192

Hubin, Y., Shuxian, Y., & Mineke, S. (2011). *China's creation and origin myths: Cross-cultural explorations in oral and written traditions*. Leiden: Brill.

Inagaki, K., & Hatano, G. (2002). *Young children's naïve thinking about the biological world*. Psychology Press.

Inagaki, K., & Hatano, G. (2006). Young children's conception of the biological world. *Current Directions in Psychological Science, 15*(4), 177–181. https://doi.org/10.1111/j.1467-8721.2006.00431.x

Järnefelt, E., Canfield, F. C., & Kelemen, D. (2015). The divided mind of a disbeliever: Intuitive beliefs about nature as purposefully created among different groups of non-religious adults. *Cognition, 140*, 72–88. https://doi.org/10.1016/j.cognition.2015.02.005

Kalish, C. W. (1998). Natural and artifactual kinds: Are children realists or relativists about categories? *Developmental Psychology, 34*(2), 376–391. https://doi.org/10.1037/0012-1649.34.2.376

Keil, F. C. (1992). *Concepts, kinds, and cognitive development*. Cambridge, MA: MIT Press.

Keil, F. C. (2003). That's life: Coming to understand biology. *Human Development, 46*(6), 369–377. https://doi.org/10.1159/000073310

Kelemen, D. (1999a). The scope of teleological thinking in preschool children. *Cognition, 70*(3), 241–272. https://doi.org/10.1016/S0010-0277(99)00010-4

Kelemen, D. (1999b). Why are rocks pointy? Children's preference for teleological explanations of the natural world. *Developmental Psychology, 35*(6), 1440–1452. https://doi.org/10.1037/0012-1649.35.6.1440

Kelemen, D. (2003). British and American children's preferences for teleological-functional explanations of the natural world. *Cognition, 88*(2), 201–221. https://doi.org/10.1016/S0010-0277(03)00024-6

Kelemen, D. (2004). Are children "intuitive theists"? *Psychological Science, 15*(5), 295–301. https://doi.org/10.1111/j.0956-7976.2004.00672.x

Kelemen, D., & DiYanni, C. (2005). Intuitions about origins: Purpose and intelligent design in children's reasoning about nature. *Journal of Cognition and Development, 6*(1), 3–31. https://doi.org/10.1207/s15327647jcd0601_2

Kelemen, D., Rottman, J., & Seston, R. (2013). Professional physical scientists display tenacious teleological tendencies: Purpose-based reasoning as a cognitive default. *Journal of Experimental Psychology: General, 142*(4), 1074–1083. https://doi.org/10.1037/a0030399

Knight, N., Sousa, P., Barrett, J. L., & Atran, S. (2004). Children's attributions of beliefs to humans and God: Cross-cultural evidence. *Cognitive Science, 28*(1), 117–126. https://doi.org/10.1016/j.cogsci.2003.09.002

Kundert, C., & Edman, L. R. O. (2017). Promiscuous teleology: From childhood through adulthood and from West to East. In R. G. Hornbeck, J. L. Barrett, & M. Kang (Eds.), *Religious cognition in China* (pp. 79–96). Cham, Switzerland: Springer.

Lombrozo, T., Kelemen, D., & Zaitchik, D. (2007). Inferring design: Evidence of a preference for teleological explanations in patients with Alzheimer's disease. *Psychological Science, 18*(11), 999–1006. https://doi.org/10.1111/j.1467-9280.2007.02015.x

Medin, D. L., & Ortony, A. (1989). Psychological essentialism. In S. Vosniadou & A. Ortony (Eds.), *Similarity and analogical reasoning* (pp. 179–195). Cambridge, UK: Cambridge University Press.

McCauley, R. N. (2011). *Why religion is natural, and science is not.* Oxford: Oxford University Press.

Newman, G. E., Keil, F. C., Kuhlmeier, V. A., & Wynn, K. (2010). Early understandings of the link between agents and order. *PNAS, 107*(40), 17140–17145. https://doi.org/10.1073/pnas.0914056107

Petrovich, O. (1997). Understanding of non-natural causality in children and adults: A case against artificialism. *Psyche en Geloof, 8*, 151–165.

Petrovich, O. (1999). Preschool children's understanding of the dichotomy between the natural and the artificial. *Psychological Reports, 84*(1), 3–27. https://doi.org/10.2466/pro.1999.84.1.3

Piaget, J. (1997). *The child's conception of the world: Selected works* (J. Tomlinson & A. Tomlinson, Trans.) (Vol. 1). London: Routledge. (Original work published in 1929).

Premack, D. (1990). The infant's theory of self-propelled objects. *Cognition, 36*(1), 1–16.

Purzycki, B. G., & Willard, A. K. (2016). MCI theory: A critical discussion. *Religion, Brain & Behavior, 6*(3), 207–248. https://doi.org/10.1080/2153599X.2015.1024915

Pyysiäinen, I. (2003). *How religion works: Towards a new cognitive science of religion.* Leiden: Brill.

Putnam, H. (1975). The meaning of "meaning." In H. Putnam (Ed.), *Mind language and reality* (Vol. 2, pp. 215–271). Cambridge, UK: Cambridge University Press.

Rosengren, K. S., Gekman, S. A., Kalish, C. W., & McCormick, M. (1991). As time goes by: Children's early understanding of growth. *Child Development, 62*(6), 1302–1320. https://doi.org/10.2307/1130808

Rottman, J., Zhu, L., Wang, W., Schillaci, R. S., Clark, K. J., & Kelemen, D. (2017). Cultural influences on the teleological stance: Evidence from China. *Religion, Brain & Behavior, 7*(1), 17–26. https://doi.org/10.1080/2153599X.2015.1118402

Simons, D. J., & Keil, F. C. (1995). An abstract to concrete shift in development of biological thought: The *insides* story. *Cognition, 56*(2), 129–163. https://doi.org/10.1016/0010-0277(94)00660-D

Slaughter, V. (2005). Young children's understanding of death. *Australian Psychologist, 40*(3), 179–186. https://doi.org/10.1080/00050060500243426

Spelke, E. (1994). Initial knowledge: Six suggestions. *Cognition, 50*(1), 431–445. https://doi.org/10.1016/0010-0277(94)90039-6

Spelke, E. S., & Kinzler, K. D. (2007). Core knowledge. *Developmental Science, 10*(1), 89–96. https://doi.org/10.1111/j.1467-7687.2007.00569.x

Sperber, D. (1996). *Explaining culture: A naturalistic approach.* Oxford: Blackwell.

Sperber, D., & Hirschfeld, L. (2004). The cognitive foundations of cultural stability and diversity. *Trends in Cognitive Sciences, 8*(1), 40–46. https://doi.org/10.1016/j.tics.2003.11.002

Wellman, H. M., Cross, D., & Watson, J. (2001). Meta-analysis of theory-of-mind development: The truth about false belief. *Child Development, 72*(3), 655–684. https://doi.org/10.1111/1467-8624.00304

Wellman, H. M., & Liu, D. (2004). Scaling of theory-of-mind tasks. *Child Development, 75*(2), 523–541. https://doi.org/10.1111/j.1467-8624.2004.00691.x

PART III

RELIGIOUS ACTIONS

CHAPTER 8

EXPLAINING AND SOLVING PRACTICAL PROBLEMS SUPERNATURALLY

RACHEL E. WATSON-JONES AND
CRISTINE H. LEGARE

Department of Psychology, The University of Texas at Austin

INTRODUCTION

SUPERNATURAL explanations are often associated with significant life events such as the death of a loved one, a severe illness, or the birth of a child. Yet they are also widely used to make sense of happenings in daily life. For example, imagine that you are running late for work. As you scramble to leave the house, you can't find the pair of shoes you want to wear. You hit your elbow on the doorframe as you exit the bathroom, and in the kitchen, you spill coffee on your shirt. When you finally make it to your car, you realize you're almost out of gas. To top it off, when you enter the freeway, you find that all the lanes are blocked. Many people in this scenario would ask themselves, "Why are all these bad things happening to me?" The number of adverse events occurring in a short period makes it unlikely that you would attribute all of them to coincidence or chance.

A negative string of events often leads us to generate explanations such as "I must have done something to deserve this," or "the universe is against me today." We tend to generate justifications of this kind—supernatural explanations—when there are no obvious natural explanations for why an adverse event happened. Natural explanations appeal to "observable and empirically verifiable phenomena of the physical or material world" (Legare et al., 2012, p. 4). For example, being near a person who was ill is a common explanation for catching a cold. Often, the natural explanation—that these events are random occurrences with physical causes—is not *satisfactory*. Explaining events by appealing to chance does not satisfy our desire to control our fate. Nor do explanations based on chance provide us with a means of averting adverse outcomes in the future. In situations like the bad-morning example, people often generate both natural explanations (e.g., "I didn't sleep well last night and am flustered today") and supernatural ones (e.g., "I am being punished for something I did wrong"). Many people may also engage in rituals to solve problems and ward off future adverse events. For example, in the southern United States some people spin a button on their clothing to protect themselves from death when a hearse (vehicle carrying a coffin) passes by.

Why are we motivated to explain events by appealing to supernatural agents or powers? We propose that one function of supernatural beliefs and behaviors is to increase the perception of control and reduce feelings of uncertainty (Legare & Souza, 2012, 2014; Legare, Watson-Jones, et al., 2016). In general, humans attempt to reduce uncertainty in life as a means of regulating emotion and maintaining homeostasis. A fundamental principle of biology, *homeostasis* refers to regulatory functions within the nervous systems of organisms. These systems are automatic and create the internal conditions for maintaining life (Bernard, 1865 Cannon, 1929). When organisms are out of homeostasis, they take action to return to that state. For example, when an animal experiences hunger, it seeks out food. In humans, at least, the motivation to return to homeostasis is experienced as feelings, both physical and emotional. Humans have a conscious and intentional means of regulation, which we experience as well-being (Damasio & Damasio, 2016, p. 126).

Experiencing something sacred or extraordinary in everyday life may increase well-being in various contexts and provide life with meaning (Doehring et al., 2009; Pargament & Park, 1997; Pargament & Mahoney, 2002). Open questions remain, however, about the nature of the relationship between supernatural beliefs and well-being. For example, why do humans seek meaning through supernatural beliefs and behaviors such as rituals? Meaning-making through supernatural explanations and practices may help people maintain psychological homeostasis.

This chapter examines how people use supernatural beliefs and practices to explain and act upon their world. We discuss why people engage in rituals and other supernatural practices that are meant to have a causal effect upon the world and to solve concrete problems in their lives. First, we examine how people use supernatural explanations to interpret outcomes and events in their lives. Second, we consider how human psychology supports the belief that rituals have a causal influence on the world. Third, we describe how the combination of supernatural explanation and practice provides a sense of control over life events and discuss the potential mechanisms underlying the connection between supernatural beliefs, rituals, and perceived control over the environment.

WHY ARE WE MOTIVATED TO EXPLAIN OUTCOMES SUPERNATURALLY?

Appealing to natural and supernatural phenomena to explain the same event is a universal cognitive experience (Campbell, 1972; Evans et al., 2010; Legare & Gelman, 2008; Misztal & Shupe, 1992; Raman & Winer, 2004). In many cases, individuals may be fully aware of *how* an event occurred (e.g., the physical causes of natural disasters). Yet the question of *why* the event occurred often remains unanswered. Anthropologist E. Evans-Pritchard (pp. 69–70) described this experience based on his observations of the Azande people in North Central Africa:

> In Zandeland, sometimes an old granary collapses. There is nothing remarkable in this. Every Zande knows that termites eat the supports over time and that even the hardest woods decay after years of service. A granary is the summerhouse of a Zande homestead, and people sit beneath it in the heat of the day. Consequently, there may be people sitting beneath the granary when it collapses who are injured, for it is a heavy structure made of beams and clay and may be stored with millet as well. That it should collapse is easily intelligible, but why should this particular granary have collapsed at the particular moment when these particular people were sitting beneath it?

The Azande fully understand the natural, or physical, causes of the collapse (i.e., termites and decaying wood) and also seek a metaphysical cause: *Why did the granary collapse at that moment and with those people sitting under it?* These kinds of why questions often prompt a supernatural explanation. Supernatural explanations appeal to phenomena that "violate, operate outside of, or are distinct from" the natural world (Legare et al., 2012, p. 5). Thus, the underlying mechanism linking action to an outcome is often not based on natural causes (Gelman & Legare, 2011; Legare & Visala, 2011). In contrast, even if we do not understand a natural process well, we assume that an expert knows how it works.

Topics of fundamental concern to humans, such as our origins, illness, and death, often motivate people to seek out both natural and supernatural explanations, a phenomenon known as *explanatory coexistence* (Busch et al., 2017; Legare et al., 2012, 2020; Watson-Jones et al., 2015, 2017). These topics share several characteristics that make people more likely to use both natural and supernatural explanations. First, they are based on unobservable, or hidden, causal mechanisms. Second, they are associated with strong emotions. Finally, they predate current scientific understanding (Evans et al., 2010). Explanatory coexistence is not limited to these topics, however. People are motivated to explain many events in their lives with natural and supernatural explanations, from the untimely death of a loved one to why their car broke down.

As the bad-morning example illustrates, people seek supernatural explanations for even innocuous adverse events. Supernatural explanations can increase the perception of control by connecting an action to an effect. Connecting an event to supernatural agency (e.g., "this happened as punishment because I was rude to the mailman yesterday"), rather than random coincidence (e.g., "this is just unfortunate"), provides a causal link between action and outcome. An agentive causal explanation may reduce our anxiety and increase our sense of well-being.

Why Do We Believe in the Efficacy of Supernatural Rituals?

Often, when we explain adverse events supernaturally, we connect those explanations with actions, or rituals, intended to alleviate anxiety and prevent future adverse outcomes. We define *ritual* as socially stipulated, causally opaque behavior (Legare & Herrmann, 2013; Legare & Nielsen, 2020; Legare & Watson-Jones, 2015; Watson-Jones & Legare, 2016; Legare, Wen, et al., 2016). Rituals are socially stipulated group conventions. People often carry them out without understanding why or how they function; it is sufficient to know that they have seen them done by others before. Most people perform rituals without understanding the connections between the physical causes (e.g., performing the ritual behaviors) and their intended effects (e.g., stopping the adverse event). For example, when someone knocks on wood after mentioning something negative that could happen, there is no clear physical-causal connection between the act of knocking on wood and averting a negative outcome. In this sense, rituals are causally opaque. Though rituals may appeal to supernatural agents in some way, there is often not an expectation of a direct physical-causal connection between actions and material outcomes (Sørensen, 2007). There is rarely a transparent connection between the specific ritual action performed (e.g., repeating a specific phrase) and the desired outcome or effect (e.g., curing an illness).

The use of rituals to treat problems is widespread in contemporary populations, including in the United Kingdom (Hutton, 1999), the United States (Crowley, 1989), Brazil (Cohen & Barrett, 2008; Legare & Souza, 2012, 2014; Souza & Legare, 2011), India (Legare et al., 2020), and South Africa (Ashforth, 2001; Legare & Gelman, 2008). Rituals are used to treat myriad problems, from asthma to unemployment. The use of rituals for problem-solving purposes dates back to ancient Egypt (*The Papyrus Ebers*, 1931, 1937). Rituals can express emotions, symbolize social relations, and represent sacred beliefs (Csordas, 2002; Ruffle & Sosis, 2003; Sax, 2010; Sax et al., 2010; Shore, 1996; Whitehouse & Lanman, 2014). Rituals encourage personal interpretations of meaning in the context of collective activities. They are examples of belief extended through action to create outcomes in the world (Rappaport, 1999).

People reason about whether ritual actions will be effective based on intuitive beliefs about causal reasoning. According to Tambiah (1979, p. 119), rituals are "patterned and ordered sequences of words and acts, . . . characterized in varying degrees by formality (conventionality), stereotypy (rigidity), and redundancy (repetition)." Information that reflects cognitive biases in causal reasoning (i.e., that repetition, number of procedural steps, and specificity of procedural detail increase the efficacy of an action) impacts the evaluation of ritual efficacy. When causal information is not available, as is common in ritual, biases in causal reasoning become especially salient to judgments of the efficacy of actions (Legare & Souza, 2012, 2014; Legare, Watson-Jones, et al., 2016).

Standard behavioral features of ritual, such as the disconnection between actions and empirical goals, compulsion, rigidity, repetition, order, and boundaries (Boyer & Liénard, 2006), are also seen on the obsessive-compulsive disorder spectrum, in routine habits, and in rituals associated with essential transition points in the life course (i.e., pregnancy, birth, childhood, adolescence, adulthood, death; Boyer & Liénard, 2006). A potential explanation for these similarities is that religious and other cultural rituals mimic the compelling and attention-grabbing aspects of ritualized behavior, such as performance frequency and emotional arousal, and thus trigger the same anxiety-reducing response (Boyer & Liénard, 2006; McCauley & Lawson, 2002).

Consider the following rituals used as remedies in ancient Egypt and in present-day Brazil. This ancient Egyptian ritual from the Papyrus Ebers was used to treat blindness:

> Crush, powder, and make into one, the two eyes of a pig (remove the water from there), true collyrium (i.e., mineral eye salve), red-lead (i.e., red oxide), and wild honey [in a clay bowl]. Inject [mixture] into the ear of the patient. When thou hast seen properly to this mixing repeat this formula: "I have brought this thing and put it in its place. The crocodile [god Sobek] is weak and powerless." Repeat twice. Thereby he will at once recover. (*The Papyrus Ebers*, 1931, p. 104)

Now consider a ritual used to find a romantic partner in Brazil:

> Buy a new sharp knife and stick it four times into a banana tree on June midnight. Catch the liquid that will drip from the plant's wound on a crisp, white paper that has been folded in two. The dripping liquid captured on the paper at night will form the first letter of the name of your future partner. (Scharf, 2010).

There are many differences in the specific content of rituals both within and across cultures. For example, rituals can involve different substances and actions, incorporate different instruments, and treat different problems. Yet there are more profound similarities: They involve procedural repetition, a large number of procedural steps, a specified time to perform the actions, and in-depth procedural detail, as well as the presence of supernatural agents or power. There is even a long-standing philosophical tradition that supports the claim that beliefs about causal connections arise from impressions of repeated instances of similar relations (Hume, 1967). Additionally, converging psychological research has demonstrated that repetition may also influence reasoning about various behaviors by making information more psychologically salient. Repetition holds a concept or action in working memory (Oppenheimer, 2008), making it familiar (Scott & Dienes, 2008) and attractive (Zajonc, 1968). The repetition of similar actions (e.g., pressing a button repeatedly to call an elevator) may be perceived to increase the likelihood of a successful outcome. The number of procedural steps and procedural specificity of the action sequence also influence perceptions of causal efficacy. A ritual with multiple procedural steps gives the impression that multiple actions may have the capacity to produce a particular effect (Depue et al., 2006). The specificity of the action sequence (i.e., the inclusion of specific, detailed information) influences perceptions of action efficacy. People are expert readers of intention. Thus, watching someone engage in a detailed course of actions (e.g., catching the liquid that will drip from the plant's wound on a crisp, white paper that has been folded in two) may give the impression that the precise details of the action sequence (i.e., time specificity, item specificity) have the potential to produce the intended outcome, even if the mechanism is unknown or unavailable (Legare & Souza, 2012, 2014; Legare, Wen, et al., 2016).

To examine the kind of information that increases perceptions of ritual efficacy, Legare and Souza (2012) asked Brazilian participants to evaluate the effectiveness of novel *simpatias* (ritualistic remedial practices used for problem-solving purposes). The *simpatias* they studied varied based on the specificity of time and place, repetition of procedures, the number of procedural steps, number of items used, and the presence or absence of a religious icon. Legare and Souza found that the rituals that included a greater number of steps, more repetition, and greater procedural specificity were evaluated as more effective. For religious believers, the presence of a religious icon (e.g., an image of the Virgin Mary for Roman Catholics) also increased efficacy evaluations. Images and icons of supernatural agents are frequently used in rituals (Cohen, 2007; Souza & Legare, 2011; Whitehouse, 2004), and thus intuitions about ritual efficacy may invoke the involvement of a supernatural agent at some level of the ritual (Barrett & Lawson, 2001; Sørensen et al., 2006). If a supernatural agenct is involved, ritualistic actions may not be as constrained as non-ritualistic actions by the same physical-causal expectations (Barrett & Malley, 2007).

How and Why Do Supernatural Beliefs and Behaviors Provide a Sense of Control?

People often use rituals to avert adverse outcomes and assert control over uncertain situations. During his time with the Trobrianders (inhabitants of the Trobiand Islands, off the east coast of New Guinea), Malinowski (1948) described the extensive ritual that preceded the uncertain and dangerous conditions of deep-sea fishing. Malinowski noted that the fishermen rarely relied on ritual when they were fishing in a familiar and safe setting such as the lagoon. In these instances, the fishermen described their successes and failures in terms of skill. Malinowski proposed that in times of uncertainty, stress, and danger, people turn to magical rituals as a means of coping and enacting some measure of control.

Ritual behavior is common in contexts in which the outcome is uncertain or some level of danger is involved (Sosis & Handwerker, 2011; Souza & Legare, 2011). From the athlete who taps his baseball three times before a game to the student who uses her "lucky" pen in an exam, ritual and uncertainty share a strong association (Bleak & Frederick, 1998; Cibrowski, 1997; Gallagher & Lewis, 2001; Todd & Brown, 2003; Van Raalte et al., 1991; Vyse, 1997; White, 2021; Womack, 1992). Engaging in ritual has also been shown to reduce stress during uncertain and dangerous times. For example, Sosis (2007) found that reciting psalms helped Israeli women cope with the stress and uncertainty of war. Because of its ability to relieve stress and cope with wartime's frightening and unpredictable nature, systematic psalm recitation may have emerged as a cultural norm for Israeli women. Rituals often entail prescriptive, rigid behavioral patterns for averting perceived danger. Threats to physical and social safety may activate mental "security systems" that result in behavioral and psychological coping strategies (Boyer & Liénard, 2006; Szechtman & Woody, 2004).

Highly uncertain situations and a perceived lack of control increase the experience of anxiety, and vice versa—anxiety can induce a sense of lack of control. When we are anxious, our psychological systems trigger responses aimed at returning to homeostasis to restore feelings of control and well-being (Lang et al., 2020; Underwood, 1996; Vaughn & Weary, 2003; Weary & Jacobson, 1997; Weary et al., 2001). Thus rituals are produced and maintained by an *illusion of control* (Langer, 1975). They may have little or no actual bearing on the success of instrumental outcomes (Lobmeyer & Wasserman, 1986). But when individuals believe or respond as if contingencies between their behavior and the outcome exist, even if the outcomes are random, they experience an illusion of control (Alloy et al., 1981; Matute, 1994). For example, when they are primed with feelings of lack of control, they detect correlations among random sets of presumably unrelated stimuli (Kay et al., 2009; Whitson & Galinsky, 2008). Priming randomness also affects the perception of a ritual's efficacy. Legare and Souza (2014) used the scrambled sentence task (Kay et al., 2010) to prime randomness. One set of participants received sentences containing words related to randomness, such as "chaotic"; another set of participants received sentences containing neutral words. The participants who had been primed with randomness rated rituals more efficacious than did the participants primed with the neutral control (Legare & Souza, 2014). Priming randomness may have activated a need to feel in control that resulted in using the ritual(s) to accomplish this goal. Even with unfamiliar content (e.g., Brazilian rituals in a US context), priming randomness increased participants' evaluations of ritual efficacy. Rituals allow individuals to exert agency through action, giving the illusion of increased control, which could also be related to emotional regulation and anxiety reduction.

One potential explanation for the influence of ritual on the perception of control is that they provide an opportunity to posit a connection between action and outcome. Research with religious participants suggests that an internal locus of control mediates the positive association between awareness of God and positive health outcomes (Ryan

& Francis, 2012). Future research could explore the relationship between the perceptions of control and actual control related to ritualistic behavior. Research of this kind has the potential to speak to the function of this behavior by determining whether the proposed psychological mechanisms produce positive behavioral outcomes and improved mental states. For instance, there is research suggesting that ritualization of the administering of medical treatment appears to affect patient confidence, thereby increasing the healing power of the treatment (Kaptchuk et al., 2010; Miller et al., 2009).

CONCLUSION

Humans seek to maintain a homeostatic state by attempting to predict what might happen next and then reacting in a way that is in their best interests. When we are in a dangerous situation, unsure of the outcome, we become anxious—indicating to our internal systems that we are no longer in homeostasis and need to remedy the situation and regain control. In ambiguous and uncertain situations, supernatural beliefs often provide psychologically satisfying explanations for consequential outcomes and events. Ritualized behaviors allow us to exert individual agency over our environment in socially sanctioned ways. Supernatural beliefs and behaviors make the world seem more meaningful, understandable, and predictable. The human tendency to explain and solve practical problems supernaturally is a psychological consequence of our desire to predict future events and exert control over the world around us.

QUESTIONS FOR FUTURE RESEARCH

1. What are the psychological processes by which ritual practice alleviates anxiety?
2. How early in development is the connection between ritual and perceived control evident?
3. What predicts individual differences in supernatural belief and behavior?
4. What predicts cultural differences in supernatural belief and behavior?

REFERENCES

Alloy, L. B., Abramson, L. Y., & Viscusi, D. (1981). Induced mood and the illusion of control. *Journal of Personality and Social Psychology, 41*, 1129–1140.

Ashforth, A. (2001). An epidemic of witchcraft? The implications of AIDS for the post-apartheid state. In H. Moore & T. Sanders (Eds.), *Magical interpretations, material realities* (pp. 184–225). London: Routledge.

Barrett J., & Lawson, T. (2001). Ritual intuitions: Cognitive contributions to judgments of ritual efficacy. *Journal of Cognition and Culture, 1*, 183–201.

Barrett, J., & Malley, B. (2007). A cognitive typology of religious actions. *Journal of Cognition and Culture, 7*, 201–211.

Bernard, C. (1865). *Introduction à l'étude de la Médecine Expérimentale.*. In J. B. Baillière et Fils, Paris, (pp. 88–89) English Translation by H. C. Greene, New York, NY: Dover Publications, Inc.

Bleak, J. L., & Frederick, C. M. (1998). Superstitious behavior in sport: Levels of effectiveness and determinants of use in three collegiate sports. *Journal of Sport Behavior, 21*, 1–15.

Boyer, P., & Liénard, P. (2006). Why ritualized behavior? Precaution systems and action-parsing in developmental, pathological, and cultural rituals. *Behavioral and Brain Sciences, 29*, 1–56.

Busch, J. T. A., Watson-Jones, R. E., & Legare, C. H. (2017). The coexistence of natural and supernatural explanations within and across domains and development. *British Journal of Developmental Psychology, 35*, 4–20.

Campbell, J. (1972). *Myths to live by*. New York: Viking Press.

Cannon, W. B. (1929). Organization for physiological homeostasis. *Physiology Review, 9*, 399–431.

Cibrowski, T. (1997). Superstition in the collegiate baseball player. *Sport Psychologist, 11*, 305–317.

Cohen, E. (2007). *The mind possessed: The cognition of spirit possession in Afro-Brazilian religious tradition*. Oxford: Oxford University Press.

Cohen, E., & Barrett, J. (2008). When minds migrate: Conceptualizing spirit possession. *Journal of Cognition and Culture, 8*(1–2), 23–48.

Crowley, V. (1989). *Wicca: The old religion in the new age*. London: Aquarian Press.

Csordas, T. J. (2002). *Body/meaning/healing*. New York: Palgrave Macmillan.

Damasio, A., & Damasio, H. (2016). Exploring the concept of homeostasis and considering its implications for economics. *Journal of Economic Behavior & Organization, 126B*, 125–129.

Depue, B. E., Banich, M. T., & Curran, T. (2006). Suppression of emotional and nonemotional content in memory effects of repetition on cognitive control. *Psychological Science, 17*(5), 441–447.

Doehring, C., Clarke, A., Pargament, K. I., Hayes, A., Hammer, D., Nikolas, M., & Hughes, P. (2009). Perceiving sacredness in life: Correlates and predictors. *Archives for the Psychology of Religion, 31*, 55–73.

Evans, E. M., Legare, C. H., & Rosengren, K. S. (2010). Engaging multiple epistemologies: Implications for science education. In M. Ferrari & R. Taylor (Eds.), *Epistemology and science education: Understanding the evolution vs. intelligent design controversy* (pp. 111–139). New York: Routledge.

Gallagher, T. J., & Lewis, J. M. (2001). Rationalists, fatalists, and the modern superstitious: Test-taking in introductory sociology. *Sociological Inquiry, 71*, 1–12.

Gelman, S. A., & Legare, C. H. (2011). Concepts and folk theories. *Annual Review of Anthropology, 40*, 379–398.

Hume, D. (1967). *A treatise of human nature*. Oxford: Oxford University Press. (Original published in 1740).

Hutton, R. (1999). *The triumph of the moon: A history of modern pagan witchcraft*. Oxford: Oxford University Press.

Kaptchuk, T. J., Friedlander, E., Kelley, J. M., Sanchez, M. N., Kokkotou, E., Singer, J. P., Kowalczykowski, M., Miller, F. G., Kirsch, I. & Lembo, A. J. (2010). Placebos without deception: A randomized controlled trial in irritable bowel syndrome. *PloS One, 5*(12), e15591.

Kay, A., Moscovitch, D., & Laurin, K. (2010). Randomness, attributions of arousal, and belief in God. *Psychological Science, 12*, 1–3.

Kay, A., Whitson, J. A., Gaucher, D., & Galinsky, A. D. (2009). Compensatory control: Achieving order through the mind, our intuitions, and the heavens. *Current Directions in Psychological Science, 18*, 264–268.

Lang, M., Krátký, J., & Xygalatas, D. (2020). The role of ritual behaviour in anxiety reduction: An investigation of Marathi religious practices in Mauritius. *Philosophical Transactions of the Royal Society B, 375*, 1805, 20190431.

Langer, E. J. (1975). The illusion of control. *Journal of Personality and Social Psychology, 32*, 311–328.

Legare, C. H., & Gelman, S. A. (2008). Bewitchment, biology, or both: The coexistence of natural and supernatural explanatory frameworks across development. *Cognitive Science, 32*, 607–642.

Legare, C. H., & Visala, A. (2011). Between religion and science: Integrating psychological and philosophical accounts of explanatory coexistence. *Human Development, 54*, 169–184.

Legare, C. H., & Souza, A. L. (2012). Evaluating ritual efficacy: Evidence from the supernatural. *Cognition, 124*, 1–15.

Legare, C. H., & Herrmann, P. A. (2013). Cognitive consequences and constraints on reasoning about ritual. *Religion, Brain & Behavior, 3*, 63–65.

Legare, C. H., & Souza, A. L. (2014). Searching for control: Priming randomness increases evaluations of ritual efficacy. *Cognitive Science, 38*, 152–161.

Legare, C. H., & Watson-Jones, R. E. (2015). The evolution and ontogeny of ritual. In D. M. Buss (Ed.), *Handbook of evolutionary psychology* (pp. 829–847). Hoboken, NJ: Wiley & Sons.

Legare, C. H., & Nielsen, M. (2020). Ritual explained: Interdisciplinary answers to Tinbergen's four questions. *Philosophical Transactions of the Royal Society B: Biological Sciences, 375*, 20190419. doi:10.1098/rstb.2019.0419

Legare, C. H., Evans, M. E., Rosengren, K. S., & Harris, P. L. (2012). The coexistence of natural and supernatural explanations across cultures and development. *Child Development, 83*, 779–793.

Legare, C. H., Watson-Jones, R. E., & Souza, A. L. (2016). A cognitive psychological account of reasoning about ritual efficacy. In H. De Cruz & R. Nichols (Eds.), *Advances in religion, cognitive science, and experimental* philosophy (pp. 85–102). London: Continuum International.

Legare, C. H., Wen, N. J., & Watson-Jones, R. E. (2016). Ritual. In M. H. Bornstein (Ed.), *The Sage encyclopedia of lifespan human development*. Thousand Oaks, CA: Sage Publications.

Legare, C. H., Akhauri, S., Chaudhuri, I., Hashmi, F., Johnson, T., Little, E. E., Lunkenheimer, H. G., Mandelbaum, A., Mandlik, H., Mondal, S., Mor, N., Saldanha, N., Schooley, J., Sharda, P., Subbiah, S., Swarup, S., Tikkanen, M., & Burger, O. (2020). Perinatal risk and the cultural ecology of health in Bihar, India. *Philosophical Transactions of the Royal Society B: Biological Sciences, 375*. doi:10.1098/rstb.2019.0433

Lobmeyer, D. L., & Wasserman, E. A. (1986). Preliminaries to free throw shooting: Superstitious behavior? *Journal of Sport Behavior, 9*, 70–78.

Malinowski, B. (1948). *Magic, science and religion*. Garden City, NY: Doubleday Anchor. (Original work published in 1925).

Matute, H. (1994). Learned helplessness and superstitious behavior as opposite effects of uncontrollable reinforcement in humans. *Learning and Motivation, 25*, 216–232.

McCauley, R. N., & Lawson, E. T. (2002). *Bringing ritual to mind: Psychological foundations of cultural forms*. Cambridge, UK: Cambridge University Press.

Miller, F., Colloca, G. L., & Kaptchuk, T. J. (2009). The placebo effect: Illness and interpersonal healing. *Perspectives in Biology and Medicine, 52*, 518–539.

Misztal, B., & Shupe, A. (1992). Making sense of the global revival of fundamentalism. In B. Misztal & A. Shupe (Eds.), *Religion and politics in comparative perspective* (pp. 3–9). Westport, CT: Praeger.

Oppenheimer, D. M. (2008). The secret life of fluency. *Trends in Cognitive Science, 12*, 237–241.

The Papyrus Ebers. (1931). (C. P. Bryan, Trans.). New York: D. Appleton and Company.

The Papyrus Ebers. (1937). (B. Ebbell, Trans.). Copenhagen, Denmark: Levin & Munksgaard.

Pargament, K. I., & Park, C. L. (1997). In times of stress: The religion-coping connection. In B. Spilka & D. McIntosh (Eds.), *Theoretical advances in the psychology of religion* (pp. 43–53). Boulder, CO: Westview Press.

Pargament, K. I., & Mahoney, A. (2002). Spirituality: Discovering and conserving the sacred. In C. R. Snyder & S. J. Lopez (Eds.), *Handbook of positive psychology* (pp. 646–659). New York: Oxford University Press.

Raman, L., & Winer, G. A. (2004). Evidence of more immanent justice reasoning in adults than in children: A challenge to traditional developmental theories. *British Journal of Developmental Psychology, 22*, 255–274.

Rappaport, R. (1999). *Ritual and religion in the making of humanity.* Cambridge, UK: Cambridge University Press.

Ruffle, B., & Sosis, R. (2003). Religious ritual and cooperation: Testing for a relationship on Israeli religious and secular kibbutzim. *Current Anthropology, 44*, 713–722.

Ryan, M. E., & Francis, A. J. P. (2012). Locus of control beliefs mediates the relationship between religious functioning and psychological health. *Journal of Religion and Health, 51*, 774–785.

Sax, W. S. (2010). Ritual and the problem of efficacy. In W. S. Sax, J. Quack, & J. Weinhold (Eds.), *The problem of ritual efficacy* (pp. 3–16). Oxford: Oxford University Press.

Sax, W. S., Quack, J., & Weinhold, J. (Eds.). (2010). *The problem of ritual efficacy.* Oxford: Oxford University Press.

Scharf, R. (2010, February 18). How to get a husband the Brazilian way. Retrieved from Deep Brazil, http://deepbrazil.com/2010/02/18/how-to-find-a-husband-the-brazilian-way/

Scott, R., & Dienes, Z. (2008). The conscious, the unconscious, and familiarity. *Journal of Experimental Psychology: Learning, Memory and Cognition, 35*, 1264–1288.

Shore, B. (1996). *Culture in mind: Cognition, culture, and the problem of meaning.* New York: Oxford University Press.

Sørensen, J. (2007). *A cognitive theory of magic.* Lanham, MD: AltaMira Press.

Sørensen, J., Liénard, P., & Feeny, C. (2006). Agent and instrument in evaluations of ritual efficacy. *Journal of Cognition and Culture, 6*, 463–482.

Sosis, R. (2007). Psalms for safety: Magico-religious responses to threats of terror. *Current Anthropology, 48*, 903–911.

Sosis, R., & Handwerker, W. P. (2011). Psalms and coping with uncertainty: Religious Israeli women's responses to the 2006 Lebanon war. *American Anthropologist, 113*(1), 40–55.

Souza, A. L., & Legare, C. H. (2011). The role of testimony in the evaluation of religious expertise. *Religion, Brain & Behavior, 2*, 1–8.

Szechtman, H., & Woody, E. (2004). Obsessive-compulsive disorder as a disturbance of security motivation. *Psychological Review, 111*(1), 111–127.

Tambiah, S. J. (1979). A performative approach to ritual. *Proceedings of the British Academy, 45*, 113–169.

Todd, M., & Brown, C. (2003). Characteristics associated with superstitious behavior in track and field athletes: Are there NCAA divisional level differences? *Journal of Sport Behavior, 26,* 168–187.

Underwood, G. (1996). *Implicit cognition.* New York: Oxford University Press.

Van Raalte, J. L., Brewer, B. W., & Nemeroff, C. J. (1991). Chance orientation and superstitious behavior on the putting green. *Journal of Sport Behavior, 14,* 41–50.

Vaughn, L. A., & Weary, G. (2003). Causal uncertainty and correction of judgments. *Journal of Experimental Social Psychology, 39,* 516–524.

Vyse, S. A. (1997). *Believing in magic.* New York: Oxford University Press.

Watson-Jones, R. E., & Legare, C. H. (2016). The social functions of group rituals. *Current Directions in Psychological Science, 25,* 42–46.

Watson-Jones, R. E., Busch, J. T. A., & Legare, C. H. (2015). Interdisciplinary and cross-cultural perspectives on explanatory coexistence. *Topics in Cognitive Science, 7,* 611–623.

Watson-Jones, R. E., Busch, J. T. A., Harris, P. L., & Legare, C. H. (2017). Does the body survive death? Cultural variation in beliefs about life everlasting. *Cognitive Science, 41,* 455–476.

Weary, G., & Jacobson, J. A. (1997). Causal uncertainty beliefs and diagnostic information seeking. *Journal of Personality and Social Psychology, 73,* 839–848.

Weary, G., Jacobson, J. A., Edwards, J. A., & Tobin, S. J. (2001). Chronic and temporarily activated causal uncertainty beliefs and stereotype usage. *Journal of Personality and Social Psychology, 81,* 206–219.

White, C. (2021). *An introduction to the cognitive science of religion: Connecting evolution, brain, cognition, and culture.* London: Routledge.

Whitehouse, H. (2004). *Modes of religiosity: A cognitive theory of religious transmission.* Walnut Creek, CA: AltaMira Press.

Whitehouse, H., & Lanman, J. A. (2014). The ties that bind us. *Current Anthropology, 55*(6), 674–695.

Whitson, J., & Galinsky, A. (2008). Lacking control increases illusory pattern perception. *Science, 322,* 115–117.

Womack, M. (1992). Why athletes need ritual: A study of magic among professional athletes. In S. Hoffman (Ed.), *Sport and Religion* (pp. 191–202). Champaign, IL: Human Kinetics.

Zajonc, R. (1968). Attitudinal effects of mere exposure. *Journal of Personality and Social Psychology Monographs, 9,* 1–27.

CHAPTER 9

MORTUARY PRACTICES

CLAIRE WHITE

INTRODUCTION

MORTUARY practices are ubiquitous features of human cultural traditions, and it is unlikely that they all derive from a single case of cultural innovation. The cross-cultural recurrence in mortuary practices, then, is a paradigmatic case of the sorts of religious cultural expressions that the cognitive science of religion has sought to explain. This chapter demonstrates why this approach is valuable.

Even early modern humans in the Paleolithic era did not merely discard their dead but deliberately buried them deep in the ground and manipulated their bodies into certain positions, accompanied by flowers, tools, and other artifacts (Brown, 1971).[1] The ethnographic record evidences the dazzling array of conventional practices that are undertaken when a community member dies. This variety is apparent in the treatment of the corpse before disposal. Corpses are washed, embalmed, anointed, pickled, dismantled, painted, adorned with jewelry, clothed, wrapped, placed in a container, moved, viewed extensively, touched, embraced, wept over, shouted at, danced over, and force-fed food, among other practices. There are also expectations concerning the mourners' appearance, behavior, and place of dwelling. These include taboos about speaking the name of the deceased; rules about shaving the mourners' heads and requirements to wear only one color of clothing, cover the mirrors or windows in the home, display flowers and other decorations outside the home, and sit on small, uncomfortable chairs. These practices can take place over days, weeks, months, or even years, typically whenever the socially delineated mourning period is over. The disposal of the body is often accompanied by a communal ceremony involving specialists, such as religious and other ritual experts, and members of the community. These ceremonies often

---

[1] This is most likely from the Upper Paleolithic era. Claims that there was deliberate burial among Neanderthals, especially that they were buried with flowers, are contested (Dibble et al., 2015).

include feasts, games, dancing, and the consumption of alcohol. How can we use evolutionary and cognitive perspectives to explain these behaviors? What function, if any, do these mortuary practices serve such that they have acquired the features that they have? Are some ways of engaging with the dead catchier to human cognitive systems?

Anthropologists have long documented rich accounts of mortuary practices, attending to particular culture regions and highlighting their striking features (e.g., Eisenbruch, 1984; Hertz, 1960; Metcalf & Huntington, 1979). They have explained the peripheral and variable aspects of these practices in terms of the meanings they hold for people. Classical theories contend that mortuary practices are a product of shared ideas about the self, the process of death, the identity of the dead in the afterlife, and the identity of the living—elements, it is claimed, that are all intrinsically related—and the researcher aims to decode such meanings (e.g., Bloch & Parry, 1982; Hertz, 1960; Metcalf & Huntington, 1979; van Gennep, 1960). However, there is inconsistent evidence for the relationship between particular afterlife beliefs, such as belief in a parallel land of the dead in another sphere of existence, and specific kinds of mortuary practices, such as double burials, placing grave goods with the dead, or the washing of the corpse before burial (e.g., Binford, 1971; Carr, 1995; Ucko, 1969). Although mortuary practices are highly regulated, they are functionally opaque; that is to say, there is no obvious physical-causal relationship between the actions and the goal. Unlike with most day-to-day actions, the causal efficacy of each step is unclear and, in terms of strict function, undermotivated.

Consequently, many mortuary practices can be more precisely characterized as mortuary rituals (Legare & Herrmann, 2013). And as with many other rituals, people's exegesis for actions following a death is often vague, circular, question-begging, mystery ridden, and highly idiosyncratic (Bloch, 1974; Boyer, 2001). Like most collective rituals, they do not convey coded meanings, except in the vaguest sense (Sperber, 1975).

Other explanations about why people perform mortuary rituals have looked beyond the details of local belief systems to account for their recurrence throughout history and across cultures. Anthropological and sociological researchers assert that mortuary rituals confer tangible benefits on the social group. Importantly, these benefits exceed their costs, which helps to explain why people engage in such time-consuming, elaborate, and often expensive practices. Postulated benefits include controlling the fear of mortality the sight of the corpse induces, reaffirming the social order (including through practicalities such as the redistribution of goods), reinforcing core group values, and redefining social relationships at a time of social uncertainty and change (e.g., Bloch & Parry, 1982; Durkheim, 1995; Goody, 1962; Hertz, 1960; Hunter, 2008; Malinowski, 1948; van Gennep, 1960). However, the evidence for these functionalist theories is almost exclusively observational. They primarily depend on ethnographic case studies, and the mechanisms that drive these effects are underspecified. Hence, such theories lack explanatory power.

However, recent research from a variety of evolutionary and cognitive sciences has provided fresh insight into the functions of mortuary practices. This chapter draws upon systematic cross-cultural comparisons of mortuary practices to demonstrate that they share core features that are not amenable to parochial explanations. Mortuary rituals are highly regulated, functionally opaque, and elaborate sets of behaviors that result in close and prolonged contact with the deceased and the social group. Viewed from a cultural-selection framework, these recurrent features reflect the winners in a constant process of generating and selecting new variants (Boyd & Richerson, 1985; Sperber, 1985), arguably, on the basis their particular fit with human cognition, as well as the functional outcomes. Based on research findings from adjacent social science disciplines, the case can be made that mortuary rituals aid in solving adaptive problems following the death of a group member.

The death of a group member threatens the stability of the social group and the adaptive benefits of social-group living (see Legare & Watson-Jones, 2015, for an overview of how rituals solve the adaptive problems of group living). Most obviously, death entails the loss of a group member, and of the benefits that particular individual brought to the group. Yet the potential impact of social loss extends well beyond the death of the individual. Other members of the group, especially the kin of the dead, are likely to withdraw at least temporarily from the daily activities of group living, which may have proven fatal to the small ancestral groups of our evolutionary past. Seeking out replacement relationships and increasing group membership—such as finding a new reproductive partner or bearing another child—may buffer the loss, but the bereaved are unlikely to be motivated to engage in behaviors associated with these outcomes until the intense negative symptoms of loss subside.

Mortuary rituals shorten and regulate the period of grief-induced disability suffered by the bereaved, enabling them to regain feelings of control in the face of threat and providing them with opportunities for form replacement relationships. They also serve important functions for the social group more generally. Following the death of a member of the community, people engage in coordinated high-risk behaviors and actions that test and strengthen their commitment to the group, and help maintain group cohesion during a period of social change. An examination of how mortuary practices are culturally transmitted will follow an outline of this theory. The existing research on ritualized behavior and cultural rituals, in general, has demonstrated that mortuary rituals are easily acquired and enjoy high-fidelity cultural transmission over time. As culturally learned practices that harness the human psychological preparedness to perform them, rituals often appear when danger is imminent, and uncertainty is high.

The ritualized structure of mortuary rituals, cultural discourse regarding negative consequences from supernatural agents, and reputational damage if rituals are not performed correctly result in orthopraxy. Intergroup competition and, in particular, the emulation of funerary practices associated with the death of high-status group members, may well have facilitated the spread of elaborate and costly funerary practices. A cognitive and functional approach to the study of mortuary rituals offers compelling explanations concerning how and why people perform them. It specifies the psychological and social mechanisms through which such behaviors emerge and are reproduced and transmitted over time. Such accounts generate testable predictions and yield valuable data, reinforcing and extending many traditional functionalist accounts of mortuary rituals.

The Functions of Mortuary Rituals

One function of mortuary rituals is that they shorten and regulate the period of grief-induced disability. The death of a valued relationship partner is a universal human experience. Although societal norms largely determine its expression, the human experience following bereavement is remarkably similar across cultures. It is characterized by a plethora of cognitive-emotional symptoms, including an extreme preoccupation with thoughts about the deceased, yearning for the deceased, rumination, and intense sadness (Cowles, 1996; Freed et al., 2009; Rosenblatt et al., 1976). These symptoms are among the most stressful experiences predictably undergone by humans, and they are also likely to be detrimental to biological fitness and can include an increased risk of mortality for the bereaved (Holmes & Rahe, 1967; Irwin & Weiner, 1987; Shuchter & Zisook, 1987; Stroebe et al., 2007). The death of an individual also significantly impacts the social group, and in the environment of evolutionary adaptation, which was characterized by small groups, may have been detrimental. When people experience grief, it is often in the context of having lost reproductive and social resources via offspring or sexual partners and the valuable social resource of having a relationship with someone whom they trust and who trusts and cooperates with them. In addition, until their negative symptoms subside, the mourner is unable to participate in the demands of group living and unlikely to engage in the pursuit of replacement relationships.

Employing cross-cultural comparison, Rosenblatt et al. (1976) found a positive association between the absence of a final ceremony and the presence of prolonged grief, measured by reports of disrupted work, troubled dreams, suicidal behavior, deviations from societal norms, and illness. This finding suggests that a functional consequence of mourning rituals is reduction of the duration of the suffering and pragmatic impairment caused by grief, an outcome that benefits the bereaved by reducing their suffering and hastening their return to productive social life, and thus the group as well. This observation raises questions about the mechanisms through which these effects are achieved. My colleagues and I have proposed that one mechanism is corpse interaction (White & Fessler, 2018; White et al., 2017). Mortuary rituals that include close and prolonged physical contact with the corpse, such as washing and dressing them, serve the compelling need to recognize the deceased person and cognitively register him or her as dead. This process has additional functional benefits, as well. The facilitation of seeing and touching the corpse in mortuary rituals plausibly aids the bereaved in the long run by diminishing the duration of grief and accelerating the recruitment of a replacement individual. In turn, the group benefits from these outcomes, gaining competitive advantage by shortening and regulating the period of grief-induced disability suffered by their members and expediting the re-formation of social bonds.

One line of support for this claim comes from a series of studies that systematically compared archival ethnographic records on the mortuary rituals of 57 representative cultures from around the globe (the Probability Sample Files [PSF]), as documented in the ethnographic database the Human Relations Area Files (HRAF), a sizeable indexed collection of anthropological writings on the world's cultural traditions (White et al., 2017). This research overwhelmingly concluded that the vast majority of mortuary rituals included visual exposure of the corpse to the participants (93%). Historically, 84% of cultures practice prolonged exposure to the corpse in a familiar dwelling place (e.g., the deceased's home), keeping the deceased for up to two weeks before disposal. Furthermore, in most mortuary rituals (90%), participants have physical contact with the corpse, most of which involves moderately intimate practices (82%), such as washing or dressing the corpse prior to disposal, compared to rituals that included low intimate contact (10%), such as briefly touching the corpse, or highly intimate contact (8%), characterized by inner body contact (i.e., penetration of natural orifices, cutting through the flesh, dismantling the corpse).

The most reliable cue that the individual is dead is, of course, the corpse. It is unsurprising that recently bereaved individuals experience a compelling desire to see the corpse and engage in contact with it, even in societies where traditional doctrines explicitly prohibit it (see McCorkle, 2010, for the case of Buddhism). Given how important social relationship are and how much effort people generally put into maintaining them, people have a (generally unconscious) skepticism regarding the death of the deceased, so that, for example, the absence of cues of agency only weakly triggers death inferences (Barrett & Behne, 2005). This disbelief is combined with the continued emotional attachment and fulfillment of social obligations toward the deceased. These are evidenced by spontaneous behaviors such as embracing and kissing the deceased loved one . In more structured mortuary rituals in which kin prepare the deceased for burial, they often engage in practices such as washing and dressing the corpse, cutting the hair and fingernails, combing the hair, rubbing the body with soap, and others (White et al., 2017).

As scholars have noted, humans are not well equipped to stop thinking about the dead person as around, even if they know on a propositional level that the person is dead (Bering, 2006; Boyer, 2001). Yet the efficiency of cognitive recategorization of the person from living to dead may well depend on the type of exposure the bereaved receive. For instance, in a series of studies with recently bereaved pet owners who had been highly attached to their pets (using pet loss as a proxy for human loss), White et al. (2016) found that seeing a non-intact corpse that exhibited reliable cues of death, such as grievous injuries or extensive disruptions to the body envelope, was associated with lower vigilance for the agent—measured by the extent to which the bereaved thought they heard or saw the deceased, even momentarily. In contrast, merely seeing a lifelike intact corpse was not. Seeing and touching a lifelike but immobile corpse of a loved one over a prolonged time may be sufficient to prompt the viewer to switch from representing the given other as a living relationship partner to representing that individual as dead.

Correspondingly, it is now generally accepted in the clinical literature that although viewing the body of a loved one may increase anxiety and distress in the short term, it is better in the long-term. Outcomes are better for those who view and even touch the body of a loved one, and doing so is thought to help people come to terms with the death (Chapple & Ziebland, 2010; Haas, 2003; Hinton, 1967; Jolly, 1987; Raphael, 1983; Wertheimer, 1991; Wright, 1991). Conversely, not seeing the body (such as in cases when the body cannot be recovered) is associated with more challenging, prolonged grief (Hodgkinson & Stewart, 1991; Kübler-Ross, 1983). Congruent phylogenetic evidence also supports this interpretation. Rudimentary urges to engage in tactile contact with a corpse are found in social birds and mammals, and naturalistic observations often report mothers carrying their dead infants, probing them, and allowing other group members to manipulate the carcass before finally abandoning it (e.g., see Archer 2001; Cronin et al., 2011). These considerations shed light on the patterns evident in White et al.'s (2017) findings, helping to explain why practices that include the close and prolonged contact with the deceased are the most widespread because the visual and tactile contact maximizes cues of death.

Other mortuary conventions beyond interacting with the corpse may also shorten the period of grief-induced disability suffered by group members. Consider that most societies have mores that remove cues of the recently deceased from the immediate environment. For example, in another study using ethnographic databases and representative cultures, Rosenblatt et al. (1976) reported that, of the 78 cultures surveyed, 91% prescribed the immediate destruction of the deceased's property; 81% stipulated the abandonment of the deceased's residence; and 59% taboo mentioning the deceased's name for the close kin and local community. Empirical research supports the theory that environmental cues may hinder the recategorization of the deceased from living to deceased. In another series of studies with pet owners, White and Fessler (2013) found that frequently visiting photographs of the deceased depicting them alive predicted increased vigilance toward cues that the deceased was in the immediate environment. Similarly, Rosenblatt et al. also found a strong positive correlation (8.0) between the practice of immediately destroying the deceased's property and high marriage rates, suggesting that the former may facilitate the rapid establishment of replacement relationships.

Regain Feelings of Control in the Face of Threat

There appear to be some consistent features in mortuary practices involving the corpse. People engage in highly regulated, functionally opaque, and elaborate sets of behaviors with the deceased. For example, White et al. (2017) found that interaction with the corpse was characterized as structured and ritualized in the majority of cultures, as opposed to being spontaneous and idiosyncratic. Typically, people do not explain to anthropologists why they perform rituals in a specific manner (i.e., washing their hands three times, walking counter-clockwise around the corpse), yet they perform them with painstaking accuracy. Anthropological insights and psychological research suggest that performing scripted behaviors may be an automatic and compensatory strategy to provide the social group with a regained feeling of control over the uncertainty of death through the association between actions and outcomes.

Corpses elicit two sources of perceived threat. First, they elicit psychological distress. One source of this distress is disgust at the sight of the decaying corpse. The strength of this reaction is likely tempered by the social closeness of the bereaved to the deceased, since feelings of disgust differ depending on the source of the disgusting material. That is, disgusting stimuli that emanate from oneself and familiar others elicit less disgust than those which come from strangers (the "source effect"; see Peng et al., 2013; McCorkle, 2010). Even a moderated disgust reaction, however, can generate ambivalence in the bereaved—they want to see the body in order to "believe" that the person is actually deceased, but simultaneously experience distress at the prospect of seeing the corpse (e.g., Boyer, 2001; Davies, 2005). Correspondingly, anthropologists have reported that the bereaved both fear and love the recently deceased corpse (e.g., Freud, 1960; Bloch & Parry, 1982; Hertz, 1960; Opler, 1936; van Gennep, 1960).

Second, physical contact with a corpse poses a health risk, especially when disease prevalence is high. Direct, nonintimate physical contact is a significant means through which a large proportion of infectious diseases are spread (e.g., Healing et al., 1995; Salathé et al., 2010; Taylor et al., 2001), and contact with human cadavers in the immediate postmortem period carries risk for the transmission of certain blood-borne and gastrointestinal pathogens (e.g., Morgan, 2004); these dangers would be heightened with invasive corpse procedures. Indeed, highly intimate mortuary rituals that reprocess or destroy the corpse (e.g., dismemberment, mummification) or involve any form of cannibalism are quite rare, comprising less than 10% of the sample in White et al.'s (2017) study. Although these practices have the advantage of entailing additional exposure to death cues that could facilitate reclassifying the deceased as dead, it is probably a case of diminishing returns—the experience of manipulating a cold, unresponsive, and immobile corpse, which may be in a state rigor mortis or emitting odors of putrefaction, would likely provide conclusive evidence of death, but the information provided by, say, dismemberment would be largely superfluous.

The ritualized behavioral patterns in mortuary practices plausibly reduce the anxiety associated with ambivalence about seeing corpses and the uncertainty of death. As mentioned in the chapter introduction, Malinowski (1948) observed that the extent to which Trobriand fishermen engaged in rituals was associated with the unpredictability of the terrain. When fishing in turbulent, shark-infested waters, they performed rituals for their safety and protection. By contrast, when they fished in the calm waters of a lagoon, they did not perform rituals. Malinowski asserted that rituals functioned to relieve people's anxiety over uncertainty when the outcome was important and beyond human control (Malinowski, 1948). His work remains a cornerstone of the anxiety-reduction explanation of ritual behavior. As was also mentioned in the introduction, scholars have asserted that rituals performed after the death of a member of the social group serve similar functions (e.g., Bloch & Parry, 1982; Durkheim, 1995; Goody, 1962; Hertz, 11960; Hunter, 2008; van Gennep, 1960). Yet until relatively recently, quantitative evidence for these conjectures was scarce. Now research has begun to emerge to support these claims. For instance, the extent to which athletes and fishermen engage in rituals is related to the unpredictability and danger of their jobs (Gmlech, 1971; Malinowski, 1948; Whitson & Galinsky, 2008). In another series of studies, Norton and Gino (2013) found that participating in a set of ritualized behaviors after writing about the death of a loved one, increased participants' feelings of control and lessened their reported feelings of grief, whereas sitting in silence did not.

Boyer and Liénard (2006) have provided an explanation of the psychological mechanisms that produce these anxiety-reducing effects. They proposed a model in which perceived threats, such as psychological distress and contamination risks of being near corpses, are thought to activate mental security systems, resulting in security-related behavior. Specifically, they argue that ritualized behavior emerges spontaneously because it triggers an evolved "Hazard Precaution System" that is geared toward the detection of and reaction to inferred fitness threats, which lowers anxiety by subjectively containing it through scripted action. Participants focus on the action they are performing, not on the goal of each behavior, and this focus swamps working memory. In other words, attention is readily deployed toward concern with performing the actions correctly, precluding atomized performance. Performing these behaviors eliminates unwanted thoughts, at least temporarily, and so they are repeated, repeatedly. Experimental work supports this theory. For instance, during a ritual that involved cleaning an object, Lang et al. (2015) found that participants' anxiety significantly predicted the number of movements they made and the time they spent cleaning. Lang et al. explained these findings in light of the anxiety-reduction model of ritual. Specifically, to cope with uncertainty, participants adopted familiar and predictable behavioral sequences and performed them repetitively to gain a sense of regularity and control over the situation. On these accounts, regulated corpse interaction results in regained feelings of control or the containment of anxiety in the face of potential hazards (e.g., Boyer & Liénard, 2006).

Identifying Group Members, Demonstrating Commitment to the Group, and Facilitating the Formation of New Social Bonds

White et al. (2017) found that almost every culture they surveyed officially marked the death of a community member with a public ceremony. These ceremonies often included key members of the community, but which members, and why? Atkinson & Whitehouse's (2011) analysis of data from the Human Relations Area Files based on a representative subset of mortuary rituals in 39 cultures provides an answer to this question. A minority of public ceremonies in their sample included only immediate kin or the extended kin group. A few cultures included all or most members of the community, and even fewer cultures included members of other communities in their ceremonies. Thus, funerals seem to function to serve members of the extended social group. By attending a funerary ceremony, people are doing more than simply "paying their respects" to the deceased. They are demonstrating their continued commitment to shared beliefs and behaviors, a mark of cooperation and trustworthiness at a time of social change and potential social instability (Cosmides & Tooby, 2013; McElreath et al., 2003). But what about cultures where the size of the extended group is well beyond 150 people, the approximate number that can be tracked in a social group (Dunbar, 1992)? In these contexts, people often freely participate in funerals of those they did not personally know, such as public funerals for monarchs, public figures, religious leaders, and those killed through war or acts of terrorism. Their behavior also signals group affiliation to the extended social group.

In terms of their social functions, another vital question concerns what happens during mortuary practices prior to disposal, and during public ceremonies? Crucially, mortuary rituals enable people to act in ways that elicit resources and provide the opportunity for people to demonstrate their commitment to the group. They also enable the bereaved to formulate new social bonds, and even to find potential replacement relationships. Rosenblatt et al. (1976) recorded public displays of emotion by the bereaved in almost all of the cultures surveyed. Public displays of grief by the bereaved signal distress, which serves to elicit resources from locals at a time when they are needed most. Grief and mourning behaviors are often costly and prolonged and can be detrimental to physical and psychological well-being. The deceased cannot repay these costs, and it may therefore seem that they are wasted expenditures. Yet the fact that such acts of devotion cannot be repaid means that the behavior acts as an honest indicator of the commitment to the deceased and signals the ability of the bereaved person to form strong bonds with others more generally (Winegard et al., 2014). As a consequence, people are more likely to judge those who display sadness at a funeral as reliable and trustworthy relationship partners (Reynolds et al., 2015).

Experiencing emotion in a group context is likely to provide more psychological benefits than grieving alone. Research has shown that affiliation and affiliate behavior buffer and moderate stress in loss and correlate positively with return to a healthy and stable psychological state 13 months after bereavement (Cobb, 1976; Parkes & Prigerson, 2013). These emotional expressions are also likely to elicit support and resources from the community, such as companionship, food, and help with childcare. Additionally, the experience of shared physiological states and the signaled support from key members of the community through ritual participation also serves to enhance social cohesion at a time of social uncertainty (Norton & Gino, 2013; Xygalatas et al., 2011), especially for high-ordeal rituals—such as those that cause pain or fear—that entail excessive costs (Xygalatas et al., 2013).

The benefits of participation are especially evident for the community members who handle the contaminating corpse. By putting time and energy into a proper burial, they are effectively communicating their commitment to the deceased and to the broader social group, their cooperative intentions, and thus their trustworthiness as social partners (e.g., see Nesse, 2005; Purzycki & Sosis, 2009; Reynolds et al., 2015; Winegard et al., 2014). The effects are heightened given the potential costs of corpse interaction, including the actual and perceived risks of handling the dead body, a debt that cannot be repaid by the deceased. Clearly, performing the duties oneself signals the willingness to engage in potentially hazardous behaviors for the benefit of the deceased. Thus, even when ritual specialists became widely available, most preparation was still carried out by the bereaved themselves, who are likely to reap the rewards (see Laderman, 1996; Parkes et al., 2003; Walter, 2005). Further, people also engage in close and prolonged contact with the corpse across cultures, even when the prevalence of disease is high (Murray et al., 2017). The extent to which fulfilling their duties to provide a "proper burial" for the deceased is thus a form of "costly signaling," an elaborate show of group commitment, performed not despite their costs but because of them (Sosis, 2004).

Acquisition and Cultural Transmission of Mortuary Practices

High-Fidelity Transmission of Functionally Opaque Behaviors

Mortuary practices are functionally opaque, culturally learned, and reproduced. As Boyer and Liénard (2006) propose, they are compelling and readily emerge in the face of perceived threat. As we have seen, thoughts about the contamination of the corpse are likely to trigger hazard-precaution systems and corresponding behaviors, such as washing and cleansing the corpse and ritual participants. These behaviors then become part of a series of prescribed behaviors surrounding the corpse. Themes of cleanliness and washing, involving the practice washing both the corpse and the corpse handlers before the burial, are especially common to funerary practices. In many ceremonies, the central theme is the pollution of the corpse and danger of contamination, which can only be prevented by extensive washing (e.g., see Boyer, 2001, p. 213).

How are these complex ritual behaviors culturally transmitted if they do not follow common-sense causal reasoning? Research in the developmental and cognitive sciences has demonstrated that even young children are well equipped to adopt behaviors when there is an arbitrary relationship between actions and stated goals. Consider, for example, studies by Csibra and Gergely (2009). When infants observed an adult switching on a light by pressing the button with her head, not her hand, and the action was communicated as though it were a ritual, they imitated it. Contrariwise, when the same action was repeated but presented as peculiar but functional, because the adult's hands were tied or they were otherwise unable to press the button, the infants used their hands to switch on the light, presumably because it was a more efficient means (pressing with the hand) to achieve the end goal (switching on the light). These and other findings suggest that children are attuned to faithfully imitate behaviors when they are part of a conventional ritual and the proper way of doing something, if not the most expedient.

In fact, research with children and adults by Legare and colleagues has demonstrated that the combination of causal opacity and social stipulation actually inhibits individual-level innovation, which leads to high-fidelity cultural transmission over time (Legare & Nielsen, 2015; Legare & Watson-Jones, 2015; Legare et al., 2015). As Legare and colleagues have argued, from an evolutionary perspective, given the variability and limitations of personal experience and intuition and the cognitive effort required to infer intentions and goals, natural selection ought to favor a social learning strategy of high-fidelity imitation of ritualized behaviors. This is especially likely when there is uncertainty in the environment, including potential hazards, and prestigious individuals (those with long-standing reputations as trustworthy and/or leaders or, for children, adults) are performing the actions (Richerson & Boyd, 2005; Henrich & Gil-White, 2001). Mortuary practices with corpses are elaborate and time-consuming and act as credibility-enhancing demonstrations for those performing them, which provides salient behavioral displays of fidelity and fosters the cultural transmission of commitment to others (Henrich, 2009). The adoption of such behaviors is also made likely through the risk of social ostracism for not conforming (Legare et al., 2015). Throughout evolutionary history, social ostracism was akin to a death sentence (e.g., see Gruter & Masters, 1984), and social affiliation and one's reputation are likely one of the most motivating forces explaining the participation in cultural rituals today. One only has to imagine the negative and potentially detrimental reputational consequences for a member of the community who refused to participate in funerary customs. In modern-day America, consider the hypothetical example of reactions to a father who refused to help carry his adolescent son's coffin on his shoulder because it was uncomfortable. One mechanism that motivates and sustains orthopraxy, especially in traditional cultures, is fear of the recently deceased—and particularly, fear of supernatural harm from the noncorporeal aspect of the person that survives biological death (e.g., spirit, ghost, ancestor). Anthropologists have painstakingly documented such beliefs (e.g., Bloch & Parry, 1982; Frazer's tome, 1966; Hertz, 1960; Opler, 1936; Rosenblatt et al., 1976), and many have argued for this interpretation (e.g., Bellah, 2011; Boyer, 2001), but until recently, there was little systematic cross-cultural support for these claims. However, White et al. (in preparation) have found evidence for the perceived relationship between fear of supernatural punishment by the recently deceased and mortuary practices cross-culturally, using a representative sample of 57 cultures in the Human Relations Area Files. Their findings suggest that representations give rise to particularly fearsome concepts of supernatural agents that logically reinforce ritualized mortuary practices. In particular, the recently deceased are represented as self-interested and motivated to harm those who do not give them what they want and, most importantly, as having the power to harm the living through a number of domains, such as biological illness or psychological torment. Further, the reasons supernatural agents will do harm is represented in the ethnographic literature as predictable in the majority of cultures, but when and how they will do such harm is not predictable. This combination is likely to give rise to orthopraxy in mortuary rituals (to ensure that the agents do not harm) and to provide the conditions for fear-based protective behaviors to spread widely and efficiently.

For these reasons, people believe that they are capable of protecting themselves from supernatural agents' harm. They can do so in a number of ways, the most common of which is following the correct ritualized practices. Such practices have two aims. The first is to limit the spirit's agency, for example, by binding the corpse before burial so that it cannot move or harm them. The second is to appease them by, for example, rubbing substances on the corpse or placing food items beside them. As anthropologists have long noted, the event of biological death moves people from the category of ordinary to extraordinary in the minds of others. Given that the recently deceased are believed to be powerful, exerting influence on the physical and biological health and even the personal events of the living, it is understandable that we find few instances of people trying to trick the deceased out of harming them. These findings add to a body of research in the cognitive science of religion suggesting that fear of supernatural punishment from these moralistic agents who are both willing and able to inflict punishment effectively modifies human behavior in ways that promote group cooperation, thereby perpetuating such beliefs (e.g., Boyer, 2001; Johnson, 2016; Shariff & Norenzayan, 2007; Purzycki, 2013). Fear of punishment from the recently deceased may also suppress cheating in individuals who would not otherwise perform mortuary practices, reducing the number of defectors within a group, which then bolsters cooperation (Johnson & Krüger, 2004; Bering & Johnson, 2005; Schloss & Murray, 2011).

Although there is a paucity of archaeological and ethnographic records, some general patterns have been observed that suggest that sociocultural mechanisms may also explain how these mortuary behaviors became widespread.

Prestige Bias, Cultural Learning, Intergroup Competition, and Social Display

Ever since deliberate burial emerged among early modern humans, as early as 300,000 years ago, it has been the case that when corpse preparation was adopted into a culture, it was selectively employed. Archaeological evidence strongly suggests that the elaborate treatment of corpses was initially reserved for high-status individuals and the wealthy (see Peebles, 1971). Reserving the extravagant treatment of the deceased for the rich and those who occupied important social roles persisted cross-culturally in modern humans (see Brown, 1971; Earle, 1987). Comparative historical analyses of mortuary behaviors in different cultures have shown that cultural learning and intergroup competition facilitated the spread of these practices. Whereas increased affluence made the initial elaboration of mortuary practices possible, it was inter-group conflict that made them widespread in many contexts (e.g., Cannon, 1989; Chapman et al., 1981; Parkes et al., 2003). But even though in many cultures, elaborate burials (including complicated corpse preparation, such as adornment) were initially reserved for wealthy and high-status individuals, lower-status group members—likely guided by the psychological tendency to learn from prestigious individuals, to whom others preferentially attended (Henrich & Gil-White, 2001)—emulated them, even if it meant neglecting their own well-being to ensure provision for burial funds. Perhaps a group member's death provided lower-status groups with an opportunity for social advancement by using funerary practices as a form of social display of their equality with higher status groups. This led to continued innovation among the high-status groups because their previous ostentatious mortuary practices ceased to be a mark of high-status distinction (Cannon, 1989; Morley, 1971). Thus, corpse preparation and adornment serves important functions, not only by showcasing and strengthening the commitment of people within groups, but also between groups.

CONCLUSION

Recent quantitative research demonstrates cross-cultural regularities in mortuary rituals. These recurrent features are demonstrated by taking account of the selection pressures incurred by the death of a group member. Specifically, cultural evolution has favored the development of practices that stipulate interaction with the corpse and participation in public ceremonies. These practices provide the bereaved with efficacious cues of death, which shortens and regulates the period of grief-induced disability and facilitates engagement in replacement social relationships while also enabling group members to demonstrate their value as social partners, and displaying a commitment to the group at a time of potential vulnerability. Orthopraxy and the high-fidelity transmission of mortuary practices over time result from the nature of ritualized behavior itself, the context of perceived imminent danger, cultural discourse regarding negative consequences from supernatural agents, and the actual reputational consequences of nonconformity. Archaeological and historical evidence also suggests that the social aspirations of lower-status groups contributed to the initial spread of these elaborate corpse practices.

A number of important questions remain. The broadest line of inquiry aims at pinpointing the relationship between the various psychological mechanisms and cultural-learning biases that have been proposed to account for mortuary practices. As has been suggested throughout the chapter, it may well be that the most common mortuary practices were once part of a larger repertoire of behaviors following death, but few variants became culturally widespread because of their lack of adaptive benefits for the individual and the social group. Another related line of inquiry concerns the potential relationship between the assortment of cognitive foundations and cultural-learning biases underpinning the cross-cultural success of mortuary practices. In other words, do some psychological mechanisms give rise to particular behaviors that then have implications for the social group? Consider the following example: Bodies trigger hazard-precaution systems that result in repetitive and redundant behaviors aimed at reducing the contamination of the corpse by cleaning and preparing it. One unforeseen consequence of these high-risk behaviors is that they signal a commitment to the deceased, and therefore to the social group, at a time of social change. There are, of course, many potential relationships between the cognitive and cultural components of mortuary practices, and future research could first propose and then test the plausibility of each configuration by drawing from experimental studies and the historical and contemporary record.

Although this chapter has focused mainly on the cross-cultural regularities of mortuary practices, there is equal merit in revisiting classic anthropological questions concerning cultural variations with a new empirical tool-kit. For example, how do environmental contexts shape the expression of mortuary practices? Moreover, what is the relationship between beliefs about the deceased and the afterlife and the evolution of mortuary practices? Systematic analyses of the ethnographic and historical record could yield more precise answers to these age-old questions and complement existing research findings on the cognitive constraints of cultural forms. Indeed, future research in the evolutionary, cognitive, and social sciences is likely to lead to a more precise understanding of the psychological and sociocultural mechanisms through which mortuary rituals are acquired and transmitted. So far, at least, we can say with a degree of certainty that mortuary rituals are not for the dead but, rather, serve the living.

Questions for Future Research

1. What is the precise relationship between the various psychological mechanisms and cultural learning biases proposed to account for mortuary practices?
2. How do the environmental contexts within which mortuary practices occur shape their expression?
3. What is the relationship between beliefs about the deceased, the afterlife, and the evolution of mortuary practices?

References

Archer, J. (2001). Grief from an evolutionary perspective. In M. S. Stroebe, R. O. Hansson, W. Stroebe, & H. Schut (Eds.), *Handbook of bereavement research: Consequences, coping, and care* (pp. 263–283). Washington, DC: American Psychological Association.

Atkinson, Q. D., & Whitehouse, H. (2011). The cultural morphospace of ritual form: Examining modes of religiosity cross-culturally. *Evolution and Human Behavior, 32*, 50–62.

Barrett, H. C., & Behne, T. (2005). Children's understanding of death as the cessation of agency: A test using sleep versus death. *Cognition, 96*(2), 93–108.

Bellah, R. N. (2011). *Religion in human evolution*. Cambridge, MA: Harvard University Press.

Bering, J. M. (2006). The cognitive science of souls: Clarifications and extensions of the evolutionary model. *Behavioral and Brain Sciences, 29*(5), 486–493.

Bering, J. M., & Johnson, D. D. P. (2005). "O Lord . . . You perceive my thoughts from afar": Recursiveness and the evolution of supernatural agency. *Journal of Cognition and Culture*, 5(1), 118–142.

Binford, L. R. (1971). Mortuary practices: Their study and their potential. *Memoirs of the Society for American Archaeology*, 25, 6–29.

Bloch, M. (1974). Symbols, song, dance and features of articulation: Is religion an extreme form of traditional authority? *European Journal of Sociology/Archives Européennes de Sociologie*, 15(1), 54–81.

Bloch, M., & Parry, J. (1982). (Eds.). *Death and the regeneration of life*. Cambridge, UK: Cambridge University Press.

Boyd, R., & Richerson, P. J. (1985). *Culture and the evolutionary process*. Chicago: University of Chicago Press.

Boyer, P. (2001). *Religion explained: The evolutionary origins of religious thought*. New York: Basic Books.

Boyer, P., & Liénard, P. (2006). Precaution systems and ritualized behavior. *Behavioral and Brain Sciences*, 29(6), 635–641.

Brown, J. A. (Ed.). (1971). *Approaches to the social dimensions of mortuary practices*. Washington, DC: Society for American Archaeology.

Cannon, A. (1989). The historical dimension in mortuary expressions of status and sentiment. *Current Anthropology*, 30(4), 437–458. Retrieved from http://www.clas.ufl.edu/users/davidson/Arch%20of%20Death/Week%2013/Aubrey%20Cannon%201989.pdf

Carr, C. (1995). Mortuary practices: Their social, philosophical-religious, circumstantial, and physical determinants. *Journal of Archaeological Method and Theory*, 2(2), 105–200.

Chapman, R., Kinnes, I., & Randsborg, K. (Eds.). (1981). *The archaeology of death*. Cambridge, UK: Cambridge University Press.

Chapple, A., & Ziebland, S. (2010). Viewing the body after bereavement due to a traumatic death: Qualitative study in the UK. *BMJ*, *340*, c2032.

Cobb, Si. (1976). Social support as a moderator of life stress. *Psychosomatic Medicine*, 38(5), 300–314.

Cosmides, L., & Tooby, J. (2013). Evolutionary psychology: New perspectives on cognition and motivation. *Annual Review of Psychology*, 64, 201–229.

Cowles, K. V. (1996). Cultural perspectives of grief: An expanded concept analysis. *Journal of Advanced Nursing*, 23(2), 287–294.

Cronin, K. A., Van Leeuwen, E. J. C., Mulenga, I. C., & Bodamer, M. D. (2011). Behavioral response of a chimpanzee mother toward her dead infant. *American Journal of Primatology*, 73(5), 415–421.

Csibra, G., & Gergely, G. (2009). Natural pedagogy. *Trends in Cognitive Sciences*, 13(4), 148–153.

Davies, R. (2005). Mothers' stories of loss: Their need to be with their dying child and their child's body after death. *Journal of Child Health Care*, 9(4), 288–300.

Dibble, H. L., Aldeias, V., Goldberg, P., McPherron, S. P., Sandgathe, D., & Steele, T. E. (2015). A critical look at evidence from La Chapelle-aux-Saints supporting an intentional Neandertal burial. *Journal of Archaeological Science*, *53*, 649–657.

Dunbar, R. I. M. (1992). Neocortex size as a constraint on group size in primates. *Journal of Human Evolution*, 22(6), 469–493.

Durkheim, É. (1995). *The elementary forms of religious life*. New York: Free Press. (Original work published in France in 1912).

Earle, T. K. (1987). Chiefdoms in archaeological and ethnohistorical perspective. *Annual Review of Anthropology, 16*(1), 279–308.

Eisenbruch, M. (1984). Cross-cultural aspects of bereavement. II: Ethnic and cultural variations in the development of bereavement practices. *Culture, Medicine and Psychiatry, 8*(4), 315–347.

Frazer, J. G. (1966). *The fear of the dead in primitive religion.* New York: Biblo and Tannen Publishers. (Original work published in 1933-1936).

Freed, P. J., Yanagihara, T. K., Hirsch, J., & Mann, J. J. (2009). Neural mechanisms of grief regulation. *Biological Psychiatry, 66*(1), 33–40.

Freud, S. (1960). *Totem and taboo: Resemblances between the psychic lives of savages and neurotics.* [Authorized English translation and introduction by A. A. Brill]. New York: Vintage Books. (Original work published in 1913).

Gmelch, G. J. (1971). Baseball magic. *Transaction, 8*(8), 39–41.

Goody, J. (1962). *Death, property and the ancestors: A study of the mortuary customs of the Lodagaa of West Africa.* Stanford, CA: Stanford University Press.

Gruter, M., & Masters, R. D. (1984). Ostracism as a social and biological phenomenon. *Ethology & Sociobiology, 7(3-4), 149–158.*

Haas, F. (2003). Bereavement care: Seeing the body. *Nursing Standard, 17*(28), 33–37.

Healing, T. D., Hoffman, P. N., & Young, S. E. (1995). The infection hazards of human cadavers. Communicable *Disease Report: CDR Review, 5*(5), R61–68.

Henrich, J. (2009). The evolution of costly displays, cooperation and religion: Credibility enhancing displays and their implications for cultural evolution. *Evolution and Human Behavior, 30*(4), 244–260.

Henrich, J., & Gil-White, F. J. (2001). The evolution of prestige: Freely conferred deference as a mechanism for enhancing the benefits of cultural transmission. *Evolution and Human Behavior, 22*(3), 165–196.

Hertz, R. (1960). *Death and the right hand* (R. Needham & C. Needham, Trans.). Glencoe, IL: Free Press. (Original work published in 1901).

Hinton, JJ. (1967). *Dying.* Baltimore: Penguin Books.

Hodgkinson, P. E., & Stewart, M. (1991). *Coping with catastrophe: A handbook of disaster management.* London: Routledge.

Holmes, T. H., & Rahe, R. H. (1967). The social readjustment rating scale. *Journal of Psychosomatic Research, 11*(2), 213–218.

Hunter, J. (2008). Bereavement: An incomplete rite of passage. *OMEGA: Journal of Death and Dying, 56*(2), 153–173.

Irwin, M., & Weiner, H. (1987). Depressive symptoms and immune function during bereavement. In *Biopsychosocial Aspects of Bereavement* (pp. 159-174). Washington, DC: American Psychiatric Press.

Johnson, D. (2016). *God is watching you: How the fear of God makes us human.* New York: Oxford University Press.

Johnson, D., & Krüger, O. (2004). The good of wrath: Supernatural punishment and the evolution of cooperation. *Political Theology, 5*(2), 159–176.

Jolly, J. (1987). *Missed beginnings: Death before life has been established.* London: Austen Cornish.

Lang, M., Krátký, J., Shaver, J. H., Jerotijević, D., & Xygalatas, D. (2015). Effects of anxiety on spontaneous ritualized behavior. *Current Biology, 25*(14), 1892–1897.

Legare, C. H., & Nielsen, M. (2015). Imitation and innovation: The dual engines of cultural learning. *Trends in cognitive sciences, 19*(11), 688–699.

Kübler-Ross, E. (1983). *On children and death: How children and their parents can and do cope with death*. New York: Touchstone.

Laderman, G. (1996). *The sacred remains: American attitudes toward death, 1799–1883*. New Haven, CT: Yale University Press.

Legare, C. H., & Herrmann, P. A. (2013). Cognitive consequences and constraints on reasoning about ritual. *Religion, Brain & Behavior, 3*(1), 63–65.

Legare, C. H., & Nielsen, M. (2015). Imitation and innovation: The dual engines of cultural learning. *Trends in Cognitive Sciences, 19*(11), 688–699.

Legare, C. H., & Watson-Jones, R. E. (2015). The evolution and ontogeny of ritual. In D. M. Buss & D. Conroy-Beam (Eds.), The *handbook of evolutionary psychology* (Vol. 2, pp. 829–847). Hoboken, NJ: Wiley.

Legare, C. H., Wen, N. J., Herrmann, P. A., & Whitehouse, H. (2015). Imitative flexibility and the development of cultural learning. *Cognition, 142*, 351–361.

Malinowski, B. (1948). Magic, *science and religion, and other essays.* (Selected and with an introduction by R. Redfield). Boston: Beacon Press.

McCorkle, William W., Jr. (2010). *Ritualizing the disposal of the deceased: From corpse to concept.* New York: Peter Lang.

McElreath, R., Boyd, R., & Richerson, P. J. (2003). Shared norms and the evolution of ethnic markers. *Current Anthropology, 44*(1), 122–130.

Metcalf, P., & Huntington, R. (1979). *Celebrations of death: The anthropology of mourning ritual.* Cambridge, UK: Cambridge University Press.

Morgan, O. (2004). Infectious disease risks from dead bodies following natural disasters. *Revista panamericana de salud pública, 15*, 307–312.

Morley, J. (1971). *Death, heaven, and the Victorians.* Pittsburgh, PA: University of Pittsburgh Press.

Murray, D. R., Fessler, D. M. T., Kerry, N., White, C., & Marin, M. (2017). The kiss of death: Three tests of the relationship between disease threat and ritualized physical contact within traditional cultures. *Evolution and Human Behavior, 38*(1), 63–70.

Nesse, R. M. (2005). An evolutionary framework for understanding grief. In D. Carr, R. M. Nesse, & C. B. Wortman (Eds.),Spousal bereavement in late life (pp. 195–226). New York: Springer.

Norton, M. I., & Gino, F. (2014). Rituals alleviate grieving for loved ones, lovers, and lotteries, *Journal of Experimental Psychology: General, 143*(1): 266–272.

Opler, M. E. (1936). An interpretation of ambivalence of two American Indian tribes. *Journal of Social Psychology, 7*(1), 82–116.

Parkes, C. M., Laungani, P., & Young, B. (2003). Culture and religion. In C. M. Parkes, P. Laungani, & B. Young (Eds.), *Death and bereavement across Cultures* (pp. 18–32). New York: Routledge.

Parkes, C. M., & Prigerson. H. G. (Eds.). (2013). *Bereavement: Studies of grief in adult life*. New York: Routledge.

Peebles, C. S. (1971). Moundville and surrounding sites: Some structural considerations of mortuary practices II. *Memoirs of the Society for American Archaeology, 25,*68–91.

Peng, M., Chang, L., & Zhou, R. (2013). Physiological and behavioral responses to strangers compared to friends as a source of disgust. *Evolution and Human Behavior, 34*(2), 94–98.

Purzycki, B. G. (2013). The minds of gods: A comparative study of supernatural agency. *Cognition, 129*(1), 163–179.

Purzycki, B. G., & Sosis, R. (2009). The religious system as adaptive: Cognitive flexibility, public displays, and acceptance. In E. Voland & W. Schiefenhövel (Eds.), *The biological evolution of religious mind and behavior* (pp. 243–256). Berlin: Springer.

Raphael, B. (1983). *The anatomy of bereavement*. New York: Basic Books.

Reynolds, T., Winegard, B. M., Baumeister, R. F., & Maner, J. K. (2015). The long goodbye: A test of grief as a social signal. *Evolutionary Behavioral Sciences, 9*(1), 20.

Richerson, P. J., & Boyd, R. (2005). *Not by genes alone: How culture transformed human evolution*. Chicago: University of Chicago Press.

Rosenblatt, P. C., Walsh, R. P., & Jackson, D. A. (1976). *Grief and mourning in cross-cultural perspective*. New Haven: HRAF Press.

Salathé, M., Kazandjieva, M., Lee, J. W., Levis, P., Feldman, M. W., & Jones, J. H. (2010). A high-resolution human contact network for infectious disease transmission. *Proceedings of the National Academy of Sciences, 107* (51), 20–25.

Schloss, J. P., & Murray, M. J. (2011). Evolutionary accounts of belief in supernatural punishment: A critical review. *Religion, Brain & Behavior, 1*(1), 46–99.

Shariff, A. F., & Norenzayan, A. (2007). God is watching you: Priming God concepts increases prosocial behavior in an anonymous economic game. *Psychological Science, 18*(9), 803–809.

Shuchter, S. R., & Zisook, S. (1987). A multidimensional model of spousal bereavement. In S. Zisook (Ed.), Biopsychosocial *aspects of bereavement* (pp. 35–48). Washington, DC: American Psychiatric Press.

Sosis, R. (2004).The adaptive value of religious ritual: Rituals promote group cohesion by requiring members to engage in behavior that is too costly to fake. *American Scientist, 92*(2), 166–172.

Sperber, D. (1975). *Rethinking symbolism* (A.L. Morton, Trans.). Cambridge: Cambridge University Press.

Sperber, D. (1985). Anthropology and psychology: Towards an epidemiology of representations. *Man, 20* 73–89.

Stroebe, M., Schut, H., & Stroebe, W. (2007). Health outcomes of bereavement. *The Lancet, 370*(9603), 1960–1973.

Stroebe, M. S., Stroebe, W., & Hansson, R. O. (Eds). (1993). *Handbook of bereavement: Theory, research and intervention*. New York: Cambridge University Press.

Taylor, L. H., Latham, S. M., & Mark, E. J. (2001). Risk factors for human disease emergence. *Philosophical Transactions of the Royal Society of London B: Biological Sciences, 356*(1411), 983–989.

Ucko, P. J. Ethnography and archaeological interpretation of funerary remains. *World Archaeology, 1*(2), (1969): 262–280.

van Gennep, A. (1960). *The rites of passage* (M. B. Vizedom & G. L. Caffee, Trans.) Paris: Emile Nourry. (Original work published in French in 1909).

Walter, T. (2005). Three ways to arrange a funeral: Mortuary variation in the modern West. *Mortality, 10*(3), 173–192.

Wen, N. J., Herrmann, P. A. , & Legare, C. H. (2016). Ritual increases children's affiliation with in-group members. *Evolution and Human Behavior, 37*(1), 54–60.

Wertheimer, A. (1991). *A special scar: The experiences of people bereaved by suicide*. London: Routledge.

White, C., & Fessler, D. M.T. (2013). Evolutionizing grief: Viewing photographs of the deceased predicts the misattribution of ambiguous stimuli by the bereaved. *Evolutionary Psychology, 11*, 1084–1100.

White, C., & Fessler, D. M. T. (2018). An evolutionary account of vigilance in grief. *Evolution, Medicine, and Public Health, 1*, 34–42.

White, C., Fessler, D. M.T., & Gomez, P. (2016). The effects of corpse viewing and corpse condition on vigilance for deceased loved ones. *Evolution and Human Behavior, 37*, 517–522.

White, C., Marin, M., & Fessler, D. M. T. (2017). Not just dead meat: An evolutionary account of corpse treatment in mortuary rituals. *Journal of Cognition and Culture, 17*(1–2), 146–168.

White, C., Marin, M., & Fessler, D, M. T. *The dead may kill you: Do ancestor spirit beliefs promote cooperation in traditional small-scale societies?* (Manuscript in preparation).

Whitson, J. A., & Galinsky, A. D. (2008). Lacking control increases illusory pattern perception. *Science, 322*(5898), 115–117.

Winegard, B. M., Reynolds, T., Baumeister, R. F., Winegard, B., & Maner, J. K. (2014). Grief functions as an honest indicator of commitment. *Personality and Social Psychology Review, 18*(2), 168–186.

Wright, B. (1991). *Sudden death: Intervention skills for the caring professions.* Edinburg, NY: Churchill Livingstone.

Xygalatas, D., Konvalinka, I., Bulbulia, J., & Roepstorff, A. (2011). Quantifying collective effervescence: Heart-rate dynamics at a fire-walking ritual. *Communicative & Integrative Biology, 4*(6), 735–738.

Xygalatas, D., Mitkidis, P., Fischer, R., Reddish, P., Skewes, J., Geertz, A. W., Roepstorff, A., & Bulbulia, J. (2013). Extreme rituals promote prosociality. *Psychological Science, 24*(8), 1602–1605.

PART IV

RELIGIOUS OBJECTS

CHAPTER 10

SCRIPTURALISM

A theory

BRIAN MALLEY

INTRODUCTION

AMONG the oldest texts in continuous use are the sacred texts or scriptures—the Muslim Qur'an, the Hindu Vedas, the Jewish Torah, the Christian Bible, and others. Such scriptures influence people not only individually, as readers, but also socially, as a community orientation, a framework for discourse, and a ground of authority. Scripturalist communities enshrine a sacred text with fine materials, exquisite artwork, miraculous stories, formalized dogma, respectful handling, ritualized performance, and—most importantly—a continuous search to discover the text's implications for their lives.

These "scriptures of the world" invite comparison. People from various religious traditions, upon becoming aware of one another's sacred texts, intuit that there is something comparable about them, as if they might somehow be more parallel to one another than to the other literature of their native communities. Scholars, too, sensing a distinctive phenomenon, have suggested that the various scriptures are members of some distinctive class—a literary genre or cultural type—that has developed independently in different parts of the world.

I propose that scripturalism is in fact a distinctive type of cultural tradition: a traditional means of establishing community, a complex of mutually supporting traditions, and a method of adaptation for both communities and individuals. The functional architecture of a scripturalist tradition is approached from the viewpoint of cultural reproduction, an epidemiology-of-beliefs perspective (Sperber, 1985, 1996). A tradition's functional architecture is the set of processes, both social and psychological, that go into reproducing a scripturalist tradition in a community. The naturalistic perspective of the epidemiology of beliefs comports with embodied, performative, and dialogical approaches to culture in focusing on people's practices—especially their interactions—because it is in and by these that cultural patterns are displayed, propagated, and disputed.

A scripturalist tradition includes a set of elements that interact to produce a distinctive form of community. A scripturalist community is one in which a scripture is normatively authoritative for community members, and community participation normatively involves distinctive rhetorical practices that, taken individually, appear to enact scriptural authority.

What makes scripturalism a *type* of tradition is that its beliefs and practices are partly defined by their formal properties. Formal properties are information-bearing distinctions—that is, differentiae that propagate, or, in the words of Gregory Bateson (1979), "differences that make a difference" (p. 228). For such properties, what is causally important is not the differentiae themselves but rather the information they communicate (Shannon & Weaver, 1948; cf. Floridi, 2011). All differentiae that communicate the same distinction are formally equivalent: they convey the same information and thus form a functional analogue between traditions. In scriptures' origin stories, for instance, what often matters is not the narrative details—about which informants are seldom much concerned—but rather the implied contrast between scripture's special origin and the normal origin of all other literature (about which informants are usually emphatic). The functional elements of scripturalist traditions must be understood, not semantically, in terms of their overt content, but rather in informational terms, in their implications for community members.

From an epidemiology-of-beliefs perspective (Sperber, 1996), a scripturalist tradition is defined by the processes that reproduce it. Scripturalist traditions must induce people to produce *just such artifacts* and to perform *just such actions* that at least some observers will go on to *do the same all over again*. They do this by a uniquely scripturalist way of making community such that the continuing life of the community reproduces at least the core elements of the scripturalist tradition. If scripturalist traditions offer communities a stable but flexible means of adaptation, one can see why scripturalism might be relatively stable within a community, and spread to others.

In the interest of clarity, *scripturalism* is described as a set of named hypotheses. So little information is available about day-to-day practices of scripturalism "on the ground" that, for examples, I have had to rely heavily upon my own fieldwork among evangelical Christians in a medium-sized Midwestern American church (Malley, 2004). The discussion of magical and mantic uses of scriptures draws upon two surveys of English-language folklore related to such uses (Malley, 2006, 2015). But the examples are intended only to be illustrative, and the empirical adequacy of the present model—its fit or lack of fit with observed practice—must be adjudged by others. An enormous amount of research remains to be done, but I take heart that, sometimes, scientific understanding is advanced more by the failure of bold proposals than by the success of timid ones.

QUESTIONS

The parallel development of scriptures in different traditions raises two basic problems: the definitional, comparative problem of what exactly makes a scripture, and the explanatory, anthropological problem of how such texts can remain in use so long.

The Definitional Problem

The last century or so has seen a number of anthologies of sacred texts, the most comprehensive of which is F. Max Mueller's fifty-volume series *Sacred Books of the East* (Winternitz & Müller, 1879–1910). In contrast to Mueller's encyclopedic endeavor, most anthologies are single-volume affairs that incorporate short selections from the better-known scriptures. Each such project raises afresh the thorny questions of (a) what exactly distinguishes "sacred texts" from other literature, and (b) what exactly justifies their inclusion in a common category. The various editors of these works have offered different criteria to explain their selections, their endeavor being to find a rational basis for a category that they *intuit* but do not really *understand*.

In wrestling with this difficulty, Miriam Levering (1989, pp. 8–9) developed the following characterization of the intuitive notion of scripture, shared by many scholars:

- There are often beliefs that the text is of divine origin, or the product of special insight.
- Whatever their origin, they are regarded and treated as sacred, that is, powerful and inviolable, to be treated with respect.
- They are regarded and consulted as normative, authoritative for a community in various aspects of its religious life: for worship, doctrine, and behavior.
- The texts, whether written or oral, are regarded as closed and fixed, not to be added to or subtracted from. In other words, they are treated as a canon.
- When the sacred text is in the form of a book, it is considered complete. It contains everything of importance, and can be applied to all aspects of human life.
- The texts are used by members of the community in religious and ritual contexts.
- Sacred texts testify to that which is ultimate.

Levering proceeded to describe the difficulty with this conception:

These are intuitively appealing generalizations, yet they are curiously misleading. I suspect that these characterizations are so intuitively appealing because all but one of them belong to the widely shared common sense characterization of the Bible. But a fully formed comparative study casts considerable doubt on the universal applicability and fruitfulness of these characterizations. Characterizations that are strongly true and significant about the Bible or the Qur'an at certain historical moments turn out to be only weakly true, and far less significant (or significant in a different sense), as statements about other scriptural texts.

As Levering notes, the common-sense notion of scripture is not exactly wrong, but neither does it capture what is common to the different scriptural traditions.

Levering, following W. C. Smith, suggested that what unites the "sacred texts of the world" has to do not with the texts but with the human belief and practice surrounding them. In *What is Scripture?*, Smith wrote:

> On close inquiry, it emerges that being scripture is not a quality inherent in a given text, or type of text, so much as an interactive relation between that text and a community of persons (though such relations have been by no means constant). One might even speak of a widespread tendency to treat texts in a "scripture-like" way: a human propensity to scripturalize. (1993, p. ix)

Smith's ultimate proposal is that "being scripture" is an existential attitude (p. 239): "[Scripture] is best characterized as . . . a relation—an engagement—among humans, the transcendent, and a text"—this text being a kind of global uber-scripture in which the various existing scriptures are mere strands. Perhaps because of this grand design, Smith's discussion offers little insight into the actual practices of scripturalism. Nonetheless, Levering's and Smith's shift of focus from scriptural texts to the cultural beliefs and practices surrounding them effectively recasts a literary problem of genre as an anthropological one of tradition.

The Explanatory Problem

James Fieser and John Powers (1998), introduce their anthology *Scriptures of the World's Religions* with what seems a simple observation about the place of scriptures in religious traditions:

> The present text introduces the world's religions through selections from their scriptures. There are special benefits to this avenue of exploration. In most cases the sacred texts are the oldest written documents in the tradition, and one gains a sense of immediate connection by studying the same documents that followers have been reading for millennia. The texts are also foundational to a religion's important doctrines, rituals, and social and ethical positions. Thus, they explain the authoritative basis of traditions that might otherwise seem incomprehensible, or even groundless. (p. xix)

This observation about the relative age of scriptures resonates with the belief of many religionists in the eternality of scripture. In human terms, however, however, such longevity presents a puzzle.

It may seem that written texts endure because of the resilience of the media upon which they are inscribed—they do not dissipate as does the sound of speech. This is indeed an advantage of literacy, and has import for the formation of some scriptures. But in fact, fixity presents a challenge to a text's longevity.

Our spoken texts are generally unique productions, motivated by a speaker's agenda, formulated for a particular audience in a particular situation. Most of our speech is *improvised* rather than *rehearsed* because our agendas, audiences, and situations are constantly changing. Scripts—planned utterances—can be and are used in situations that are highly recurrent, such as greetings, customer-service communications, legal procedures, and so forth, but scriptures are (relatively) fixed texts facing circumstances that have changed dramatically over their lengthy histories. Is not their fixity a serious hindrance to their continued use?

The fixity of texts presents a grave difficulty for functionalist explanations of scripturalism. Consider a hypothesis to the effect that the Bible continues in use because of its legitimation of male authority. This hypothesis certainly explains some rhetorical uses of the Bible, but it presupposes rather than explains Biblical authority: the Bible can be used to legitimize male authority only because it was *already* considered authoritative. The utility is derived from the authority rather than explaining it.

Might not a text rise to authoritative status because of its uses? Yes. But *that* text would not be the text of the Bible, or the Qur'an, or any other actual scripture. No actual scripture is optimized for any particular rhetorical purpose, or even for any specifiable set of purposes. Existing scriptural texts have mostly been written and compiled through a combination of writers' occasional needs, material availability, rhetorical art, historical accident, individual ambition, and political compromise. In the case of the Bible, the resulting text has never been perfectly suited even for Christian doctrine and practice!

The one thing that a fixed text might plausibly do is to convey a fixed message, a static "meaning." Might not the function of a *fixed text* be to establish and maintain a *fixed set* of beliefs and practices? In fact, is this not a reason that informants explicitly give for reading, reciting, and studying scripture?

Belief that a community's doctrine and practice represent that community's interpretation of scripture has underlain the publication of most of the sacred-text anthologies. Chung Hwan Kwak gives it voice in his preface to *World Scripture: A Comparative Anthology of Sacred Texts*:

> These sacred scriptures contain essential truths. And they have immeasurably great historical significance, for they have influenced the minds, hearts and practices of billions of people in the past. They continue to exert tremendous impact in the present, and we have every reason to believe that such influence will continue into the future. The words of truth in sacred scriptures form the core beliefs of religion and thus, of civilization. (Wilson, 1991, p. xiii)

The supposition is that by reading a religion's scripture, the student of a religion is "reading over the shoulders" of the religionists (cf. Geertz, 1972), acquiring an understanding of their beliefs from the same source they do—and in those beliefs' definitive, scriptural form.

Implicit in statements like these is an epistemological model, *scriptural foundationalism* (Keller, 2005; Malley, 2004, 2011). Scriptural foundationalism consists of two hypotheses:

1. *The interpretive-belief hypothesis.* The beliefs and practices of a religion stand in an interpretive relationship to a scripture; the scripture is the text, and the religious beliefs and practices are interpretations of the text.
2. *The authoritative-text hypothesis.* The semantic relationship is established by the text's authority; the community regard for the text is a basis on which one can legitimize or justify beliefs and practices.

Both of these hypotheses are so intuitive as to seem indubitable, but let us doubt them anyway.

Empirically, scriptural foundationalism is supported by three basic kinds of observations, commonplace in scripturalist communities:

1. *Statements of scriptural authority.* Community members say—quite readily and explicitly—that the text is authoritative for their beliefs and practices. Not only do community members say it, but institutions explicitly avow the text's authority in their published self-descriptions, and it has often been the subject of reflection within traditions.
2. *Scriptural explanation.* Community members explain—again, readily and explicitly—their beliefs and practices by appeal to the scripture. They say that the scripture's instruction and authority are the reason they believe and behave as they do.
3. *Conformity.* There are clear points of correspondence between the semantic content of scripture and the beliefs and practices of community members. At least some of the time, people do what the text says they should.

Scriptural foundationalism thus seems a self-evident case of people doing exactly what they say they are doing.

Yet, since when do people go about describing their normal behavior? Why would anyone do that? The articulation of scriptural foundationalism as a part of normal practice ought to cause suspicion. Let us take a closer look at the three lines of evidence just discussed:

1. *Statements of scriptural authority.* To say that scripture is authoritative for a community is to repeat what its members say about it. Moreover, these self-reports are often themselves traditional: community members have been

taught to describe their communities in terms of scriptural authority, and they often do so using fairly standardized language. Of all the community's many attributes, why should this particular one be singled out and articulated? And why traditionally?

2. *Scriptural explanation.* Scriptural explanations are justifications rather than autobiographical accounts of how the individuals have come to those beliefs and practices. When I asked informants specific questions about how they had learned their beliefs and practices, they easily distinguished this question of personal history from the question of scriptural justification, and were perfectly willing to relay how they had learned them in Sunday school or from their parents. Significantly, *the scriptural justification was itself part of what they were taught*: beliefs were true and practices obligatory because they were from the Bible. So when people explain their behavior by appeal to scripture, they are relating a traditional behavior along with a traditional justification. I do not doubt that scriptural authority provides some people with genuine motivation for behaving as they have been taught. But in general, people's explanations of their behaviors by appeal to scripture are *not* evidence that they behave as they do because the scripture says to do so; this shows only that people have been *taught* to explain their behavior in this way. But why do they explain their behavior in this relatively circuitous way?

3. *Conformity.* People may perform actions enjoined by scripture simply because the actions themselves are normative. The coincidence of practice with scriptural teaching is evidence of scriptural authority only when (a) alternative practices are equally effectual and available and (b) the influence of other authorities can be excluded. And what about nonconformity? In the community I studied, the straightforward instruction "Greet one another with a holy kiss" was simply ignored. I have seen wealthy donors treated with special consideration—exactly as is forbidden in the Epistle of James. Similar cases of neglect and even outright contradiction may be observed in many scripturalist communities, but these have largely been ignored despite the problems they pose for scriptures' alleged authority.

When evaluated as an explanation of actual Scripturalist practice, scriptural foundationalism is not so impressive after all. Scriptural foundationalism clearly does represent some communities' understanding of their own practices. This self-understanding structures much of their discourse and formal epistemology. I developed an outline of this model in my analysis of evangelical Biblicism in the United States (Malley, 2004), and Eva Keller (2005) independently discovered the same structure underlying Seventh-Day Adventist practice on Madagascar. The mistake comes in taking scriptural foundationalism as the explanation for rather than as part of the phenomenon to be explained.

DISTINCTIONS

An understanding of scripturalist traditions requires distinguishing between artifacts, texts, and performances.

Text

A *text*, as I shall use the term, is an ordered set of words. This definition seems simple but requires some explanation.[1]

Given that evangelical Christians regularly reference "the Bible" and that they use a variety of particular Bibles, I inquired into the relationship between "the Bible" and these particular books. Systematic questioning revealed that my informants expected "the Bible" to be a text in the sense used here, as an ordered set of words. Those words could be written, spoken, audio-recorded, impressed in braille, or beamed across the galaxy on radio waves, but they had to be words—not pictures, enactments, tunes, or anything else. "The Bible" is a *text*.

The tendency to conceptualize linguistic performances as texts may be traceable to the organization of working memory, specifically the role of a phonetic loop in which the order of speech sounds is preserved. This, combined with the lexical organization of languages, almost guarantees that in any society some public representations will take the form of texts, even if they are performed only for citation and mockery.

Although the words of a text must be ordered, they need not be grammatical or have any other internal organization. Magical spells are often aggregations of words, nonsense syllables, and names with no semantic content in any normal sense of the term. Other texts, such as signatures and some receipts, serve as evidence of events without respect to their semantic content. A text may be *no more* than an ordered set of words.

No distinction is necessary between written scriptures and oral sacred texts. If it really is a *text* that is sacred—not a plot or style or story—then it remains a text whether it is inscribed or not. Conversely, if what is sacred is not a text but an oratory *style* or *narrative*, then writing down a corresponding text does not create a sacred text but merely a textual example of the sacred style or sacred narrative. The Iliad and the Odyssey, for example, have a distinctive vocabulary, meter, and narrative that are thought to be part

---

[1] The use of the term *text* in the humanities has been greatly confused owing to its adoption as a model for social action (Ricoeur, 1971), and *reading* as a model for the observation and analysis thereof (Geertz, 1973). One cannot use this model for the explanation of scripturalist traditions, in which the hermeneutic relationship is itself part of the explanandum, without begging important questions.

of their performance, and their texts should not be mistaken for scriptures just because someone put stylus to parchment.

Oral texts may well be scriptures. Even in highly literate societies some texts exist only in oral form. During my fieldwork, members of Creekside Baptist Church recited the Lord's Prayer fairly regularly, in a standard form:

> Our Father, Who art in heaven, Hallowed be Thy name, Thy kingdom come, Thy will be done, On earth as it is in heaven, Give us this day our daily bread. And forgive us our sins, As we forgive those who have sinned against us. And lead us not into temptation, But deliver us from evil. For Thine is the kingdom, and the power, and the glory forever. Amen.

This text does not appear in *any* version of the Bible. It is most similar to the text of the Revised Standard Version, with the longer ending of the King James Version, but the change from "trespasses" to "sins" was directed from the pulpit and thereafter followed without comment. In this community, the Lord's Prayer had always existed as an oral tradition, transmitted independently of any particular Bible translation.

Writing does, of course, make a difference. In a society without literacy, texts can be associated with artifacts but not inscribed on them, and this limits their length. Going forward, I will refer to the texts of scriptures, as opposed to their artifacts and performances, as *scripture-texts*.

Text-Artifact

In "The Natural Histories of Discourse," Michael Silverstein and Greg Urban (1996) describe a text-artifact as follows: "The text-artifact is the physical medium that seems, on the face of it, to carry an organization of information, sometimes narrative information, that we decontextualize as the denotational text we are reading" (p. 5). Their caution is well measured, because it is in fact difficult to identify precisely what it is about a text-artifact that allows it to be recognized (read, interpreted) as an inscribed text. Fortunately, this uncertainty seldom arises in scripturalist traditions, so we can simply stipulate that any physical expression or instantiation of a text is a text-artifact. When an artifact bears a scriptural text, I shall refer to it as a *scripture-artifact*.

It has often been observed that scripture-artifacts are the focus of special effort in reproduction, decoration, distribution, and handling. Ritual actions performed upon scripture-artifacts include bringing a Bible to church, placing a Qur'an upright on a shelf, or bowing to the Adi Granth. Such acts are generally conceived to be within the power of the performer.

Greater effects are purportedly achievable by means of scripture-artifacts. E. Thomas Lawson and Robert N. McCauley (Lawson & McCauley, 1990; McCauley & Lawson, 2002) point out that acts performed by means of special objects are often said to produce superhuman effects. Thus, rituals to heal or harm sometimes involve the production and manipulation of scripture-artifacts, for example:

> If a woman is forsaken by her lover, she has but to write out the CIX Psalm, send the copy of it to him, and he will never thrive. (Gregor, 1881, p. 87)

And:

> A farmer near Clun had an animal suffering from a bad knee joint. The charmer wrote a verse from the Bible on a piece of paper and put it into the boosey (or manger) for the animal to eat with its hay. The animal recovered. (Hayward, 1938, p. 230)

The use of scripture-artifacts to achieve superhuman effects is widely reported but quite difficult to explain. If the text-artifact is just going to be eaten by a horse, why should its semantic content matter?

Text-Performance

A text-performance is an oral performance of a text, such as in the example of the congregation's recitation of the Lord's Prayer. I will refer to performances of scriptural texts as *scripture-performances*.

The most common ritual action upon a scripture-text is reading or recitation. These are usually carried out in a stylized manner, as when, on May 31, 1934, Muhammad Rif'at became the first person to recite the Qur'an on Egyptian Cairo Radio, performing it in the style *tasweer al-mana*. The reading of the Torah by Jewish men—at bar Mitzvahs and in study—is another example of this type.

In other rituals people perform actions *by means of* scripture-performances, such as protecting oneself against fairies, exorcising ghosts, or relieving a curse:

> When Mr. Jones was curate of Llanyblodwel a parishioner sent to ask the "parson" to come to see her. . . . In the course of conversation Mr. Jones ascertained that the woman had sent for him to counteract the evil machinations of her enemy. "I am witched," she said, "and a parson can break the spell." The clergyman argued with her, but all to no purpose. She affirmed that she was witched, and that a clergyman could withdraw the curse. Finding that the woman was obdurate he read a [Bible] chapter and offered up a prayer, and wishing the woman good day with a hearty "God bless you," he departed. Upon a subsequent visit he found the woman quite well, and he was informed by her, to his astonishment, that he had broken the spell. (Owen, 1896, pp. 244–245)

Many folklore reports suggest that reading the Bible or reciting specific Biblical texts is efficacious for protection, healing, and more. What we lack is an explanation of why scripture-artifacts and scripture-performances are reported to have such uses. Might it have something to do with the conceptualization of scriptures?

SCRIPTURE-CONCEPTS
=

What do people have in mind when they refer to scripture-concepts, such as the Bible, the Qur'an, or the Long Discourses of the Buddha? Do these scripture-concepts have any special properties, different from the ways in which people think of other texts? I suggest three hypotheses—unification, recognition, distinctiveness—concerning the structure and dynamics of scripture-concepts.

Unification

It ought to be a striking fact that scripture-texts are so often *named* collections. In modern, highly literate societies, we are accustomed to texts having titles, by which we might refer to them, but many ancient texts—in fact, most scripture-texts—have no original titles: they were named only after composition, by readers who wanted to reference them. Scripture names like the Bible, Qur'an, or Tripitaka designate not individual texts but collections of independent works. The *unification hypothesis* proposes a historical tendency among scripturalist communities to gather their scripture-texts into a single named collection—a *canon* of scripture, to use the traditional but ambiguous term. It holds that where a plurality of scripture-texts are in use—whether different works or different collections of works—scripturalist communities will collect them into a single category designated by a simple name. The unification hypothesis does not suggest the elimination of other names for scripture texts—the prediction is simply that there will develop a single term for the entire scriptural library.

Recognition

Scripture-concepts need not necessarily define the categories they name; one need not know the defining features of the Bible to recognize Bibles, or the precise definition of a Qur'an to recognize a "copy" of it. The *recognition hypothesis* holds that everyday recognition of scripture-artifacts relies on a set of formal recognition features rather than a definition. Christian evangelicals need not define the Bible so long as they can reliably *recognize* Bible artifacts. To identify the criteria used in recognition, I asked informants how they would determine whether a given artifact was a Bible. Once the title was taken out of consideration, they looked to stereotyped characteristics—leather binding, a brown or black cover, two-column text, fine paper, enlarged capital letters, column headers, a ribbon marker, and so forth—to decide. This reliance on recognition criteria rather than verbiage afforded them a convenient textual eclecticism. But even when definitions of scripture are culturally available, as in the Islamic case, they are not essential, because the recognition of scripture-artifacts depends on readily observable features—formal properties—rather than a definition.

Distinctiveness

Scripturalists' understanding of their scriptures—whether as a unified corpus or as individual works—requires that they be understood as instances of some higher or superordinate taxon, as species of some genus. The *distinctiveness hypothesis* holds (a) that scriptures will be understood as relatively distinct from other taxa at the same level of abstraction, and (b) that scriptures will be considered atypical members of their superordinate taxon. My informants classified the Bible as a text, comparable to other texts and not comparable to things other than texts, such as giraffes or Tuesdays. In the terms of the distinctiveness hypothesis, they regarded the Bible as relatively distinct from other texts—more different from other texts than other texts are from one another—and as an atypical—indeed, unusual or special—instance of its superordinate category, text.

The recognition and distinctiveness hypotheses together facilitate the specialization of scripture production. Given the small capacity of working memory, it is efficient for the day-to-day recognition of scripture-artifacts and scripture-performances to be based on a relatively small number of highly evident formal characteristics, and for the production of scripture-artifacts and scripture-performances to be entrusted to specialists. It is, then, in the interest of the specialists, who derive their influence and perhaps livelihoods from the esteem people have for their products, to make those products highly recognizable. To that end, scripture-artifacts are often specially decorated because such marking (a) helps community members to recognize them as instances of their scripture and (b) lends substance to members' sense that the scriptures are unique. Both are critical for the role of scripture in the community.

TRADITIONS ABOUT SCRIPTURES

The traditions concerning scriptures are famously varied in form and content. However varied, such scriptural lore—stories, doctrines, legal prescriptions, and other discourse about scripture—must convey (a) the *principle of scriptural authority*—that the scripture is authoritative for the community—and (b) the *principle of scriptural uniqueness*—that the scripture is distinctive, quite different from other literature. These principles guide reasoning, discourse, and practice in scripturalist communities.

The Principle of Scriptural Authority

Statements about scriptural authority convey important features of a scripturalist community's *normative self-understanding*: that is, community members (a) regard their (ideal) beliefs and practices as the (true) meaning or (correct) interpretation of scripture and (b) rationalize and legitimize this relationship by appeal to the scripture's authority. This self-understanding is at the heart of scripturalism—in part because it does *not* describe actual practice.

Authority in Principle

Philosophers have long noted that any proposition may be understood as a statement about the world or as a statement about language. In much the same way, statements about scripture may serve as statements about the cosmos or about the scripturalist community. So it is with statements about scriptural authority: although formally they are statements about a text, they function as statements *about the scripturalist community*. To say that a scripture is authoritative is (a) to identify with the (real or imagined) community that recognizes the scripture's authority and (b) to invite the audience to join that community, either explicitly by stating agreement, or tacitly, by going along with the supposition. In being expressed, statements of scriptural authority reproduce the very authority they purport to describe.

The nature of scriptural authority is different from normal literary authority. Scriptures are authoritative *in principle*. This is most clearly evident in community members' open-ended commitment to the scriptural authority. Biblicists believe what the Bible says, even if they *don't know* what all it says. This contrasts starkly with normal literature, where agreement with the text can be decided only *after* it is read.

Authority and Unification

The principle of scriptural authority attributes authority to the scriptural corpus as a whole. It is therefore the engine driving the unification hypothesis, the source of communities' tendency to gather all their scripture-texts under a single name.

Unification can have a significant consequence for the interpretation of scriptural self-reference. In 2 Timothy 3:16, Paul writes: "All Scripture is inspired by God and profitable for teaching, for reproof, for correction, for training in righteousness so that the man of God may be adequate, equipped for every good work." In the original context, "all Scripture" referred to the Jewish scriptures of the time, constituting—at most—the Septuagint canon of the Old Testament. But today, this statement is commonly used as a description of the authority of the entire Christian Bible, including the New Testament.

Unification creates an asymmetry that is important for scriptural authority: the authority of the scriptural corpus can potentially, but need not actually, devolve upon any particular passage therein. The authority of the entire corpus is logically available to be rhetorically applied to any constituent text, but need not automatically be so applied. This affords the community a flexibility in the practice of scriptural authority that belies the generality of the principle of scriptural authority.

Authority Grounded

The principle of scriptural authority is what Roy Rappaport (1999) called an *ultimate sacred postulate*. Rappaport proposed that all communities have at their conceptual core a small set of statements that are regarded as sacred and unquestionable. These postulates are *ultimate* in that they provide the (ostensible) basis for community discourse. Ultimate sacred postulates (USPs) are different from mere presuppositions in three ways.

Explicit transmission. USPs are explicitly communicated as statements of great importance. USPs are explicitly communicated because the acceptance of the description as true *reproduces the community's self-conception* in any listener who identifies with the community, such as a child or new convert.

Symbolism. Unlike presuppositions, USPs function symbolically—associatively, evocatively—rather than propositionally. Statements like "the Bible is the word of God" are used not for their (often modest or trivial) propositional content but because they represent, in a looser, more associative fashion, assumptions that are important for the community. Dan Sperber (1975) has noted that the propositional vacuity of such enigmatic statements grabs listeners' attention and triggers a search for associations that might illuminate their relevance. The public expression of USPs makes them potent symbols of the community and its norms.

Generativity. Without much relevant propositional content, seldom can the USPs logically generate the specific set of principles that guide community practice, but they are nonetheless *thought* to do so by community members. The authority of the principles guiding community practice is attributed to the UPSs when in fact the guiding principles are normative in their own right.

The principle of scriptural authority functions as a USP in scripturalist communities. In the community I studied, biblical authority was communicated emphatically to children in Sunday school curriculum and to adults in the church-membership process. It's reinforced by regular reference to the Bible as "God's word." Yet the sense of this phrase is vague: in discussing it, my informants often echoed 2 Timothy 3.16, describing the Bible as "inspired by God" or "God-breathed." They were uncertain what these phrases might mean, but certain that they entail that God is the ultimate author of the Bible, and that the Bible is true and authoritative. Such enigmatic talk functioned not semantically but formally, as a signal of commitment to Biblical authority.

Scriptural authority is often attributed to and purportedly derived from some other authority or event. Such derivations present the authority or event as logically more fundamental than scriptural authority, but they are psychologically secondary: it is scriptural authority that is primary, and the purported derivations rationalize this fact. The real force of scriptural authority comes from the shared understanding that *if you are one of us, then you will regard the scripture as authoritative.* Acceptance of scriptural authority is tied to community membership because the community understands itself in terms of scriptural authority (among other things). The principle of scriptural authority is that we—the participants in *this* community or *this* tradition—recognize the scripture's authority, in contrast to others—outsiders or defectors—who do not. The scriptural foundationalism they espouse does not describe Scripturalist practice: it *conditions, evokes, causes* that practice.

As many have intuited, the ostensible derivation of scriptural authority from some more fundamental event or source is a result rather than the cause of scriptural authority, the *rationalization* of scriptures' authority. It is for this reason that variations in different revelatory accounts or alternative theories of scriptural authority are normally of merely academic interest to members of scripturalist communities. So long as scriptural authority is maintained, members sense intuitively that nothing important depends on such details. It is only when a narrative distinction signals a social difference that people sit up and take notice.

The community basis for the principle of scriptural authority may be one reason the authority is often regarded as an *inherent property* of the scripture: from the viewpoint of a community member, there is little difference between the description of reality and the statement of an accepted social understanding. The reification of social authority in a scripture justifies community tradition and naturalizes scriptural behaviors as rational responses to cosmic reality.

The Principle of Scriptural Uniqueness

The second key proposition essential to scripturalist traditions is that their scriptures are unique, distinctive among texts. This principle is the social, motivational engine that drives the distinctiveness of the scripture's taxon relative to its coordinate taxa. Because the principle of scriptural authority serves to define a community, the distinction between members and nonmembers implies the uniqueness of scripture among texts.

The *principle of spiritual uniqueness* is that a scripture is unique among all texts—those that exist now and those that may be discovered or created. As a claim about texts, this quite problematic: given any text, it is always possible to create another text that is almost arbitrarily similar. The *Wicked Bible*, for instance, differs from other Bibles by one small word: *not*, specifically in "Thou shalt [not] commit adultery." No scripture-text can really be all that different from other texts. The principle of spiritual uniqueness, then, attempts to project a *social distinction* onto a *verbal continuum*.

Lore about scriptures often communicates their uniqueness formally. Probably the most common way of communicating a scripture's uniqueness and rationalizing its authority is the origin story. Scriptures' origin stories often occur in varied forms even within a given community, but they all share a common implication: that the scripture is special, distinctive among texts, *because of the event narrated*. The scripture stands apart from other texts not because the scripture's origin is different in its narrative details but because the scripture's origin is of *a different kind entirely* from those of other texts. Likewise, doctrines of scripture, theories of inspiration, and stories about scripture miracles communicate that scripture is quite different from all other texts.

The principle of spiritual uniqueness is reinforced by the decoration and handling of scripture-artifacts. The lavish decoration of and artistic investment in scripture-artifacts are intended to show that the scriptures are uniquely valuable to the community. So too, ritual: To swear on a Bible, to properly handle a Qur'an, to bow before the Adi Granth—each practice implies the uniqueness of scripture. The principle of spiritual uniqueness thus explains the special treatment of scriptures as artifacts or performances. Such practices not only reflect the reverence participants feel for their scriptures but also reproduce the scripturalist tradition, by lending substance to scriptures' distinctiveness.

Scripture Citation and Interpretation

Whatever else people may do with scriptures, they read them. To understand scripturalist reading, it is essential to distinguish four phenomena:

1. *Interpretation.* An interpretation is a statement that is attributed to a text. An interpretation consists of (a) some concept or statement and (b) the attribution of this concept or statement to the scripture. Statements are often assertions (propositions about the universe) or exhortations (injunctions for or against some action). They may be in a semipropositional form, in which case there is often discussion about what the proposition actually is or what specific action is enjoined. The attribution may be to the scripture-text as a whole, "the Bible says . . ."; to some portion of the text, "John 3.16 says . . ."; or to some person or event reported in the text, "St. Paul says . . ." or "Jesus showed us by ___ that . . ."

2. *Traditional interpretation.* A tradition in which ideas are communicated *as interpretations,* that is, paired with an attribution to a text. In many cases particular *points of relevance* are also transmitted, implicitly or explicitly, alongside the interpretation. In these cases the interpretation is passed on as an interpretation relevant to some question or topic. Traditional points of relevance can exert a very strong constraint on the socially acceptable uses of a traditional interpretation.

3. *Interpretive process.* The mental process of producing an interpretation from a text. It is the reading process triggered when a person perceives a text-artifact and adopts a *semantic stance* toward it. The semantic stance is the assumption that some features of the text-artifact can be treated as a verbal signal.

4. *Hermeneutic prescription.* Some—not all—scripturalist traditions include descriptions of and prescriptions for the interpretive process. As descriptions, these are psychological propositions: claims about how a person infers a meaning from a scripture-text. As is the case in traditional logic, hermeneutic prescriptions are formally a mixture of description and prescription, but their rhetorical deployment is almost always *prescriptive.* Even brief inspection reveals that these traditions are not so much scientific as normative. It is unclear how often, and to what degree, hermeneutic prescriptions actually affect interpretive processes.

With these phenomena distinguished, let us take a look at the elements of scripturalist tradition.

Interpretive Traditions

A scripturalist community has, as a part of its culture, a mental library of interpretations. This important part of a scripturalist tradition is its interpretive tradition—that is, the entire set of interpretations passed down *as* interpretations. A community's interpretive tradition is the set of traditional interpretations known by any member of the community. The entirely mental library need not—in fact, cannot—be shared by all community members: there will always be individual variations, but what members do share is the expectation that some sets of traditional interpretations are shared, and a respect for a common authority.

Vitally, not all interpretations are the result of an interpretive process, of *any* actual reading of the scripture. One interpretation I observed being drawn in a Sunday school class was a proposition originally deduced from theological argumentation and only later—centuries later—attributed to Bible passages. In this case, the interpretive tradition was passing on, not the product of any interpretive process, but a rationalization for a proposition already established on other grounds. (I have occasionally heard Christian scholars refer to such rationalizations as *eisagesis*—"reading into"—the opposite of exegesis.) In my lifetime I have seen many trends in belief or practice—most impressively, aerobics and recycling—come to be attributed to the Bible, as if they were authentic teachings somehow overlooked for millennia.

Interpretive Process

It has sometimes been assumed that scripturalists derive their interpretations from their interpretive processes, so that differences in beliefs and practices are explained by differences in the *methods* by which readers interpret a scripture. But as so often happens in social and psychological analysis, our intuitive understanding is backward.

If one simply sets, side by side, scripture texts and their alleged interpretations, it quickly becomes evident that no deductive process can possibly produce the latter from the former. Table 10.1 lists a few of the interpretations I observed among American evangelical Christians, along with the texts to which they were attributed at church events I witnessed.[2]

---

[2] Many interpretations are attributed to more than one passage, though seldom are all those passages supporting any particular idea marshaled together. Interestingly, the possibilities for interpreting a text

184 BRIAN MALLEY

Table 10.1. Some Bible interpretations

	Biblical attribution	Proposition
(1)	Thou shalt not kill.	We should not kill [people, except in self-defense or in military service].
(2)	Jesus cared for the poor.	We should care for the poor.
(3)	You should not eat meat sacrificed to idols if it causes your brother to stumble.	You should not drink alcohol if doing so angers a fellow Christian.

Consider the rules required to turn the Biblical texts into their observed interpretations.

1. Thou shalt not kill. → We should not kill [people, except in self-defense or in military service].

It is not difficult to see how one might take "Thou shalt not kill" and derive from it the belief "I should not kill." In the event I observed, the preacher interpreted this rule collectively, for himself and his audience, making it "We should not kill."

The only interpretive inference here is to assume that the reader is a member of the text's intended audience, a person addressed by the deictic "Thou." Yet readers do not keep the Sabbath, enjoined in a parallel way in the same passage.

2. Jesus cared for the poor. → We should care for the poor.

Here the text—Jesus cared for the poor— is a declaration, not an instruction. To conclude from this that "we should care for the poor" requires a background assumption along the lines of "we should do what Jesus did." Yet to introduce this background assumption creates many difficulties, because Christians do not in fact try to reproduce most of Jesus's actions.

3. You should not eat meat sacrificed to idols if it causes your brother to stumble. → You should not drink alcohol if doing so angers a fellow Christian.

The third example introduces the kinds of metaphor that are so important in scripturalist interpretation. Here the problem is that any interpretive process capable of these transformations must also generate many other, equally imaginative interpretations, presumably from even the most prosaic passages. To be sure, there are many imaginative interpretations in the history of Christianity and other scripturalist traditions,

are never foreclosed: any given interpretation can *always* be supported by some other passage, if some connection can be established.

but it is hard to see how any process sufficiently flexible to generate them could generate *only* the imaginative interpretations we actually find. If these are regular outputs of some inferential process, how can it fail to produce many tens of thousands more bizarre interpretations?

These examples illustrate the general problem. It has never been shown, for any scripturalist tradition, that texts and their purported interpretations are related in any systematic manner. At most, researchers have found that in some communities there are hermeneutic prescriptions and that these are sometimes followed. But claims to the effect that sizable communities are really using prescribed interpretive processes for reading scripture have little empirical support. Any prescribed hermeneutic, or regular interpretive process, would be far too restrictive for life in a scripturalist community.

One might reasonably ask whether scripturalist communities are really engaged in the interpretation of scripture-texts at all. Scripturalists certainly read their scriptures, and are eager to connect them to their lives. But instead of interpretation, what we see is the *practice of scriptural authority*.

The Practice of Scriptural Authority

The practice of scriptural authority is the logical and rhetorical grounding of belief and practice in scripture. It requires the establishment of *transitivity* between a scripture-text and the thought-world of community members. It is by transitivity that the normative authority of scripture is extended to people's beliefs and practices.

What Bible readers actually do in reading the Bible is to search for relevant connections between the Biblical text and their beliefs or behaviors (cf. Bielo, 2009). It is this goal—not the "meaning" of the text, but a relevant connection to it—that structures their actual practice of Bible reading. The limits of attention being what they are, the only ways to establish such a connection—in literature, in preaching, in discussion, even in personal reading—is to constrain one side of the search or the other: to proceed either from some delimited scripture-text to life or from some delimited part of life to the scripture-text. Each direction has its own assumptions and requirements.

The Textual Study

The purpose of a textual study is to establish the relevance of some scripture-text to the lives of community members. In the community I studied, this process often began with the selection of a scripture-text for reading or study.

In the group Bible studies I observed, participants took turns making interpretive proposals—a particular reading of the scriptural passage and a suggested take-away from it—for others to consider. Participants would begin by reading a portion of the text aloud, adding intonation and stress in accord with their proposed understanding, and possibly drawing on textual alternatives (from the margin) or translation alternatives (from other Bible versions) for variants. These variants were understood not as true alternatives—disjunctive sets from which a single reading must be selected—but rather as *sets of optional renderings* of different phrases, from which any combination of selections could constitute the scripture text under discussion. Even when only one Bible text is considered, different readings are afforded by the semantic range of specific words and the ambiguities of grammatical form. Most texts can be read in a variety of ways, and scripturalist traditions have often made use of this flexibility.

The presentation of a proposed reading is often followed by discussion involving two types of consideration: (a) comparison with other Biblical texts or doctrines and (b) anecdotes from the media or participants' experiences to illustrate its practicability. Comparison with other Biblical passages or doctrines results from an implicit expectation of rationality: consistency is support; inconsistency, an objection. Practicality seems a weaker consideration but one that is nevertheless perceived as relevant. Ideally—and in fact, most of the time—the discussion concludes with one or two points of relevant connection between the scripture-text and the issues that are important to readers. Such issues form the point of departure for a topical study.

The Topical Study

The purpose of a topical study is to establish a relevant connection between some concern in the lives of community members and any scripture-text. The structure and dynamics of topical studies are most manifest when the studies are carried out by groups.

Among evangelical Christians, topical studies begin with the suggestion of a topic or issue, and Bible study or Sunday school–class participants are invited to consider what the Bible might have to say about the topic. Significantly, the whole of the Bible is considered potentially relevant to any topic. There is no a priori restriction on the passages that might be relevant to a general topic, and the assumption is that the Bible speaks to almost any modern topic consistently throughout. Neither is there any restriction on the kind of connection that might be drawn between a text and a topic: a coincidence of vocabulary, thematic relevance, analogy of situation, generality of principle—any type of connection may be cited.

As the discussion begins, individual participants suggest a variety of scripture passages: each proposal involves a particular Biblical text and some indication of its relevance to the topic at hand. Once an interpretive proposal is made, other participants may take it up—or not—depending on the implication for the topic at hand. The same criteria—consistency with other Bible passages or doctrines, practicality of the implication—are adduced in favor of or against the suggested connection. In such contexts, participant-proposed biblical connections are seldom rejected on the grounds of the Biblical text's context, or because the passage is addressing some other topic. Ideally, the topical study concludes with "applications" of a variety of scripture-texts to the subject of interest.

Transitivity

What often gets described as scriptural interpretation is really a *search* process, and one guided not by interpretation—discovery of the text's "meaning"—but by the logical and practical requirements of connecting scripture to life.

Whether it begins with the text or a life concern, the interpretive process is a concurrent search through two fields: possible readings of scripture-texts and permissible implications for real life. It is driven by relevance, the same as the rest of our communicative efforts (Sperber & Wilson, 1995). Presented with an authoritative text, readers naturally—intuitively—look for its semantic relevance to their lives. It is for this reason that scripture interpretation can be carried out without any special instruction as to its procedure: it is just regular reading. Among less literate people, other types of relevance—such as the potential efficacy of scripture-artifacts for healing—may have seemed equally obvious.

The object of the search is the establishment of transitivity between scripture and life, such that a reading is connected to a socially acceptable course of action. To establish a connection between the text and one's life, one need only find some link—*any* link: verbal, logical, analogical, whatever—between the text and an issue or concern (actual or potential) in one's life. The major constraint is not on the link to scripture but on its implications.[3]

Interpretive proposals face tacit expectations about the kinds of things the scripture might enjoin. In the community I studied, suggested implications, to be plausible, were expected to be prosocial and polite, to affirm traditional beliefs, and to not ask anything obviously impractical or, in fact, seriously threatening to a middle-class American way of life. Proposed implications that ran counter to acceptable behavior were rejected. The most common response (in social settings, anyway) was simply to ignore the offending suggestion: it was met with silence, and after a moment's pause the discussion moved on.

Transitivity is the legitimization that results from relevant connections with acceptable implications. It is the logical basis of authority, extending the authority of a scripture to a specific idea or action. Once accepted, the belief or action is established as a "teaching" of the scripture—and added to the interpretive tradition. Ultimately, it is transitivity that makes scripturalism work, because it enables a scripture's authority to be extended far beyond its literal contents. It enables scriptures to be relevant in situations quite different from those for which they were originally intended, and is, I think, one of the features that has made the historical proliferation of scripturalist traditions possible.

---

[3] It is the constraint of acceptable implications that ultimately prevents any widespread use of prescribed hermeneutics. For people to adhere to prescribed hermeneutics, they would have to (a) reject otherwise acceptable interpretations simply on methodological grounds—something I have occasionally seen in written works but never in normal social interaction—and (b) adopt socially unacceptable interpretations simply because they were generated by the prescribed hermeneutic. The same considerations, I suggest, make it unlikely that any large community will rely upon an interpretive process more determinate than a search.

CONCLUSION

With the invention of writing came history, and historical time is largely a story of the increasing inscription of human communication: receipts, contracts, records, stories, missives, declarations, constitutions, and websites. Even death has a certificate. In a broad sense, scripturalism might be understood as the notion that one can organize a community around an authoritative text. In this perspective, the history of religious and many other kinds of communities have increasingly gravitated toward this structure. Why? Three factors, I suggest, make scripturalism an especially successful form of culture.

First and foremost, people seem to have difficulty recognizing the implications of textual authority. To propose the appointment of (or consent to) an authoritative person immediately raises an alarm, fears of what that person might do with that authority. In comparison, a text seems innocuous. It would seem there could be no hidden motive, no secret agenda, for all that it says is known in advance. The attribution of authority to a text thus appears neutral. Indeed, the potential to read a text in various ways means that it is often easier for interested parties to agree on particular verbiage than a particular idea or proposition. This is evident in the wrangling about verbiage that is the specialty of legal experts and speech writers. Textual authority does not set off the same cognitive and emotional red flags as does human authority, and people seem to agree more readily to textual authority than to human authority.

A second advantage of textual authority is the perceived longevity of the text. A text long in use gives the impression of institutional continuity and consistency, tending to hallow it with ancestral authority. The ongoing relevance of such a text can then be seen as an indication of its divine origin or eternal nature. The ongoing relevance of an ancient text creates a powerful rhetorical appeal.

But this perceived longevity also has a functional importance. Adaptability, whether of an organism or institution, requires rigidity *and* flexibility. For an organization to adapt, it must change but still remain itself. Some part of it must be conserved, to serve as a frame on which the changes may hinge. When what must be conserved is a community's sense of identity, continuity perceived is continuity achieved. Thus the apparent conservation of texts is, in fact, an important part of a scripturalist tradition.

The actual conservation of the text is much less important than the perceived conservation, and in fact, between the text-concept and the text-artifacts that constitute its extension there can be some flexibility, as in the case of the Bible. Conservation of the principle of scriptural authority can serve as the frame within which the practice of scriptural authority permits extensive adaptability to different times and circumstances. The text and its authority thus seem part of a long-standing tradition, even as the actual implications of that scriptural authority are highly adaptable.

This adaptability is, I suggest, an important consideration in understanding the proliferation of scripturalist traditions. Although the story of the Bible is often told as one continuous, widespread tradition, its history has always been one of local communities adapting their particular brand of Biblicism to their local circumstances. What the many communities really share is the Biblicist framework for adaptation: the Bible remains authoritative (in principle), while (in practice) its implications for readers' lives are changed to fit local circumstances.

Finally, one must not forget that scriptures can be a tremendously powerful aid to individual reflection and maturation. Regardless of how it comes about, the attempt to articulate the observations, warnings, and instructions of an alien text with one's own particular circumstances and perspective is likely to generate inferences that, precisely because they take one's mind in new directions, become useful tools of reflection. Comparing an alien perspective with one's own is almost bound to lead to new observations and insights.

And in the main, scriptures are genuinely great literature. In considering the power of the institutional processes described here, I often asked myself whether an old-fashioned phone directory might not, in some way, come to serve as a scripture. I think not. I think the scriptural texts that we see today are works of genuine quality in their own right, and their influence is due not only to the institutions that adopt them but also to their own literary excellencies.

QUESTIONS FOR FURTHER RESEARCH

1. Do participants in scripturalist communities intuit that their communities are characterized by recognition of scriptural authority?
2. Are there any clear cases of a community acting on the basis of scriptural authority when all other considerations—practical, social, ethical—are against it?
3. When considering variants or potential variants in stories of their scripture's origin, do scripturalists consider variations bearing on scriptural distinctiveness more important than other types of variations?
4. Are performances of scriptures more different from performances of nonscriptures than performances of nonscriptures are from one another?
5. Do scripturalists consider their scripture more distinct from other literary works than those other works are from one another?
6. Do scripturalist communities have mechanisms for resolving the cognitive dissonance caused when readers discover that what the scripture says differs from what the community normatively practices?
7. In scripturalist communities where a scripture-artifact is officially (doctrinally) regarded as just an artifact, are participants nonetheless more susceptible to suggestions that the scripture-artifact is indeed special than they are to suggestions that other text-artifacts are special?

REFERENCES

Bateson, G. (1979). *Mind and nature: A necessary unity.* New York: Dutton.
Bielo, J. S. (2009). *Words upon the Word: An ethnography of evangelical group Bible study.* New York: New York University Press.

Fieser, J., & Powers, J. (1998). *Scriptures of the world's religions*. Boston: McGraw Hill.

Floridi, L. (2011). *The philosophy of information*. Oxford: Oxford University Press.

Geertz, C. (1972). Deep play: Notes on the Balinese cockfight. *Daedalus, 101*(1), 1–37.

Geertz, C. (1973). *The interpretation of cultures*. New York: Basic Books.

Gregor, W. (1881). *Notes on the folk-lore of the north-east of Scotland*. London: Pub. for the Folk-lore society by E. Stock.

Hayward, L. H. (1938). Shropshire folklore of yesterday and to-day. *Folklore, 49*(3), 223–243.

Keller, E. (2005). *The road to clarity: Seventh-Day Adventism in Madagascar*. New York: Palgrave Macmillan.

Lawson, E. T., & McCauley, R. N. (1990). *Rethinking religion: Connecting cognition and culture*. Cambridge, UK: Cambridge University Press.

Levering, M. (1989). Rethinking scripture. In M. Levering (Ed.), *Rethinking scripture: Essays from a comparative* perspective (pp. 1–17).. Albany: State University of New York.

Malley, B. (2004). *How the Bible works: An anthropological study of evangelical Biblicism*. Walnut Creek, CA: AltaMira Press.

Malley, B. (2006). The Bible in British folklore. *Postscripts, 2*(2–3), 241–272.

Malley, B. (2011). Biblical authority: A social scientist's perspective. In C. Bovell (Ed.), *Interdisciplinary perspectives on the authority of scripture: Historical, Biblical, and theoretical perspectives* (pp. 303–322). Eugene, OR: Pickwick.

Malley, B. (2015). The Bible in North American folklore. In V. L. Wimbush (Ed.), *Scripturalizing the human: The written as the political* (pp. 34–77). New York: Routledge.

McCauley, R. N., & Lawson, E. T. (2002). *Bringing ritual to mind: Psychological foundations of cultural forms*. Cambridge, UK: Cambridge University Press.

Owen, E. (1896). *Welsh folk-lore: A collection of the folk-tales and legends of North Wales; being the prize essay of the national Eisteddfod, 1887*. Oswestry and Wrexham, UK: Woodall.

Rappaport, R. A. (1999). *Ritual and religion in the making of humanity*. Cambridge, UK: Cambridge University Press.

Ricoeur, P. (1971). The model of the text: Meaningful action considered as a text. *Social Research, 38*, 529–562.

Shannon, C. E., & Weaver, W. (1948). *The mathematical theory of communication*. Urbana: University of Illinois Press.

Silverstein, M., & Urban, G. (1996). The natural history of discourse. In M. Silverstein & G. Urban (Eds.), *Natural histories of discourse* (pp. 1–20).. Chicago: University of Chicago Press.

Smith, W. C. (1993). *What is scripture? A comparative approach*. Minneapolis, MN: Fortress Press.

Sperber, D. (1975). *Rethinking symbolism* (A. L. Morton, Trans.). Cambridge, UK: Cambridge University Press.

Sperber, D. (1985). *On anthropological knowledge: Three essays*. Cambridge, UK: Cambridge University Press.

Sperber, D. (1996). *Explaining culture: A naturalistic approach*. Oxford: Blackwell.

Sperber, D., & Wilson, D. (1995). *Relevance: Communication and cognition* (2nd ed.). Oxford: Blackwell.

Wilson, A. (1991). *World scripture: A comparative anthology of sacred texts*. New York: Paragon House.

Winternitz, M., & Müller, F. M. (1879–1910). *Sacred books of the East*. Oxford: Clarendon Press.

CHAPTER 11

SPECIAL OBJECTS

TYLER S. GREENWAY

INTRODUCTION

HOLY water and the Eucharist are both considered special objects in the Orthodox Christian tradition. Orthodox priests treat both with special care, and both possess special properties, but the way priests use holy water is different from their use of the wine and bread of the Eucharist. A priest may throw holy water on members of the church, but a priest would never throw the wine of the Eucharist on members. In fact, items that touch the bread and wine, such as the chalice that holds the wine and the plate that holds the bread, also become sacred and cannot be used for any other purposes. If the chalice or plate falls on a rug or touches an article of clothing, the item it touched must be burned. Other items near the chalice or plate become sacred, even if they do not come in contact with the chalice or plate. The Eucharist requires additional special objects, such as an altar, which is typically consecrated along with the church building, and an antimension, a cloth blessed by a bishop and containing a relic. The same is not true for holy water.

People across cultures and religious traditions maintain beliefs about certain objects they consider sacred or special. They treat these objects differently than other objects, though they may look the same and function similarly. A sacred text may look like an ordinary book, but it is treated with a care not given to other books. Likewise, holy water is only used in special circumstances and is not handled in the same way as ordinary water.

Why? What makes these objects special, and why are they treated differently from the ordinary objects they may resemble? Some objects are special simply because they have been special for hundreds or thousands of years—the history of an object designates that it be treated differently than other objects. Other objects are special because a group of people considers them to be; social pressures dictate that they be treated with special care, and such care is provided as long as the group maintains such beliefs. Historical or social factors are certainly important for understanding why some objects are special and others are ordinary, but what if other factors can also predict—or better predict—the likelihood that an object will be regarded as special? Can cognitive science identify variables that predict whether an object will be considered special or how special objects will be treated differently than ordinary objects? If so, what are the implications? Can we identify pancultural patterns based on natural cognition and cultural deviations from these patterns?

This chapter considers the existing research addressing the cognitive processes that surround special objects by exploring answers to three questions: (a) what are special objects, (b) where do special objects come from, and (c) what do special objects do? The empirical research investigating answers to these questions is limited. The chapter provides a summary of the available research, connects it to findings from related areas of the cognitive science of religion (CSR), and suggests avenues for future empirical inquiry.[1]

WHAT ARE SPECIAL OBJECTS?

Special objects require definition. What is—and just as importantly, what is not—a special object? A broad overview of religions reveals several possibilities. A gold statue, made to resemble a divine being, signifying or embodying the presence of a god, worshiped by many, and cared for by a religious leader seems a likely candidate. But what made that object—the gold form itself—special, and could it lose its special qualities, becoming ordinary or profane?

The specialness of other objects is less clear. What about the temple housing this idol? What about the surrounding area—the temple grounds, special lakes or pools, or other landmarks—to which pilgrims travel to offer sacrifices and collect relics? What about those sacrifices or relics and the texts that specify how religious followers should conduct these activities? Are all copies of this text special or only those connected to a specific leader? Do religious leaders need to perform special actions to make objects special, or is contact with the leader sufficient? What about the ordinary objects used in special religious rituals? When, if at all, do these objects become special? There are several possible answers to these questions. The next section (see "Objects and Agents") seeks to answer them by defining and examining special objects; it begins by examining the cognition used to distinguish "objects" from "agents."

Importantly, this chapter approaches these questions using insights from the CSR. Although the history of an object and the social or cultural beliefs surrounding it are important and influence how it is treated, the present chapter considers how cognition may

---

[1] The concern throughout the chapter is not whether the objects in question in fact possess special ontological status, but whether they are conceptualized and treated as if they do. Thus, when I consider why, how, and when objects are deemed special, I mean from the perspective of believers, but for the sake of linguistic economy I do not include such qualifiers.

inform and constrain beliefs about special objects. This approach is based on the work of scholars who argue that the developmentally natural cognitive architecture of the human mind results in the formation of certain beliefs or types of beliefs across cultures (e.g., Sperber & Hirschfeld, 2004; Barrett, 2011; Boyer, 2001; McCauley, 2011). Certain aspects of this cognition produce patterns across religious traditions that are revealed in beliefs about supernatural beings, rituals, the origins of the universe, death, the afterlife, and—perhaps also—special objects. In particular, this chapter (see "Ordinary and Special Objects") considers (a) objects with counterintuitive properties and (b) objects with counterschematic causal effects as two means of distinguishing ordinary and special objects.

Objects and Agents

Before we can distinguish ordinary objects from special objects, we need to clarify three things: (a) the distinction between objects and nonobjects—namely, agents; (b) the means by which humans make this distinction; and (c) the implications of this distinction.

Identifying objects is typically simple: objects lack agency. They cannot act or do anything by themselves and require an agent or outside force to move or change them. Objects also respond to movement or action mechanistically (e.g., a thrown ball will follow a predictable trajectory). Agents, by contrast, are able to move with intentionality and can therefore act upon objects (Greenway & Barrett, 2017). A coffee mug is an object, as is the coffee inside the mug. Neither the coffee nor the mug can move unless they are acted upon by an agent. The adult drinking the coffee or the child tipping the mug over are both agents, acting upon these objects in accordance with their own goals or desires.[2]

The distinction between objects and agents may seem trivial, but the capacity to make the distinction is important for everyday life and even for survival. Crying out to a tree for help makes little sense and fails to bring aid, but identifying an agent that can respond to cries for help may bring some assistance. Children begin to distinguish objects from agents in the first year of life (Spelke et al., 1995), and they interact with agents and objects differently (Legerstee, 1994). This foundational ability helps children interact with agents that will secure necessities for them (e.g., my mother can bring me my cereal), instead of endlessly coaxing objects that will fail to respond (e.g., the bowl holding

---

[2] I recognize another distinction between bounded objects (e.g., coffee mugs and other solid objects), masses of substances (e.g., coffee and other liquids), and unbounded, nonagential, object-like substances (e.g., flames, waves, shadows). These three types share certain properties in that they are nonagential; but they are also distinct: they do not move in bounded wholes, may pass through solid objects, and so forth. In this chapter, I focus on bounded objects rather than substances or unbounded object-like things, both for the sake of simplicity and because previous research (e.g., Barrett, 2008) has primarily focused on bounded objects.

my cereal will not move toward me on its own, no matter how much I yell). Lawson and McCauley (1990) describe this capacity to distinguish objects and agents as "the object agency filter" (p. 98).

Beyond this object-agent dichotomy, Barrett (2008) draws on cognitive developmental psychology to identify five tacit ontological categories that it appears humans use to generate inferences about different sorts of things: SPATIAL ENTITIES, SOLID OBJECTS, LIVING THINGS, ANIMATES, and PERSONS.[3] These cognitively intuitive ontological categories allegedly emerge from the differential activation of six intuitive expectation sets: universals, spatiality, physicality, biology, animacy, and mentality. Expectation sets typically build upon one another so that knowledge from more basic expectation sets carries forward.[4]

Though both objects and agents share several properties (e.g., both occupy a spatial and temporal location), the placement in an ontological category triggers additional knowledge derived from these expectation sets (Barrett, 2008). For instance, SPATIAL ENTITIES are understood to occupy a specific place in time and space, but if something is identified as a SOLID OBJECT, additional knowledge is typically also inferred (e.g., cohesion, continuity, tangibility). The same is true of LIVING THINGS, ANIMATES, and PERSONS. If something is identified as an ANIMATE, certain beliefs shared with SPATIAL ENTITIES, SOLID OBJECTS, and LIVING THINGS are typically still inferred (e.g., consistency, cohesion, tangibility, growth, and development) but additional knowledge specific to ANIMATES is also inferred: ANIMATES are self-propelled and act according to goals. If something is identified as a PERSON, all knowledge related to SPATIAL ENTITIES, SOLID OBJECTS, LIVING THINGS, and ANIMATES is inferred and additional knowledge is also added—namely, mentality: the belief that persons are self-aware and possess representational mental states (Barrett, 2008). For the purposes of distinguishing between objects and agents, all SPATIAL ENTITIES, SOLID OBJECTS, and LIVING THINGS (i.e., those ontological categories that lack agential qualities) may be considered objects, and all ANIMATES and PERSONS (i.e., those ontological categories that possess agential qualities) may be considered agents.

Though identifying objects and agents is typically simple and done without conscious effort, the correct identification may at times be difficult, particularly when individuals are under stress or required to make quick decisions. Computers, phones, vending machines, and other electronic objects are often treated as agents (e.g., a frustrated office worker may ask a computer, "Why are you doing this to me today?"), and agents may sometimes be treated as objects (e.g., an impatient or rushed person may shove people or animals aside as if they were objects; Greenway & Barrett 2017).

---

[3] Following Barrett, I am using capital letters to identify ontological categories and to distinguish them from expectation sets. These ontological categories are not meant to be exhaustive. Similar earlier work suggesting both intuitive cognitive domains similar to Barrett's "expectation sets" and tacit ontologies can be found in Keil (1979), Boyer (1994), and Sperber et al. (1995).

[4] Barrett (2008) notes some exceptions to this progression, which are often associated with mentality and animacy.

The distinction between objects and agents may be even more difficult in religious settings when various objects seem to possess agential qualities. Most trees, which fall within the LIVING THINGS ontological category, are considered objects (they do not act according to their own will, are not self-propelled, etc.).[5] However, some trees seem to possess special qualities: sacrifices are presented to the tree (Dafni, 2007), fruit eaten from the tree results in special knowledge (e.g., the tree of the knowledge of good and evil; Genesis 2–3), or branches of the tree are important for special rituals (e.g., sakaki tree branches in the Shinto religion). Are these trees still objects, or are they agents? The following sections build upon the distinction between objects, which typically lack agency, and agents, who are able to act according to their will, by considering another distinction: the difference between ordinary objects and special objects.

Ordinary and Special Objects

If objects are distinguished from agents by their lack of agency, how, then, are special objects distinguished from ordinary objects? How do religious practitioners come to recognize that some statues or containers of water are different than others? Several possible cognitive pathways to such a distinction may exist. Religions traditions may record that some objects were created directly by supernatural action. Other objects may result from rituals. Still other objects may come in contact with a special agent and take on some of the agent's properties.

Each of these types of objects may share a common quality in that they deviate from the properties of ordinary objects in some way. Holy water is different from ordinary water because holy water is thought to have special properties. The Black Stone located inside the Kaaba is different from other stones because it, too, is thought to have special properties. How may cognitive science help identify when properties are special and when they are ordinary?

Counterintuitiveness. One useful means by which such special properties may be identified is by attending to any properties it possesses that are cognitively intuitive and counterintuitive.[6] Ordinary objects are believed to possess certain

---

[5] Some readers may take issue with the inclusion of the LIVING THINGS ontological category in this definition of special objects. A separate category may certainly be considered and utilized (perhaps designated *special living things*), such that special trees and other plants may have their own category, but for the purposes of this chapter, SPATIAL ENTITIES, SOLID OBJECTS, and LIVING THINGS will be considered together. In other words, this distinction between special objects and supernatural agents hinges on whether or not the ontological category ordinarily possesses agency.

[6] Here "counterintuitive" is used as a technical term: counterintuitive concepts violate one or more domain-specific intuitive assumptions. These intuitive assumptions are tied to the aforementioned ontological categories and intuitive expectation sets (sometimes referred to as *template-level cognition*), and differ from schema-level cognition, which is built on personal experience. By this definition, an invisible rabbit is counterintuitive because it violates intuitive assumptions about visibility. A 600-pound rabbit, though remarkable and surprising, is counterschematic but not counterintuitive because it

qualities: they occupy a specific location in time and space; they cohere and move by contact consistently; and they are solid, tangible, and visible (Barrett, 2008). Special objects, by contrast, may be understood to violate one or more of these expected beliefs (Sørensen, 2005b). A rock that remains still until it is acted upon by an agent, continues to move along a predictable trajectory when acted upon, cannot pass through walls, and is readily visible is just an ordinary object—there is nothing special about it. But a rock that moves itself (a property of ANIMATES), speaks (a property of PERSONS), or is invisible (has lost a property associated with SOLID OBJECTS) is certainly not ordinary. But if possessing counterintuitive properties increases the likelihood that objects are identified as special within religious traditions, it does not follow that objects with counterintuitive properties are necessarily so identified. Gregory et al. (2019) note that counterintuitive concepts may be common (helium-filled balloons, magnets) or popular in culture (e.g., Mickey Mouse) though not religious.

A definition of special objects that incorporates counterintuitive properties is not entirely novel; it relates to the definition of supernatural agents—otherwise termed "gods"—that is common to the CSR. Boyer (2001) and Barrett (2011) argue that these agents are counterintuitive in that they violate domain-specific knowledge concerning agents. Invisible elves (e.g., the *huldufólk* of Iceland) may be considered supernatural agents in part because they violate intuitive assumptions concerning physicality. An omniscient person may be considered supernatural because he or she violates intuitive assumptions concerning the limitations of human mentality. These agents are considered supernatural because they do not conform to the knowledge expected of their ontological category. Special objects violate their own domain-specific knowledge. A phone booth that can travel in time or be in more than one place at a time may be considered special because it violates intuitive assumptions concerning its spatiality. A hat that has the power to read minds and speak to the wearer violates assumptions concerning mentality. Both objects, though different in their abilities, may be considered special because they violate the knowledge intuitively expected of their ontological category.

Counterschematic causal effects. Another useful means by which special properties may be identified is to attend to special causal effects or powers. Holy water may not be counterintuitive in the technical sense: it does not violate a domain-specific intuitive assumption. Holy water maintains the normal ontological properties expected of water. Holy water is, however, believed to possess the ability to produce special or nontypical effects; it violates schematic knowledge (knowledge based on personal experience) concerning its causal effects. Normal water may produce certain effects (cleansing, hydration), but holy water confers blessings. Holy oil, special clothing, and relics may all fall into this category of special objects.

---

only violates schema-level knowledge based on typical experience with rabbits, and not template-level knowledge based on a rabbit's ontological category (LIVING THING; Gregory et al., 2019).

Beyond only identifying counterintuitive properties that violate domain-specific knowledge related to an object's ontology, special counterschematic causal properties may also be important for distinguishing ordinary objects and special objects. The normal effects resulting from coming into contact with or ingesting water, oil, or bread are well understood, but the effects of holy water, holy oil, or the Eucharist are thought to be different. Objects may also be considered special because they are both counterintuitive and possess counterschematic causal effects. A weeping or bleeding icon is one example. Icons are thought to produce certain counterschematic causal effects (they can produce miracles, or have a property that is not typical of other objects that appear similar) and may also violate intuitive ontological properties (some icons weep or bleed, which are both counterintuitive properties of objects).

Special Objects and Special Agents

It is also necessary to go beyond these initial distinctions. A rock that does not violate any intuitive expectations is just an ordinary rock; an invisible rock, a hungry rock, a walking rock, and a talking rock (SOLID OBJECTS exhibiting a breach of physicality and transfers of biology, animacy, and mentality, respectively) might all readily be considered special objects. But what about a rock that walks and talks, or a rock that walks, talks, and is also hungry (SOLID OBJECTS with two or three transfers)?[7] Are these rocks still best considered special objects, or would they be better considered supernatural agents?

These cases point to an important issue that requires clarification. How are objects that have agential qualities and agents that look or function as objects best categorized? One possible solution is to identify the ontological category in which something is typically classified. Special objects could be classified as such using the categories into which they would typically fall if they possessed no domain-specific intuitive-assumption violations (those categories that ordinarily lack agency: SPATIAL ENTITIES, SOLID OBJECTS, or LIVING THINGS). Another solution is to consider any counterintuitive object or being with any agential qualities a supernatural agent and any counterintuitive object or being without some agential qualities a special object. Accordingly, any transfer of mentality or animacy to SPATIAL ENTITIES, SOLID OBJECTS, or LIVING THINGS would render them supernatural agents, and any breaches of mentality or animacy that resulted in ANIMATES or PERSONS lacking some aspects of mentality or animacy would render them special objects.

Both of these solutions yield complications that require further clarity. The first solution will still result in hungry, walking, talking rocks that are labeled special objects

[7] A *transfer* refers to the addition of "properties from a 'non-native' set of intuitive expectations" (Barrett, 2008, p. 322). A *breach* refers to the absence of properties from a native set of intuitive expectations.

though they may be intuitively treated as supernatural agents. The second solution will result in moving rocks that are labeled supernatural agents though they may be intuitively treated as special objects (depending on the nature of their movement). Given these problems, another solution is needed. Concerning mental representations of counterintuitive objects and agents, Barrett (2008) describes a "Simplicity Principle," arguing that human minds tend to represent counterintuitive concepts in their simplest form. An invisible rock or a talking cat are simply understood as an object and an agent that each possess a counterintuitive property (i.e., a domain-specific intuitive-assumption violation). When additional counterintuitive properties are added, however, it may be simpler to represent these objects and agents differently. The hungry, walking, talking rock, for instance, might be better considered a PERSON with a biology breach (an agent composed of rock). Similarly, using the simplicity principle, a bronze statue that can move on its own, is self-aware, can speak, and has mental states may be better understood as a PERSON made of bronze (one breach of an intuitive assumption) than a SOLID OBJECT with a transfer of animacy and several transfers of mentality. If that bronze statue could not move and did not speak, however, it may still be best considered a SOLID OBJECT with two transfers of mentality.[8]

Still, further clarification is required for objects such as magnets or helium-filled balloons. These objects are not typically considered special in that most people in the modern world understand the natural, physical properties that enable magnets to attract metals and balloons to float. However, using the aforementioned distinction between ordinary and special objects, these objects would still be considered special in that they are most simply represented as SOLID OBJECTS that violate a domain-specific intuitive assumption. These and similar natural objects motivate some modification of this definition to incorporate beliefs about them. There is precedent for including reflective beliefs in such definitions. As mentioned previously, Barrett's (2011) definition of supernatural agents or gods specifies that such agents are counterintuitive, but his definition also specifies that the term "gods" refers to beings

> that a group of people reflectively believes exists; that have a type of existence or action (past, presence, or future) that can in principle, be detected by people; and whose existence motivates some differences in human behavior as a consequence. (p. 96)

This definition highlights the importance of belief in and reaction to gods or supernatural agents. In this sense, magnets or balloons are not special objects because their existence does not motivate nonnatural differences in behavior. In their discussion of

---

[8] Further empirical work may help to identify how many or what type of expectation-set violations motivate a shift in thinking and behavior (i.e., what agential qualities motivate thinking of an object as an agent).

religious rituals, Barrett and Lawson (2001) similarly emphasized that "religious rituals are also a particular type of action. In such representations someone does something to someone in order to bring about some non-natural consequence" (p. 184). These authors emphasize that religious beings and religious rituals are distinct from ordinary agents and actions in that they are believed to have the capacity to effect nonnatural change. Accordingly, a definition of special objects should emphasize similar beliefs and reactions. Akin to Barrett's (2011) definition of gods, we may thus define special objects as objects that

- are most simply represented as SPATIAL ENTITIES, SOLID OBJECTS, and LIVING THINGS (using the simplicity principle);
- are (1) counterintuitive (i.e., violate a domain-specific intuitive assumption), or (2) possess counterschematic causal properties;
- are reflectively believed to exist by a group of people;
- have a type of existence or action (past, present, or future) that is, in principle, detectable by people; and
- whose existence motivates some differences in human behavior as a consequence.

It should also be stated here that this definition of special objects focuses on intuitive notions concerning these objects, and not on beliefs supported by the high degrees of cultural scaffolding often found in theological works. In other words, a special object that is intuitively treated as an object will still be considered a special object, even if religious experts have written about it and argued that it is, in fact, an agent. This position aligns with the limitations and focus of cognitive science and religion.

Types of Special Objects

The nature of a special object's counterintuitiveness—the assumptions that are missing from or added to the typical ontological category—may also bear important implications for representations of and interactions with special objects. For example, an invisible tree will be treated much differently than a tree that provides instructions and predicts the future (e.g., the burning bush of Exodus 3).[9] Special medicine that heals regardless of the user's intent will be treated much differently than special medicine that causes harm to the user if the user's intentions are malicious (Sørensen, 2005b). Here a distinction between two types of special objects may be helpful. *Agential* special objects

---

[9] Invisible and intangible objects (non-agents) are not of primary concern in this chapter. Generally, such objects are absent or marginal in the religious beliefs and practices of people across traditions for good reason: if you cannot see an object or feel an object, you do not know where it is, and you cannot easily use it in rituals or as an object of devotion.

are those SPATIAL ENTITIES, SOLID OBJECTS, or LIVING THINGS that are counterintuitive in part or whole due to a transfer of animacy or mentality. *Nonagential* special objects are those SPATIAL ENTITIES, SOLID OBJECTS, or LIVING THINGS that are counterintuitive due solely to a breach of their intuitive assumptions or a transfer of nonagential qualities, or that are not counterintuitive but are still considered special because they possess counterschematic causal effects.

Special objects that possess some agency (keeping in mind that too many transfers of agential qualities may make them better considered supernatural agents) may be used in particular aspects of rituals, whereas special objects that lack agency may be restricted to other aspects of rituals. Lawson and McCauley (1990) note: "Those entities which are incapable of agency from the perspective of common sense, but which are, within the framework of a religion's conceptual system, capable of ritual agency, are categorized before the operation of the action representation system as (ritual) agents" (p. 102). More specifically, it may be that special objects that possess some agency function most often as patients in rituals, whereas special objects that lack agency may function most often as instruments in rituals. Importantly, Lawson and McCauley (1990) note that

> unless an object has already undergone the necessary ritual alteration investing it with agency, its presence in the agent's position will yield a structural description of inappropriate form that the object agency filter will either modify or eradicate. Without having earlier undergone this ritual transformation, ritual objects are no more capable of acting in ritual contexts than non-human entities are in the everyday world. (p. 104)

These agential special objects are not to be confused with nonagential objects or instruments (special or ordinary), even if these instruments are required within religious rituals (McCauley & Lawson, 2002).

Further empirical work is needed to determine which types of objects are most common in religious systems. Research investigating the mnemonic advantages of counterintuitive concepts found that minimally counterintuitive PERSON concepts were better remembered than other intuitive or counterintuitive concepts (Gregory et al., 2019). Given the enhanced memorability of counterintuitive PERSON concepts, agential special objects associated with certain agents may share similar mnemonic advantages, though further empirical work is required to confirm this hypothesis. Furthermore, agential special objects (e.g., special medicine that affects different changes based on the user's intent) may influence the morality or values of those interacting with the object in a way that nonagential special objects do not, although empirical investigation is required to confirm this hypothesis as well. Interestingly, the nature of the special object may very well be connected to how that object is generated. Agential special objects may require direct action by a god or ritual action by special agents, whereas simple contact with a special agent may result in the generation of nonagential special objects.

WHERE DO SPECIAL OBJECTS COME FROM?

Building on this definition of special objects leads us to another outstanding question, Where do special objects come from? More specifically, How do individuals within religious traditions believe these objects become special or acquire supernatural qualities? The next section ("Direct Supernatural Action") will consider three possible avenues of special-object generation: (a) direct action by a supernatural agent, (b) ritual action, and (c) contagion. These categories may overlap (e.g., ritual action can at times be considered direct supernatural action), and they may not be mutually exclusive (e.g., some objects are generated one way but are then affected by or changed in another way later), but they are distinct enough cognitively to merit independent consideration.

Direct Supernatural Action

The most direct means by which special objects are thought to take on supernatural qualities may be through the immediate action of a supernatural being. A supernatural agent, which is believed to possess supernatural abilities, may alter objects in important ways. For instance, the Black Stone of Kaaba, central to Islamic pilgrimages to Mecca, is thought to have fallen from the sky or been given directly by the angel Gabriel. The two stone tablets containing the law of the covenant, important to Judaism, are thought to have been written by the finger of God. The specialness of these objects may be considered the direct and unmediated result of a supernatural agent's action.

Accordingly, the special properties these objects possess may be considered the direct result of this supernatural action. It is believed, for example, that the Black Stone was originally white but has since turned black from absorbing the sins of those who touch it. If the stone's special quality is that it can atone for sins, then it may be considered special because of its unique causal effects. Objects do not typically absorb sins or other nonmaterial qualities, nor do they typically operate or act in the nonmaterial realm of mental states. The two tablets of stone, and the Ark of the Covenant that housed them, are also thought to possess unique causal power. According to tradition, individuals who touched or looked inside the Ark of the Covenant died.

The Black Stone and the Ark of the Covenant are examples of powerful special objects generated via direct supernatural action, and further work is needed to determine if they are considered more powerful than objects generated in other ways. McCauley and Lawson (2002) argue that the fewer the number of rituals required to connect an object or agent to a supernatural agent, the more central a ritual is to that tradition (for more discussion of their principle of superhuman immediacy, see the section "Power or Efficacy in Special Objects"). It may also be that the fewer the rituals required to connect an object to a supernatural agent, the more powerful that object is. If this is the case, direct supernatural action involves no rituals, and the objects are immediately connected to the agent and may, accordingly, be considered the most powerful. Further work is also needed to investigate intuitive beliefs concerning how these objects take on their special qualities, and the degree to which direct supernatural action is related to contagion as a means of generation (see "Contagion" section).

Ritual Action

A related means of generating special objects is via religious rituals. McCauley and Lawson (2002) outline their *ritual form hypothesis* in which they distinguish three categories of rituals: special agent rituals (SARs), special patient rituals (SPRs), and special instrument rituals (SIRs). Religious rituals typically involve an agent, an action (sometimes with an instrument), and a patient on which the agent is acting. The presence of a special supernatural agent determines the type of ritual (i.e., a SAR involves a supernatural agent acting as an agent; McCauley & Lawson, 2002).

To generate a special object (to change an ordinary object into something special), requires SARs or SIRs, because the patient—in this case an ordinary object—is being acted upon to instill in it certain counterintuitive qualities. Lawson and McCauley (1990) note two examples of such rituals. The first is the Hindu and Taoist "opening of the eyes" ritual. When a new statue is brought into a temple, the priests consecrate it and paint various features on it, including the eyes. It is believed that the statue possesses agency after the ritual is performed, and is capable of acting in subsequent rituals. A second ritual noted by Lawson and McCauley (1990) is the Vedic Agnyadhana ritual in which fire is made special. In this case, a priest ritually prepares a fire in such a way that Agni, a god, is represented in the fire. Both of these rituals are SARs in which a special agent (a priest) acts to change an ordinary object (a statue or fire) into an agential special object.

Rituals might also produce nonagential special objects. Holy water, blessed by a priest, is one example. A special agent—a priest—acts in such a way that ordinary water takes on a special property, the ability to bless others. Here again, a special agent is acting, but in this case a nonagential special object is generated. The action of the special agent is important—were it not for the agent's specialness, the water would remain ordinary (McCauley & Lawson, 2002). Special objects might also be generated via SIRs, in which an otherwise ordinary agent acts upon an otherwise ordinary object using a special instrument (e.g., holy water, a relic) to make that object special (see also the next section, "Contagion," for discussion of contagion as a means of generating special objects).

Further research is needed to determine whether special objects generated by ritual action are believed to be less powerful or efficacious than those generated by direct supernatural action. Because rituals involve prior enabling rituals (e.g., a priest is special because the church declared him special through ordination, and the church is special because Christ declared it so; see McCauley & Lawson, 2002, for embedding framework), they may be perceived as less directly connected to the supernatural agent whose special ability renders these objects special. Future research might also investigate the frequency by which special objects are thought to be generated via SARs and SIRs, and the frequency by which SIRs involve agential special objects or nonagential special objects. As with special objects generated by direct supernatural action, further work may investigate intuitive beliefs concerning how these objects take on their special qualities.

Contagion

A third means of generating special objects is via contagion. *Contagion* refers to the transfer of the essence or properties of one being or object to another being or object (Rozin et al., 1986), often through contact, though not necessarily (Kim & Kim, 2011; also see the section, "Means of Change," for a discussion of contagion as a means of bringing about change). When something special or supernatural touches an object or a place, the object or place may become special. Special objects generated in this way may in part be conflated with those generated by direct supernatural action or with SIRs in which an ordinary person uses a special instrument such as holy water to produce some supernatural effect. However, nonritual examples may also be envisioned. The prophet Elisha, important in Judaism, Christianity, and Islam, is believed to have been buried in a tomb in which another man was later placed. Upon touching Elisha's bones, the dead man was, reportedly, brought back to life (2 Kings 13:20–21). Similarly, objects that had been touched by the apostle Paul, central to Christianity, were reported to bring healing and drive out evil spirits (Acts 19:11–13). These examples portray no formalized or repeated ritual, but they do demonstrate supernatural change by which an object brings about healing via contagion. Vestments, special clothing worn by priests, and relics, such as the bones or clothing of saints, are examples of this type of special object. In Orthodox Christian churches, a relic may be sewn into an antimension or be sealed in the altar. The antimension and the altar are special in part because of their contact with the relics.

Nordin (2009) provides another example. He describes the collection of objects from pilgrimage sites, noting that one particularly important object was *jal*, or holy water:

> Most pilgrims believed in a "dosage effect" that meant *jal* could be diluted almost endlessly. *Jal* has miraculous qualities, such as preserving its purity and freshness while contained in bottles for fifty years and it has the power to make other things *pavitra* [sacred/pure] and pure. Keeping *jal* indoors purified the pilgrims' homes. Dropping *jal* on the lips of a family member at the moment of death and purifying the corpse with the liquid ensured a "good death." (p. 208)

Nordin's examples reveal special properties of *jal* (endless dilution and purity) and the power of contagion that special objects can have on both people and objects.

Here again, further empirical work is needed to understand the perceived efficacy of these objects compared to those directly generated by supernatural agents and those generated by rituals. Given their direct contact with special agents, these objects may be more powerful than objects created by rituals but perhaps less powerful than those created purposefully by supernatural agents due to the lack of intentionality. Further work is also needed to better understand the degree to which contagion effects are believed to occur in direct supernatural action and rituals. Indeed, it may be that contagion is central to the generation of all or a majority of special objects. A catalog of special objects and the means by which they were generated would aid such investigation. If such data exist, both the nature of the special object and its origin may be examined to determine the degree to which they are interrelated. Finally, further investigation is needed to better understand the circumstances in which contagion occurs. Does an object coming into contact with something believed to be supernatural always become a special object? (For example, do my shoes become special if I walk into a holy temple or spill holy water on them?) If this is not the case, further work may uncover the specific circumstances in which special objects or supernatural effects do and do not occur via contagion.

Interpretation of Origin and Agency

One further interpretative issue must be addressed. Many of the objects that become special instruments are believed to have the ability to act in some way, but as Nordin (2009) has noted, "It is an empirical question as to whether the people who use sacred instruments believe that divine agents act through these objects or whether the instrument itself is ascribed independent agency" (p. 205). The means by which nonagential special objects are thought to have acquired their special properties or by which they use their properties represent outstanding questions as well.

Several factors must be considered when addressing these questions, and the examination of agency is a principal one: Do the special qualities derived from an agent become independent of that agent, or do they remain connected to the agent in some way? Does the agent continue to act through the object? Several experiments may be envisioned. Participants may be asked whether the power of a special object is lost or diminished if the supernatural agent who generated the object dies. Participants may also be asked whether the special object can be used for purposes contrary to the will or desires of the generator of the object. Further investigation may address the degree to which answers to these questions vary across objects. Perhaps certain objects maintain more connection, or certain types of connection, to the supernatural agent than others, and perhaps the degree of connection is determined by the means of generation, the agent, or some other factor.

Further questions also remain concerning the difference between the theological accounts of an object's agency and lay accounts. It may be that religious experts maintain certain beliefs concerning these objects that differ from those of lay religious practitioners because they deviate from intuitive cognition (see Cohen, 2007, for example). Sørensen (2005a) notes a related concern about a distinction between notions of magic and religion:

> Some participants will represent objects as containing magical agency by virtue of their mere appearance in a ritual setting... This, of course, threatens a conceptual distinction between magic and religion based on types of rituals (i.e., whether or not their power is represented as stemming from a god, spirit, ancestor, or by necessity). It is, however, possible to maintain a distinction between magic and religion as different modes of interpretation (i.e., how people use and understand the rituals they participate in). (p. 176)

It may very well be that lay practitioners possess little knowledge of the agent who provided the special object, despite the knowledge possessed by religious experts or contained within religious texts. Accordingly, the interpretation of rituals may be influenced by the histories passed down by religious leaders. Further work is required to identify the degree to which lay religious practitioners understand these ritual histories and to which this understanding affects their perceptions of the rituals. If lay practitioners believe objects are simply magical and have no sense of the supernatural agent who generated them, does it affect the practitioner's perception of the objects in important ways? Additional anthropological work may help identify different special objects whose origins are known and unknown, and investigate how these objects are perceived.

Another outstanding question related to the origin of special objects concerns the frequency with which special objects are believed to be generated. Objects generated by contagion could, hypothetically, be created almost endlessly, whereas objects generated directly by supernatural agents may be much less common. To address this question, it might be helpful to have a broad database of the special objects present within various religious systems. Objects could be classified according to their means of generation to determine how often special objects are generated in various ways and whether other factors are related to their perceived origin.

Finally, the connection between the origins of special objects and the type of object they become is an important, open empirical question. Investigation across religious traditions might reveal that objects may only become agential special objects via direct supernatural action or by ritual (and perhaps only by SAR). Contagion, and perhaps direct supernatural action, which may be related to contagion, may primarily produce special objects with counterschematic causal effects. And further investigation may focus on objects that are a part of rituals and are also considered special because of contagion.

What Do Special Objects Do?

A natural question that follows a discussion of special objects and their origins is, "What do special objects do?" The "What do Special Objects Do?" section will consider the role of special objects in rituals, the power of special objects, their perceived means of producing effects, the types of effects they are perceived to produce, and the degree to which their origins influence these factors.

Special Objects in Rituals

Special objects are often key elements in religious rituals, though the role they play may vary from ritual to ritual. McCauley and Lawson's (2002) ritual form hypothesis identifies three different types of rituals—SARs, SPRs, and SIRs. As previously discussed, these three ritual forms provide opportunities for the generation of special objects, but they are also useful for understanding what special objects do.

In attempting to understand which ritual role special objects might serve, the distinction between agential and nonagential special objects becomes important. Agential special objects can, hypothetically, serve as agents, instruments, or patients. A statue that is believed to possess agency following a Taoist "opening of the eyes" ritual may serve as the agent in a SAR if it is believed to confer blessings of some sort. This statue might also be the patient in a SPR to whom sacrifices are offered. Special fire representing a god, such as the fire following the Vedic Agnyadhana ritual, may, hypothetically, be used in an SIR.

Nonagential objects may serve as instruments or patients. Holy water is one example often used in SIRs. An ordinary person may cleanse or protect him or herself from evil using this special water. Holy Communion, at least in the Roman Catholic and Eastern Orthodox traditions, is an SPR in which people act on the body and blood of Christ.[10]

Although agential special objects may serve as agents, instruments, or patients, these objects may theoretically appear most often in SPRs. Agential special objects may often represent the presence or essence of a supernatural being, which might lead religious practitioners to use them less frequently as instruments, and within Lawson and McCauley's (1990) ritual framework, an action must be observable to trigger the action representation system, which might lead religious practitioners to use both agential and nonagential special objects less frequently as agents in SARs. By contrast, nonagential special objects may be most often used in SIRs, given their lack of agency. The frequency with which agential and nonagential special objects occur in various ritual forms is an open empirical question that requires further examination. It may be that some special objects, such as masks or special clothing, are used in SARs or that some agential objects are used within SIRs. Experimental studies may investigate intuitions concerning natural beliefs about the appropriate places for these different objects, and a catalog of special objects across religious traditions may provide helpful data as well. Such data may be examined to determine the frequency with which various special and ordinary objects are used within each ritual form.

---

[10] At least in the Roman Catholic tradition, the bread and wine involved in the Eucharist or Holy Communion are believed to be the body and blood of an agent and to be connected to that agent, Jesus Christ. However, the elements themselves are not agential in the sense that they are able to move themselves.

Power or Efficacy in Special Objects

The power or efficacy of special objects is also an interesting topic that requires further empirical work. Certain objects are certainly considered more powerful, special, or central to various religious traditions, but why is this? McCauley and Lawson (2002) articulate a Principle of Superhuman Immediacy. They argue that the number of enabling rituals required to connect an object or agent to a supernatural agent determines the ritual's centrality to the religious tradition. The fewer rituals required, the more central to the tradition the ritual. They use the examples of Holy Communion and baptism. Holy Communion involves the body and blood of Christ, so a supernatural agent is directly involved in the ritual. Baptism must be performed by a priest who has been ordained by the Church, which is usually represented by another priest or higher-ranking official, such as a bishop, who has been given authority through ordination by someone who had been ordained, and so on, back to Christ ordaining Peter (requiring many enabling rituals). They predict that folk intuitions will point toward Holy Communion being more central than baptism to the Catholic tradition because it requires fewer enabling rituals.

A similar argument could be made for the power or efficacy of a special object. Theoretically, it may be that objects requiring more enabling rituals are believed to be less powerful or efficacious than objects requiring fewer enabling rituals. Objects delivered directly from a supernatural agent may, accordingly, be considered more powerful than those delivered by an agent made special by a supernatural agent (e.g., a priest who blesses holy water).

The power or efficacy of special objects may also be compared with the power or efficacy of supernatural agents. Two studies have shed light on how essential special objects and supernatural agents are to perceived ritual efficacy (Barrett & Lawson, 2001; Sørensen et al., 2006). Barrett and Lawson (2001) conducted two experiments. In Experiment 1, participants judged the efficacy of various fictitious ritual actions as compared to a prototype named as effective. The results indicated that changing the action within the ritual was considered less problematic for the ritual's efficacy than changing the agent or instrument. They also found that participants judged the inclusion of some "special label" (e.g., special person, special trumpet) as important for the ritual's efficacy even when the prototype, which was named as effective, contained no special labels. Interestingly, they found no significant differences in perceived effectiveness between special instruments and special agents. In other words, the presence of something special (defined as "someone or something that has been given special properties or authority by the gods"; Barrett & Lawson, p. 187) "was judged as more important for the success of the ritual than using the original instrument or performing the proper action" (Barrett & Lawson, p. 192). Furthermore, rituals in which two special labels were present (a special instrument and special agent) were judged to be even more effective.

In Experiment 2, Barrett and Lawson (2001) employed a condition similar to Experiment 1 and found similar results: changing the special agent lowered judgments of ritual efficacy more than changing the action. Based on the results of Experiments 1 and 2, they concluded that "having 'special'-markers was more important than any other component of the action sequence" for judgments of ritual efficacy (Barrett & Lawson, p. 197).

Building on the findings of Barrett and Lawson (2001), Sørensen et al. (2006) conducted a similar experiment to more closely examine the cognitive effects of changing the agents and instruments in rituals. Their study differed from Barrett and Lawson (2001) in that their prototypes had two "special" labels and alternative ritual examples that contained either a special agent or a special instrument (every example had at least one special label). They found that changing the specialness of an instrument ("sacrificial axe" compared to "axe") was less detrimental to judgments of efficacy than changing the form or substance of the instrument ("sacrificial axe" compared to "sacrificial hoe"). This finding contrasts with the changes in judgments of efficacy related to agents, in which the removal of status ("shaman" compared to "man") was more detrimental to judgments of efficacy than changing the category of the agent ("medicine-man" compared to "medicine-woman"; Sørensen et al., 2006, p. 465). Sørensen et al. argue that this finding may be the result of a focus on both the function of the instrument, which changes when the form or substance of the object is changed, and the continued specialness of the ritual, even when the special label was removed from the instrument, because a special agent was still present in these examples.

Taken together these studies demonstrate that the presence of some special marker is important for judgments of ritual efficacy and that changes in ritual actions are less important to these judgments than the presence of a special agent or instrument. Sørensen et al. (2006) further demonstrated that when a special agent is present, changes in the form or substance of an instrument are more detrimental than changes in the special status of the instrument to judgments of efficacy. Further work is needed to determine whether the presence of a special instrument or of a special agent is more important for judgments of efficacy, and the scenarios in which this may vary. Though Sørensen et al. found no support for their hypothesis that the special status of instruments would be more important for the perceived efficacy of rituals with instrumental or pragmatic goals (e.g., a good harvest) rather than social goals (e.g., reconciliation or peace between two parties), further work may examine the degree to which the nature of the instrument does influence these judgments.

Means of Change

Related to the power and efficacy of special objects are the means by which these objects are thought to produce change. In describing the transfer of supernatural agency from pilgrimage sites to various objects and agents, Nordin (2009) described three types of change by which this transfer occurs: essence change, forward contagion, and backward contagion. *Essence change* occurs when something ordinary becomes supernatural or special, or when core qualities of the object change (e.g., ordinary bread becomes the body of Christ in the Eucharist). Bread ordinarily provides physical nourishment, but because of the change in essence believed to occur, Holy Communion is believed to provide spiritual nourishment (Sørensen, 2005b). *Forward contagion* occurs when "a past history of contact affects the contacted entity in the present" (Rozin et al., 2018, p. 441).

For example, *jal*, or holy water, from pilgrimage sites is used to cleanse other objects. Something supernatural or special from these sites comes into contact with a person or object and results in special change. Beliefs related to this type of forward contagion are analogous to beliefs concerning the transmission of disease or germs (i.e., an object that touches someone with an illness may then transmit that illness to another person; Rozin et al., 2018). *Backward contagion* occurs when "actions on an object formerly owned by an individual influence that individual in the present" (Rozin et al., 2018, p. 441). Such change is believed to occur because some aspect of the individual's essence remains connected to the individual through an object (e.g., hair, clothes). Accordingly, these objects may be used to influence that individual. For example, something connected to a family member may be brought to a pilgrimage site and result in special change for that family member (Nordin, 2009) or a voodoo doll tied to an individual in some way may be used to harm that individual (Sørensen, 2005b).

Research investigating contagion effects suggests that contact with an object may result in a permanent change (sometimes expressed as "once in contact, always in contact"; Rozin et al., 1986). Other research suggests that the size and volume of an object (e.g., a small piece of clothing) or the amount of contact (e.g., brief or light contact) does not necessarily determine the effects—even small objects that briefly come into contact with an individual may be thought to transfer a great amount of the object's essence and produce widespread effects (Huang et al., 2017). Research also finds that a wide variety of nonphysical qualities may transfer by contagion: morality, traits, abilities, luck, and even emotions (Huang et al., 2017). Furthermore, direct contact is not always necessary to transfer some qualities; proximity to an object or even occupying a space an object previously occupied may produce effects similar to direct contact (Huang et al., 2017).

These three means of change—essence change, forward contagion, and backward contagion—may be dependent on or the result of the nature of the objects themselves and the means by which they were generated. It may be that an object created by contagion produces change via contagion. Objects generated in other ways, either via direct supernatural action or by SARs or SIRS, may have other effects. For example, it may be that a tree directly endowed with agency by a supernatural agent is not limited to power by contagion; rather, this tree may have a capacity for influence that is more closely linked to the supernatural agent that created it.

CONCLUSION

This chapter has addressed three questions: (a) what are special objects, (b) where do special objects come from, and (c) what do special objects do? Special objects are defined as objects with counterintuitive properties or counterschematic causal effects that a group of people reflectively believes exist, that have a type of existence or action that can, in principle, be detected by people, and whose existence motivates some differences in human behavior as a consequence. A meaningful distinction between agential and nonagential special objects has also been made. Three means of generating special objects have been identified: direct supernatural action, ritual action, and contagion. Implications of these means of generation have also been discussed. Finally, the effects of special objects within rituals, the power of these objects, and the means by which they bring about change have also been addressed.

The study of special objects is ripe for further investigation because many empirical questions remain. This chapter has outlined several lines of inquiry that may prove fruitful. In particular, further work must investigate the prevalence of various special objects across religious traditions, their uses, and their types. Such work will aid investigations of beliefs concerning the generation and efficacy of special objects as well.

QUESTIONS FOR FUTURE RESEARCH

1. Which types of special objects are most common in religious systems?
2. How are special objects most typically generated?
3. What variables influence the power or effects of special objects?

ACKNOWLEDGMENTS

The author thanks Justin Barrett for his advice, support, and suggestions; Gregory Foley for his examples of special objects in the Orthodox Christian tradition; and Sarey Martin for her editorial assistance.

REFERENCES

Barrett, J. L. (2008). Coding and quantifying counterintuitiveness in religious concepts: Theoretical and methodological reflections. *Method & Theory in the Study of Religion, 20*, 308–338. https://doi.org/10.1163/157006808X371806

Barrett, J. L. (2011). *Cognitive science, religion, and theology: From human minds to divine minds.* West Conshohocken, PA: Templeton Press.

Barrett, J. L., & Lawson, E. T. (2001). Ritual intuitions: Cognitive contributions to judgments of ritual efficacy. *Journal of Cognition and Culture, 1*(2), 183–201.

Boyer, P. (1994). *The naturalness of religious ideas: A cognitive theory of religion.* Berkeley: University of California Press.

Boyer, P. (2001). *Religion explained: The evolutionary origins of religious thought.* New York: Basic Books.

Cohen, E. (2007). *The mind possessed: The cognition of spirit possession in an Afro-Brazilian religious tradition.* New York: Oxford University Press.

Dafni, A. (2007). Rituals, ceremonies and customs related to sacred trees with a special reference to the Middle East. *Journal of Ethnobiology and Ethnomedicine, 3*(28). https://doi.org/10.1186/1746-4269-3-28

Greenway, T. S., & Barrett, J. L. (2017). Evolutionary developmental psychology of children's religious beliefs. In J. R. Liddle & T. K. Shackelford (Eds.), *The Oxford handbook of evolutionary psychology and religion*. Oxford: Oxford University Press. doi:10.1093/oxfordhb/9780199397747.013.7

Gregory, J. P., Greenway, T. S., & Keys, C. (2019). Gods and talking animals: The pan-cultural transmission advantage of supernatural agent concepts. *Journal of Cognition and Culture*, 19(1–2), 97–130.

Huang, J. Y., Ackerman, J. M., & Newman, G. E. (2017). Catching (up with) magical contagion: A review of contagion effects in consumer contexts. *Journal of the Association for Consumer Research*, 2(4), 430–443.

Keil, F. C. (1979). *Semantic and conceptual development: An ontological perspective*. Cambridge, MA: Harvard University Press.

Kim, L. R., & Kim, N. S. (2011). A proximity effect in adults' contamination intuitions. *Judgment and Decision Making*, 6(3), 222.

Lawson, E. T., & McCauley, R. N. (1990). *Rethinking religion: Connecting cognition and culture*. Cambridge, UK: Cambridge University Press.

Legerstee, M. (1994, June). Patterns of 4-month-old infant responses to hidden silent and sounding people and objects. *Early Development and Parenting*, 3, 71–80. https://doi.org/10.1002/edp.2430030204

McCauley, R. N. (2011). *Why religion is natural, and science is not*. New York: Oxford University Press.

McCauley, R. N., & Lawson, E. T. (2002). *Bringing ritual to mind: Psychological foundations of cultural forms*. Cambridge, UK: Cambridge University Press.

Nordin, A. (2009). Ritual agency, substance transfer and the making of supernatural immediacy in pilgrim journeys. *Journal of Cognition and Culture*, 9(3–4), 195–223. https://doi.org/10.1163/156770909X12489459066228

Rozin, P., Dunn, C., & Fedotova, N. (2018). Reversing the causal arrow: Incidence and properties of negative backward magical contagion in Americans. *Judgment and Decision Making*, 13(5), 441–450.

Rozin, P., Millman, L., & Nemeroff, C. (1986). Operation of the laws of sympathetic magic in disgust and other domains. *Journal of Personality and Social Psychology*, 50(4), 703–712.

Sørensen, J. (2005a). Charisma, tradition, and ritual: A cognitive approach to magical agency. In H. Whitehouse & R. McCauley (Eds.), *Mind and religion: Psychological and cognitive foundations of religiosity* (pp. 167–186). Walnut Creek, CA: AltaMira Press.

Sørensen, J. (2005b). The problem of magic—or how gibberish becomes efficacious action. *Semiotic Inquiry*, 25(1/2), 93.

Sørensen, J., Liénard, P., & Feeny, C. (2006). Agent and instrument in judgements of ritual efficacy. *Journal of Cognition and Culture*, 6(3), 463–482.

Spelke, E. S., Phillips, A., & Woodward, A. L. (1995). Infants' knowledge of object motion and human action. In D. Sperber, D. Premack, & A. J. Premack (Eds.), *Causal cognition: A multidisciplinary debate* (pp. 44–78). New York: Oxford University Press.

Sperber, D., & Hirschfeld, L. A. (2004). The cognitive foundations of cultural stability and diversity. *Trends in Cognitive Sciences*, 8(1), 40–46. https://doi.org/10.1016/j.tics.2003.11.002

Sperber, D., Premack, D., & Premack, A. J. (Eds.). (1995). *Causal cognition: A multidisciplinary debate*. New York: Oxford University Press.

PART V

RELIGIOUS EXPERIENCES

CHAPTER 12

CONCEIVING RELIGIOUS DREAMS AND MYSTICAL EXPERIENCES

A Predictive Processing Investigation

ROBERT E. SEARS

INTRODUCTION

PSYCHOLOGY and anthropology are two of the historic disciplines that contributed to the development of the cognitive science of religion (CSR) in the 1990s (see Barrett, 2011a; and Lawson, this volume). William James (1842–1910), who is generally regarded as one of the founders of psychology, the psychology of religion in particular, grounded his theory of religion in "mystical experience" (James, 2012; Barnard, 1997; Sears, 2017a). By contrast, the founder of anthropology, E. B. Tylor (1832–1917), developed his theory of religion in close connection with dreams and, relatedly, visions (Tylor, 2016; Kracke, 2003). Despite the early (and ongoing) attempts to study dreams and mystical experiences within psychology and anthropology, they did not receive substantial attention in early CSR investigations. In fact, personal religious experience was largely neglected by early CSR investigations in favor of ritual and concept analyses (Taves & Asprem, 2017).[1] In recent years, however, there has been a growing interest in personal religious experience among CSR researchers, and both dreams and mystical experience have been accorded special consideration (e.g., Nordin, 2011; Petrican & Burris, 2012; Andersen et al., 2014; Hornbeck & Sears, 2015; McNamara & Bulkeley, 2015; Bulkeley, 2016; Sears, 2016, 2019; Nordin & Bjälkebring, 2019). Nevertheless, there have been relatively few CSR analyses tailored to dreams and mystical experience, and a variety of

---

[1] For an exception to this general rule, see Andresen (2001).

issues are in need of attention given the previous oversight and advances in the field. By and large, these issues pertain to how such experiences are processed and what function they serve. Though the conclusion will briefly address some broader functional implications of dreams and mystical experience, the chapter is primarily concerned with offering a cognitive processing account of these phenomena based on recent theoretical developments in CSR and cognitive science more broadly.

The fundamental backdrop to this analysis is *hierarchical predictive coding* ([HPC]; Friston & Kiebel, 2009; Hobson & Friston, 2012, 2014; Clark, 2013, 2016; Hermans, 2015; Taves & Asprem, 2017; Schjoedt & Andersen, 2017). According to a generic rendering of HPC, the mind-brain corresponds to a hierarchical arrangement of systems that send signals to each other. Among any pair of levels within the hierarchy, the higher-level system uses available cognitive resources to construct models of the information it expects to be conveyed at the lower level. Higher-level models supply predictions that are fed backward to the adjacent lower level, where they are compared with actual model parameters at that level. Deviations between expected and actual model parameters result in error signals that function as a form of feedback to the higher level. "Good" predictions essentially cancel error, whereas failed predictions result in an amplification of the error signal; this, moreover, tends to induce a higher-level search for information to revise predictions (for a detailed technical discussion of the foregoing, see Clark, 2013, 2016; Friston & Kiebel, 2009).

While HPC describes the relationship between individual levels of the cognitive hierarchy, it also undergirds a broad understanding of the mind-brain as an instrument that proactively uses previously stored information to construct models of its environment, including the body and what lies beyond it. Hence, HPC models of perception differ from those suggesting that perception is a passive activity that amounts to the accumulation and repackaging of sense data. According to HPC, sensory input functions as a corrective to cognitive predictions (Andersen et al., 2014; Clark, 2013, 2016; Hobson & Friston, 2012); the mind uses preexisting information to *predict* sensory input and revises those predictions when they fail to accommodate the "driving signal" associated with sense data. Discrepancies between sense data and basic model predictions result in error signals that are propagated up the cognitive hierarchy, reforming higher-level predictions along the way (Friston & Kiebel, 2009; Clark, 2013, 2016). Predictions associated with higher levels of the cognitive hierarchy do not directly interact with sense data; instead, they interact with perceptual representations at the adjacent lower level *via* error units that supply feedback (Clark, 2013, p. 12). These lower-level representations are themselves sensitive to error signals that are ultimately traceable to sensory input. Whereas HPC has indeed been influential as a model of low-level cognitive activities such as perception (see Clark, 2013), the general framework of using available information resources to form predictions and then revising predictions based on lower-level feedback appears to be applicable to higher-level cognitive operations, such as (re-)forming narrative judgments (Schjoedt et al., 2013; Taves & Asprem, 2017).

At base, my claim is that both basic and abstract elements of religious dreams and mystical experiences are explainable in terms of prediction casting and error signaling within a functioning cognitive hierarchy. Prior examinations of dreams and mystical experiences have explicitly relied on variations of HPC for analysis (Andersen et al., 2014; Hobson & Friston, 2012). However, these studies have largely overlooked religious components of dreams and classical varieties of mystical experience. They also focus primarily on the basic/perceptual characteristics of the phenomena they consider rather than the abstract/cognitive features. Although their proposals offer some applications to the basic phenomenology of the experiences I consider, they are problematic in certain respects. I will address shortcomings of prior processing analyses; ultimately, however, my goal is to provide a constructive account of how the basic features and abstract religious appraisals of dreams and mystical experiences are formed. Fulfilling this aim first requires an elaboration of HPC in relation to *event cognition* (Radavansky & Zacks, 2014; Taves & Asprem, 2017) and *complexity-based reasoning* (Fortier & Kim, 2017). The discussion of dreams and mystical experiences thereafter will introduce additional principles that aim to reinforce or complement the predictive processing analysis of these phenomena.

For the purposes of this chapter, *dreams* are taken to be personal "imaginative experiences that may include thoughts, feelings, visions, auditions, and other sensations" (Sears, 2015a, p. 134) and coincide with the activity of the mind-brain during sleep. This definition distinguishes between dreams and phenomenologically similar visions or hallucinations in that the latter occur during waking states.

Unlike dreams, *mystical experiences* can occur during sleep or wakefulness (Bulkeley, 2009a; Marshall, 2005, pp. 19, 95–96; Sears, 2015a; Sears & Hood, 2016). The precise components and varieties of mystical experience have inspired voluminous debate (cf. James, 2012; Otto, 2016; Zaehner, 1957; Stace, 1960; Katz, 1978; d'Aquili & Newberg, 1993; Hood, 2001a; Marshall, 2005; Andersen et al., 2014; Taves, 2020). Although it has attracted significant criticism, Walter Stace's (1960) treatment of mystical experience remains one of the most influential.[2] Stace considered the sense of "unity" or "oneness" to be the quintessential feature of mystical experience, though he and others have also recognized other potential aspects such as awe, bliss, profound knowledge, timelessness/spacelessness, and luminosity (cf. Stace, 1960, pp. 62–133; Marshall, 2005, pp. 24–29; Taves, 2020). Additionally, Stace divided mystical

---

[2] Stace's work serves as the basis for Ralph Hood's (1975) M Scale, perhaps the most widely used psychological instrument in studies of mystical experience. Both the M Scale and Stace's original typology have faced considerable criticism of late (see Taves, 2020). Given space constraints, it is not possible to offer a substantial response to this criticism here. However, it is worth noting that construct validity for each of the M Scale's basic facets (which were originally based on Stace's descriptions of mystical experience) was confirmed in a study of non-Western participants (Chen et al., 2011). Although the extrovertive/introvertive classification of these facets has proven somewhat malleable and limiting, it remains a useful means of characterizing some non-ordinary experiences in terms of the self's relationship to the world.

experience into two varieties or "species": extrovertive and introvertive. Generalizing from Stace and others who have used his terminology, extrovertive mystical experience involves a perceived relationship between the self and objects beyond the self or, rather, between the objects themselves (while the self remains an observer).[3] Again, such experiences are often typified by union and other nonordinary qualities. Franklin's (2000) autobiographical account of extrovertive experience provides a useful illustration of some common features:

> [W]atching the flickering sun-light through the leaves of the lime tree, my mind went blank—I suddenly found myself surrounded, embraced, by a white light, which seemed both to come from within me and from without, a very bright light but quite unlike any ordinary physical light. I was filled with an overwhelming sense of Love, of warmth, peace and joy . . . I had the feeling of being "one" with everything, and "knowing" all things—whatever I wanted to know, I "knew" instantly and directly.[4]

In contrast with the outward orientation of extrovertive experiences, introvertive experiences are inward oriented; in other words, during an introvertive experience, the individual engages with his or her consciousness rather than (perceived) external conditions. "Pure consciousness," regarded by some as the paradigmatic introvertive experience, is an allegedly "contentless" state of consciousness. It corresponds to awareness without reference: thoughts and other sensations are supposedly held in abeyance, which (may) result in a profound sense of oneness/unity (cf. Deikman, 2010; Forman, 2007; Stace, 1960, pp. 85–111). Forman (2007) describes his experience of pure consciousness as follows:

> Sometimes during meditation my thoughts drift away entirely, and I gain a state I would describe as simply being awake. I'm not thinking about anything. I'm not particularly aware of any sensations, I'm not aware of being absorbed in anything in particular, and yet I am quite certain (after the fact) that I haven't been asleep. (p. 77)

Although introvertive and extrovertive experiences are distinctive in important respects, several scholars consider them to be related. Common explanations of the relationship refer to overlapping phenomenology and/or progression from one type of experience to the next (cf. Stace, 1960; Deikman, 2010; Hood, 1989; d'Aquili & Newberg, 1993; Forman, 2007; Chen et al., 2011). This study treats introvertive and extrovertive experience as two "species" of a single mystical "genus." Though other "species" have been proposed (and rejected), the just-described introvertive/extrovertive typology will largely steer the remaining discussion of mystical experience.

---

[3] The self's "external" environment is essentially projected without the aid of sensory input in the case of dreaming mystical experience.

[4] Quoted in Marshall (2005, p. 24).

Predictive Processing and Religious Experience

To better understand the relationship between perception and higher-level processes that deal with causal attribution and narrative understanding, I will briefly discuss Radavansky and Zack's theory of *event cognition* (summarized by Taves & Asprem, 2017). Event cognition refers to the mind's processing of events. "Events" refer to discrete experiences—that is, experiences with a beginning and end (Taves & Asprem, 2017, p. 46). While the mind is constantly generating percepts—corresponding to "the brain's current best hypothesis for the driving sensory input"—it simultaneously relies on working memory and "event schemata" (procedural and semantic memory, which includes concepts and beliefs) to create "event models" that aim to describe/predict the relationships between percepts over time (Taves & Asprem, 2017, pp. 45–47). Event models can include both basic information about percepts (such as type(s) and number of objects, agents, behaviors, etc., over time) as well as inferences about causes, reasons, and meaning (Taves & Asprem, 2017, p. 50).

In consonance with HPC, event models supply predictions and are sensitive to error feedback from accumulating percepts (Taves & Asprem, 2017, pp. 45–47). Though the mind may briefly settle on a particular event model for a set of percepts by virtue of its relevant predictions, the constant updating of perceptual information ensures that these predictions will eventually fail; the corresponding amplification of the error signal will then result in model revision or replacement. "Event segmentation," associated with spikes in prediction error, entails the creation of a new event model in working memory; the old event model will potentially be stored as an episodic memory, however, enabling recall and further processing (Taves & Asprem, 2017, pp. 45–46). In the case of dreams, event segmentation reliably occurs when an individual begins to wake. Dream content, which is essentially equivalent to percepts generated while awake, rapidly gives way to strikingly different percepts with the onset of waking. The event model associated with the prior dream sequence fails to predict these novel percepts, and the resulting amplification of the error signal causes the mind to search for and adopt a new event model ("I'm awake").

Although waking reliably triggers event segmentation, dream sequences may give rise to a series of short event models in conjunction with changes in content. In fact, event cognition takes place on multiple timescales within a hierarchic system (Radavansky & Zacks, 2014, p. 28). Thus, shorter and longer events are processed simultaneously; moreover, the former may function as subevents of the latter. Hence, a dream sequence can be considered a single event that comprises several subevents. Models for both short (sub) events and longer (super)events are sensitive to bottom-up error signals associated with perceptual representations (see Radavansky & Zacks, 2014, esp. pp. 49–52).

To summarize, event models, representing discrete experiences, stand atop a chain of perceptual processing that recruits preexisting information to predict underlying conditions or input. Event models comprise both basic/perceptual characteristics and more abstract cognitive inferences about causes, reasons, and meaning. Similarly, "religious" events or experiences can be divided into more basic perceptual characteristics and more abstract appraisals (cf. Spilka et al., 1985; Sears, 2016; Taves, 2009; Taves & Asprem, 2017). Making sense of these religious appraisals will benefit from an understanding of the concept of complexity drop and its relationship to supernatural attribution.

Complexity drop is related to the concept of unexpectedness, which has served a number of researchers examining religious experience (see, e.g., Hood, 1978; Taves, 2009; Hermans, 2015; Sears, 2016, 2019; Fortier & Kim, 2017). Generally speaking, researchers have argued that situations that defy initial expectations facilitate religious interpretations. Fortier and Kim (2017) developed this claim vis-à-vis drops in complexity between expected and actual circumstances (cf. Dessalles, 2007, 2008). Complexity refers to the "size of the shortest program that generates a given string; the longer the program (the higher the number of instructions a program needs to generate a given string), the more complex the program. . . . A random string such as (4, 7, 3, 5) demands more instructions because it is not compressible" (Fortier & Kim, 2017, p. 283). To illustrate complexity, consider the following scenarios: driving along the highway and encountering multiple vehicles of various colors and shapes versus driving along the highway and encountering only vehicles of the same color and shape. The latter situation/event is much less complex than the former because it requires fewer cognitive resources to describe or represent. According to Fortier and Kim, the latter would be unexpected because it is *less complex* than what one typically expects to find while driving (events that are more complex than expectations do not result in complexity drops and corresponding "unexpectedness"; see Fortier & Kim, 2017, p. 284).

As the foregoing indicates, complexity and randomness are interrelated concepts (randomness amounts to maximum complexity). Recognizing this relationship, Fortier and Kim bridged the subject of complexity drops with research from developmental psychologists concerning apparent violations of randomness. The latter essentially demonstrates "that very early on, humans explain the absence of randomness (i.e., high simplicity) by postulating the interference of an agency" (Fortier & Kim, 2017, p. 284). Combining this observation with the complexity drop concept enables Fortier and Kim to formulate the complexity drop model of the supernatural (CDMS). Accordingly, complexity drops between expected conditions and actual conditions produce unexpectedness, which drives agency attribution; furthermore, supernatural agency attribution will ensue when nonsupernatural concept alternatives are unavailable or unable to account for what happened (Fortier & Kim, 2017, p. 286). The attribution of a given event to a supernatural agent is essentially what makes the event "religious" (cf. Taves, 2009; Hermans, 2015; Sears, 2016; Nordin & Bjälkebring, 2019). Situations likely to entail complexity drops and supernatural attribution are those involving familiar people or places, redundant features, and atypical phenomena (see Fortier & Kim, 2017, pp. 287–288, for examples and discussion; the investigation of dreams and mystical experience that follows will illustrate the last two scenarios in particular). It requires few cognitive resources to represent these situations, which explains their tendency to trigger complexity drops and associated ramifications.

Like HPC, the CDMS trades on the principles of expectation (or prediction) and actual circumstance or input. Since unexpectedness begets reconceptualization (Fortier & Kim, 2017), it should be associated with prediction error (cf. Clark, 2013, pp. 2–3, 12). Furthermore, (supernatural) agency explanations for unexpected circumstances can be regarded as attempts to minimize unexpectedness/prediction error (cf. Dessalles, 2008, 2013). In short, though Fortier and Kim do not explicitly situate their discussion of the CDMS within the context of HPC, their model of supernatural agency attribution could be regarded as an application of HPC to the phenomenon of religious cognition.

Finally, it is important to understand that religious (and nonreligious) appraisals are liable to change. Given more time and evolving circumstances, new information may become available that enables subjects to reframe past events (Spilka et al., 1985; Barrett, 2004; Taves, 2009; Sears, 2016). Complexity drops may trigger the attribution of supernatural agency initially; however, subjects may ultimately decide that the situation they encountered does not merit this distinction. This investigation will focus on initial complexity drop situations and potential ramifications rather than the evolution of subjective interpretation after the event has transpired.

Mystical Experience

Relying on an HPC framework similar to what has been described, Andersen et al. (2014) offer what may be the most detailed predictive coding account of "mystical experience"[5] to date:

> [W]e define mystical experiences as perceptions embedded in a religious or spiritual framework, which are caused by a dominance of the brains [sic] internal models. In a more pragmatic sense, this definition seeks to capture phenomena such as visions, epiphanies, holistic experiences, and the sensed presence of supernatural beings or entities. (p. 224)

Moreover, they suggest that the brain's internal models for mystical experience will dominate perception when activated by contextual circumstances and prediction-error feedback permits their continued application. In particular, they claim that sensory-deprived conditions play an important role in facilitating mystical experience by minimizing prediction error stemming from sensory input (Andersen et al., 2014, p. 223).

To support their theoretical claims, Andersen et al. (2014) designed an experiment to test the effects of highly suggestive circumstances and sensory deprivation on subjects

---

[5] Due to space constraints, I focus on waking mystical experiences rather than dreaming ones in this section.

with varying levels of prior religious/spiritual experience. Subjects were ultimately placed in a dark room, blindfolded, and fitted with an electromagnetic helmet that emitted a random, very weak magnetic field, which was not likely to substantially affect brain functioning (cf. Persinger, 1987; Granqvist et al., 2005). Subjects recorded any unusual experience they felt during the approximately one hour they were under these conditions by pressing a button; afterward, they were given an opportunity to describe their experiences in an interview setting. Prior to encountering the test conditions, the subjects were informed about them and about the types of experiences they might undergo while wearing the helmet (awareness of a presence in the room, unusual visions, voices, haptic sensations, etc.). Equipped with this referent-specific "religious" knowledge, subjects exposed to the aforementioned conditions indeed registered "unusual sensory" and "sensed presence" experiences. Specifically, the researchers found that persons with prior spiritual or meditation experiences were substantially more likely than persons without such experiences to undergo mystical experiences in the laboratory setting. Nonetheless, inexperienced persons (who nonetheless possessed referent-specific religious knowledge) reported some of the same types of mystical experiences as the adepts. On the whole, however, religious adepts reported stronger experiences than novices (Andersen et al., 2014, pp. 231–232).

Although Andersen et al.'s (2014) predictive coding framework offers a possible interpretation of their findings, it is important to note that their findings do not obviously include mystical experiences of the sort discussed in the introduction. In fact, their framework is problematic in light of the phenomenology of introvertive experience and, especially, extrovertive experience. Extrovertive experience generally entails sensory openness to the natural world and can occur "spontaneously," that is, without the subject possessing a conscious expectation for the experience prior to its onset (Hood, 2001b, p. 159; Marshall, 2005; cf. Andersen et al., 2014, pp. 226–228). Moreover, subjects without prior extrovertive experiences or an approximate conceptual framework for the experience itself may nonetheless undergo dramatic versions of the experience (see Marshall, 2005, pp. 191–193).

If the phenomenology of extrovertive experience seemingly challenges Andersen et al.'s findings and discussion, the phenomenology of introvertive experience is generally more consistent with their report. Unlike the spontaneous circumstances of some extrovertive experiences, introvertive experiences tend to follow apophatic meditation (cf. Egan, 1978; Forman, 2007; Hood, 2001b; Luhrmann, 2012). Those who adopt a meditation posture generally do so with the expectation/intention of facilitating meditation-related effects. Moreover, certain apophatic practices, such as shutting the eyes, entail sensory deprivation. One therefore might be tempted to argue a la Andersen et al. (2014, p. 224) that individuals who practice apophatic meditation activate a general expectation for introvertive experience that, combined with the lack of prediction error following meditation-related sensory deprivation, results in experiential fulfillment.

Although some may find the foregoing explanation of introvertive experience broadly acceptable, it fails to address common phenomenological accounts of "pure consciousness," which describe the experience as devoid of discrete thoughts and images. A more robust explanation of this experience can potentially be derived from Deikman's (2010) discussion of "de-automatization" and Schjoedt et al.'s (2013) description of "cognitive resource depletion" in rituals involving goal demotion and causal opacity. Both studies seemingly refer to the same essential process, but I focus on Schjoedt et al.'s discussion here.[6] It begins with the observation that the mind processes action sequences in a hierarchical system that combines lower-level action units into higher-level action narratives according to intentional and causal specification. The hierarchical arrangement normally allows the mind to conserve attention by relying on higher-level action narratives to predict lower-level action units. However, certain ritualized forms of behavior, for example, apophatic meditation, may entail obscure goals and causal relationships.[7] These can prevent the mind from automatically assigning an action narrative to the ritualized behavior, demanding reallocation of cognitive resources to attend to "low-level perceptual detail" (Schjoedt et al., 2013, p. 45). The resulting cognitive arrangement amounts to a *less differentiated* psychological experience (cf. Deikman, 2010).[8] Put in terms of HPC, apophatic meditation creates a dynamic source of prediction error that could interfere with cognitive/higher-level specification of percepts (cf. Schjoedt et al., 2013, pp. 45–46).

Following Schjoedt et al., one consequence of cognitive-resource depletion during apophatic meditation/mystical experience is an inferential gap at the executive level of cognition. While the ritual context of introvertive experience may encourage subjects to seek the interpretive help of religious authorities (Schjoedt et al., 2013, p. 46), subjects will undoubtedly engage in personal reflection initially, which would result in an understanding of the experience that could make the counsel's explanation seem more or less plausible (see Barrett, 2004, pp. 13–14). The causal opacity of the apophatic ritual may initially cause a subject to interpret the introvertive experience as unintended (i.e., not the product of the subject's action). Following Malle (1999, 2004) and Taves (2009, pp. 100–111), the unintended nature of the event will orient the subject to extrinsic causal explanations.

Additionally, the subject may have reason to believe that an agent is responsible for the event because of its simplicity vis-à-vis other conscious experiences and the expectations derived from those experiences (Fortier & Kim, 2017). Common descriptions of introvertive experience emphasize its lack of features associated with general conscious

---

[6] The term "cognitive resource depletion" refers to the reduction of cognitive resources for executive functioning following an increased load from attention (Schjoedt et al., 2013, p. 41). "De-automatization" refers to the undoing of "automatic" cognitive processing (Deikman, 2010, p. 58), which the former term implies.

[7] Apophatic goals such as entering "the cloud of unknowing" (Luhrmann, 2012), attaining "watchful stillness of the spirit" (Gavrilyuk, 2013), and "quieting the mind" differ from more conventional goals such as "drinking a cup of coffee" or "writing a paper" in terms of animacy and intentionality (see Schjoedt et al., 2013, p. 45). Moreover, the causal relationship between these goals and concrete meditative actions such as repeating a simple word or phrase, breathing at regular intervals, and so forth, does not appear to be intuitive.

[8] By definition, differentiation contrasts with oneness. Arguably, then, focusing attention on lower-level perceptual details during cognitive-resource depletion contributes to the oneness that is frequently reported by mystics.

functioning; hence, introvertive experience has been described as nondiscursive, contentless, void, thought-free, and so on (e.g., see Deikman, 2010; Forman, 2007). Descriptions of introvertive experience even contrast with cognitive situations that lack clear goals or external tasks—as is the case with apophatic meditation generally—during which the self's natural inclination is to daydream discrete images, recall memories, and formulate abstract ideas (cf. Bulkeley, 2016, pp. 139–140; Forman, 2007; Schjoedt et al., 2013).[9] From these descriptions, it would appear that expectations derived from "normal" consciousness, as well as from the situation that typically precedes the introvertive experience, assume greater complexity than the experience actually entails, which satisfies the conditions for a complexity drop. Additionally, Fortier and Kim (2017)—following Dessalles (2007)—cite "atypical" objects or circumstances as one of the causes of complexity drops.[10] In light of the foregoing descriptions, introvertive experience can indeed be regarded as an atypical conscious experience, which, following the logic of Fortier and Kim, results in a complexity drop and search for agency. Without the self to vie for explanation initially (on account of the causal opacity of the ritual leading up to the experience), God or some comparable supernatural agent may seem to be the most likely cause of the event.

The foregoing description of causal attribution would seemingly apply to extrovertive experiences as well. Like introvertive experience, extrovertive experience may be regarded as unintended initially. This seems especially valid when extrovertive experience occurs spontaneously. However, if an extrovertive experience were to occur during or after ritual attempts to provoke it, the subject may nonetheless regard the experience as unintentional if the causal relationship between the ritual means and experiential ends remains subjectively vague. Additionally, features of extrovertive experience— such as unity between objects—could occasion complexity drops by virtue of atypicality or simplicity. Thus, both of the conditions for supernatural causal attribution in the case of introvertive mystical experience appear to be satisfied by extrovertive experience, generally considered.

Besides abstract processing, the basic/perceptual processing of extrovertive phenomena also requires attention from researchers. There are a few considerations to bear in mind when addressing this issue—namely, whether the experience is spontaneous

---

[9] Thus, cognitive-resource depletion (de-automatization) needs to be understood in dynamic/ progressive terms and introvertive experience should be regarded as the eventual result of sustained apophatic meditation.

[10] Although Jean-Louis Dessalles and Fortier and Kim have somewhat different definitions of complexity drops, Dessalles's discussion of atypicality and complexity complements Fortier and Kim's definition. According to Dessalles, "objects or situations that are close to the centre of the prototype for a multi-attribute resemblance are maximally complex, as discrimination is most difficult there... the complexity of discrimination is expected to decrease... until it reaches zero for items that are regarded as unique in their own kind" (2007, p. 9; cf. Fortier & Kim, 2017, p. 287). Certain characteristics of introvertive experience differ greatly from those associated with the typical or mundane experiences that serve as event schemata, rendering introvertive experience easy to delineate even if difficult to put into words ("ineffability" is a frequently mentioned aspect of mystical experience).

or consciously sought, and whether it precedes or follows introvertive experience (cf. Stace, 1960, pp. 41–133; Hood, 1989; Forman, 2007; Marshall, 2005, pp. 167–172). If it follows introvertive experience, an episodic memory of that experience may be triggered during the processing of sensory input. The combination of this memory and the sensory information conveyed through the driving signal might result in an event/experience model that corresponds to a sense of oneness with the natural world. Although this explanation may apply to some cases of extrovertive experience, it remains abstract. Researchers will need to specify how an introvertive experience memory gets triggered during ordinary, daytime conditions and, more importantly, how this would dominate the *perceptual* features of the experience (cf. Andersen et al., 2014; Schjoedt & Andersen, 2017). It is one thing for subjects to be reminded of prior experiences while continuing to process sensory data normally, and another for memories of prior experiences to control how sensory data is perceived.

Alternatively, extrovertive experience may result from conscious focus on normally unconscious aspects of one's perception or thought (Deikman, 2010; Schjoedt et al., 2013). Some subjects may acquire the unique ability to attend to basic mental processes via meditative training, which, in accordance with Deikman's (2010) reasoning, could facilitate introvertive experience under certain conditions (such as sensory deprivation) and extrovertive experience under other conditions (such as exposure to ordinary, daytime conditions). Whereas certain individuals may purposely "tune in" to the characteristic phenomena of extrovertive experience via meditation, research suggests that other individuals experience extrovertive states spontaneously and without having a prior background in introvertive experience (Marshall, 2005). One possible explanation for these spontaneous cases is that abnormal bodily circumstances (e.g., microseizures of the brain; see Alston & Fales, 2004, p. 154; Marshall, 2005, pp. 101, 226–232) create "noise," which functions as a source of prediction error during the handling of sense data. Prediction error disrupts automatic perceptual processing, causing attention to shift to the cognitive activities or structures responsible for mystical experience.

In summary, the principles of predictive coding, cognitive-resource depletion/de-automatization, extrinsic causal reasoning, and complexity drops provide possible means of explaining the basic features and religious interpretations of mystical experiences. The foregoing analysis has been brief and hypothetical, however, implying the need for future research.

Dreams

Although Andersen et al.'s (2014) predictive coding scheme is problematic with respect to certain varieties of mystical experience, it appears to be quite applicable to dream content, that is, what the mind dreams about (Bulkeley, 2016, p. 121). Accordingly, dream content derives from the mind's available models/schemata under (bodily) conditions that compromise access to the sensorium (cf. Hobson & Friston, 2012, 2014). The general lack of access to sensory—particularly exteroceptive—input during dreaming is widely accepted by researchers (e.g., see Hobson & Friston, 2012; Taves & Asprem, 2017, pp. 47–48). Since the mind is largely deprived of exteroceptive input during sleep, external sources of information operating contemporaneously to the dreaming mind have little impact on the forms of content that are experienced by the dreamer; hence, preexisting schemata "dominate" oneiric experience (cf. Andersen et al., 2014, pp. 223–224).[11]

The previous notion is consistent with some understandings of continuity theory. *Continuity theory* is perhaps the most widely discussed cognitive/psychological theory of dreaming. Although the precise definition of continuity theory continues to be debated (cf. Domhoff, 2017; Schredl, 2017), it essentially aims to describe dream content and reasoning in relation to waking experience (Bulkeley, 2016, pp. 119–122; Kahan & LaBerge, 2011). Dream content, in particular, is understood by some to reflect both "overt behavior" and "covert thoughts, feelings, and fantasies" enacted during waking-life (Schredl, 2017, p. 352). What is implicit in this description, and more-or-less explicated in other descriptions of continuity theory (e.g., Schredl, 2003; Paquette, 2018), is that oneiric events are essentially dependent on the dreamer's waking-life experiences. In other words, the dreaming mind generally makes use of schemata that are formed and reformed while the individual was previously awake. This is not to deny the idea that dreaming may introduce refinements to preexisting schemata or even result in novel schemata that influence future waking and dreaming behavior (Lohmann, 2003b); nevertheless, it is commonly accepted that dream content is contingent on an individual's prior waking experience.[12] Consistent with this notion, Lohmann (2000, 2003b) argues that the Asabano, an originally animistic tribe from the highlands of Papua New Guinea, only began to have dreams with overtly Christian content after missionaries first introduced Christianity.

Although dreams largely depend on preexisting schemata, the question of why certain schemata but not others are activated during dreaming is an important one for researchers to consider. Related to this issue, there is some research to suggest that during dream cognition an individual's "preoccupations" or "concerns" are generally more active than more trivial concepts, beliefs, events, or behaviors (Domhoff, 2017). This claim seems plausible and, together with the above notion of conceptual continuity between waking and dreaming, may offer a rudimentary means of doing psychological assessment (see, e.g., Bulkeley, 2009b; Domhoff, 2017); however, it is not so precise as to enable reliable prediction of an individual's next dream. Indeed, the likelihood of particular schemata undergoing activation during dreaming sleep is a matter that continues to deserve critical inquiry (Schredl, 2003, 2017).

[11] Though external sources of information generally appear to have minimal influence on dream content, they may nonetheless affect dream content when their stimulation of sensory pathways exceeds threshold conditions (Dement & Wolpert, 1958; Koulack, 1969; Nielsen et al, 1993; Schredl, 2017). According to the HPC framework advocated here, sensory information would be translated into a driving (error) signal that reforms higher-level models recruited by the dreaming mind.

[12] Occasionally, researchers have argued that some dreams may be the product of telepathy or quantum entanglement (e.g., Smith, 2013; Paquette, 2018), in which case an individual's preexisting schemata would seemingly play a minimal role in dream content production.

As indicated previously, sensory deprivation goes hand-in-hand with the idea that preexisting schemata are largely responsible for the dreamer's experience. As a consequence of sensory deprivation, higher-level cognitive models generally have to contend with less prediction error, which Hobson and Friston (2012) suggest as an explanation for dream content that is bizarre or fantastic (as compared with typical waking content/percepts). Their explanation for bizarre or fantastic dream content may double as an explanation for certain forms of religious dream content, such as the appearance of gods, ghosts, heavenly realms, etc. Individuals may "think" about God, heaven, and so forth, during waking consciousness, but they typically do not "see" or "hear" these things as they might during dreaming. One explanation for the mundane perceptual characteristics of typical waking consciousness during daytime conditions is that incoming sensory information prohibits the application of perceptual models that do not align with the physical features of the external environment; without sensory information acting as a "corrective" (during dreaming or other cognitive situations), the mind is essentially free to construct content/percepts that do not correspond to physical features of one's external environment (cf. Hobson & Friston, 2012, pp. 88–89, 92–93; Andersen et al., 2014, pp. 223–224).

Additionally, the lack of prediction error stemming from the reduced sensory input during sleep arguably contributes to an individual's sense of the dream's veridicality (Hobson & Friston, 2012, p. 88). The veridical sense is important when thinking about a dream's lasting significance on an individual's belief system. Religious experiences involving heaven, ghosts, gods, etc.—experiences that would be either unlikely or impossible under typical waking conditions—occur during dreaming sleep and may be granted as much credence as waking experiences, if not more (see Morewedge & Norton, 2009).

Dream content provides fodder for cognitive appraisal both during and after the oneiric event has transpired. Additionally, certain forms of dream content are more common in dreams deemed religious than in other dream types, which suggests that the implicated content facilitates religious interpretation (see Sears, 2016, pp. 96–121). Here I briefly focus on the case of good fortunes, which have been positively associated with spiritual/religious dreams in several studies (Casto, 1995; Bulkeley, 2007, 2009a; Bulkeley & Hartmann, 2011; Sears, 2016).

"Good fortunes" is the name of a category of dream content according to the widely used Hall and Van de Castle (1966) scheme for coding dream reports. The original "good fortunes" definition referred to "adventitious" positive circumstances that occurred within the dream (see Domhoff, 1996, p. 243), though a more specific typology of good fortune phenomena has since been created (Bulkeley, 2006) and used by researchers (e.g., Bulkeley & Hartmann, 2011; Sears, 2016). The original definition, subsequent typology, and related examples offer clues as to possible mechanisms for religious interpretation. As the term *adventitious* implies, good fortunes generally refer to oneiric events that were not intended by the dreamer or other characters known to the dreamer prior to the event. Thus, good fortunes typically challenge the dreamer to look for a cause beyond the actions of the self and other previously recognizable agents (cf. Taves, 2009, pp. 100–102; Malle, 1999, 2004).

If a good fortune event entails (a) a substantial drop in complexity, or (b) violation of domain-specific folk beliefs for natural objects, subjects would be expected to entertain divine or supernatural explanations (Fortier & Kim, 2017; Sears, 2016).[13] Flying human characters and (re-)animation of dead characters or inanimate objects, two varieties of good fortunes found in dreams (see Bulkeley, 2006), appear to meet these qualifications. Good fortunes can also refer to the spontaneous remission of illness or deliverance from threatening characters. These may occasion complexity drops by virtue of atypicality or feature loss. For instance, one of my interviewees described the following scenario: "[a male 'person'] comes with a very shiny sword and then he says this word 'slash'. . . and *all the people who have come to attack us vanish.*"[14] A situation involving no or few people is simpler than a situation involving several. Additionally, the dreamer would not have expected physical persons to instantaneously vanish during the dream, as there is practically no precedence for such during waking life. In other words, the sudden loss of characters amounts to a complexity drop. Furthermore, in keeping with CDMS predictions, this event was part of a dream that the dreamer, a Christian, regarded as being from God. In sum, good fortunes have several qualities that seem to make them prime subjects for religious attribution. There are multiple types of good fortunes, however, and further detailed analysis of their relationship to religious attribution is needed.

Both online and post hoc interpretive processing of dreams depends on basic content as well as the preexisting information that is available to memory. Examples of the latter include beliefs about religious and nonreligious things and event memories. In other words, events besides the dream under consideration may be instrumental in the religious interpretation of the dream. Relatedly, research suggests that dream repetition and dream fulfillment facilitate religious/spiritual interpretation of implicated dreams (Sears, 2016, 2018). *Dream repetition* essentially refers to a situation involving two or more dreams that subjectively resemble one another (Sears, 2016, pp. 131–133, 197). *Dream fulfillment* refers to a waking experience with one or more features bearing a subjective resemblance to the dream content or its associated meaning (Sears, 2016, pp. 187–188; 2018, pp. 192–194). Both dream repetition and (literal) dream fulfillment appear to satisfy conditions for a Type 1 complexity drop by virtue of redundancy (Fortier & Kim, 2017, p. 287).[15] That is, if the subject encounters a dream or a waking event that resembles

---

[13] Fortier and Kim (2017, pp. 279–282) distinguish domain-specific/ontological violations from domain-general/prototypical ones (cf. Purzycki & Willard, 2015; Sears, 2017a, pp. 89–93). Although Fortier and Kim acknowledge the potential of the former to elicit supernatural explanations, they do not consider such violations to be instances involving complexity drops. I am skeptical of this assessment, however, in light of their claim that *atypical* objects entail complexity drops (Fortier & Kim, 2017, p. 287; cf. Dessalles, 2007).

[14] This quote comes from a collection of interviews that served as data for Sears (2016) and is not found in the dissertation itself.

[15] See Sears (2016) for the distinction between literal versus symbolic dream fulfillment. In the discussion here I mainly have literal dream fulfillment in mind, though a similar mechanism of religious interpretation may apply to cases of symbolic dream fulfillment.

a prior dream, the subject will have the impression that he or she is experiencing a nonrandom event. Most dreams are discursive with respect to one another and subsequent waking experiences. Hence, dream fulfillment and dream repetition tend to defy subjects' prior expectations for discursivity/randomness. Moreover, the seemingly nonrandom state of affairs drives agency detection (Fortier & Kim, 2017), which, in the case of dream repetition or dream fulfillment, is likely to entail supernatural attribution (after all, what other agent would be able to disclose a future state of affairs to the individual?; see Sears, 2016, pp. 197–199). Though this appraisal process appears to be intuitive, some individuals reflexively grasp the relationship between randomness and spiritual/religious interpretation of dreams and corresponding events. To summarize this relationship, consider the following statement from one of my informants:

> I think the only way to know [if a dream is spiritual/religious] is if it is recurring and similar to the scripture and similar to what I heard from [the] pulpit and others. If I see those kinds of things in my dreams then I know that it is spiritual and God is giving me insight through dreams, but if it is just *random* then I think it is not from God. (Sears, 2016, p. 132; emphasis mine)

CONCLUSION

Although dreams and mystical experiences are separate (though possibly overlapping) phenomena, this chapter has demonstrated that both can be analyzed through the same set of cognitive theories. The previous processing descriptions of these phenomena relied extensively on the principles of hierarchical predictive coding (HPC) and event cognition, though additional concepts and principles were introduced to make sense of particular features. Most notably, complexity and intentionality-based principles provided expedient means of understanding the formation of abstract religious appraisals. While the foregoing discussion examined both the perceptual and abstract processing of dreams and mystical experiences, analysis was typically brief and several possible features of these experiences were left unattended. Therefore, much concerning the processing of religious dreams and mystical experiences awaits development and exploration.

Apart from its concise portrayal of experiential processing, this chapter has not considered the functional implications of dreams and mystical experiences for religion in general. Though this topic deserves significant attention from CSR researchers, I can offer only a few comments in closing. Tylor (2016) and James (2012) were willing to credit dreams and mystical experience, respectively, as the primary source of religious thought and behavior (see Kracke, 2003; Sears, 2017a). Cognitive scientists have generally advocated a different "source" understanding. One of the more popular theories of religion that cognitive scientists have forwarded claims instead that religion is a byproduct of "maturationally natural" beliefs and processes for inferring one's environment (see, e.g., Boyer, 2003; Barrett, 2004, 2011b). These include naturalistic *folk beliefs* and processes for *detecting agency* and *deducing intentions* (see, e.g., Gallagher, 2001; Atran & Norenzayan, 2004; Spelke & Kinzler, 2007; Taves, 2009; Barrett, 2004, 2011b). All of these maturationally natural beliefs/processes are necessary for navigating the physical world but may, under certain conditions, give rise to religious beliefs (and subsequent behaviors). Consistent with this byproduct understanding of religious thought, the foregoing review of dreams and mystical experiences demonstrates that *both* phenomena engage these fundamental beliefs/processes in the actualization of religious beliefs.

While mystical experiences and dreams may provide reliable platforms for the activation of religious belief, there are certainly other experiences/phenomena that can recruit basic mental resources for religious ends (see Barrett, 2004, 2011b; Taves, 2009). Given this, it may be possible to envision a world where religions exist without the aid of dreams or mystical experience. Nonetheless, it is prudent to consider whether dreams and mystical experience have made or continue to make "signature" contributions to religious thought or practice. With regard to dreams in particular, researchers continue to affirm the Tylorian notion that they provide a foundation for beliefs in souls, spirits, and supernatural agents (Lohmann, 2003a; Willerslev, 2004; McNamara & Bulkeley, 2015; Forstmann & Burgmer, 2017; Nordin & Bjälkebring, 2019). Although I concur with this notion, I hasten to note that beliefs about these things are nourished by other types of experience as well (see Barrett, 2004, 2011b; Forstmann & Burgmer, 2017). Nonetheless, dreams are a particularly important contributor to spirit/soul beliefs because of their pervasiveness, frequency, and realism due to the lack of prediction error. When individuals dream, they (typically) experience themselves in a realistic setting that differs dramatically from the bedroom they encounter upon waking. Waking consciousness, moreover, comes with bodily sensations that are typically absent in dreams. Taken together, these conditions provide a strong basis for thinking that the mind or soul is capable of existing apart from the body. The animistic belief in dreaming as an occasion of soul flight is a testament to this intuitive line of thinking (see Lohmann, 2003a, 2007; Sears, 2016).

In addition to their propensity to foster beliefs in body/soul dualism, dreams can also support beliefs in ghosts, deities, and other supernatural agents by virtue of their physiological conditions and psychological content (McNamara & Bulkeley, 2015; Nordin & Bjälkebring, 2019; Sears, 2019). Dreams provide a platform for theorizing about the actions of supernatural agents and envisioning them (Lohmann, 2000, 2003a; McNamara & Bulkeley, 2015; Nordin & Bjälkebring, 2019; Sears, 2016, 2019). Although visual "encounters" with supernatural agents can occur during other conscious states (Lohmann, 2003b; Wiebe, 2000), dreaming may be the most common platform for visionary interaction with supernatural agents. Such oneiric experiences may have played—and perhaps continue to play—a significant role in the creation of religious iconography (cf. Bulkeley, 2008, pp. 93–94, 139–140; Lewis-Williams, 2011, p. 248ff.).

Although affect may sometimes contribute to the religious significance of dreams (Bulkeley, 2007; Sears, 2016), their religious significance generally seems to owe more to imagery than affect. By contrast, affect rather than imagery appears to be the most salient dimension of mystical experience (James, 2012; Stace, 1960; Hood, 2001a). The affective characteristics of mystical experience (namely, union, peace, ego loss, and timelessness/ spacelessness) are markedly consistent with affective descriptions of personal salvation in various religious traditions (Sears, 2015b; Sears, 2017b, p. 17). Descriptions of mystical experience and personal salvation are so similar that some regard the former as a typological precursor or foretaste of the latter (Heim, 2001). To what extent mystical experiences involving ego loss, union, etc., nourish or underwrite salvation beliefs is a matter requiring further attention, however.

Despite being subjected to more than a century of scientific investigation, dreams and mystical experiences continue to necessitate critical inquiry. How these experiences are processed and what roles they serve in individual and corporate religion are two basic issues that deserve ongoing attention from cognitive scientists. Beyond these issues, ontological questions remain. For example, are the spirits that appear in dreams and the profound sense of oneness that occurs during mystical experience merely the peculiar affordances of cognitive processes operating under specific physical constraints, or is a transcendent entity/order somehow also responsible for these events? James (2012) once distinguished between a "hither" and "farther" side of religious experience (cf. Bulkeley, 2016, pp. 219–220). The former corresponds to the purview of psychology, while the latter—hypothetically spiritual or transcendent dimension of religious experience—is essentially beyond psychology's powers to describe, let alone confirm or deny. Though CSR may be regarded as significantly more advanced than the psychological science James was familiar with, the same basic limitations seemingly apply to both.

QUESTIONS FOR FURTHER RESEARCH

1. What are the limits of a de-automatization/cognitive resource depletion framework for mystical experience? Can it explain qualitative aspects such as awe, bliss, timelessness/spacelessness, luminosity, and "inner subjectivity" (see Hood, 1975)?
2. What is the role of complexity drops in mystical experiences that have nontheistic or monistic appraisals?
3. What are the various types of complexity drops found in dreams, and are certain types more likely than others to engender religious interpretations?
4. What is the prevalence of complexity drops in religious vs. nonreligious dreams? What factors, if any, modulate the frequency of complexity drops?
5. How would personal and institutional religion be different if there were no dreams or mystical experiences—in other words, what are the precise consequences of dreams and mystical experiences for religion, and are any of these unique?
6. What are the ontological/theological implications of a predictive processing explanation of dreams and mystical experiences?

REFERENCES

Alston, W. P., & Fales, E. (2004). Does religious experience justify religious belief? In M. L. Peterson & R. J. VanArragon (Eds.), *Contemporary debates in philosophy of religion* (pp. 135–163). Malden, MA: Blackwell.

Andersen, M., Schjoedt, U., Nielbo, K. L., & Sørensen, J. (2014). Mystical experience in the lab. *Method & Theory in the Study of Religion, 26*, 217–245. doi:10.1163/15700682-12341323

Andresen, J. (Ed.). (2001). *Religion in mind: Cognitive perspectives on religious belief, ritual, and experience*. Cambridge, UK: Cambridge University Press.

Atran, S., & Norenzayan, A. (2004). Religion's evolutionary landscape: Counterintuition, commitment, compassion, communion. *Behavioral and Brain Sciences, 27*, 713–730. doi:10.1017/S0140525X04000172

Barnard, G. W. (1997). *Exploring unseen worlds: William James and the philosophy of mysticism*. Albany: State University of New York Press.

Barrett, J. L. (2004). *Why would anyone believe in God?* Lanham, MD: AltaMira Press.

Barrett, J. L. (2011a). Cognitive science of religion: Looking back, looking forward. *Journal for the Scientific Study of Religion, 50*(2), 229–239. doi:10.1111/j.1468-5906.2011.01564.x

Barrett, J. L. (2011b). Cognitive science, religion, and theology: From human minds to divine minds. West Conshohocken, PA: Templeton Press.

Boyer, P. (2003). Religious thought and behaviour as by-products of brain function. *Trends in Cognitive Sciences, 7*(3), 119–124. doi:10.1016/s1364-6613(03)00031-7

Bulkeley, K. (2006). Revision of the good fortune scale: A new tool for the study of "big dreams." *Dreaming, 16*(1), 11–21. doi:10.1037/1053-0797.16.1.11

Bulkeley, K. (2007). Sacred sleep: Scientific contributions to the study of religiously significant dreaming. In D. Barrett & P. McNamara (Eds.), *The new science of dreaming: Vol. 3. Cultural and theoretical perspectives* (pp. 71–94). Westport, CT: Praeger.

Bulkeley, K. (2008). *Dreaming in the world's religions: A comparative history*. New York: New York University Press.

Bulkeley, K. (2009a). Mystical dreaming: Patterns in form, content, and meaning. *Dreaming, 19*(1), 30–41. doi:10.1037/a0014788

Bulkeley, K. (2009b). The religious content of dreams: A new scientific foundation. *Pastoral Psychology, 58*(2), 93–106. doi:10.1007/s11089-008-0180-8

Bulkeley, K. (2016). *Big dreams: The science of dreaming and the origins of religion*. New York: Oxford University Press.

Bulkeley, K., & Hartmann, E. (2011). Big dreams: An analysis using central image intensity, content analysis, and word searches. *Dreaming, 21*(3), 157–167. doi:10.1037/a0024087

Casto, K. L. (1995). *Contemporary spiritual dream reports: Their content and significance* (Order No. 9608737) [Doctoral dissertation, Saybrook Institute]. ProQuest Dissertations and Theses Global.

Chen, Z, Wen, Q., Hood, R. W., Jr., & Watson, P. J. (2011). Common core thesis and qualitative and quantitative analysis of mysticism in Chinese Buddhist monks and nuns. *Journal for the Scientific Study of Religion, 50*(4), 654–670. doi:10.1111/j.1468-5906.2011.01606.x

Clark, A. (2013). Whatever next? Predictive brains, situated agents, and the future of cognitive science. *Behavioral and Brain Sciences, 36*(3). doi:10.1017/S0140525X12000477

Clark, A. (2016). *Surfing uncertainty: Prediction, action, and the embodied mind*. New York: Oxford University Press.

d'Aquili, E. G., & Newberg, A. B. (1993). Religious and mystical states: A neuropsychological model. *Zygon, 28*(2), 177–200.

Deikman, A. J. (2010). De-automatization and the mystic experience. In J. L. Barrett (Ed.), *Psychology of religion* (Vol. 2, pp. 51–71). New York: Routledge. (Originally published in 1966 in *Psychiatry 29*, 324–338).

Dement, W., & Wolpert, E.A. (1958). The relation of eye movements, body motility, and external stimuli to dream content. *Journal of Experimental Psychology, 55*, 543–553.

Dessalles, J.-L. (2007). *Spontaneous assessment of complexity in the selection of events.* [Technical Report (ParisTech-ENST 2007D011)]. Paris: École Nationale Supérieure des Télécommunications.

Dessalles, J.-L. (2008). Coincidences and the encounter problem: A formal account. In B. C. Love, K. McCrae, & V. M. Sloutsky (Eds.), *Proceedings of the 30th Annual Conference of the Cognitive Science Society* (pp. 2134–2139). Austin, TX: Cognitive Science Society.

Dessalles, J.-L. (2013). Algorithmic simplicity and relevance. In D. L. Dowe (Ed.), *Algorithmic probability and friends—LNAI 7070* (pp. 119–130). Berlin: Springer Verlag.

Domhoff, G. W. (1996). *Finding meaning in dreams: A quantitative approach.* New York: Plenum Press.

Domhoff, G. W. (2017). The invasion of the concept snatchers: The origins, distortions, and future of the continuity hypothesis. *Dreaming, 27*(1), 14–39. doi:10.1037/drm0000047

Egan, H. D. (1978). Christian apophatic and kataphatic mysticisms. *Theological Studies, 39*(3), 399–426. doi:10.1177/004056397803900301

Forman, R. K. C. (2007). What does mysticism have to teach us about consciousness? *AntiMatters, 2*, 71–89. (Originally published in 1998 in *Journal of Consciousness Studies, 5*(2), 185—201).

Forstmann, M., & Burgmer, P. (2017). Antecedents, manifestations, and consequences of belief in mind-body dualism. In C. M. Zedelius, B. C. N. Müller, & J. W. Schooler (Eds.), *The science of lay theories: How beliefs shape our cognition, behavior, and health* (pp. 181–205). Cham: Springer.

Fortier, M., & Kim, S. (2017). From the impossible to the improbable: A probabilistic account of magical beliefs and practices across development and cultures. In C. M. Zedelius, B. C. N. Müller, & J. W. Schooler (Eds.), *The science of lay theories: How beliefs shape our cognition, behavior, and health* (pp. 265–315). Cham: Springer.

Franklin, J. (2000). A spiritual biography: An account of spiritual/religious experiences from a small child to the present moment. *De Numine, 28*, 14–17.

Friston, K., & Kiebel, S. (2009). Predictive coding under the free-energy principle. *Philosophical Transactions of the Royal Society, 364*, 1211–1221. doi:10.1098/rstb.2008.0300

Gallagher, S. (2001). The practice of mind: Theory, simulation, or primary interaction? *Journal of Consciousness Studies, 8*(5–7), 83–108.

Gavrilyuk, P. L. (2013). Nineteenth- to twentieth-century Russian mysticism. In J. A. Lamm (Ed.), *The Wiley-Blackwell companion to Christian mysticism* (pp. 489–500). West Sussex, UK: Wiley-Blackwell.

Granqvist, P., Fredrikson, M., Unge, P., Hagenfeldt, A., Valind, S., Larhammar, D., & Larsson, M. (2005). Sensed presence and mystical experiences are predicted by suggestibility, not by the application of transcranial weak complex magnetic fields. *Neuroscience Letters, 379*, 1–6.

Hall, C. S., & Van de Castle, R. L. (1966). *The content analysis of dreams.* New York: Appleton-Century-Crofts.

Heim, S. M. (2001). *The depth of the riches: A trinitarian theology of religious ends*. Grand Rapids, MI: William B. Eerdmans.

Hermans, C. A. M. (2015). Towards a theory of spiritual and religious experiences: A building block approach of the unexpected possible. *Archive for the Psychology of Religion, 37*, 141–167. doi:10.1163/15736121-12341306

Hobson, J. A., & Friston, K. J. (2012). Waking and dreaming consciousness: Neurobiological and functional considerations. *Progress in Neurobiology, 98*, 82–98. doi:10.1016/j.pneurobio.2012.05.003

Hobson, J. A., & Friston, K. J. (2014). Consciousness, dreams, and inference. *Journal of Consciousness Studies, 21*(1–2), 6–32.

Hood, R. W., Jr. (1975). Construction and preliminary validation of a measure of reported mystical experience. *Journal for the Scientific Study of Religion, 14*(1), 29–41. doi:10.2307/1384454

Hood, R. W., Jr. (1978). Anticipatory set and setting: Stress incongruities as elicitors of mystical experience in solitary nature situations. *Journal for the Scientific Study of Religion, 17*(3), 279–287.

Hood, R. W., Jr. (1989). Mysticism, the unity thesis, and the paranormal. In G. K. Zollschan, J. F. Schumaker, & G. F. Walsh (Eds.), *Exploring the paranormal* (pp. 117–130). New York: Avery Publishing Group.

Hood, R. W., Jr. (2001a). *Dimensions of mystical experiences: Empirical studies and psychological links*. Amsterdam: Rodopi.

Hood, R. W., Jr. (2001b). Epilogue and prospects: The empirical study of mysticism. In *Dimensions of mystical experiences: Empirical studies and psychological links* (pp. 153–163). Amsterdam: Rodopi.

Hornbeck, R. G., & Sears, R. E. (2015). Mysticism and mind: Using cognitive science to explore religious experience. *European Journal for Philosophy of Religion, 7*(2), 59–80. doi:10.24204/ejpr.v7i2.120

James, W. (2012). *The varieties of religious experience: A study in human nature* (M. Bradley, Ed.). Oxford: Oxford University Press. (Original work published in 1902).

Kahan, T. L., & LaBerge, S. P. (2011). Dreaming and waking: Similarities and differences revisited. *Consciousness and Cognition, 20*, 494–514. doi:10.1016/j.concog.2010.09.002

Katz, S.T. (1978). Language, epistemology, and mysticism. In S. T. Katz (Ed.), *Mysticism and philosophical analysis* (pp. 22–74). London: Sheldon Press.

Koulack, D. (1969). Effects of somatosensory stimulation on dream content. *Archives of General Psychiatry, 20*, 718–725.

Kracke, W. (2003). Afterword: Beyond the mythologies; a shape of dreaming. In R. I. Lohmann (Ed.), *Dream travelers: Sleep experiences and culture in the Western Pacific* (pp. 211–235). New York: Palgrave Macmillan.

Lewis-Williams, D. (2011). *The mind in the cave: Consciousness and the origins of art*. London: Thames & Hudson. (Originally published in 2002).

Lohmann, R. I. (2000). The role of dreams in religious enculturation among the Asabano of Papua New Guinea. *Ethos, 28*(1), 75–102.

Lohmann, R. I. (Ed.). (2003a). *Dream travelers: Sleep experiences and culture in the Western Pacific*. New York: Palgrave Macmillan.

Lohmann, R. I. (2003b). Supernatural encounters of the Asabano in two traditions and three states of consciousness. In R. I. Lohmann (Ed.), *Dream travelers: Sleep experiences and culture in the Western Pacific* (pp. 189–210). New York: Palgrave Macmillan.

Lohmann, R. I. (2007). Dreams and ethnography. In D. Barrett & P. McNamara (Eds.), *The new science of dreaming: Vol. 3. Cultural and theoretical perspectives* (pp. 35–69). Westport, CT: Praeger.

Luhrmann, T. M. (2012). *When God talks back: Understanding the American evangelical relationship with God.* New York: Alfred A. Knopf.

Malle, B. F. (1999). How people explain behavior: A new theoretical framework. *Personality and Social Psychology Review, 3*(1), 23–48. doi:10.1207/s15327957pspr0301_2

Malle, B. F. (2004). *How the mind explains behavior: Folk explanations, meaning, and social interaction.* Cambridge, MA: MIT Press.

Marshall, P. (2005). *Mystical encounters with the natural world: Experiences and explanations.* New York: Oxford University Press.

McNamara, P., & Bulkeley, K. (2015). Dreams as a source of supernatural agent concepts. *Frontiers in Psychology, 6*(283). doi:10.3389/fpsyg.2015.00283

Morewedge, C. K., & Norton, M. I. (2009). When dreaming is believing: The (motivated) interpretation of dreams. *Journal of Personality and Social Psychology, 96*(2), 249–264. doi:10.1037/a0013264

Nielsen, T. A., McGregor, D. L., Zadra, A., Ilnicki, D., & Ouellet, L. (1993). Pain in dreams. *Sleep: Journal of Sleep Research and Sleep Medicine, 16*, 490–498.

Nordin, A. (2011). Dreaming in religion and pilgrimage: Cognitive, evolutionary and cultural perspectives. *Religion, 41*(2), 225–249. doi:10.1080/0048721X.2011.553141

Nordin, A., & Bjälkebring, P. (2019). Measuring counterintuitiveness in supernatural agent dream imagery. *Frontiers in Psychology, 10*, 1728. doi:10.3389/fpsyg.2019.01728

Otto, R. (2016). *Mysticism East and West: A comparative analysis of the nature of mysticism* (B. L. Bracey & R. C. Payne, Trans.). Eugene, OR: Wipf & Stock. (Original work published in 1932).

Paquette, A. (2018). The interpretation of independent agents and spiritual content in dreams. *International Journal of Dream Research, 11*(2), 86–105.

Persinger, M. A. (1987). *Neuropsychological bases of God beliefs.* New York: Praeger.

Petrican, R., & Burris, C. T. (2012). Am I the stone? Overattribution of agency and religious orientation. *Psychology of Religion and Spirituality, 4*(4), 312–323. doi:10.1037/a0027942

Purzycki, B. G., & Willard, A. K. (2015). MCI theory: A critical discussion. *Religion, Brain & Behavior, 6*(3), 207–248. doi:10.1080/2153599X.2015.1024915

Radavansky, G. A., & Zacks, J. M. (2014). *Event cognition.* Oxford: Oxford University Press.

Schjoedt, U., & Andersen, M. (2017). How does religious experience work in predictive minds? *Religion, Brain & Behavior, 7*(4). doi:10.1080/2153599X.2016.1249913.

Schjoedt, U., Sørensen, J., Nielbo, K. L., Xygalatas, D., Mitkidis, P., & Bulbulia, J. (2013). Cognitive resource depletion in religious interactions. *Religion, Brain & Behavior, 3*(1), 39–86. doi:10.1080/2153599X.2012.736714

Schredl, M. (2003). Continuity between waking and dreaming: A proposal for a mathematical model. *Sleep & Hypnosis, 5*(1), 26–39.

Schredl, M. (2017). Theorizing about the continuity between waking and dreaming: Comment on Domhoff (2017). *Dreaming, 27*(4), 351–359. doi:10.1037/drm0000062

Sears, R. E. (2015a). The construction, preliminary validation, and correlates of a dream-specific scale for mystical experience. *Journal for the Scientific Study of Religion, 54*(1), 134–155. doi: 0.1111/jssr.12169

Sears, R. E. (2015b). *One or many? How the psychology of religion and emotion can help us understand mystical experience and critique the typological debate within the theology of religions*. [Unpublished presentation]. Center for Missiological Research, Fuller Theological Seminary, Pasadena, CA.

Sears, R. E. (2016). *Spiritual dreams and the Nepalese: Attribution theory and the dream-related cognition of Nepali Christians and Hindus* (Order No. 10104552) [Doctoral dissertation, Fuller Theological Seminary]. ProQuest Dissertations and Theses Global.

Sears, R. E. (2017a). The naturalness of religious ideas: Soundings from the cognitive science of religion. *Epistemology and Philosophy of Science, 54*(4), 82–98. doi:10.5840/eps201754474

Sears, R. E. (2017b). The nature of experience: Empirical considerations and theological ramifications. *Perspectives on Science & Christian Faith, 69*(1), 13–26.

Sears, R. E. (2018). Dreams and Christian conversion: Gleanings from a Pentecostal church context in Nepal. *Mission Studies, 35*(2), 183–203. doi:10.1163/15733831-12341566

Sears, R. E. (2018). Dreams and Christian conversion: Gleanings from a Pentecostal church context in Nepal. *Mission Studies, 35*(2), 183–203. doi:10.1163/15733831-12341566

Sears, R. E. (2019). Commentary: Measuring counterintuitiveness in supernatural agent dream imagery. *Frontiers in Psychology, 10*, 2855. doi:10.3389/fpsyg.2019.02855

Sears, R. E., & Hood, R. W., Jr. (2016). Dreaming mystical experience among Christians and Hindus: The impact of culture, language, and religious participation on responses to the Dreaming Mysticism Scale. *Mental Health, Religion & Culture, 19*(8), 833–845. doi:10.1080/13674676.2016.1266472

Smith, C. (2013). Can healthy, young adults uncover personal details of unknown target individuals in their dreams? *Explore, 9*(1), 17–25. doi:10.1016/j.explore.2012.10.003

Spelke, E. S., & K. Kinzler, D. (2007). Core knowledge. *Developmental Science, 10*(1), 89–96. doi:10.1111/j.1467-7687.2007.00569.x

Spilka, B., Shaver, P., & Kirkpatrick, L. A. (1985). A general attribution theory for the psychology of religion. *Journal for the Scientific Study of Religion, 24*(1), 1–20. doi:10.2307/1386272

Stace, W. T. (1960). *Mysticism and philosophy*. Los Angeles, CA: Jeremy P. Tarcher.

Taves, A. (2009). *Religious experience reconsidered: A building block approach to the study of religion and other special things*. Princeton, NJ: Princeton University Press.

Taves, A. (2020). Mystical and other alterations in sense of self: An expanded framework for studying nonordinary experiences. *Perspectives on Psychological Science, 15*(3), 669–690. doi:10.1177/1745691619895047

Taves, A., & Asprem, E. (2017). Experience as event: Event cognition and the study of (religious) experiences. *Religion, Brain & Behavior, 7*(1), 43–62. doi:10.1080/2153599X.2016.1150327

Tylor, E. B. (2016). *Primitive culture: Researches into the development of mythology, philosophy, religion, language, art, and custom* (Vol. 1, 2nd ed.). Mineola, NY: Dover. (Original published in 1873).

Wiebe, P. H. (2000). Critical reflections on Christic visions. *Journal of Consciousness Studies, 7*(11), 119–144.

Willerslev, R. (2004). Spirits as "ready to hand": A phenomenological analysis of Yukaghir spiritual knowledge and dreaming. *Anthropological Theory, 4*(4), 395–418. doi:10.1177/1463499604047918

Zaehner, R. C. (1957). *Mysticism, sacred and profane: An inquiry into some varieties of praeternatural experience*. London: Oxford University Press.

CHAPTER 13

....

EXTREME RITUALS

....

DIMITRIS XYGALATAS

INTRODUCTION

....

THE term "extreme ritual" does not imply rituals involving deviant or pathological behaviors, nor is it meant as a value judgment. Instead, it is used to describe the types of ritual that, compared to most other ceremonies, are high in intensity and entail significant levels of pain, stress, physical risk, or trauma. By way of analogy, consider the term "extreme sports"—activities such as parachuting, rock-climbing, and the Ironman Triathlon, that involve exceptional effort or risk but are not considered aberrant behaviors. Contrary to what many might expect, extreme rituals are not rare, and they have been thoroughly documented historically and cross-culturally across numerous contexts (Rossano, 2015). In fact, anthropologists who study extreme rituals find that within these contexts they tend to be performed widely by people of all socioeconomic backgrounds.

Examples of extreme rituals abound (Xygalatas, 2022). In Greco-Roman times, devotees of Cybele and Attis performed ecstatic rituals that involved self-flagellation, the slashing and cutting of the skin, and other forms of mutilation. Similar actions are involved in the contemporary rituals performed by many Shia Muslims on the day of Ashura to mourn the martyrdom of Imam Hussein, when devotees slash their flesh with knives and flog themselves with razors attached to chains. In the initiation rituals performed among some Amazonian tribes, agitated, venomous bullet ants are used to inflict excruciating stings on the hands of initiates. On the other side of the world, Catholics in the Philippines have their hands nailed to crosses on Good Friday to commemorate the passion of Christ. In Vanuatu, young men jump from tall towers headfirst with vines tied around their ankles, risking serious injury or even death. And in Thailand, Taoists gather in the thousands to celebrate the Feast of the Nine Emperor Gods with bloodletting and self-mutilation. Such extreme rituals are not confined to religious traditions alone. For instance, the practice of piercing the body with hooks, needles, or skewers is found among secular groups of "suspenders" (people who practice body suspension through hooks attached to their skin) around the world (Klement et al., 2017). Similarly, fire- or glass-walking rituals are performed by various secular organizations (Danforth, 1989).

The widespread existence of these customs presents a puzzle: Why do people engage in practices that appear to be painful, stressful, risky, or dangerous but have no obvious benefits? Of course, many painful rituals are performed without the participants' consent, such as circumcision and other forms of genital mutilation. This, too, raises intriguing questions, since inflicting deliberate harm upon one's offspring, especially in ways that may compromise their reproductive potential, is not behavior we typically expect from parents. But in many (and perhaps the most widespread) cases, extreme rituals are performed voluntarily. It is then a reasonable question: Why are millions of people around the world willing to suffer to participate in these ceremonies?

Social theorists have long proposed various answers to the puzzle of extreme rituals, suggesting that these practices may serve important functions for individual participants as well as for society at large. However, for a variety of reasons, these events are hard to study scientifically. Extreme rituals usually take place annually or less frequently, so repeated observations take time and commitment. Moreover, field observations in the midst of frenetic collective activities are difficult to carry out, and researchers' ability to control confounding variables is limited or even impossible. Devotees can be reluctant to discuss their participation for fear of being misunderstood or misportrayed by the ethnographer (Xygalatas, 2011). At the same time, extreme rituals are impossible to study in a laboratory setting—not only because of practical and ethical limitations but also because sacred ceremonies do not make any sense to participants once they have been taken outside of their natural context (Xygalatas, 2019). For these and various other reasons, early scholars did not have the methodological tools that would allow them to test their intuitions.

Recent methodological advances have made it possible for researchers in the cognitive science of religion (CSR) to study extreme rituals in more systematic ways. These methodologies typically involve a combination of qualitative and quantitative techniques, anchored in expert knowledge of particular ritual traditions. Rather than try to move these rituals to the more controlled environment of the laboratory, researchers sometimes bring laboratory methods into the field or move back and forth between laboratory and field settings (Xygalatas, 2016). To deal with the complexity of the social world, they typically follow a fractionating approach, focusing on particular ritual components to study their effects independently, one at a time (Taves, 2009). To manage the increased demands of these designs, cognitive scientists of religion have been moving toward ever-stronger forms of interdisciplinarity, shifting from a traditional single-scholar paradigm to a new model of collaborative, team-based research (Xygalatas, 2013a, 2018a, 2013b). Thanks to these methodological advances, in recent years cognitive scientists of religion have been able to test long-standing claims about the psychological and social functions of extreme rituals, shining new light on this age-old puzzle.

Extreme Rituals and the Individual

Much of the research on extreme rituals has focused on the individual participation experience because these ceremonies are commonly perceived to be deeply meaningful and to play a crucial role in shaping people's personal and collective identities. Ethnographic observations suggest that although practitioners of extreme rituals are often not provided with official theological interpretations for their participation, the emotional and physiological arousal involved in these events triggers a spontaneous search for reflection (Whitehouse, 2002; Xygalatas & Mano, n.d.). For example, most novices might say, vaguely, that their decision to participate was based on custom, but later re-evaluate that decision as having a specific purpose and meaning all along (Xygalatas, 2012). Cognitive scientists of religion have studied various factors that may contribute to this meaning-making process.

Episodic Memory

Various cognitive scientists of religion have stressed the role of memory in the meaning-making process (McCauley & Lawson, 2002; Whitehouse, 2004). Extreme rituals involve high levels of arousal and sensory pageantry that can include bright lights and fires, the smell of incense or the blood of animals, the deafening sounds of vibrating drums and the cheers of the crowd, the burning sensation of walking on glowing embers, and the taste of special drinks and meals. Extravagant displays and prolonged exhaustion hyperstimulate all the senses. Everything in the environment is telling the brain that this is a special moment, which is worth paying attention to and remembering. Rituals are designed to feel special, and extreme rituals feel *extremely* special, which is why they result in vivid, long-lasting memories. Crucially, after their performance, the subsequent vindication of the experience through constant retellings and symbolic reminders helps consolidate these memories as utterly significant (McCauley & Lawson, 2002).

These memories are very different from the recollections people typically have of more ordinary rituals. Instead of sensory arousal, most rituals rely on frequent repetition and official doctrines for transmission (which is why they are often called *doctrinal*). But when the same ceremony takes place again and again, it is hard to remember any specific instance of it. Instead, the various occurrences tend to blend together to produce *semantic* memories, which are generic schemas of what usually happens during a ritual, without much specificity (Whitehouse, 2004). If you ask congregants to describe what happened at a certain Mass one year ago, for example, they will probably tell you what typically takes place at church every Sunday, but not what happened on any particular Sunday (unless something exceptional happened on that occasion).

In contrast, extreme rituals comprise the kinds of practices Harvey Whitehouse (2004) calls *imagistic*. They are, as noted, infrequently performed and particularly intense. They stand out as special and rely on extravagance to create *episodic* memories—that is, detailed representations of specific important events in our lives. Although research shows that episodic memories are often malleable and prone to error (Xygalatas, Schjoedt, et al., 2013; Loftus & Kaufman, 1992), they are nonetheless experienced as true and consistent. They play an instrumental role in creating and maintaining our narrative self—our sense of identity, continuity, and unique life history—which is why they are also called *autobiographical* memories.

The extraordinary events that unfold in the context of extreme rituals beg for explanation. However, because extreme rituals often lack official exegesis, it is up to performers to find their own spontaneous interpretations of the events. Indeed, these rituals tend to trigger a persistent search for meaning, which also helps to increase the motivation to maintain and transmit them (Whitehouse, 2001). As we will see later, this has important implications for the social effects of extreme rituals.

Effort Justification

A related view, which stems from social psychology, focuses on how extreme rituals create the need for effort justification: people tend to attribute value to an outcome based on how much it costs to achieve it. When we engage in an action that is very costly (e.g., financially, physically, or emotionally) but has no obvious benefits, we feel uncomfortable or anxious. Leon Festinger (1957) called this feeling "cognitive dissonance." To reduce this feeling of dissonance, then, people often come to reinterpret the action as more meaningful, pleasurable, or important.

One of the first and best-known empirical demonstrations of this phenomenon is an experiment conducted by Aronson and Mills (1959), in which three groups of women were invited to join a discussion group. As part of the process, one group had to go through an innocuous initiation, while another underwent an initiation that was designed to cause embarrassment. The third group did not undergo any initiation. All the subjects then went on to participate in the discussion group, which had been intentionally set up to be boring and unappealing. In the words of the experimenters, it involved "one of the most worthless and uninteresting discussions imaginable" (Aronson & Mills, 1959, p. 179). At the end of the activity, the experimenters asked the subjects to rate the group and its members along a number of attributes, such as how interesting they found the discussion and how intelligent and likeable the other participants were. The researchers found that the participants who had paid a steeper price to join the group provided higher ratings.

Similarly, because some our most important rituals (e.g. initiations, weddings, coronations) require a lot of effort, our intuitive assumption is that if something if very effortful, it must also be very important and meaningful. Anthropologists have documented this effort justification in the context of extreme rituals. For example, my ethnographic research in the context of a fire-walking ritual in Greece showed that while novice performers were unable to provide specific reasons for participating, more seasoned fire-walkers did offer more specific justifications. Critically, an examination of the ethnographic record showed that this was not an effect of age or generational differences. After their first time, most fire-walkers reported that they were not fully aware of the reason they had done it, typically referring to tradition (e.g., "this is just what we do") or some inexplicable urge. But several years later, the same participants had re-evaluated that first time and reported that it had been driven by a specific purpose, such as healing or fertility (Xygalatas, 2007).

This process of post-hoc justification of ritual practice may be the rule rather than the exception. Few people partake in their first ritual because they are motivated by any deep intrinsic reason. Most people initially participate because they have been asked to or encouraged to by their parents, relatives, or educators, or because their peers do it, or merely out of curiosity. But after investing substantial time and effort in their participation, they intuitively associate all that time and effort with something valuable and meaningful. Because extreme rituals by definition involve greater effort, this effect will be even stronger.

Health and Healing

This link between effort and value may be one of the reasons behind the paradoxical association between extreme rituals and healing. In spite of the high levels of stress and suffering involved, as well as various health risks such as injury, trauma, or infection, in many contexts such rituals are often culturally prescribed remedies for a variety of conditions, especially ones related to mental health. Those who suffer from chronic illness are often particularly likely to engage in them (Jilek, 1982). A field study examined the health effects on people who had performed the *kavadi* ritual, which involves severe bodily mutilation and other forms of intense suffering, and compared them to a control group (Xygalatas et al., 2019). For two months, the experimenters monitored subjects' physiological health by measuring their blood pressure, heart rate, electrodermal activity, and sleep efficiency, and also obtained psychometric assessments of subjective well-being. The results revealed that even though the participants experienced exceptionally high levels of physiological stress during the ritual, they did not experience any long-term physical harm. On the contrary, during the weeks following the ritual they showed an improvement in their psychological well-being and quality of life. In fact, the participants who had endured more pain and suffering during the ritual were the ones who showed the greatest benefits of participation.

These intriguing effects may be due to a variety of factors. At a top-down level, the cultural beliefs and expectations surrounding ritual may bring about placebo effects, which can help practitioners cope with stress and have a positive impact on the immune system (Rabin, 1999). Structural properties of ritual, too, such as repetition and rigidity, can trigger intuitive expectations about ritual efficacy (Xygalatas, Maňo, & Baranowski-Pinto, 2021) and help provide a sense of control and reduce anxiety (Lang et al., 2015,

2020). Moreover, participation may boost performers' confidence and perceived fitness. Importantly, those rituals can help foster social interactions, strengthen communal bonds, and provide a sense of belonging, all of which can provide important psychological benefits (Hobson et al., 2017).

On the bottom-up level, the physiological stimulation involved in extreme rituals can trigger processes stemming from neurological responses to the ordeal. A study of another Hindu ceremony that involved prolonged exhaustion found that the devotees who had put more physical effort into the ritual felt less tired and experienced stronger feelings of happiness after the ceremony (Fischer et al., 2014). This is reminiscent of the phenomenon known as the "runner's high," the feeling of elation and euphoria marathon runners experience when running long distances, which is attributed to alterations in endogenous chemicals such as endorphins or endocannabinoids. Indeed, studies have found that communal activities involving chanting, dancing, and other common aspects of ritual can result in a boost in endorphin levels (Tarr et al., 2015). Endorphins are opioid chemicals produced naturally in the body by the central nervous system and the pituitary gland. They serve a variety of functions, including regulating aversive states. They can have analgesic, anxiolytic, and euphoric effects—that is, they help numb pain, reduce stress, and produce feelings of bliss or ecstasy, and can even cause hallucinations. As we will see later, they also have important social implications. In the context of an extreme ritual, where intense pain, suffering, or terror may be eventually replaced by such pleasurable feelings, the sudden relief can be experienced as a life-changing event (Xygalatas, 2008).

Altered States of Consciousness

Because of these neurophysiological effects and the concomitant overwhelming of mental functioning, extreme rituals are frequently associated with altered states of consciousness. Phenomenological reports and psychological measurements suggest that participants often experience cognitive depletion, amnesia, and dissociation from external stimuli (Schjoedt et al., 2013; Jegindø et al., 2013; Lee et al., 2016), symptoms that participants often attribute to possession by a supernatural agent (Ward, 1984).

Hallucinogens are used in some rituals to induce altered states of consciousness; however, similar outcomes can be achieved through vigorous physiological arousal alone. After hours or days of intense activity (e.g., dancing, shaking, or self-flagellating), often accompanied by hardships such as fasting and sensory deprivation or hyperstimulation, devotees often report vivid visions, hallucinations, and other revelatory experiences (Xygalatas, 2012). Triggered by this hyperarousal, the brain's mesolimbic pathway plays a crucial role in how these experiences are interpreted. As in schizophrenia, increased dopamine release mediates the representation of external stimuli (real or imagined), assigning them an aura of factuality and salience (Deeley, 2004). But unlike in schizophrenia, the hallucinations produced in a ritual context can be soothing rather than scary, because schemas for their interpretation are readily available. Thus, rather than unwelcome aberrations, these experiences are typically seen as signs of charisma, supernatural intervention, and divine favor.

Social context is also important with regard to altered states of consciousness. Although the structure of the ritual and individual personality factors (such as susceptibility) are crucial to the ability to reach such a state, falling into a trance or some other state of absorption is a process that can to some extent be learned and encouraged (Luhrmann et al., 2010). In many cases, the observer can see these states spread from one person to the next in the context of the same ritual in a process of emotional contagion (Xygalatas, 2022).

EXTREME RITUALS AND SOCIETY

Extreme rituals are usually social affairs, that is, they are typically performed collectively. It is therefore unsurprising that early anthropologists of religion stressed the important role these rituals might play in fostering social solidarity (Durkheim, 1995), regulating psychosocial states (Rappaport, 1967), and maintaining social order (Turner, 1967). But as insightful as these observations may have been, they lacked precise operationalization (e.g., how do we measure social cohesion?), and consideration of the relevant mechanisms (e.g., how exactly do rituals achieve these effects?). Recent research in the CSR has tried to address these limitations by testing and expanding these early theories.

Social Cohesion

For example, a study conducted in Mauritius examined the effects of participation in the Thaipusam *kavadi* ritual (Xygalatas et al., 2013) on prosocial behavior. This ceremony, which is practiced by millions of Tamil Hindus around the world, involves piercing the body with numerous metallic objects, such as needles, hooks, and skewers. Once these piercings are in place, devotees embark barefooted on a pilgrimage to the temple of Lord Murugan, carrying their *kavadi* (heavy, ornate structures decorated with icons, flowers, and peacock feathers) on their shoulders. The ordeal, which takes place under the tropical sun, lasts several hours and culminates with carrying the *kavadi* 242 steps up a hill before finally reaching the temple.

The *kavadi* ritual is part of the Thaipusam festival, a 10-day celebration that includes different rituals of varying intensity. Because these rituals are attended by the same people, in similar numbers, and at the same temple, researchers were able to compare the effects of participation in both high-intensity rituals and low-intensity rituals. Comparing how much money people donated to charity after each type of ritual, they found that devotees were significantly more generous after the high-intensity ritual. Importantly, these effects were not limited to the active participants (those who suffered the piercings), but to the entire community—merely attending the *kavadi* was enough to increase prosocial behaviors. Moreover, when the researchers looked at how much pain the participants had experienced during the ritual, they found that the more they had suffered, the more generous they were toward the community.

These findings accord with the above-mentioned psychological evidence that effortful activities are perceived as more meaningful (Olivola & Shafir, 2013), and when they are shared with others they can increase social bonding and cooperation (Bastian et al., 2014). Moreover, they are supported by historical evidence that ritual intensity increases when cooperation is most needed and that communities that have more costly rituals tend to be more successful in the long run. For example, an archival study of ethnographic records looked at cross-cultural variation in the intensity of male initiation rituals. The results showed that in societies that engaged in warfare more frequently, males tended to endure costlier initiation rites (Sosis et al., 2007). Another study examined historical data on rituals practiced in nineteenth-century communes in the United States. The researchers found that the communes with more costly ritual requirements tended to survive longer than those with more relaxed rules (Sosis & Bressler, 2003). But how exactly do extreme rituals achieve these social effects?

Shared Identity

Extreme rituals can forge powerful social identities, a topic that has been the subject of much CSR research. Here too, the role of episodic memory has been highlighted. The intense, often traumatic, experiences involved in extreme rituals are carved in memory as vivid episodes, becoming a core and permanent part of one's autobiographical self—closely associated with a deep sense of personal identity. Participants in a collective ritual share these unique memories, and the sense of having been through the experience with all the other members of the group can lead to the formation of strong bonds between them.

It has been argued that sharing such transformative experiences with other group members triggers intuitive notions of shared essence related to kinship psychology (Whitehouse, 2018). Group members perceive other members of the group as psychological kin, which might explain why those who undergo the same initiation ritual often use terms such as "brother" to refer to their peers. This phenotypic matching produces visceral feelings of oneness with the group as a whole, creating a sense of strong alignment between personal and group interests that is often referred to as "identity fusion" (Whitehouse & Lanman, 2014; Whitehouse et al., 2017). Psychological studies find that fused individuals report being more willing to fight or die to defend their group, although it is unknown whether these statements correspond to actual self-sacrificial behavior (Whitehouse, 2018; Xygalatas, 2018b).

Emotional Alignment

Other CSR research has examined some of the potential mechanisms involved in this process. For example, a study of a fire-walking ritual (Konvalinka et al., 2011) examined Émile Durkheim's claim that these rituals produce "collective effervescence" (Durkheim 1995). Durkheim used this term to describe a process of emotional alignment that occurs during the performance of collective rituals and results in a feeling of oneness that bonds participants together. This is similar to that feeling of awe and ecstasy that causes the goosebumps at the back of your neck that you might get from being part of an exhilarated large crowd moving in unison (such as at a concert, demonstration, or a sports stadium). However, it was unclear how this feeling could be quantified.

To measure this emotional alignment, researchers looked at a fire-walking ritual performed annually in the small Spanish village San Pedro Manrique. After mapping the social network of the village, the researchers used biometric devices to monitor heart-rate activity among both the performers of the ritual and the spectators. They found that people's heart-rate patterns—that is, fluctuations in arousal—became synchronized during the ritual. This effect extended beyond the performers to the other members of the community who were present, regardless of their role or position in the ritual—for example, whether they were walking on the hot embers, waiting for their turn, or merely watching as spectators. However, it did not extend to outsiders—that is, those who had come from other towns to watch the ritual. Moreover, this emotional alignment was neither automatic nor indiscriminate: the intensity of the phenomenon was proportional to the degree of social relatedness. The more closely two people were related, whether through blood or friendship, the higher the synchrony observed in their patterns of arousal. In other words, the physicality of the ritual interacts in important ways with its sociocultural context, bringing those who share the same values and experiences into a deeper communion (Xygalatas, 2015; Xygalatas et al., 2011). This is in accordance with the observations of Durkheim, who noted that these rites do not merely generate emotions but also create a more intimate and dynamic relationship among participants.

A more direct way to achieve emotional alignment is by engaging in synchronous actions. Coordinated rhythmic movements and vocalizations are a recurrent component of many extreme (and other) rituals, and the shared feelings those synchronized actions evoke may play a crucial role in producing the powerful bonding effects of those rituals (McNeill, 1995). Research shows that the matching of movement can create interpersonal rapport and promote prosocial behaviors (Valdesolo et al., 2010; Wiltermuth & Heath, 2009; Reddish et al., 2013), and recent work has explored some of the mechanisms responsible for this phenomenon. Across a variety of contexts, synchrony has been found to increase participants' sense of cooperation and similarity with one another and to elevate endorphin levels (Cohen et al., 2010; Lang et al., 2015; Tarr et al., 2015), and these factors independently mediate prosocial attitudes and behaviors (Lang et al., 2017). Besides inducing feelings of well-being (see Health and Healing section above), endorphins are implicated in interpersonal bonding and can play an instrumental role in fostering group cohesion (Shultz & Dunbar, 2010; Weinstein et al., 2016).

Costly Signals and CREDS

The high costs involved in extreme rituals make them efficient communicative devices. An evolutionary perspective that has explored the communicative functions of rituals is costly signaling theory ([CST]; see Whitehouse and Kavanagh, this volume). According to CST, some seemingly wasteful behaviors can in fact be beneficial because they convey useful information about an individual's underlying qualities. A classic example is a peculiar trait observed among gazelles, which often spring into the air after spotting a predator (a behavior called *stotting*). It is a risky move, because it wastes valuable energy and makes the animal more conspicuous. But precisely because of these costs, it also communicates an important message to the predator. A low-fitness gazelle would not be able to jump very high and could not afford to get tired before a potential attack. A stronger gazelle, on the other hand, can use this behavior to advertise its fitness to predators, informing them that they would be better off turning their attention to other, more vulnerable prey (Zahavi & Zahavi, 1997). By communicating information that can be beneficial to both senders and receivers, such signals can result in evolutionarily stable equilibria and become fixed in a population (Grafen, 1990).

Extreme rituals can function in similar ways by signaling important underlying traits to the performer's group. In addition to displaying physical prowess, participation allows adherents to publicly communicate their commitment to the group and its values, because only those truly committed to these values would be willing to pay the steep price of membership (Cronk, 1994; Iannaccone, 1994; Sosis, 2000; Sosis & Alcorta, 2003). In other words, participation provides performers with opportunities to demonstrate to their peers that they are willing to go to great lengths to reaffirm their group membership, even if that means enduring substantial physical harm.

By signaling their commitment in this way, participants gain reputational benefits and increased status. This is why individuals of lower social status put more effort into their participation (Xygalatas et al., n.d.), which in turn helps to increase their social standing, as illustrated by empirical studies showing that those who engage in extreme rituals are recognized as more trustworthy and prosocial by their peers and manage to build stronger social connections (Power, 2017b, 2017a). This can have cascading consequences for the group, as it provides a mechanism for enhancing trust, facilitating cooperation among group members (Sosis & Ruffle, 2003; Xygalatas et al., 2017), and deterring free-riders who would not be willing to bear the costly requirements of group membership (Bulbulia, 2004).

Finally, participation in extreme rituals can function as a credibility-enhancing display (Henrich, 2009), based on the premise that "actions speak louder than words." Merely attesting one's commitment to the group and its values is cheap and can easily be faked, but engaging in costly rituals is expensive and hard to fake. As cultural learners, humans are particularly attuned to such displays in deciding whether a particular belief is worthwhile and honestly held. Thus, by engaging in costly behaviors, practitioners function as role models and help propagate these rituals and the beliefs associated with them to others.

IMPLICATIONS

Extreme rituals have properties that make them attractive to individuals around the world, who engage in them to experience extraordinary sensations, find healing, or feel part of a group. Religions and other cultural systems can then co-opt those practices, adding layers of symbolism and ideology to make them useful vehicles for social group formation and maintenance. Once these practices become the established order—once they become the norm—participation becomes a token of group membership in itself, bringing social benefits to the performers and contributing to the maintenance of social order.

Thus, extreme rituals are powerful social technologies (Fischer & Xygalatas, 2014) that can help address the key adaptive problem of coordinating human action by providing reliable markers of group membership and commitment, fostering cohesion, and facilitating cooperation (Watson-Jones & Legare, 2016). This, presumably, is why they have been used in numerous contexts since time immemorial (Rossano, 2015). These contexts extend far beyond religion. Militaries incorporate high-intensity rituals in their training regimes. Indeed, specialist units such as the US Navy SEALs tend to have the toughest rituals, and their intensity tends to increase when the stakes are higher (Sosis et al., 2007); college fraternities use hazing to boost the loyalty of their members; sports fans engage in high-arousal rituals to create affiliation and raise the team's morale; and corporations take their employees through team-building rituals to improve productivity.

However, as with all technologies, these rituals can be used for better or for worse. Groups that build, or even come to worship, their own social identities often begin to see themselves in direct opposition to other groups and outsiders (Tajfel et al., 1971). Therefore, the flip side of facilitating group cooperation and cohesion can often be elevated hostility towards out-groups. When talking about collective effervescence, one might be reminded of Nazi parades, which utilized the effects of synchrony, arousal, and symbolism to fuel hatred and nationalism. When discussing initiation ceremonies, one might also include the initiations regularly used by criminal gangs and paramilitary organizations to further dark causes. And when thinking of how shared dysphoric experiences create identity fusion, one cannot overlook terrorist organizations, which may use such experiences to promote self-sacrificial behaviors among their members (Whitehouse & McQuinn, 2013). These far-reaching implications of extreme rituals mean that it is imperative to get a better scientific understanding of these behaviors, including their effects, mechanisms, benefits, and dangers. CSR scholars have taken some important first steps in this direction, but there is still much that we do not know.

Because of the high risks they impose and the physical and emotional expenditure they require, extreme rituals have often been discussed in the context of costly signaling theory. However, though several studies have tried to explore the benefits of participation, the costs have been hard to quantify. Moreover, because extreme rituals are social affairs, we need a better understanding of how socioeconomic factors may modulate their costs and benefits. Similarly, more research is needed to clarify their potential benefits at the individual level. As we have seen, there is some evidence that such rituals may have beneficial effects on participants' subjective well-being (Tewari et al., 2012; Xygalatas et al., 2019), but understanding the conditions in which this occurs and the mechanisms that may be responsible for it requires further investigation.

We also know little about gender-specific forms of participation in extreme rituals. Some bloody practices, such as self-flagellation and crucifixion, are performed exclusively by males; however, many rituals, including fire-walking, are attended equally by men and women (Xygalatas, 2012); still others, such as those of various orgiastic cults, seem to be a predominantly female domain (Kraemer, 1979). Moreover, significant gender differentiation can often be observed within the same ritual. For example, in the context of the kavadi ritual, the most physically painful activities are carried out by males, but women are more likely to be involved in the emotionally intense displays, such as those involving trance and possession states (Xygalatas et al., 2021). Whether this is due to personality or genetic factors, such as a higher pain threshold for men or hypnotic susceptibility for women, or to social factors such as conformity to gender roles or the need to advertise different qualities, is a matter that requires further investigation.

To answer these questions, researchers need to study extreme rituals in their natural contexts, which requires the use of mixed methodologies that combine ethnographic depth and experimental rigor. Archival research and the systematic analysis of big data may help us gain a better understanding of the historical development and the cross-cultural distribution of extreme rituals. One question that arises with regard to this distribution is the relationship between religious and secular extreme ritual practices. Focusing on the former, one might get the impression that these practices are rare today and mostly present in small-scale societies. But if we look at rituals of similar quality and intensity performed outside the context of organized religion, we might get a very different picture. From military units and college fraternities to corporate team-building organizations and New Age festivals, physically and emotionally intense rituals are abundant in large-scale societies. Is it possible that all these rituals are simply different forms of fulfilling similar basic human needs, such as to feel connected or be part of a collective, or to experience ecstasy and catharsis? These are broad questions that can only be answered in small, incremental steps. To tackle them, CSR scholars proceed to fractionate their object of study into smaller and more manageable components that can be studied one at a time. As more and more of those studies accumulate, so will our knowledge and understanding of these puzzling but widespread human practices.

Questions for Future Research

1. Do extreme rituals serve the same functions in secular contexts as in religious contexts?
2. What is the role of women in extreme rituals that seem to be dominated by men?
3. What is the role of extreme rituals in out-group hostility and intergroup conflict?

References

Aronson, E., & Mills J. (1959). The effect of severity of initiation on liking for a group. *Journal of Abnormal and Social Psychology*, 59(2), 177–181.

Bastian, B., Jetten, J., & Ferris, L. J. (2014). Pain as social glue: Shared pain increases cooperation. *Psychological Science*, 25(11), 2079–2085. https://doi.org/10.1177/0956797614545886

Bulbulia, J. (2004). Religious costs as adaptations that signal altruistic intention. *Evolution and Cognition*, 10(1), 19–42.

Cohen, E., Ejsmond-Frey, R., Knight, N., & Dunbar, R. I. M. (2010). Rowers' high: Behavioural synchrony is correlated with elevated pain thresholds. *Biology Letters*, 6, 106–108.

Cronk, L. (1994). Evolutionary theories of morality and the manipulative use of signals. *Zygon*, 29(1), 81–101. https://doi.org/10.1111/j.1467-9744.1994.tb00651.x

Danforth, L. M. (1989). *Firewalking and religious healing: The Anastenaria of Greece and the American firewalking movement*. Princeton, NJ: Princeton University Press.

Deeley, P. Q. (2004). The religious brain: Turning ideas into convictions. *Anthropology and Medicine*, 11(3), 245–267. https://doi.org/10.1080/1364847042000296554

Durkheim, É. (1995). *The elementary forms of religious life*. New York: Free Press. (Original published in 1915).

Festinger, L. (1957). *A theory of cognitive dissonance*. Stanford, CA: Stanford University Press.

Fischer, R., & Xygalatas, D. (2014). Extreme rituals as social technologies. *Journal of Cognition and Culture*, 14, 345–355. https://doi.org/10.1163/15685373-12342130

Fischer, R., Xygalatas, D., Mitkidis, P., Reddish, P., Tok, P., Konvalinka, I., & Bulbulia, J. (2014). The fire-walker's high: Affect and physiological responses in an extreme collective ritual. *PLoS One*, 9(2). https://doi.org/10.1371/journal.pone.0088355

Grafen, A. (1990). Biological signals as handicaps. *Journal of Theoretical Biology*, 144(4), 517–546.

Henrich, J. (2009). The evolution of costly displays, cooperation and religion: Credibility enhancing displays and their implications for cultural evolution. *Evolution and Human Behavior*, 30(4), 244–260. https://doi.org/10.1016/j.evolhumbehav.2009.03.005

Hobson, N. M., Schroeder, J., Risen, J. L., Xygalatas, D., & Inzlicht, M. (2017). The psychology of rituals: An integrative review and process-based framework. *Personality and Social Psychology Review*, 25(1). https://doi.org/10.1177/1088868317734944

Iannaccone, L. R. (1994). Why strict churches are strong. *American Journal of Sociology*, 99(5), 1180. https://doi.org/10.1086/230409

Jegindø, E. M. E., Vase, L., Jegindø, J., & Geertz, A. W. (2013). Pain and sacrifice: Experience and modulation of pain in a religious piercing ritual. *International Journal for the Psychology of Religion*, 23(3), 171–187. https://doi.org/10.1080/10508619.2012.759065

Jilek, W. G. (1982). Altered states of consciousness in North American Indian ceremonials. *Ethos, 10*(4), 326–343.

Klement, K. R., Lee, E. M., Ambler, J. K., Hanson, S. A., Comber, E., Wietting, D., Wagner, M. F. et al. (2017). Extreme rituals in a BDSM context: The physiological and psychological effects of the "Dance of Souls." *Culture, Health & Sexuality, 19*(4), 453–469.

Konvalinka, I., Xygalatas, D., Bulbulia, J., Schjødt, U., Jegindø, E. M., Wallot, S., Van Orden, G., & Roepstorff, A. (2011). Synchronized arousal between performers and related spectators in a fire-walking ritual. *Proceedings of the National Academy of Sciences of the United States of America, 108*(20), 8514–8519. https://doi.org/10.1073/pnas.1016955108

Kraemer, R. (1979). Ecstasy and possession: The attraction of women to the cult of Dionysus. *Harvard Theological Review, 72*(1–2), 55–80. doi:10.1017/S0017816000029783

Lang, M., Bahna, V., Shaver, J. H., Reddish, P., & Xygalatas, D. (2017). Sync to link: Endorphin-mediated synchrony effects on cooperation. Biological Psychology, *127*. https://doi.org/10.1016/j.biopsycho.2017.06.001

Lang, M., Krátký, J., Shaver, J., Jerotijević, D., & Xygalatas, D. (2015). Effects of anxiety on spontaneous ritualized behavior. *Current Biology, 25*, 1–6.

Lang, M., Krátký, J., & Xygalatas, D. (2020). The role of ritual behavior in anxiety reduction: An investigation of Marathi religious practices in Mauritius. Philosophical Transactions *of the Royal Society* B: *Biological Sciences, 375*, Article 20190431.

Lang, M., Shaw, D. J., Reddish, P., Wallot, S., Mitkidis, P., & Xygalatas, D. (2015). Lost in the rhythm: Effects of rhythm on subsequent interpersonal coordination. *Cognitive Science*, 1–19. https://doi.org/10.1111/cogs.12302

Lee, E. M., Klement, K. R., Ambler, J. K., Loewald, T., Comber, E. M., Hanson, S. A., Pruitt, B., & Sagarin, B. J. (2016). Altered states of consciousness during an extreme ritual. *PloS One, 11*(5), Article e0153126. https://doi.org/10.1371/journal.pone.0153126

Loftus, E. F., & Kaufman, L. (1992).Why do traumatic experiences sometimes produce good memory (flashbulbs) and sometimes no memory (repression)? In E. Winograd & U. Neisser (Eds.), *Affect and accuracy in recall* (pp. 212–224). Cambridge, UK: Cambridge University Press. https://doi.org/10.1017/CBO9780511664069.011

Luhrmann, T. M., Nusbaum, H., & Thisted, R. (2010). The absorption hypothesis: Learning to hear God in evangelical Christianity. *American Anthropologist, 112*(1), 66–78. https://doi.org/10.1111/j.1548-1433.2009.01197.x

McCauley, R. N., & Lawson, E. T. (2002). *Bringing ritual to mind: Psychological foundations of cultural forms*. Cambridge, UK: Cambridge University Press.

McNeill, W. (1995). *Keeping together in time: Dance and drill in human history*. Cambridge, MA: Harvard University Press.

Olivola, C. Y., & Shafir, E. (2013). The martyrdom effect: When pain and effort increase prosocial contributions. *Journal of Behavioral Decision Making, 26*(1), 91–105.

Power, E. A. (2017a). Discerning devotion: Testing the signaling theory of religion. *Evolution and Human Behavior, 38*(1), 82–91.

Power, E. A. (2017b). Social support networks and religiosity in rural South India. *Nature Human Behavior, 1*(3), 1–6.

Rabin, B. S. (1999). Religion and medicine. *The Lancet, 353*(9166), 1803–1804.

Rappaport, R. A. (1967). Ritual regulation of environmental relations among a New Guinea people. *Ethnology, 6*(1), 17. https://doi.org/10.2307/3772735

Reddish, P., Fischer, R., & Bulbulia, J. (2013). Let's dance together: Synchrony, shared intentionality and cooperation. *PLoS One, 8*(8). https://doi.org/10.1371/journal.pone.0071182

Rossano, M. J. (2015). The evolutionary emergence of costly rituals. *PaleoAnthropology, 2015*, 78–100. https://doi.org/10.4207/PA.2015.ART97

Schjoedt, U., Sørensen, J., Nielbo, K. L., Xygalatas, D., Mitkidis, P., & Bulbulia, J. (2013). Cognitive resource depletion in religious interactions. *Religion, Brain & Behavior, 3*(1), 39–55. https://doi.org/10.1080/2153599X.2012.736714

Shultz, S., & Dunbar, R. (2010). Bondedness and sociality. *Behaviour, 147*(7), 775–803. https://doi.org/10.1163/000579510X501151

Sosis, R. (2000). Costly signaling and torch fishing on Ifaluk atoll. *Evolution and Human Behavior, 21*(4), 223–244. https://doi.org/10.1016/S1090-5138(00)00030-1

Sosis, R., & Alcorta, C. (2003). Signaling, solidarity, and the sacred: The evolution of religious behavior. *Evolutionary Anthropology, 12*(6), 264–274. https://doi.org/10.1002/evan.10120

Sosis, R., & Bressler, E. R. (2003). Cooperation and commune longevity: A test of the costly signaling theory of religion. *Cross-Cultural Research, 37*(2), 211.

Sosis, R., Kress, H. C., & Boster, J. S. (2007). Scars for war: Evaluating alternative signaling explanations for cross-cultural variance in ritual costs. *Evolution and Human Behavior, 28*(4), 234–247. https://doi.org/10.1016/j.evolhumbehav.2007.02.007

Sosis, R., & Ruffle, B. J. (2003). Religious ritual and cooperation: Testing for a relationship on Israeli religious and secular kibbutzim. *Current Anthropology, 44*(5), 713–722.

Tajfel, H., Billig, M. G., Bundy, R. P., & Flament, C. (1971). Social categorization and intergroup behaviour. *European Journal of Social Psychology, 1*(2), 149–178. https://doi.org/10.1002/ejsp.2420010202

Tarr, B., Launay, J., Cohen, E., & Dunbar, R. I. M. (2015). Synchrony and exertion during dance independently raise pain threshold and encourage social bonding. *Biology Letters, 11*, 20150767. https://doi.org/10.1098/rsbl.2015.0767

Taves, A. (2009). *Religious experience reconsidered: A building block approach to the study of religion and other special things.* Princeton, NJ: Princeton University Press.

Tewari, S., Khan, S., Hopkins, N., Srinivasan, N., & Reicher, S. (2012). Participation in mass gatherings can benefit well-being: Longitudinal and control data from a North Indian Hindu pilgrimage event. *PLoS One, 7*(10), 3–7. https://doi.org/10.1371/journal.pone.0047291

Turner, V. (1967). *The forest of symbols: Aspects of Ndembu ritual.* Ithaca, NY: Cornell University Press.

Valdesolo, P., Ouyang, J., & DeSteno, D. (2010). The rhythm of joint action: Synchrony promotes cooperative ability. *Journal of Experimental Social Psychology, 46*(4), 693–965. https://doi.org/10.1016/j.jesp.2010.03.004

Ward, C. M. (1984). Thaipusam in Malaysia: A psycho-anthropological analysis of ritual trance, ceremonial possession and self-mortification practices. *Ethos, 12*(4), 307–334.

Watson-Jones, R. E., & Legare, C. H. (2016). The social functions of group rituals. *Current Directions in Psychological Science, 25*(1), 42–46.

Weinstein, D., Launay, J., Pearce, E., Dunbar, R. I. M., & Stewart, L. (2016). Singing and social bonding: Changes in connectivity and pain threshold as a function of group size. *Evolution and Human Behavior, 37*(2), 152–158. https://doi.org/10.1016/j.evolhumbehav.2015.10.002

Whitehouse, H. (2001). Transmissive frequency, ritual, and exegesis. *Journal of Cognition and Culture, 1*(2), 167–181. https://doi.org/10.1163/156853701316931399

Whitehouse, H. (2002). Religious reflexivity and transmissive frequency. *Social Anthropology, 10*(1), 91–103. https://doi.org/10.1017/S0964028202000071

Whitehouse, H. (2004). *Modes of religiosity: A cognitive theory of religious transmission.* Walnut Creek, CA: Altamira Press.

Whitehouse, H. (2018). Dying for the group: Towards a general theory of extreme self-sacrifice. *Behavioral and Brain Sciences, 41,* e192. https://doi.org/10.1017/S0140525X18000249

Whitehouse, H., Jong, J., Buhrmester, M. D., Gómez, Á., Bastian, B., Kavanagh, C. M., Newson, M. Matthews, M., Lanman, J. A., McKay, R. & Gavrilets, S. (2017). The evolution of extreme cooperation via shared dysphoric experiences. *Scientific Reports,* 7:44292.

Whitehouse, H., & Lanman, J. A. (2014). The ties that bind us. *Current Anthropology, 55*(6), 674–695. https://doi.org/10.1086/678698

Whitehouse, H., & McQuinn, B. (2013). Ritual and violence: Divergent modes of religiosity and armed struggle. In M. Juergensmeyer, M. Kitts, & M. Jerryson (Eds.), *Oxford handbook of religion and violence,* pp. 597–619. Oxford Univeristy Press.

Wiltermuth, S. S., & Heath, C. (2009). Synchrony and cooperation. *Psychological Science, 20*(1), 1–5.

Xygalatas, D. (2007). *Firewalking in Northern Greece: A cognitive approach to high-arousal rituals.* Belfast: Queens University Belfast.

Xygalatas, D. (2008). Firewalking and the brain: The physiology of high-arousal rituals. In J. Bulbulia, R. Sosis, E. Harris, R. Genet, C. Genet, & K. Wyman (Eds.), *The evolution of religion* (pp. 197–203). Santa Margarita, CA: Collins Foundation Press.

Xygalatas, D. (2011). Ethnography, historiography, and the making of history in the tradition of the Anastenaria. *History and Anthropology, 22*(1), 57–74. https://doi.org/10.1080/02757206.2011.546855

Xygalatas, D. (2012). *The burning saints: Cognition and culture in the fire-walking rituals of the Anastenaria.* London: Routledge.

Xygalatas, D. (2013a). Přenos Laboratoře Do Terénu: Využití Smíšených Metod Během Terénního Studia Náboženství [Bringing the lab into the field: Using mixed methods to study religion in the wild]. *Sociální Studia, 10*(2), 15–25.

Xygalatas, D. (2013b). Special issue on the experimental research of religion. *Journal for the Cognitive Science of Religion, 1*(2), 137–139. https://doi.org/10.1558/jcsr.v1i2.137

Xygalatas, D. (2015). The biosocial basis of collective effervescence: An experimental anthropological study of a fire-walking ritual. *Fieldwork in Religion, 9*(1), 53–67. https://doi.org/10.1558/fiel.v9i1.53

Xygalatas, D. (2016). Bridging the gap between laboratory and field: Commentary on David Sloan Wilson and Harvey Whitehouse, "Developing the Field Site Concept for the Study of Cultural Evolution." *Cliodynamics, 7*(2), 267–270.

Xygalatas, D. (2018a). Bridging the gap: The cognitive science of religion as an integrative approach. In J. Sinding Jensen, J. Sørensen, A. Klostargaard, I. Sælid Gilhus, & L. Martin (Eds.), *Evolution, cognition, and the history of religion: A new synthesis; festschrift in honour of Armin W. Geertz* (pp. 255–272). Leiden: Brill.

Xygalatas, D. (2018b). What fuses sports fans? *Behavioral and Brain Sciences, 41,* Article e221. https://doi.org/10.1017/S0140525X18001814

Xygalatas, D. (2019, April 16). Strong interdisciplinarity and explanatory pluralism in social scientific research. *Items.* https://items.ssrc.org/insights/strong-interdisciplinarity-and-explanatory-pluralism-in-social-scientific-research/

Xygalatas, D. (2022). *The power of ritual.* London: Profile Books.

Xygalatas, D., Khan, S., Lang, M., Kundt, R., Kundtová-Klocová, E., Kratky, J., & Shaver, J. (2019). Effects of extreme ritual practices on health and well-being. *Current Anthropology, 60*(5): 699–707.

Xygalatas, D., Konvalinka, I., Roepstorff, A., & Bulbulia, J. (2011). Quantifying collective effervescence heart-rate dynamics at a fire-walking ritual. *Communicative and Integrative Biology*, 4(6), 735–738.

Xygalatas, D., Kotherová, S., Maňo, P., Kundt, R., Cigán, J., Klocová, E. K., & Lang, M. (2017). Big Gods in small places: The random allocation game in Mauritius. *Religion, Brain & Behavior*, 8(2): 243–261. https://doi.org/10.1080/2153599X.2016.1267033

Xygalatas, D., & Mano, P. (forthcoming). Ritual exegesis among Mauritian Hindus.

Xygalatas, D., Maňo, P., Bahna, V., Kundtová-Klocová, E., Kundt, R., & Shaver, J. (2021) Social status and costly signaling in an extreme ritual. *Evolution and Human Behavior*. DOI: 10.1016/j.evolhumbehav.2021.05.006

Xygalatas, D., Maňo, P., & Baranowski-Pinto, G. (2021). Ritualization increases the perceived efficacy of instrumental actions. *Cognition* 215, 104823.

Xygalatas, D., Mitkidis, P., Fischer, R., Reddish, P., Skewes, J. Geertz, A. W., Roepstorff, A., & Bulbulia, J. (2013). Extreme rituals promote prosociality. *Psychological Science*, 24(8), 1602–1605. https://doi.org/10.1177/0956797612472910

Xygalatas, D., Schjødt, U., Konvalinka, I., Jegindø, E. M. E., Roepstorff, A., & Bulbulia, J. (2013). Autobiographical memory in a fire-walking ritual. *Journal of Cognition and Culture*, 13(1–2), 1–16. https://doi.org/10.1163/15685373-12342081

Zahavi, A., & Zahavi, A. (1997). *The handicap principle: A missing piece of Darwin's puzzle*. New York: Oxford University Press.

PART VI

FORMING RELIGIOUS SYSTEMS

CHAPTER 14

KEY INGREDIENTS FOR A WORLD RELIGION

Insights from Cognitive and Evolutionary Science

JAMES VAN SLYKE AND D. JASON SLONE

INTRODUCTION

IMAGINE you want to start a religion, and you want it to spread widely throughout the world and last for many generations. What would your religion need to be like to have a good chance of success? Is there a recipe of some kind you could follow? One activity of the cognitive science of religion (CSR) has been to explore the foundational ingredients that lie beneath the various cultural expressions of religion. In this chapter, we argue, based on insights from cognitive and evolutionary science, that contemporary world religions (e.g., Christianity, Islam, and Hinduism) tend to follow the same basic recipe. And as with all successful recipes—those shared among friends and family and passed down through generations—the reason they have become *world* religions is that they fit the expectations, biases, and preferences of the human mind formed through our shared evolutionary heritage.

The three key ingredients the chapter describes are not intended as an exhaustive list, but rather, they are key elements that have produced considerable empirical evidence in the development of CSR and these ingredients have been found in several different domains of contemporary world religions. The first ingredient, the *cognitive foundations of gods and rituals*, refers to the cognitive tendencies that influence the formation and spread of god concepts and rituals. The second ingredient, *supernatural monitoring and intuitive morality*, refers to the use of religion as a form of social monitoring and the ways in which religious morality reflects aspects of evolved moral intuitions. The third and final ingredient is *mating strategies*, in that religion enhances aspects of long-term mating strategies at both the individual and cultural level.

First Ingredient: Cognitive Foundations of Gods and Rituals

One of the first major contributions to CSR came from anthropologist Stewart Guthrie's book *Faces in the Clouds* (1993). In *Faces*, Guthrie noted that one cross-culturally recurrent feature of religion is anthropomorphism—perceiving humanlike characteristics in the world where there are none, such as seeing faces in the clouds or regarding a wisp of smoke as a spirit. Guthrie's explanation for why this is a recurrent cross-cultural phenomenon laid a foundation for what would become a central theory in CSR: humans have a cognitive capacity to identify agents in their environment, which has evolved with a bias toward finding this agency even with scant or ambiguous evidence—that is, toward false positives. Because humans find agents and agency even when humans and animals are not present, this cognitive capacity or mechanism supports the postulation of superhuman agents. Eventually, this evolved cognitive capacity was dubbed the *hypersensitive agency-detection device* ([HADD]; Barrett, 2004). The logic is that selection pressures favored the evolution of brains prone to false positives regarding agency because it is much better, in terms of costs and benefits, to see an agent where none exists than to *not* see an agent where there is one. For instance, in terms of survival, it is much better to mistake a stick for a snake than vice versa. The former can scare you; the latter can kill you.

Early cognitive science research demonstrated basic forms of agency bias, where persons tended to ascribe agency to nonhuman objects. In an early experiment in which participants were shown a movie of geometrical shapes circling a square and performing various actions, they tended to ascribe intentional agency to the shapes. This included describing an entire narrative wherein the shapes were in love or two men were fighting over a woman (Heider & Simmel, 1944). Babies show a preference for objects that resemble human faces very soon after birth, and face-to-face contact is one of the primary channels for mirroring between parents and children; these interactions become the foundations of early attachment (Bowlby, 1969; Johnson et al., 1991; Valenza et al., 1996). These tendencies indicate a preference for interacting with and understanding agents. Thomas the Tank Engine would not be so popular if it were just a train; the addition of a face highlights its agentic qualities, matching the biases and preferences of early childhood cognition.

Agency detection is related to theory of mind, which is a basic aspect of human cognitive development. By some lights, theory of mind develops by about age 3 or 4, when children are able to differentiate their own thoughts and intentions from those of others, and to realize that those thoughts may at times be mistaken based on the vantage point of the other (Callaghan et al., 2005). Cross-cultural studies have shown similarities in the developmental trajectories of this ability in both US and Chinese preschoolers (Sabbagh et al., 2006). The advantage of this form of cognition is evident in the intensely social world occupied by our species.

Research on the relationship of theory of mind, anthropomorphism, and religious belief has generated considerable experimental support for Guthrie's initial claim. By probing young children's intuitions through the use of precultural and noncultural information, psychologists, including Jesse Bering and others, have shown that religious beliefs, for example, "when you die, your soul lives on," are based on cognitive biases that emerge developmentally in very young children. Specifically, Bering and Bjorklund (2004) showed that young children have the bias that living agents (in this case, animals) comprise two parts: a biological body, which ceases to work at death, and a psychological mind or "soul" that continues on after death.

To demonstrate this, Bering and Bjorklund (2004) put on a puppet show for a number of children of various ages and socioreligious backgrounds. In it, a brown mouse became separated from his family, and while wandering in search of them, he was eaten by an alligator. The researchers then asked the young children questions to elicit their thoughts about what was happening with respect to the (dead) mouse's biology and psychology. For instance, they were asked, "Will the brown mouse sleep in his bed tonight?" and "Will the brown mouse eat dinner tonight?" For these types of questions, which probed children's intuitions about the mouse's biology, most of the children answered that the mouse's biology had stopped working. However, when asked questions about the mouse's *psychology*, they answered differently. They were more likely to answer the questions, "Does the brown mouse miss his mother?" and "Is the brown mouse sad?" in the affirmative, indicating they believed that some aspect of the mouse had lived on.

Young children also acquire beliefs about fictional invisible agents very easily, and those beliefs can, with minimal reinforcement, affect their behavior. In one experiment, Bering and Parker (2006) introduced one group of children to an invisible agent, Princess Alice, and told them that she would help them with a game they were playing in the lab. A control group of children were not introduced to the agent. During the experiment, the researchers triggered an unexpected event (such as the lights going on and off or a picture falling) as the children played the game. The children who had been introduced to Princess Alice attributed the unexpected event to her trying to influence their answers in the game and would then modify their responses, in contrast to the control group. In one post-test explanation, when asked what happened during the unexpected event, a child answered, "Princess Alice did it because I chose the wrong box" (Bering & Parker, p. 253).

Teleology—the tendency to attribute purpose to different entities and events—also seems to be a human cognitive default, especially among children. (Kelemen, 1999, 2004; Kelemen & DiYanni, 2005). Testing children's *intuitions* rather than acquired cultural concepts, Kelemen (1999) asked children to infer why certain things are the way they are in the world, for instance, why rocks are pointy or animals have certain features. She found that, even when provided with options, they tended to give teleological explanations more than nonteleological explanations (such as mechanistic explanations). Rocks are pointy because animals use them for scratching, for example, and the *footle* (a fictional animal the researchers invented for the study) looked the way it did for a purpose, not because of the random processes of natural selection (Kelemen, 1999).

People do not necessarily outgrow this conceptual teleological tendency, even when they become experts in a field. Kelemen et al. (2013) demonstrated this inclination in adults by applying a cognitive load (in this case, time constraints) to a task. In a variety of different types of cognitive tasks, the application of a cognitive load causes a reversion to intuitive cognitive biases, primarily because those biases are easier to process and come to us much more quickly. For the experiment, scientists from top-ranked American universities read lists of single explanations for different types of phenomena (70 control explanations and 30 test explanations) and indicated "true" or "false" for each. The test explanations used nonscientific teleological descriptions of the phenomena, such as "the sun radiates heat because warmth nurtures life" (Kelemen et al., p. 3). Under the time constraints, the scientists affirmed more nonscientific teleological descriptions than they did when they had more time to evaluate each explanation. In a second study, scientists and humanities scholars showed the same teleological bias and at similar levels. Thus, even with specialized training in scientific methods, the cognitive tendency for teleological explanations remains in certain contexts.

The cognitive inclination toward teleological explanations of various phenomena helps to explain the attraction of various religious creation stories and the ease with which such accounts are transmitted within religions. In the United States, there has been a major disagreement between creationist accounts of the origins of human life based on a literal interpretation of the Bible and evolutionary accounts of human origins based on descent from a common ancestor in the primate lineage. This debate may be more related to differences between accounts related to cognitive intuitions such as teleology than to accounts based on the effortful, reflective products of scientific inquiry. McCauley (2011) has argued that religion (not theology) is natural in that it is based, to a larger extent, on the cognitive defaults of the human mind; whereas science is unnatural in that it tends to work against many of the intuitions of human cognition and takes considerably more effort and practice to master.

This helps us to understand why acceptance of evolutionary theory, which is based primarily on the "unnatural" practices of science, is so difficult for people to understand and accept as an explanation of human origins. Teachers often have to resort to different methods to teach evolutionary theory because the nonteleological explanations of evolutionary change over time make it difficult to teach (Bakalar, 2011). Evans and Lane (2011) argue that the problem is not lack of information but differences in the susceptibility to the ideas offered in creationist accounts versus evolutionary accounts. Creationist ideas are not easily extinguished and often tenaciously resist amendment even with repeated exposure to evolutionary explanations. Interestingly, most often, creationist ideas are merged with evolutionary descriptions to form hybrid explanations based on both accounts (Legare et al., 2012).

The key insight from these scholars is that part of the reason for the widespread acceptance and transmission of religious beliefs is that they fit well with our evolved cognitive inclinations toward agency detection and teleological explanation. Of course, religion is cultural in that we acquire concepts that are particular to a specific religious tradition ("Allah is God," for example, or "this occurred because of karma") and behaviors from our cultures, but those concepts become cultural because they spread easily through populations. Based on the insights offered by McCauley (2011), "religion is easy" in the sense that many of the concepts are easily understood and remembered because they match the cognitive tendencies of the human mind; whereas "science is hard" because many scientific concepts are counterintuitive and the practice of science requires extensive training (Van Slyke, 2014).

MINIMALLY COUNTERINTUITIVE CONCEPTS

A successful religion *must* have good stories. It must have stories that capture a person's attention, are memorable enough to be stored and then recalled from memory with ease and *relative* accuracy, and interesting enough to be told to others (Barrett, 1999; Slone, 2004). Boyer (2001, 2003) has shown that successful religions offer concepts that are *minimally counterintuitive* (MCI) and violate our expectations and intuitions. Because they only minimally violate our expectations and intuitions, the concepts grab our attention, and because they are not massively counterintuitive, they are easy enough to imagine, visualize, store in memory, and recall later. This is a winning recipe, especially when the concepts involve MCI *agents* such as gods, angels, demons, ghosts, and more. Indeed, this recipe for creating a culturally successful concept is so effective that it shows up not just in religions but in many cultural products—folk tales, comic books, cartoons, films, songs, and so forth.

Boyer's research draws on a robust body of research in cognitive psychology on memory and learning concepts. For instance, Eleanor Rosch (1975) showed that when people encounter novel objects, they tend to categorize those objects based on various prototypes. So, when a person sees an animal that has wings and a beak and can fly, she categorizes it as a "bird." The speed and confidence with which they categorize the novel thing in an established category depends on the degree to which the novel thing shares features with the prototype.

Importantly, the properties of categories are *hierarchical* starting from the most general (e.g., objects) to the more specific (living thing, animal, dog). Although there are various differences in the concepts associated with these categories, the hierarchical structure seems to be consistent across cultures (Atran, 1998; Boyer & Barrett, 2005). For example, a robin is a bounded physical object (as is a rock), which is also living (unlike a rock, but like a plant), and is an animal and a self-moving, goal-directed agent (unlike a plant). Once something is categorized, a significant amount of information consistent with different levels in the hierarchy is assumed to be also true of the object you have just categorized (Boyer & Barrett, 2005). So, when a person sees a bird she has never seen before and recognizes (categorizes) it, she automatically assumes that it is an animal, and thus an agent, a living thing, and a physical object. She also assumes that the new bird possesses all the properties of other birds: it has wings, a beak, and can fly. This cognitive system allows us to make sense of the types of things in our world with relative accuracy. It is not perfect, however, and we are constantly adjusting our categories as we learn new information (for example, an ostrich is a bird but doesn't fly). This system has been described as a *folk ontology system* because it allows us to make fast and efficient sense of the things in our world.

Drawing on this body of literature, Boyer noted that the types of concepts we see in religious systems tend to be *minimally counterintuitive* (MCI) in the sense that religious agents and objects, among other cultural concepts, tend to violate one or two major property expectations (Boyer & Ramble, 2001). More specifically, Boyer noted, MCI concepts involve one of just two types of expectation violations: *transfer* violations, and *breach* violations. For example, an angel is a type of human person who can *fly*. This concept is interesting because it transfers expectations from one category (birds) to another (humans). But consider the popular story in the Judeo-Christian tradition of the "burning bush," which catches fire but does not burn. This concept involves a *breach* of our expectations about bushes in relation to fire. Boyer argues that these types of expectation-violating concepts and stories achieve a cognitive optimum because they are attention-grabbing, memorable, and interesting enough to motivate people to share them with others, but do not have so many counterintuitive features that they are hard to understand, remember, and communicate. Over time, all else being equal, MCI concepts outcompete other types of concepts, which is why they spread widely across cultures (horizontal transmission) and eras (vertical transmission).[1]

Boyer's account explains why certain religious concepts recur across cultures. For example, in the theology of the three major world religions, when you "die" you may not entirely die. In common folk conceptions in Christianity and Islam, your "soul" goes to heaven/paradise or hell. In Hinduism, your soul (atman) is reincarnated in another form. That agents (humans, in this case) don't die is a breach of expectations but perhaps a modest one. Our natural default bias about people may be that we have two substances, a body and a mind (or "soul"; Bering, 2006). This inclination seems to indicate a type of folk dualism, which is the default cognitive expectation even in young children and appears to be cross-cultural, also showing up in ancient Chinese texts (Bloom, 2004; Slingerland & Chudek, 2011).

Religious texts act as a form of cultural scaffolding that helps to ease the burden on individual memory systems by externalizing certain types of religious ideas, and thus facilitates the transmission of religious concepts that are more than minimally counterintuitive (Clark, 1996; McCauley, 2011). However, texts may be more important for legitimating the authenticity of the religion—and the authority of the guilds who run them—than for transmitting the concepts themselves because the concepts are typically easy to remember through oral transmission. Common stories include creation

---

[1] Boyer (2001) notes that other factors play a role in religious transmission, including the inferential richness of religious concepts and their relationship to basic human fitness. Thus things aren't always necessary equal in the distribution and adoption of religious beliefs.

and afterlife myths, which provide accounts of where the world came from and what happens after we die. These stories are a combination of agency detection, teleological reasoning, and MCI concepts. We tend to think that things exist for a reason. Thus, when we are thinking about the origins of the universe, our natural default bias toward teleology gives us the intuition that it was created purposefully. Creation myths contain MCI characters who create the world, and afterlife myths, in which our bodies die but our souls live on (in heaven/hell or through reincarnation), which are able to achieve a cognitive optimum that promotes the spread of the religious concept. They are attention-grabbing but understandable and believable. This gives them a cultural-transmission advantage that allows them to circulate widely in human populations.

RITUALS AND MCI CONCEPTS

Successful world religions must have more than just catchy stories populated with MCI concepts. To become a world religion, they must also give people something to do, such as rituals. *Religious rituals* are prescribed behavioral action sequences that involve, in various ways, the MCI concepts from the religion's conceptual scheme. And importantly, well-designed ritual systems also achieve a cognitive optimum, just like well-designed religious stories and concepts. One of the most important works in CSR came from two pioneers of the field, E. Thomas Lawson and Robert N. McCauley. In their book, *Rethinking Religion: Connecting Cognition and Culture,* they outlined a cognitive theory of religious rituals (Lawson & McCauley, 1990). Inspired by Noam Chomsky's work in linguistics, Lawson and McCauley note that ritual systems, like languages, are symbolic systems and can be analyzed accordingly. Like languages, religious ritual systems have a "syntactic" structure of sorts that follows certain patterns that are predictable because they are based on biases in human cognition.

Lawson and McCauley note that because rituals are behavioral action sequences they are constrained by the way our brains represent all action sequences: actions are *transitive* or *intransitive*. That is, in every human action sequence, either someone is doing something, often to something or someone, or, something is being done to someone, often with something and/or by someone. Despite the surface-level diversity we see in religious rituals across the globe, structurally, all rituals take one of these two forms: either a person is doing something, or something is being done to the person.

Consider these religious rituals from two world religions: the Hindu puja and Christian baptism. First, the puja in Hinduism is a ritual offering to a deity, such as Shiva or Vishnu. Puja can be done by a lay person at a simple home shrine or by a guru or priest in a lavish temple. But regardless of who initiates the action, the deity is the *recipient* of the ritual action. Lawson and McCauley (1990) dub these *special patient rituals.* Akin to special patient rituals are *special instrument rituals,* which require the use of a special object (e.g., a relic, holy water, sacred text), which is usually deemed necessary for the success of the ritual. In special instrument rituals, as in special patient rituals, the deity is not the agent. In contrast, consider Christian baptism. In this ritual, a "special agent" (a priest) does something to someone, as in "priest baptizes baby." Lawson and McCauley dub these *special agent rituals* because the deity from the religion's conceptual scheme (God) is represented by the agent. That is, the deity, usually acting through a surrogate, such as the priest, is the agent, not the patient.

To summarize: rituals take one of two basic forms: those in which the god initiates the action (special agent rituals), and those in which an ordinary human initiates the action (special patient and special instrument rituals).[2] The action occurs as follows:

Special agent ritual: SPECIAL AGENT → PATIENT
Special patient ritual: AGENT → SPECIAL PATIENT
Special instrument ritual: AGENT → PATIENT BY MEANS OF SPECIAL INSTRUMENT

In their follow-up book, *Bringing Ritual to Mind: Psychological Foundations of Cultural Forms*, McCauley and Lawson (2002) extended this analysis to the macrolevel, noting that well-designed ritual systems have an optimal balance of special agent and special patient rituals. Special agent rituals are typically done only once in a lifetime, are emotionally charged, and involve high (often expensive) sensory pageantry. Examples include weddings, ordinations, and baptisms, each of which typically occur rarely or infrequently and often features displays of resources and/or status.

In contrast, special patient (and special instrument) rituals are often performed repeatedly, even daily, are typically not as emotionally charged, and involve relatively little sensory pageantry. Special agent rituals are exciting and often emotionally arousing but can't be performed on a regular basis because the increased frequency would make them less memorable and because most people don't have the resources to sustain the level of extravagant pageantry. Special patient rituals give people something to do with a minimal level of emotional arousal, but don't require the extravagance necessary for special agent rituals. An example of this would be reciting a special prayer during a Christian church service. However, special patient rituals can become monotonous if they are repeated too often, so they may need to be augmented with a special religious retreat or other ritual that contains more elements of a special agent ritual, which are more unique and emotionally arousing. So, the ideal, cognitively optimal ritual system has a balance of enough special patient rituals to give people something to do on a regular basis, punctuated by a few very important and very exciting special agent rituals throughout the life span. A religion with only special agent rituals wouldn't spread widely because it would be too resource intensive (including emotional resources), and a religion with only special patient rituals wouldn't spread widely because it would not be emotionally arousing enough to sustain attention and commitment from religious members.

---

[2] See also Lawson, this volume.

SECOND INGREDIENT: SUPERNATURAL MONITORING AND INTUITIVE MORALITY

Around 10,000 years ago, human life changed significantly when humans discovered how to farm, which provided a stable and reliable food source (Mithen, 1996). This agricultural revolution changed humanity, and our religions, forever (Cauvin, 2000). Having a reliable food supply extended human life spans and increased group sizes; human cognition and behavior shifted from fast-life concerns (survival) to slow-life concerns (longevity and social living in large groups) (Del Giudice et al., 2015). In turn, the focus of religions changed during this era from the immediate concerns of life and death to concerns with the *social challenges* of living in highly populated areas for a greater number of years. Prior to the rise of agriculture, group sizes were likely limited to around 150 people because that's all a hunting-gathering culture that lacked a hierarchical organizational structure could sustain (Dunbar, 1992). With the invention of farming, however, community sizes grew to thousands. This created unique challenges for humans, specifically how to live among lots of people whom you do not know and therefore may not trust.

Morality is an important concern of many contemporary world religions. Concern with morality may have developed as a form of cultural evolution, in that aspects of religiosity function as a form of social monitoring to ensure moral behavior and enable cooperation and trust within and among larger social groups (Coogan, 2003; Norenzayan, 2013). A basic aspect of human psychology is that people behave differently when they are being watched or observed by someone else. Cues or proxy signals for this psychological experience of observation can be as simple as a pair of eyes looking out from a picture on a computer screen. Research studies indicate that these kinds of cues can have an impact on prosocial behaviors. For example, eyes on a computer screen increased monetary payouts during economic games and a picture of eyes pasted above a sign asking for money for coffee in a break room increased donations to the common fund (Bateson et al., 2006; Haley & Fessler, 2005). This effect seems to be related to reputation and social evaluation. A meta-analysis of seven similar studies showed that watching eyes increased the probability of giving a donation of some amount, but they did not increase the mean amount of the donation (Nettle et al., 2012).

Religions build on this psychological propensity to modify behavior based on perceived observation by others by creating gods who can monitor by proxy, acting as internalized representations of observers, who monitor social behavior. The presence of internalized representations of religious agents who could monitor behavior allowed for the expansion of group size to go beyond what could be accomplished through direct person to person observation. For example, implicitly activating religious concepts increased monetary offers towards partners in an economic game (Shariff & Norenzayan, 2007). Implicit exposure to the *athan*, the Islamic call to prayer, increased honesty on a math test in comparison to controls (Aveyard, 2014). In Mauritius, a small island nation in the Western Indian Ocean, participants played a bargaining game in two different settings, one religious (a Hindu temple) and another secular (a local restaurant). The participants in the religious setting were more cooperative and used more terms related to fairness to justify their decisions in comparison to the secular (Xygalatas, 2013). A meta-analysis of 93 studies showed that religious priming has a robust effect on a number of different outcome measures, including prosociality (Shariff et al., 2016).

A research team investigated how religious beliefs that supernatural agents see us, judge us, and will punish us is related to cognitive biases (Piazza et al., 2011). Piazza and colleagues did this by bringing a group of children into a room that contained a ball-dart game. They were told that they had to stand behind a line a certain distance from the wall and then throw the balls at the dartboard backward over their shoulders. If they hit the target, they were told, they would win a prize. Then the experimenters left the room, while a hidden camera recorded the children's behavior. Not surprisingly, many of them cheated by walking up to the dartboard and placing balls on it when no one was in the room to watch them. Then Piazza and colleagues brought a second group of children into the same room but explained to them that the invisible "Princess Alice" was in the room, watching them. Strikingly, when the children were told that they were being watched by an invisible agent, the amount of cheating was significantly reduced.

In addition to policing antisocial behavior, religious communities often establish membership requirements that involve hard-to-fake signals of commitment to the group. For example, by willingly undergoing painful or expensive initiation rituals (see Whitehouse & Kavanagh, this volume; Xygalatas, this volume), as well as other public on-going membership commitments, individuals could signal to others that that they were committed to the religious group and the morality that it condoned (Bulbulia, 2004; Sosis & Alcorta, 2003). Being a member of a religious group is a strategic means of advertising one's trustworthiness, potentially increasing one's reputation and social status. The flip side of strong in-group solidarity based on hard-to-fake signals of commitment is that people who *do not* belong to the group may be seen as suspicious and dangerous; they are not to be trusted. This can trigger the brain's threat-detection bias and lead to out-group hostility and possibility violence (Atran & Ginges, 2015; Atran & Henrich, 2010).

Models of the evolution of cooperation in groups often presuppose a situation similar to the prisoner's dilemma, in which persons must maximize individual gains and minimize the potential for defection, usually at some cost to the exchange partner (Axelrod, 1984). However, an important variable was missing from this model: partner choice, which allowed for a more equitable exchange of goods because persons could signal their value as potential cooperators through reputation (André & Baumard, 2011b; Baumard et al., 2013). When partners are chosen, exchanges become more proportional and mutually beneficial for both participants (André & Baumard, 2011a). In variations of economic games (e.g., the prisoner's dilemma) that occur over successive interactions between players, participants often prefer cooperative strategies over simply defecting, while also paying attention to fairness (Fehr & Camerer, 2007). Indeed, selection pressures for group living most likely contributed to the evolution of moral emotions that underwrite social cooperation, such as empathy (de Waal, 2008).

Baumard and Boyer (2013) have argued that the emergence of moralizing religions in recent history is based on these evolved moral dispositions toward fairness in cooperative exchanges. Several moral religions, including Buddhism, Hinduism, Confucianism, Christianity, and Islam, contain religious moral codes that are often variations on the golden rule or are related to forms of supernatural justice, with an emphasis on fairness and reciprocity in human relationships (Neusner & Chilton, 2009). Religious moral systems outcompeted secular moral systems because they matched the evolved intutions favoring agents with supernatural access to human actions relevant to moral behavior, and evaluated those actions based on reasons that matched intutive forms of morality (Baumard & Boyer, 2013).

Contemporary world religions are "successful" for a variety of reasons, which are illuminated by the cognitive and evolutionary sciences. Supernatural agents and religious rituals match important aspects of the evolved human cognitive architecture making them easy to remember, transmit to others, and motivational for different types of actions. Pairing these supernatural agents and rituals with religious moral codes that match evolved intutions about fairness and reciprocity increases their salience and effectiveness in motivating moral behavior and the ease with which moral beliefs are acquired. Aspects of religious beliefs in supernatural agents and rituals function as a form of social monitoring based on psychological mechanisms related to changes in behavior when persons know they are being observed. Finally, demonstrations of adherence to particular religious beliefs and rituals serve as hard-to-fake signals of group commitment and increase individual reputational status as being trustworthy and a good exchange partner.

THIRD INGREDIENT: MATING STRATEGIES

Darwin recognized that reproductive success was as important as survival because a reliable mechanism was required to transmit adaptive traits to successive generations (Darwin, 1871; Geher & Kauffman, 2013). He was initially perplexed by the beautiful plumage of male peacocks, which seemed to decrease their fitness in avoiding potential predators. The answer to his quandary came in the form of sexual selection, in that certain types of adaptations contribute to male and female competition for high-quality mates. Thus, it is not surprising that every world religion contains teachings that help to manage this adaptive challenge. That is, every world religion contains teachings that promote pair-bonding (a.k.a. "marriage"), and parental investment (the so-called family values; Buss, 2002; Slone, 2008; Slone & Van Slyke, 2015). Contemporary world religions enhance long-term mating success at both the individual and cultural levels by promoting hard-to-fake signals of long-term mating potential and rules and values that help to manage the challenges of mating in groups (Van Slyke, 2017; Van Slyke & Szocik, 2020).

Human sexual dimorphism creates specific reproductive challenges for each biological sex—namely, how to attract and hold onto a desirable mate—that successful religions help to manage. Because human offspring have a long period of development, we have the added challenge of high-cost parental investment, which are not shared equally by sexes (Trivers, 1972). Females have higher reproductive costs than males because of pregnancy and nursing. Females also have fewer reproductive opportunities due to their smaller number of sex cells (eggs) and shorter window of fertility interrupted by pregnancy. Human females have to make each opportunity for reproduction count, and therefore, they tend to be the choosier sex. This leads to both intra- and intersexual competition. Males compete with females, females compete with other females, and males compete with other males for sexual access to desirable mates.

Research on mating cognition has shown that across cultures, women tend to prefer males who show an ability to acquire resources and willingness to invest those resources in offspring (Buss, 1989; Buss & Shackelford, 2008; Shackelford et al., 2005). This leads to male-male intrasexual competition. Males try to outcompete males in domains like hunting and, in the modern world, high-paying jobs. Males can also outcompete other males by displaying behaviors that signal to potential mates that they will be good fathers and faithful long-term mates. Being a committed member of a world religion is a particularly effective strategy for displaying these qualities. Through his commitment to a religion that preaches fidelity and parental investment, a male can signal to a potential mate that he has "family values."

The competition for mates, among both males and females, can be understood along a continuum of short-term and long-term strategies (Buss, 2006; Buss & Schmitt, 1993). Short-term strategies focus on higher numbers of mating partners, higher frequency of sexual activity, and shorter duration of relationships (Easton et al., 2015). Long-term strategies focus on higher fertility through multiple mating opportunities with the same person, parental investment over time, and increased certainty about paternity. On average, females are inclined toward long-term strategies and men are inclined toward short-term strategies based on sex differences in reproductive costs, and both sexes demonstrate various adaptations toward their strategy inclination. However, these tendencies are not fixed, and both males and females engage in strategies to maximize reproductive success in both short-term and long-term relationships.

Religions can support long-term mating strategies through two routes: at the individual level by influencing decisions regarding mate potential, and at the cultural level, by placing constraints on behavior and managing various problems associated with inter- and intrasexual competition (Van Slyke, 2017). Several studies indicate a relationship between higher levels of religiosity and more restrictive forms of sexual activity and values, consistent with a long-term strategy. Religiosity has been associated with more conservative views of human sexual activity, such as not condoning premarital intercourse, and has been associated with a lower frequency of premarital intercourse (Beckwith & Morrow, 2005; Pluhar et al., 1998). Higher frequency of attendance at religious services and self-reported religiosity has been associated with delayed coital debut among adolescents and emerging adults (Hardy & Raffaelli, 2003; Hull et al., 2011; Rostosky et al., 2003). Conservative Protestant women were shown to be less likely to have engaged in "hooking up" behaviors, those involving various types of sexual activities with less familiar partners, consistent with short-term strategies (Burdette et al., 2009).

Weeden et al. (2008) have suggested the reproductive religiosity model as an explanation for the relationship between religiosity and sexual behavior, in that people affiliate with religious groups as a way to support their mating strategies. This reverses the common assumption that people acquire their sexual morality by joining a religious group; instead, they seek out sexual values that match already established mating strategies by joining particular religious groups. Several studies indicate this relationship based on the relative value placed on sexual morality compared to other forms of morality. Among a sample of over 21,000 from the General Social Survey (GSS), sexual behaviors were the best predictors of attendance at religious services, even when the variables of age and gender were controlled (Weeden et al., 2008). When sexual morality was compared to the morality involved in cooperative behavior in the World Values Survey and European Values Study, sexual morality was a better predictor of individual differences in religiosity; whereas the predictive power of cooperative morals was relatively weak (Weeden & Kurzban, 2013). Among a sample of college students at an evangelical university, lower scores on the Sociosexual Orientation Inventory - Revised (lower scores are more characteristic of individuals engaged in a long-term strategy) were associated with higher scores on two measures of religiosity (Van Slyke & Wasemiller, 2017). Perceptions of long-term mating strategies (described in a narrative) were more likely to be associated with religiosity, while perceptions of short-term mating strategies (described in a separate narrative) were more likely to be associated with being nonreligious (Van Slyke, 2021).

At this point, evidence for the relationship between religiosity and mating strategies has been primarily correlational, but some studies have started to tease out a more causal story in which religiosity is used more strategically in mating contexts. For example, Li et al., (2010) found that both heterosexual males and females reported higher levels of religiosity when exposed to a pool of physically attractive same-sex persons in online dating profiles, in contrast to a second group that viewed dating profiles of attractive persons of the opposite sex. The higher levels of religiosity after exposure to attractive members of the same sex may be due to the enactment of a particular mating strategy based on the current pool of mating competitors. If several physically attractive rivals of the same sex are detected in a mating pool, it may be more advantageous to promote a different attractive feature, such as commitment to a religion, as a more effective long-term mating strategy. In a second study, participants associated religious individuals with long-term mating strategies and viewed them as more trustworthy; their mating strategy was a primary mediating factor in determining trust. Interestingly, when persons had more direct knowledge of the target's mating strategy, religiosity played a less significant role in perceiving trust. Thus, individuals appear to use religiosity strategically as a type of signal to determine mating strategy and the possibility of trust (Moon et al., 2018).

World religions support factors associated with long-term strategies over short-term strategies, which is helpful for both males and females. Paternity certainty is a much larger concern for males than females since there are fewer direct signs that can identify their progeny. Engagement in long-term strategies increases paternity certainty through exclusive reproductive access to a single female, and long-term commitments increase the chances that a female will remain faithful. Females increase the chances of both resource and parental investment by their male partners over time by becoming involved in long-term commitments. Women often show preferences for mates who signal resource-acquisition potential—namely, earning capacity, ambition, and social status—as well as good parenting skills such as kindness, emotional stability, dependability, and general interest in children (Easton et al., 2015). Increased fertility helps both males and females since conception may face a variety of potential obstacles including fertilization, miscarriage, and various teratogens. Increased mating frequency with a single partner may overcome these potential hurdles and increase overall reproductive success. Several studies indicate that religiosity is associated with higher fertility rates (Rowthorn, 2011). An analysis of the New Zealand Attitudes and Values Survey showed that greater church attendance and higher frequency of weekly prayer were associated with higher fertility; and in a similar study of the World Values Survey (1981–2004) highly religious individuals had higher average numbers of children (Blume, 2009; Bulbulia et al., 2015).

Evaluating potential mates can be difficult because of the need to make predictions about future behaviors and attitudes; there is always a chance that mate value or commitment to the relationship will be misrepresented during the courtship process. Religions establish a context for evaluating a long-term mate value by providing various hard-to-fake beliefs and through rituals that can signal fidelity to the religious group and serve as a proxy for the qualities sought after in a potential mate. Especially among major world religions, there is an emphasis on morality that is focused on fidelity in marriage, parental investment in child-rearing, and maintaining the sanctity of family life. Many churches invest considerable time, energy, and financial resources in family-life education and marriage-enhancement retreats. Evangelical colleges often serve as the primary setting for trying to find a marriage partner (especially for female students); the goal was characterized by one student as "ring by spring or your money back!" (Freitas, 2015, p. 114).

Interestingly, in several decades of research on the measurement of religiosity, it has been found that females tend to be more religious than males (Trzebiatowska & Bruce, 2012). Females report higher levels of religious attendance (especially those belonging to more conservative religious groups) and tend to get more out of religious services and experiences (Kosmin & Keyser, 2009; Woolever et. al., 2006). This gender difference may be related to preferences in mating strategies. Since females are the choosier sex and show preferences for long-term strategies, religious affiliation may be an effective measure for evaluating potential mates. Commitment to a particular religion may function as a proxy, signaling the mate qualities associated with a long-term relationship, such as relationship fidelity and parental investment (i.e., commitment to family values), and relationships with others involved in long-term strategies (i.e., marriage small groups).

Another important characteristic of many world religions is that they discourage infidelity and encourage chastity. Finding a mate, especially for those engaged in a long-term strategy, gives rise to a new problem, that of holding onto the mate, sometimes referred to as *mate guarding* or *mate retention*. Mate guarding can take two forms: either *prohibitive* (restricting a mate's behaviors to prevent or diminish the mate's contact with other potential mates) or *persuasive* (paying more attention to or buying gifts for the mate) (Pillsworth & Haselton, 2006). A candidate for prohibitive mate guarding distinctive for some forms of Islam is veiling, where females are encouraged or required to cover parts of their head, body, and/or face.

In short-term mating strategies, males often pay more attention to attributes of the female body, such as the waist-to-hip ratio ([WHR]; Confer et al., 2010). Males show a preference for an optimal WHR of about .7, which is associated with a curvaceous hourglass shape and activates reward centers of the brain (Spicer & Platek, 2010; Singh, 1993). During an eye-tracking study, conservative religious clothing decreased visual access to curvaceous features of the female body associated with WHR and increased focus on the face region, in contrast to more liberal clothing, where visual fixations focused more on curvaceous features (Pazhoohi et al., 2017). When males view females in various levels of religious veiling, they prefer those with less veiling and rate them as more attractive. Thus, clothing can serve a mate guarding function by decreasing the perception of female attractiveness, which reduces potential advances from other males (Pazhoohi & Hosseinchari, 2014). Interestingly, the use of religious veiling in different cultures varies based on ecological conditions. In more harsh environments, where there is a higher need for biparental investment, there is an increase in levels of religiosity and the use of veiling as form of mate guarding to decrease the chances of mate poaching (Pazhoohi et al., 2016).

Henrich et al. (2012) argue that monogamous marriage has been favored by cultural evolutionary processes because it promoted a variety of group-level benefits such as reduced crime, reduced sexual and physical abuse, and increased child investment and economic productivity. By managing various forms of inter- and intrasexual competition and increasing commitment to monogamous marriage and family, religion may function as a form of cultural evolution that produced group-level benefits for many of its members.

Conclusion

There are obvious and important differences in the major world religions, but CSR is interested in looking at religion at the level of universal human cognitive structures and our shared evolved psychology (Van Slyke, 2016). World religions develop based on a common recipe with three major ingredients: *cognitive foundations of gods and rituals, supernatural monitoring and intuitive morality*, and *mating strategies*. Gods develop in world religions based on certain cognitive defaults and biases that make these religious beliefs easy to acquire and spread effortlessly within cultures because they build on natural inclinations of the human mind (McCauley, 2011; Sperber, 1996). World religions develop morality based on evolved aspects of social cognition, intuitive aspects of morality, and the adaptive problems of living in groups. These religions provide an effective means for social monitoring in large groups, increasing group cohesion, and for managing group competition through both cooperation and rivalry. Mating is an important aspect of social living and world religions help to facilitate mating strategies by providing a means for evaluating potential mates, different forms of mate guarding, and social structures that encourage aspects of long-term mating and parental investment. Our argument is that the reason world religions are so successful is that they manage these key ingredients so well, despite their differences, and we are hopeful that CSR will continue to expand and delineate these ingredients through further empirical research.

Questions for Future Research

1. Are there other ingredients that play a decisive role in the development of world religions?
2. Are there other aspects of sexual selection that have an important role in the functioning of world religions?
3. What is the relative contribution of cognitive defaults and cultural novelty in the formation of god concepts?
4. How flexible are moral intuitions as they emerge in different cultures and religions?

Acknowledgments

Dr. Van Slyke's contribution to this chapter was partially sponsored by a grant given by Bridging the Two Cultures of Science and the Humanities II, a project run by Scholarship and Christianity in Oxford, the UK subsidiary of the Council for Christian Colleges and Universities.

References

André, J., & Baumard, N. (2011a). The evolution of fairness in a biological market. *Evolution*, 65(5), 1447–1456. doi:10.1111/j.1558-5646.2011.01232.x

André, J., & Baumard, N. (2011b). Social opportunities and the evolution of fairness. *Journal of Theoretical Biology*, 289, 128–135. doi:10.1016/j.jtbi.2011.07.031

Atran, S. (1998). Folk biology and the anthropology of science: Cognitive universals and cultural particulars. *Behavioral and Brain Sciences, 21*(4), 547–609.

Atran, S., & Ginges, J. (2015). Devoted actors and the moral foundations of intractable intergroup conflict. In J. Decety & T. Wheatley (Eds.), *The moral brain: A multidisciplinary perspective* (pp. 69–85). Cambridge, MA: MIT Press.

Atran, S., & Henrich, J. (2010). The evolution of religion: How cognitive by-products, adaptive learning heuristics, ritual displays, and group competition generate deep commitments to prosocial religions. *Biological Theory, 5*(1), 18–30.

Aveyard, M. E. (2014). A call to honesty: Extending religious priming of moral behavior to middle eastern Muslims. *PLoS One, 9*(7), Article e99447.

Axelrod, R. M. (1984). *The evolution of cooperation.* New York: Basic Books.

Bakalar, N. (2011, February 7). On evolution, biology teachers stray from lesson plan. *New York Times.* Retrieved from http://www.nytimes.com.

Barrett, J. L. (1999). Theological correctness: Cognitive constraint and the study of religion. *Method and Theory in the Study of Religion, 11*, 325–339.

Barrett, J. L. (2004). *Why would anyone believe in God?* Walnut Creek, CA: AltaMira Press.

Bateson, M., Nettle, D., & Roberts, G. (2006). Cues of being watched enhance cooperation in a real-world setting. *Biology Letters, 2*, 412–414.

Baumard, N., André, J., & Sperber, D. (2013). A mutualistic approach to morality: The evolution of fairness by partner choice. *Behavioral and Brain Sciences, 36*(1), 59–78. https://doi.org/10.1017/S0140525X11002202

Baumard, N., & Boyer, P. (2013). Explaining moral religions. *Trends in Cognitive Sciences, 17*(6), 272–280. https://doi.org/10.1016/j.tics.2013.04.003

Beckwith, H. D., & Morrow, J. A. (2005). Sexual attitudes of college students: The impact of religiosity and spirituality. *College Student Journal, 39*, 357–367.

Bering, J. M. (2006). The folk psychology of souls. *Behavioral and Brain Sciences, 29*(5), 453–462. https://doi.org/10.1017/S0140525X06009101

Bering, J. M., & Bjorklund, D. F. (2004). The natural emergence of reasoning about the afterlife as a developmental regularity. *Developmental Psychology, 40*(2), 217–233. https://doi.org/10.1037/0012-1649.40.2.217

Bering, J. M., & Parker, B. D. (2006). Children's attributions of intentions to an invisible agent. *Developmental Psychology, 42*(2), 253–262. doi:10.1037/0012-1649.42.2.253

Bloom, P. (2004). *Descartes' baby: How the science of child development explains what makes us human.* New York: Basic Books.

Bowlby, J. (1969). *Attachment* (Vol. 1). New York: Basic Books.

Boyer, P. (2001). *Religion explained: The evolutionary origins of religious thought.* New York: Basic Books.

Boyer, P. (2003). Religious thought and behavior as by-products of brain function. *Trends in Cognitive Sciences, 7*(3), 119–124.

Boyer, P., & Barrett, C. (2005). Evolved intuitive ontology: Integrating neural, behavioral and developmental aspects of domain specificity. In D. M. Buss (Ed.), *The handbook of evolutionary psychology* (pp. 96–118). Hoboken, NJ: John Wiley & Sons.

Boyer, P., & Ramble, C. (2001). Cognitive templates for religious concepts: Cross-cultural evidence for recall of counter-intuitive representations. *Cognitive Science, 25*, 535–564.

Blume, M. (2009). The reproductive benefits of religious affiliation. In E. Voland & W. Schiefenhovel (Eds.), *The biological evolution of religious mind and behavior* (pp. 117–126). Heidelberg: Springer.

Bulbulia, J. (2004). Religious costs as adaptations that signal altruistic intention. *Evolution and Cognition*, 10, 19–38.

Bulbulia, J., Shaver, J., Greaves, L., Sosis, R., & Sibley, C. G. (2015). Religion and parental cooperation: An empirical test of Slone's sexual signaling model. In J. A. Van Slyke & D. J. Slone (Eds.), *The attraction of religion: A new evolutionary psychology of religion*. London and New York: Bloomsbury Academic.

Burdette, A. M., Ellison, C. G., Hill, T. D., & Glenn, N. D. (2009). "Hooking up" at college: Does religion make a difference? *Journal for the Scientific Study of Religion*, 48(3), 535–551.

Buss, D. M. (1989). Sex differences in human mate preferences: Evolutionary hypotheses tested in 37 cultures. *Behavioral and Brain Sciences*, 12, 1–49.

Buss, D. M. (2002). Sex, marriage, and religion: What adaptive problems do religious phenomena solve? *Psychological Inquiry*, 13(3), 201–238.

Buss, D. M. (2006). Strategies of human mating. *Psychological Topics*, 15, 239–260.

Buss, D. M., & Schmitt, D. P. (1993). Sexual strategies theory: An evolutionary perspective on human mating. *Psychological Review*, 100, 204–232.

Buss, D. M., & Shackelford, T. K. (2008). Attractive women want it all: Good genes, economic investment, parenting proclivities, and emotional commitment. *Evolutionary Psychology*, 6(1), 134–146.

Callaghan, T., Rochat, P., Lillard, A., Claux, M. L., Odden, H., Itakura, S., Singh, S. (2005). Synchrony in the onset of mental-state reasoning. *Psychological Science*, 16, 378–384.

Cauvin, J. (2000). *The birth of the gods and the origins of agriculture*. Cambridge, UK: Cambridge University Press.

Clark, A. (1996). *Being there: Putting brain, body, and world together again*. Cambridge, MA: MIT Press.

Confer, J. C., Perilloux, C., & Buss, D. M. (2010). More than just a pretty face: Men's priority shifts toward bodily attractiveness in short-term versus long-term mating contexts. *Evolution and Human Behavior*, 31(5), 348–353. https://doi.org/10.1016/j.evolhumbehav.2010.04.002

Coogan, M. D. (Ed.). (2003). *The illustrated guide to world religions*. Oxford: Oxford University Press.

Darwin, C. (1871). *The descent of man, and selection in relation to sex*. London: John Murray.

de Waal, F. (2008). Putting the altruism back into altruism: The evolution of empathy. *Annual Review of Psychology*, 59(1), 279–300. https://doi.org/10.1146/annurev.psych.59.103006.093625

Del Giudice, M., Gangestad, S. W., & Kaplan, H. S. (2015). Life history theory and evolutionary psychology. In D. M. Buss (Ed.), *The handbook of evolutionary psychology* (2nd ed., pp. 88–114). Hoboken, NJ: John Wiley & Sons.

Dunbar, R. I. M. (1992). Neocortex size as a constraint on group size in primates. *Journal of Human Evolution*, 22(6), 469–493. https://doi.org/10.1016/0047-2484(92)90081-J

Easton, J. A., Goetz, C. D., & Buss, D. M. (2015). Evolution of human mate choice. In J. D. Wright (Ed.), *International encyclopedia of the social and behavioral sciences* (2nd ed., pp. 340–347). Oxford: Elsevier.

Evans, M. E., & Lane, J. D. (2011). Contradictory or complementary? Creationist and evolutionist explanations of the origin(s) of species. *Human Development*, 54(3), 144–159. doi:10.1159/000329130

Fehr, E., & Camerer, C. (2007). Social neuroeconomics: The neural circuitry of social preferences. *Trends in Cognitive Sciences*, 11(10), 419–427. http://doi.org/10.1016/j.tics.2007.09.002

Freitas, D. (2015). *Sex and the soul: Juggling sexuality, spirituality, romance, and religion on America's college campuses* (Updated ed.). New York: Oxford University Press.

Geher, G., & Kaufman, S. (2013). *Mating intelligence unleashed: The role of the mind in sex, dating, and love*. New York: Oxford University Press.

Guthrie, S. (1993). *Faces in the clouds: A new theory of religion*. Oxford: Oxford University Press.

Haley, K. J., & Fessler, D. M. T. (2005). Nobody's watching? Subtle cues affect generosity in an anonymous economic game. *Evolution and Human Behavior, 26*, 245–256.

Hardy, S. A., & Raffaelli, M. (2003). Adolescent religiosity and sexuality: An investigation of reciprocal influences. *Journal of Adolescence, 26*(6), 731–739. https://doi.org/10.1016/j.adolescence.2003.09.003

Heider, F., & Simmel, M.-A. (1944). An experimental study of apparent behavior. *American Journal of Psychology, 57*, 243–249.

Henrich, J., Boyd, R., & Richerson, P. J. (2012). The puzzle of monogamous marriage. *Philosophical Transactions of the Royal Society B: Biological Sciences, 367*(1589), 657–669. https://doi.org/10.1177/1069397100003400205

Hull, S. J., Hennessy, M., Bleakley, A., Fishbein, M., & Jordan, A. (2011). Identifying the causal pathways from religiosity to delayed adolescent sexual behavior. *Journal of Sex Research, 48*(6), 543–553. https://doi.org/10.1080/00224499.2010.521868

Johnson, M. H., Dziurawiec, S., Ellis, H. D., & Morton, J. (1991). Newborns' preferential tracking of face-like stimuli and its subsequent decline. *Cognition, 40*, 1–19.

Kelemen, D. (1999). Why are rocks pointy? Children's preference for teleological explanations of the natural world. *Developmental Psychology, 35*(6), 1440–1453.

Kelemen, D. (2004). Are children "intuitive theists"? *Psychological Science, 15*, 295–301.

Kelemen, D., & DiYanni, C. (2005). Intuitions about origins: Purpose and intelligent design in children. *Journal of Cognition and Development, 6*, 3–31.

Kelemen, D., Rottman, J., & Seston, R. (2013). Professional physical scientists display tenacious teleological tendencies: Purpose-based reasoning as a cognitive default. *Journal of Experimental Psychology: General, 142*(4), 1074–1083. https://doi.org/10.1037/a0030399

Kosmin, B., & Keyser, A. (2009, March). *American religious identification survey: ARIS 2008*. [Summary report]. Trinity College, Hartford, CT.

Lawson, E. T., & McCauley, R. N. (1990). *Rethinking religion: Connecting cognition and culture*. Cambridge, UK: Cambridge University Press.

Legare, C. H., Evans, M. E., Rosengren, K. S., & Harris, P. L. (2012). The coexistence of natural and supernatural explanations across cultures and development. *Child Development, 83*(3), 779–793. doi:10.1111/j.1467-8624.2012.01743.x

Li, J., Cohen, A. B., Weeden, J., & Kenrick, D. T. (2010). Mating competitors increase religious beliefs. *Journal of Experimental Social Psychology, 46*(2), 428–431. doi:10.1016/j.jesp.2009.10.017

McCauley, R. N. (2011). *Why religion is natural, and science is not*. New York: Oxford University Press.

McCauley, R. N., & Lawson, E. T. (2002). *Bringing ritual to mind: Psychological foundations of cultural forms*. Cambridge, UK: Cambridge University Press.

Mithen, S. (1996). *The prehistory of the mind: The cognitive origins of art and science*. London: Thames & Hudson.

Moon, J. W., Krems, J., & Cohen, A. B. (2018). Religious people are trusted because they are viewed as slow life-history strategists. *Psychological Science, 29*(6), 947–960. doi:10.1177/0956797617753606

Nettle, D., Harper, Z., Kidson, A., Stone, R., Penton-Voak, I. S., & Bateson, M. (2012). The watching eyes effect in the dictator game: It's not how much you give, it's being seen to give something. *Evolution and Human Behavior*, 34(1), 1–6. https://doi.org/10.1016/j.evolhumbehav.2012.08.004

Neusner, J., & Chilton, B. (Eds.). (2009). *The golden rule: The ethics of reciprocity in world religions*. New York: Continuum.

Norenzayan, A. (2013). *Big Gods: How religion transformed cooperation and conflict*. Princeton, NJ: Princeton University Press.

Pazhoohi, F., & Hosseinchari, M. (2014). Effects of religious veiling on Muslim men's attractiveness ratings of Muslim women. *Archives of Sexual Behavior*, 43(6), 1083–1086. https://doi.org/10.1007/s10508-014-0259-5

Pazhoohi, F., Lang, M., Xygalatas, D., & Grammer, K. (2016). Religious veiling as a mate-guarding strategy: Effects of environmental pressures on cultural practices. *Evolutionary Psychological Science*, 3, 118–124. https://doi.org/10.1007/s40806-016-0079-z

Pazhoohi, F., Macedo, A. F., & Arantes, J. (2017). The effect of religious clothing on gaze behavior: An eye-tracking experiment. *Basic and Applied Social Psychology*, 39(3), 176–182. https://doi.org/10.1080/01973533.2017.1307748

Piazza, J., Bering, J. M., & Ingram, G. (2011). "Princess Alice is watching you": Children's belief in an invisible person inhibits cheating. *Journal of Experimental Child Psychology*, 109, 311–320.

Pillsworth, E. G., & Haselton, M. G. (2006). Male sexual attractiveness predicts differential ovulatory shifts in female extra-pair attraction and male mate retention. *Evolution and Human Behavior*, 27(4), 247–258. https://doi.org/10.1016/j.evolhumbehav.2005.10.002

Pluhar, E., Frongillo, E. A., Stycos, M., & Dempster-McClain, D. (1998). Understanding the relationship between religion and the sexual attitudes and behaviors of college students. *Journal of Sex Education and Therapy*, 23, 288–296.

Rowthorn, R. (2011). Religion, fertility and genes: A dual inheritance model. *Proceedings of the Royal Society B: Biological Sciences*, 278(1717), 2519–2527. http://doi.org/10.1098/rspb.2010.2504

Rosch, E. (1975). Cognitive representations of semantic categories. *Journal of Experimental Psychology: General*, 104, 192–223.

Rostosky, S. S., Regnerus, M. D., & Comer Wright, M. L. (2003). Coital debut: The role of religiosity and sex attitudes in the add health survey. *Journal of Sex Research*, 40(4), 358–367.

Sabbagh, M. A., Xu, F., Carlson, S. M., Moses, L. J., & Lee, K. (2006). The development of executive functioning and theory of mind: A comparison of Chinese and US preschoolers. *Psychological Science*, 17, 74–81.

Shackelford, T. K., Schmitt, D. P., & Buss, D. M. (2005). Universal dimensions of human mate preferences. *Personality and Individual Differences*, 39(2), 447–458. https://doi.org/10.1016/j.paid.2005.01.023

Shariff, A. F., & Norenzayan, A. (2007). God is watching you: Priming god concepts increases prosocial behavior in an anonymous economic game. *Psychological Science*, 18(9), 803–809.

Shariff, A. F., Willard, A. K., Anderson, T., & Norenzayan, A. (2016). Religious priming: A meta-analysis with a focus on prosociality. *Personality and Social Psychology*, 20(1), 27–48.

Singh, D. (1993). Adaptive significance of female physical attractiveness: Role of waist-to-hip ratio. *Journal of Personality and Social Psychology*, 65(2), 293–307.

Slingerland, E., & Chudek, M. (2011). The prevalence of mind–body dualism in early China. *Cognitive Science*, 35(5), 997–1007. https://doi.org/10.1111/j.1551-6709.2011.01186.x

Slone, D. J. (2004). *Theological incorrectness: Why religious people believe what they shouldn't.* Oxford: Oxford University Press.

Slone, D. J. (2008). The attraction of religion: A sexual selectionist account. In J. Bulbulia, R. Sosis, E. Harris, R. Genet, C. Genet, & K. Wyman (Eds.), *The evolution of religion* (pp. 181–188). Santa Margarita, CA: Collins Foundation Press.

Slone, D. J., & Van Slyke, J. A. (Eds.). (2015). *The attraction of religion: A new evolutionary psychology of religion.* New York: Bloomsbury Academic.

Sosis, R., & Alcorta, C. (2003). Signaling, solidarity, and the sacred: The evolution of religious behavior. *Evolutionary Anthropology, 12,* 264–274.

Sperber, D. (1996). *Explaining culture: A naturalistic approach.* Oxford: Blackwell.

Spicer, K. R., & Platek, S. M. (2010). Curvaceous female bodies activate neural reward centers in men. *Communicative & Integrative Biology, 3*(3), 282–283. http://doi.org/10.4161/cib.3.3.11560

Trivers, R. L. (1972). Parental investment and sexual selection. In B. Campbell (Ed.), *Sexual selection and the descent of man* (pp. 52–95). Chicago: Aldine.

Trzebiatowska, M., & Bruce, S. (2012). *Why are women more religious than men?* Oxford: Oxford University Press.

Valenza, E., Simion, F., Cassia, V. M., & Umilta, C. (1996). Face preference at birth. *Journal of Experimental Psychology: Human Perception and Performance, 22*(4), 892–903.

Van Slyke, J. A. (2014). Religion is easy, but science is hard . . . Understanding McCauley's thesis. *Zygon, 49*(3), 696–707.

Van Slyke, J. A. (2016). *The cognitive science of religion.* New York: Routledge.

Van Slyke, J. A. (2017). Can sexual selection theory explain the evolution of individual and group-level religious beliefs and behaviors? *Religion, Brain, & Behavior, 7*(4), 335–338.

Van Slyke, J. (2021). Intuitive perceptions of the relationship between mating strategies and religiosity: Participant religiosity influences perceptions, but not gender. *Evolutionary Psychological Science,* 1–11. https://doi.org/10.1007/s40806-021-00286-w

Van Slyke, J. A. & Szocik, K. (2020). Sexual selection and religion: Can the evolution of religion be explained in terms of mating strategies? *Archive for the Psychology Religion 42,* 123–141. https://doi.org/10.1177/0084672420909460

Van Slyke, J. A., & Wasemiller, A. (2017). Short-term mating strategies are negatively correlated with religious commitment: Exploring evolutionary variables for religiosity at a small Christian liberal arts college. *Evolutionary Psychological Science, 8*(170), 253–260. https://doi.org/10.1007/s40806-017-0093-9

Weeden, J., Cohen, A. B., & Kenrick, D. T. (2008). Religious attendance as reproductive support. *Evolution and Human Behavior, 29,* 327–334.

Weeden, J., & Kurzban, R. (2013). What predicts religiosity? A multinational analysis of reproductive and cooperative morals. *Evolution and Human Behavior, 34*(6), 440–445. https://doi.org/10.1016/j.evolhumbehav.2013.08.006

Woolever, C., Bruce, D., Wulff, K., & Smith-Williams, I. (2006). The gender ratio in the pews: Consequences for congregational vitality. *Journal of Beliefs and Values, 27,* 25–38.

Xygalatas, D. (2013). Effects of religious setting on cooperative behavior: A case study from Mauritius. *Religion Brain and Behavior, 3*(2), 91–102. https://doi.org/10.1080/2153599X.2012.724547

CHAPTER 15

WHAT IS THE ROLE OF RITUAL IN BINDING COMMUNITIES TOGETHER?

HARVEY WHITEHOUSE AND CHRISTOPHER M. KAVANAGH

INTRODUCTION

SOCIAL scientists have long observed that collective rituals—ranging from religious ceremonies to state rituals and military ceremonies to royal weddings—bind participants together (e.g., Kertzer, 1989). Efforts to explain how rituals generate social cohesion go back many centuries, if not millennia. The fourteenth-century Tunisian Arab historian, Ibn Khaldun (1958), argued that *asabiyya* (عصبيّة), a form of social solidarity emphasizing group unity and shared purpose, resulted from the rituals of tribalism. This idea was further developed by Victorian scholars such as William Robertson-Smith (1889) and Émile Durkheim (1965) who advanced theories about the capacity of rituals to produce collective effervescence and the *conscience collective*. But only in recent decades have cognitive scientists begun to thoroughly unpack the causal pathways through which rituals bind groups together. Research on religion has been at the forefront of such efforts because of the prominent role of ritual in most religious traditions (McCauley & Lawson, 2002; Purzycki & Sosis, 2013; Rappaport, 1999).

It seems increasingly likely that the link between ritual performance and social glue is multistranded, in part because "ritual" is an umbrella term for several quite distinct behavioral features that are rooted in different psychological systems. For example, one common feature of collective rituals is social synchrony achieved by moving (dancing, marching, swaying, etc.) or vocalizing (singing, chanting, intoning, etc.) rhythmically in time. Numerous studies have shown that moving in synchrony increases social cohesion and cooperation (e.g., Good et al., 2017; Hove & Risen, 2009; Jackson et al., 2018; Lang et al., 2017; Wiltermuth & Heath, 2009; but see Cohen et al., 2014), and there is some evidence that this bonding effect can transcend the immediate group of coparticipants and, in some cases, be extended to out-groups (e.g. Reddish et al., 2016). One possible explanation is that social synchrony blurs the boundary between self and other, creating a temporary illusion of expanded agency (Pronin et al., 2006).

Another common feature of rituals is *causal opacity*—the fact that nobody can, even in principle, provide an adequate physical-causal rationale for the action sequences prescribed in rituals (Whitehouse, 2011). Ritual procedures are simply performed a certain way because it is the convention, the "done" or the "proper" method of performing the actions (Herrmann et al., 2013; Kapitány & Nielsen, 2015, 2016; Lyons et al., 2007). There is evidence that even young children appreciate the distinction between ritualistic behavior and instrumental behavior and recognize that the former has an affiliative function (Clegg & Legare, 2015; Legare & Wen, 2014; Wen et al., 2016). Moreover, it has been shown that, when primed with the threat of ostracism, children copy causally opaque actions more faithfully and innovate less, possibly as a re-inclusion behavior (Watson-Jones et al., 2014, 2016).

Thus, both social synchrony and causal opacity contribute to group cohesion and cooperation but do so via quite different psychological processes. This illustrates how we need to fractionate the category "ritual" into its myriad component elements to understand how different elements contribute to social bonding (McKay & Whitehouse, 2015; Whitehouse & Lanman, 2014). Fractionated elements of ritual include not only social synchrony and causal opacity but also "goal demotion" (Kapitány & Nielsen 2016). Goal demotion refers to the extent to which an observer of a ritual is capable of inferring and understanding an actor's reason for a given action sequence, distinguishing it from causal opacity, which addresses whether an action sequence has an identifiable and understandable mechanism of action (Boyer & Liénard, 2006; Kapitány & Nielsen, 2016). Additionally, at a functional level, it is important to consider aspects such as costly signaling through ritual participation (Sosis & Alcorta, 2003) or the performance of credibility-enhancing displays (Henrich, 2009). In this chapter, we focus particularly on the features of frequency and emotionality in *rituals*, understood as causally opaque collective actions. We focus on these aspects in particular because both theoretical and empirical research suggests that they are fundamentally linked to the main types of social glue that rituals are capable of forging. The framework that has detailed these connections in the most detail is the theory of "divergent modes of religiosity" (hereafter, DMR theory).

DMR Theory

DMR theory originates in the observation that religions tend to cluster around two types of ritual practices when we are considering their frequency and emotional intensity: the first type are the rare but intensely emotional *imagistic* rituals, and the second are the less emotional but more frequently performed *doctrinal* rituals (Whitehouse,

1995, 2000, 2004). The low-frequency/high-arousal (hereafter, LF/HA) rituals of the imagistic mode are so called because they become seared into the memories of the coparticipants as episodic images and events. The fact that imagistic rituals are, by definition, causally opaque, as well as intrinsically memorable, means that they can trigger long-enduring processes of reflection on their meaning and significance. As such, rituals of this kind have a lasting transformative effect psychologically and can become part of a participant's essential autobiographical self. To the extent that such experiences are shared with other members of the group, they can also generate very intense social cohesion. But because these bonds are based on shared ritual experiences among those who were co-present at a ritual performance, they do not spread efficiently to larger groups. Examples of such LF/HA rituals range from initiation rites into secret societies or cults (Allen, 1967) to traumatic fire-walking ordeals (see Xygalatas, this volume; for more examples, see Whitehouse, 1996).

The doctrinal mode of religiosity, by contrast, is characterized by high-frequency/ low-arousal (hereafter, HF/LA) collective rituals. These rituals tend to be welded into the fabric of everyday life, to the extent that hardly anybody can remember when they first performed them, and consequently they are not remembered as distinct episodes but, rather, as generalized experiences constructed from the thousands of times they have been performed. These experiences blur together and exist as "semantic memories" rather than as the specific events found with "episodic memory" (Tulving, 1972). The weekly Roman Catholic mass and Protestant church services are paradigmatic examples of HF/LA rituals. High-frequency repetition enables the rituals to become deeply ingrained in procedural memory, meaning that the ritual procedures can be produced with little or no explicit reflection. Additionally, frequent repetition makes it easier to spot deviations from orthopraxy, enabling doctrinal rituals to become highly standardized and routinized. This entails the suppression of individual interpretations of ritual meanings. Rather than each participant figuring out the ritual meanings for themselves, they are told what they mean by religious experts. Religious orators (gurus, prophets, teachers, and other types of sermonizers) rise above the common herd, establishing doctrinal orthodoxies and narrative traditions that are also, along with the rituals, frequently repeated and highly standardized. Unlike in the imagistic mode, doctrinal beliefs and practices are thus able to spread very efficiently, requiring only a handful of proselytizing individuals to spread a tradition to much wider audiences. The doctrinal mode, through standardization and efficient transmission, can serve as the basis for the establishment of vast "imagined communities" (Anderson, 1983), whose members are too numerous to know each other personally but who are united by a common creed. But if the bonds of shared doctrine and practice can mobilize larger populations, the social cohesion generated by the doctrinal mode is more diffused than that resulting from shared imagistic experiences.

The DMR theory was originally inspired by the study of a so-called cargo cult in Papua New Guinea (Whitehouse, 1995, 1996)—one of many new religious movements that emerged in that region in the wake of colonization (Worsley, 1957). Some Melanesian cargo cults were modeled on the small-scale ritual systems of traditional island cultures, involving LF/HA practices that united coparticipants but either never spread to larger populations or fragmented as they did so; others took their inspiration from various forms of missionary Christianity and adopted HF/LA rituals, forming movements of unprecedented scale (Whitehouse, 2000). The doctrinal traditions that spread most effectively and persisted often incorporated an imagistic dimension, for example, in the form of sporadic splintering in local communities that raised levels of enthusiasm and then, following the failure of prophesy, rejuvenated the commitment to the mainstream doctrinal tradition (Whitehouse, 1995, 2000). Such a pattern also serves to illustrate why it is inaccurate to conceive of DMR theory as presenting a simple dichotomy of two noninteracting forms of ritual behavior. In reality, religious traditions often feature both types of rituals.

The initial publication of the DMR theory prompted a flurry of scholarship that furnished various examples of both doctrinal and imagistic practices in ethnographic regions as far apart as the Middle East (Shankland, 2004), West Africa (Berner, 2004; Højberg, 2004; Peel, 2004), and Asia (Laidlaw, 2004; Bayly, 2004; Howe, 2004) and in historical traditions as diverse as Greco-Roman cults (Beck, 2004; Gragg, 2004) and early Protestantism (Hinde, 2005; Pyysiäinen, 2004; Vial, 2004). One outcome of this extensive exploration of case-study material has been the realization that DMR theory applies not only to religious communities (i.e., those espousing beliefs in supernatural entities), but to all kinds of groups, ranging from armies and paramilitary battalions to communist cells and secessionist movements (Whitehouse, 2004).

Ritual Frequency, Emotion, Memory, Social Glue, and Prosociality

The DMR theory makes a series of predictions about the relationships between ritual frequency, emotion, memory, social cohesion, and cooperation (Whitehouse, 2004, chap. 8). To test these predictions, it has been necessary to deploy suitable measures of the relevant variables and to devise ways of examining the causal connections between them. For example, to establish how rituals produce social glue requires a reasonably precise method of conceptualizing and measuring what is meant by "social glue." Below we consider two types of social glue that have different psychological causes and different social consequences: *group identification* and *identity fusion*.

In the field of social identity theory, a long tradition of psychological research looking at how people bond with groups has suggested that group identification is depersonalizing (Rosenberg, 1987). That is, when a person highly identifies with a given group identity and when that identity is made salient, their personal identity becomes less salient (and vice versa), implying a hydraulic relationship between personal identities and group identities (Hogg, 2006; Hogg & Turner, 1987; Hornsey, 2008). Consider someone who strongly identifies with a specific political party: though this individual may have many personally distinctive characteristics (e.g., enjoys chess, was orphaned in middle childhood, has a quick temper), in the context of an intense election battle these personal-identity features fade into insignificance in comparison to political-party allegiance. What becomes most salient to the individual is not whether others also lost their parents as children or like to play board games but whether they share the same attitudes to a political in-group or out-group, positive and negative attributions are then assigned on that basis.

From the viewpoint of DMR theory, identification accurately describes the way followers of doctrinal traditions align with their groups. The beliefs and practices that define their tradition, and on the basis of which they are united with other followers, are socially learned and stored in semantic memory (see the section "DMR Theory"). As such, these beliefs and practices bear little or no relationship to the qualities that define the personal self (Whitehouse & Lanman, 2014), which have been shown across a number of studies to be strongly related to self-defining autobiographical memories (Conway et al., 2004; Rose Addis & Tippett, 2004; Thorne & McLean, 2003; Wilson & Ross, 2003). It is therefore quite understandable that thinking about group-identity markers would not activate personal identity. But one would not expect that to be the case with imagistic experiences, which are at once intensely personal but also group-defining. A more suitable construct from group psychology research that is capable of capturing this type of group alignment is "identity fusion," characterized as a visceral sense of oneness with the group, where the boundary between personal and group identities is porous (Swann et al., 2012). For fused individuals, the relationship between the self and the group is synergistic such that when the group identity is salient, it activates personal agency (and vice versa). Consequently, when the group comes under attack, those who are fused with the group take it personally and will be willing to pay very high costs to defend the group's interests; but at the same time, experiencing a threat to a personal identity can also motivate a progroup response. The hydraulic identity models of group identification that outline a *functional antagonism* between personal and social identities (Turner & Oakes, 1986: 241; Sim et al., 2014) are ill-equipped to account for these kinds of synergistic responses. Fusion is typically measured using an adapted version of the "inclusion of self in other scale" (See Figure 15.1) or from a seven-item verbal scale validated to provide a measure distinct from established group-identification scales, including statements such as "I am one with my group," "My group is me," and "I feel immersed in my group" (Swann et al., 2010, 2014).

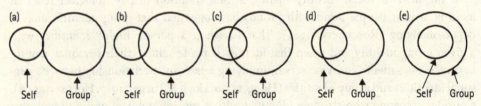

FIGURE 15.1 Pictorial measure of identity fusion.

WHAT IS THE ROLE OF RITUAL IN BINDING COMMUNITIES TOGETHER? 283

Fusion produces family-like bonds associated with feelings of shared essence. Such feelings can result from sharing life-defining experiences or from perceptions of having a common genealogy. For example, in the wake of the 2013 Boston Marathon bombings, fusion—measured using the verbal fusion scale—was predictive of willingness to help the victims. But the desire to make a personal sacrifice in order to help the victims (e.g., by giving blood or donating money) was mediated by perceptions of kinship and familial connection—measured by a kin perception scale that included items such as "I see other members of my country as brothers and sisters" (Buhrmester et al., 2014). Another study, using a sample of 256 identical and fraternal twins, showed that bonds based on both actual genetic similarity and perceptions of shared experiences independently predicted fusion with one's sibling (Whitehouse et al., 2017). These are just two examples and overall there is strong existing evidence that the bonds formed through identity fusion are linked to psychological kinship (Whitehouse & Lanman, 2014). Fusion with family typically relies on a combination of sharing phenotypic characteristics and life experiences; but we argue that culturally evolved institutions, such as imagistic rituals, are potentially able to activate the shared-experience pathway to fusion, creating family-like bonds among coparticipants who are not in fact closely related genetically.

LF/HA rituals are thought to produce fusion via a somewhat elaborate causal chain in which emotionally intense but causally opaque experiences lead, via reflection on their meaning, to a transformation of the personal self, which in the case of collective rituals produces feelings of shared essence and fusion (Whitehouse, 2018; for a developmental account, see Reese and Whitehouse, 2021). The elements in this causal chain are the subject of ongoing empirical study, via lab and field experiments and surveys conducted with a wide range of special populations. However, a substantial number of results already support the proposed model. For instance, a series of early experiments showed that emotionally arousing rituals generated deeper and more protracted reflection on their meaning than did less arousing ones (Richert et al., 2005). While Jong et al. (2015) provided correlational and experimental evidence linking shared negative experiences (the Northern Irish Troubles and the Boston Bombing) to levels of identity fusion via reflection. Similarly, Whitehouse et al. (2017) presented a diverse array of evidence that sharing painful experiences produces identity fusion, and that this, in turn, can motivate self-sacrifice. A comparable relationship has also been observed for positive (euphoric) experiences. Newson et al. (2016) found that positive and negative feelings among British football fans that were associated with crucial group-related events produced in them a sense of having been personally shaped by the experience, which consequently influenced their levels of fusion with their clubs.

Focusing specifically on ritual contexts, Páez et al. (2015) examined both negatively valenced and positively valenced ritualized gatherings and found that participating in these events "consistently strengthened . . . identity fusion, and social integration," and that "perceived emotional synchrony (collective effervescence) with others mediated these effects" (p. 711). Another recent study, which examined the experiences of more than 600 Brazilian Jiu-Jitsu practitioners during promotional rituals (Kavanagh et al., 2019), reported that subjective positive assessments of the rituals—including, by those who had endured painful events, such as belt-whipping ordeals—were associated with higher levels of identity fusion with the training group. Finally, a preregistered study conducted with over 1,300 Indonesian Muslims (Kavanagh et al., 2020) found that both the self-rated 'transformativeness' and perceived sharedness of group-defining events were predictive of levels of identity fusion with relevant group targets. Although the relationship with transformativeness was more consistent than perceived sharedness across analyses.

The link between fusion and extreme progroup behavior, including a stated willingness to fight and die for the group, has been shown to be mediated by perceptions of outgroup threat (Whitehouse, 2018). Extreme self-sacrifice poses an evolutionary puzzle; kin selection, however, provides a potential solution. Specifically, one possibility is that identity fusion originally evolved as a psychological mechanism meant to motivate closely related kinsmen to defend each other in the face of enemy attack. If so, the same mechanisms may have later been co-opted to target non-kin groups as a group-level cultural adaptation (Whitehouse & Lanman, 2014; but see also Whitehouse et al., 2017). It is noteworthy that LF/HA rituals are particularly widespread in warlike groups, especially in the initiation rites and hazing practices of tribal warriors, terrorist organizations, revolutionary insurgents, and conventional armies (Sosis et al., 2007; Whitehouse & McQuinn, 2012). Data collected during the 2011 uprising in Libya supports the view that imagistic experiences, when combined with out-group threat, not only lead people to theoretically endorse a willingness to fight and die for their group, but also translate into behaviors, with people actually risking their lives on the battlefield (Whitehouse, McQuinn, et al., 2014).

Meanwhile, research on the doctrinal mode of religiosity has been investigating the pathways from HF/LA ritual to identification and the spread of group-defining beliefs and practices to larger populations (see Figure 15.2). The central idea here is that the routinization of cultural practices enables the group's identity markers to be stored in semantic memory as a set of schemas and procedural scripts (Whitehouse, 1992, 2000). Frequent repetition not only makes possible the standardization of the practices, including rituals, but also promotes processes of identification with groups comprising large anonymous populations. This is a different kind of bond than those found with the prototypical imagistic rituals in groups that are based on networks in which everyone has a relational tie with other group members and are locally fused. Group

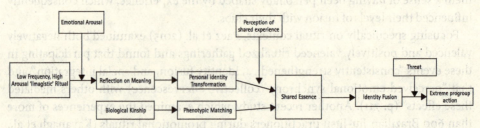

FIGURE 15.2 Pathways to fusion and extreme pro-group action.

identification has repeatedly been demonstrated to be capable of motivating both in-group preference and out-group derogation (Brown, 2006; Hornsey, 2008; Tajfel & Turner, 1985). A recent study by Hobson et al. (2017), for instance, found that to generate intergroup bias—where an individual discriminates against an out-group in favor of an in-group—novel ritual performances had to be repeated; one-off performances did not produce this effect. Yet, since this form of group alignment does not tap into personal agency, an individual's personal interests will often win out over those of the group when the two are in direct conflict, making identification a less powerful form of social glue than fusion (Whitehouse & Lanman, 2014). To illustrate the difference in the context of war: strong identification may motivate civilians to sign up for wartime military service when the risks of personal death or injury are relatively low, but it is fusion that will lead to willingness to jump on a grenade or undertake suicide missions (Whitehouse, 2018).

Imagistic practices serve to fuse members of small groups in situations or environments in which the temptation to defect is strong (e.g., when the group is under fire from the enemy), but doctrinal practices can bind together much larger groups, albeit more diffusely. Extreme group identification may also be capable of motivating extreme self-sacrifice through depersonalization processes when relevant group norms dictate extreme out-group derogation; however, in most circumstances, the identification is weaker and thus likelier to promote weaker forms of progroup actions, such as willingness to pay taxes or tribute. Yet, because the doctrinal mode is capable of bonding very large populations, even small contributions from individual members can rapidly mount up to a significant store of cumulative value. The doctrinal mode is thus capable of supporting collective action on a much larger scale than is the imagistic mode.

RITUAL AND THE RISE OF SOCIAL COMPLEXITY

In introducing DMR theory (see the section "DMR Theory"), we considered efforts to investigate the divergent modes in real-world settings based on the analysis of case-study material, both contemporary and historical. A benefit of that approach is that it has yielded detailed information on modes dynamics as they play out at particular times and places. But a limitation of this approach is that it cannot be regarded as a valid test of the core claims of the theory in any objective or systematic way, since case studies are always vulnerable to selection bias. To address this problem, Atkinson and Whitehouse (2011) constructed a large database on the world's rituals using materials extracted from the Human Relations Area Files—a vast online storehouse of ethnographic writings (Murdock et al., 2006). The database included detailed information on 644 rituals from a sample of 74 cultural groups (designed to minimize the effects of the Galton problem, that of nonindependence across sites). For each of the rituals selected, data relating to roughly a hundred variables relevant to testing the modes theory were coded, including frequency of ritual performance and emotional arousal. Analysis of the dataset confirmed that the frequency and emotionality of collective rituals are indeed negatively correlated (as predicted); but the exercise also generated some major surprises. First, the strongest inverse correlation between frequency and emotional intensity was found for negatively valenced rituals; whereas for positive euphoric rituals, there was instead a quadratic relationship. That is, while more intensely negative rituals were less frequent, the positive rituals in the dataset demonstrated a more variable relationship. Additionally, the analysis revealed that ritual frequency correlates positively with agricultural intensity, measured on a six-point scale from "no agriculture" to "intensive irrigated agriculture" (with intermediary points covering incidental agriculture, long fallow, horticulture, etc.; Atkinson & Whitehouse, 2011). This finding suggested that as human societies begin to depend more on intensive farming, and grow larger and more complex, their ritual practices become more frequent and less emotionally arousing. A recent reanalysis (Kapitány et al., 2020) of the 644 ritual dataset employing a novel factor analysis reaffirmed the euphoric and dysphoric clustering of features and noted that these appeared to be largely orthogonal. Moreover, the same study reported a similar clustering of euphoric, dysphoric, and frequency related dimensions in accounts of contemporary ritual experiences collected from 779 individuals from Japan, India, and the US.

These findings prompt speculation on whether a rise in the performance frequency of collective rituals might have helped drive the transition from foraging to farming in human prehistory. To investigate that precise question, Whitehouse established a collaboration with archaeologists at the Neolithic site Çatalhöyük in central Anatolia (Whitehouse, Mazzucato, et al., 2014; Whitehouse & Hodder, 2010), where techniques of crop cultivation and animal domestication were gradually evolving for the first time in Western Eurasia. During roughly 1800 years of settlement at Çatalhöyük, there was a steady rise in agricultural intensity as increasing varieties of animals were brought under human control and the sizes of flocks and herds increased. At the same time, there was evidence of the increasing regional homogeneity of cultural markers, such as stamp seals and pottery designs. Along with these developments came evidence of increasing frequencies of ritual performances, especially in domestic settings. Although these observations suggest the emergence and spread of a more doctrinal mode of religiosity, the same time period also witnessed a decline in imagistic rituals. Very large but infrequent feasting events, involving the manhandling and "baiting" of dangerous wild animals, had occurred during earlier periods of settlement, but the indications of these gradually declined, along with other indicators of cult activity associated with hunting. Activities that involved taking large risks, such as trading obsidian with distant groups in potentially hostile lands, also appeared less often and so, too, the more impressive projectiles associated with large-game hunting.

Although the general picture at Çatalhöyük is one in which doctrinal religiosity emerges and imagistic practices decline, it is still just one archaeological site and covers a time period of less than two millennia, falling somewhere in the middle of the initial transition from foraging to farming. So even if there was a transition from imagistic to doctrinal modes of religiosity at Çatalhöyük that drove a major shift in social morphology, it is impossible to say on the basis of this site alone whether this represented a general pattern in human history or something unique to this one, rather remarkable, civilization. It was therefore necessary to assemble data on a much larger range of sites. This has now been done for 64 sites scattered across Anatolia and the Levant, covering a much longer time period (from the Epipaleolithic to the Chalcolithic). The goal of this new regional study was to establish whether there was any broad evidence for a decline in the imagistic mode and the rise of the doctrinal mode as agriculture first appeared and became more fully established across the region as a whole. Unfortunately, variables such as ritual frequency and emotional arousal are hard to observe directly in the archaeology of most prehistoric human settlements. To get around this problem, a new technique, known as "material correlates analysis," was developed by Gantley and colleagues.

Gantley et al. (2018) began by selecting the ten most doctrinal and ten most imagistic cultures from the Atkinson and Whitehouse (2011) ethnographic database; they then identified variables in each of those cultures that had known correlates in the sixty-four archaeological sites featured in the regional sample. This generated a set of 90 ritual, subsistence, and social-complexity material correlate variables that could be examined in both the ethnographic and the archaeological records. In the archaeological sample researchers found a clear statistical separation between cultures that had indicators of predominantly practicing either imagistic rituals or doctrinal rituals, based on characteristics associated with subsistence, burial practices, storage, food preparation, resource management, communal buildings, and cemeteries. Based on this analysis, it appears that imagistic features were progressively replaced by doctrinal ones as farming intensified and societies became larger and more complex. These results are compelling, but admittedly, the study has its limitations. In particular, despite including over 60 archaeological sites, the sample still covers only a small portion of the globe, Anatolia and the Levant, and can only speak to patterns over a few thousand years of prehistory. Furthermore, as is inevitable when one is dealing with rituals in prehistory, the data used for the study have many gaps.

In an effort to overcome some of these limitations, a more ambitious project is currently being assembled, called Seshat: Global History Databank (Turchin et al., 2015). One of the major advantages of Seshat is, as its name suggests, that the coverage of the data being included is global in nature, not just regional. Furthermore, the time frame of the databank stretches back 10,000 years, so far covering more than 400 polities and involving the expertise of over a hundred historians, archaeologists, and classicists in its coding of historical data. At the time of writing, Seshat already contains over 300,000 entries. As with the rituals database that employed materials mined from the Human Research Area Files, all the data in Seshat relate to prespecified variables that were selected to test theories relating to the evolution of social complexity. These include variables that are relevant to testing the DMR theory. Among the core variables in the code book are those relating to social complexity, ritual and religion, warfare, and agriculture. To maximize diversity in the dataset, Seshat utilizes a stratified sample of thirty "natural geographic areas" (hereafter, NGAs). In each of ten specified world regions, NGAs were chosen in which social complexity emerged early, late, or somewhere in the middle (again, to maximize diversity).

To measure the rise of social complexity in world history, Seshat's researchers used 51 variables that scholars have previously linked with complexity associated with population size, hierarchy, territory, governance, money, infrastructure, information systems, and texts (Turchin et al., 2018). These different characteristics exhibited strong relationships with one another across all the NGAs. Statistical analysis also revealed that social complexity emerged at widely differing time points in different parts of the world. From the perspective of DMR theory, a key question is whether HF/LA rituals precede the rise of social complexity in all these world regions, consistent with the hypothesis that the doctrinal mode helped to drive that process by providing a mechanism for the establishment of common identity and cooperation in large groups (Whitehouse et al., 2015).

Another hypothesis with some prima facie plausibility is that moralizing high gods, referred to by some scholars as "Big Gods" (entailing beliefs in moralizing supernatural punishment) contributed to the rise of "big societies" (large-scale, complex sociopolitical formations) and provided a means of regulating cooperation as transactions became increasingly impersonal and the temptation to cheat or free ride under the cloak of anonymity became more acute (Lang et al., 2019; Norenzayan, 2013; Norenzayan et al., 2016). However, research by Watts et al. (2015), who conducted a Bayesian phylogenetic analysis of the beliefs of ninety-six Austronesian cultures, suggests that broad supernatural punishment but not moralizing high gods preceded political complexity in that region of the world. Analysis of Seshat data suggests that, throughout world history, concern with moralizing supernatural punishment only becomes a primary feature of (some) religious systems after, and not before, the sharpest rises in social complexity (Whitehouse et al., 2021). Further analyses of Seshat data, using more fine-grained measures of belief in moralizing supernatural punishment, also lend support to the late appearance of Big Gods, suggesting that moralizing religions did not play a key causal role in the rise of sociopolitical complexity, and that the more significant evolutionary drivers were warfare and agricultural intensity (see Turchin et al., 2019). Some researchers have suggested that by focusing on group-level data and coding single values for entire societies, we may be flattening important individual variation and more subtle moralistic concerns, including among societies with relatively "smaller" and more locally restricted deities (Purzycki & Watts, 2018; Purzycki et al., 2020; Singh et al., 2021). Even if that is so, however, the ramifications for the efforts to test the Big Gods hypothesis against cross-cultural or historical data have not yet been fully mapped out. To the extent that cultural systems support and amplify intuitions about supernatural monitoring, a key question is whether and how such cultural systems, in turn, contribute to the rise of big societies by scaling up relevant forms of cooperation. This requires a focus, at least in part, on group-level data. It remains to be seen whether the doctrinal mode of religiosity, if not belief in Big Gods more specifically, drove the rise of social complexity in world history, perhaps subsequently buttressed by military innovations and resource availability. This question is currently a major research topic for a wide array of scholars and scientists working with historical data.

RITUAL AND GROUP COHESION IN COMPLEX SOCIETIES

Although the imagistic mode was once the dominant way in which rituals generated social glue in human societies and the doctrinal mode was unheard of, the dominance of the two modes has now been more or less reversed worldwide. The doctrinal mode now reigns supreme in all but the most isolated human societies and has done so for centuries or, more commonly, millennia. In the process, cultural evolution has wrought a diversity of changes to the dynamics of doctrinal systems in different regions and at different times. In this section, we consider how moralizing gods and credibility-enhancing displays ([CREDs]; Henrich, 2009) or credibility-undermining displays ([CRUDs]; Turpin et al., 2018) may have strengthened or weakened beliefs in doctrinal orthodoxies and thus their ability to facilitate trust and cooperation in changing social ecologies. We also consider how factors influencing the tightness and looseness of group norms may impact the maintenance of orthodoxy and the standardization of ideology more generally. Finally, we consider how varying levels of relational mobility in different societies may have impacted the relative prevalence of doctrinal and imagistic rituals.

We have briefly discussed the possibility that moralizing gods might have been necessary to sustain cooperation in large-scale societies, especially in multiethnic empires where common overarching identities were lacking (see the section "Ritual and the Rise of Social Complexity"). But for moralizing gods to motivate prosocial action, they would have had to be believable. The idea of an "eye in the sky" watching over everyone, punishing the wicked and rewarding the pious, may have some intuitive appeal (Boyer, 1994, 2001; Johnson, 2015; Norenzayan, 2013), but religions of that kind also invite skepticism, not least because such beliefs often seem to be rather convenient for power holders (McKinnon, 2005). Seeing evidence that others truly believe, however, might help to quell doubts and skepticism. It has been suggested that CREDs constitute a culturally evolved mechanism that provides precisely that kind of hard-to-fake evidence (Henrich, 2009).

When a person acts in a way that would be costly and therefore irrational if they do not really believe what they claim, it makes their belief in their claims more convincing to others. To offer a simple example, if someone claims that a potentially poisonous mushroom is safe to eat, that claim will be far more convincing if they then proceed to eat the mushroom themselves. In the same way, it has been argued that performing

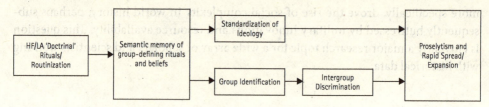

FIGURE 15.3 Pathways to group identification and rapid spread.

costly (e.g., time-consuming, physically demanding, resource-consuming) rituals makes the beliefs associated with those rituals more believable. Such rituals, serve as CREDs, increasing the believability of doctrinal beliefs, including in the belief in the existence of a moralizing god. If correct, CREDs theory can help to explain why some doctrinal traditions spread more rapidly or last longer than others (see Figure 15.3). Conversely, traditions that fail to sustain adequate CREDs will, without other compensatory mechanisms, such as state-mandated support, struggle to retain their members. This is especially true in the context of a competitive ideological landscape, where other religions or secular ideologies are also eager to recruit defectors. Worse still, religious traditions whose leaders are seen to be hypocritical, such as the Catholic clergy who sought to cover up child-abuse scandals in the church, may be seen as engaging in CRUDs that undermine credibility and contribute to a more rapid decline in belief. Indeed, such a phenomenon has recently been observed in the Republic of Ireland in the wake of Catholic Church abuse scandals (Turpin et al., 2018).

Besides variables such as CREDs and CRUDs that can strengthen or weaken the links between variables within the doctrinal mode, there are also factors external to religious institutional systems that could influence how they develop. For example, although the precise mechanisms by which the rise of agriculture could lead to an increase in the frequency of the collective rituals of the doctrinal mode is not yet clear, it seems plausible that some external third factor (i.e., one that is neither agriculture nor HF/LA ritual but related to both) somehow triggered the whole process. One such candidate would be increasing population densities and the spread of infectious diseases (Fincher et al., 2008). The heightened risk may have triggered emotional and behavioral routines that evolved to combat such invisible environmental hazards, dubbed "hazard precaution systems," and, as a result, an increased desire to engage in ritualistic behaviors (Boyer & Liénard, 2006). Another factor may have been the rise in routinized activities of all kinds, as part of the emergence of a farming lifestyle and behavioral toolkit. Many of these activities likely incorporated ritualistic elements, such as high-frequency repetition to facilitate learning processes (Whitehouse, Mazzucato, et al., 2014). These are currently speculative hypotheses, and certainly, it is likely that a variety of other factors exerted an influence on the processes discussed to different degrees at different locations. Whatever the environmental variables (including demographic, ontogenetic, and social factors) were that originally triggered the emergence of LF/HA rituals along with the emergence and spread of agriculture, it is clear that some of those variables may

WHAT IS THE ROLE OF RITUAL IN BINDING COMMUNITIES TOGETHER?

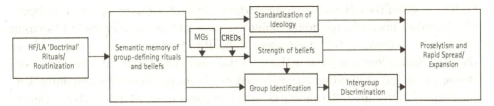

FIGURE 15.4 Moralizing gods (MGs) and credibility-enhancing displays (CREDs) may strengthen doctrinal beliefs.

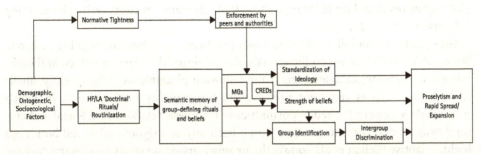

FIGURE 15.5 Normative tightness promotes social enforcement, increasing standardization.

also have had an ongoing and interactive impact on the nature of the doctrinal mode and how it functions.

A growing body of empirical research suggests that when environments become harsher, for example, due to natural disaster or out-group conflict, social norms are more tightly enforced (Gelfand et al., 2011). Doctrinal traditions are also normative systems, and we would expect any effects on tightness-looseness to play a significant role in their functioning. In particular, an increase in normative tightness would strengthen peer-to-peer enforcement of conformist behavior, as well as support for the suppression by religious leaders of unauthorized deviations from the orthodox canon. This in turn would help to ensure the standardization of the tradition as a whole, necessary to ensure shared identity and cooperation (see Figure 15.4).

RELATIONAL MOBILITY AND DMR THEORY

Another socioecological factor that is likely to play an important role in determining what kind of ritual practices are able to flourish is *relational mobility*. Relational mobility refers to the ability of individuals within a society to voluntarily form new relationships or to dissolve dissatisfying ones (Kavanagh & Yuki, 2017; Yuki & Schug, 2012; Yuki et al., 2007). In the contemporary world, the United States is a prototypical high-relational-mobility society, in which there is a strong culture of individualism and people are relatively free and encouraged to seek out new relationships, both in terms of friends and romantic partners. In contrast to this pattern, in Japan, which ranked lowest in relational mobility in a recent 39-country study (Thomson et al., 2018), individuals find it extremely difficult to form new relationships or leave old ones. Such a low-relational-mobility environment has broader implications, with strong social and cultural emphasis placed on the importance of maintaining harmonious relationships and avoiding actions that could result in irreversible social ostracism. Levels of relational mobility have also been shown to be inversely correlated with levels of historical threat, as well as highly correlated with subsistence practices. Specifically, societies that historically have a greater reliance on animal husbandry display higher relational mobility than those that rely more on cooperative rice farming (Thomson et al., 2018).

How relational mobility relates to ritual practices is a subject of ongoing research, but notable parallels between the growth of agriculture, doctrinal practices, and high-relational- mobility societies suggest the following plausible hypothesis: early small-scale tribal societies represent prototypical, low-mobility environments in which individuals have very limited opportunities to form new relationships. Social and cultural systems that serve to preserve group harmony and tighten relational bonds are highly adaptive (Schug et al., 2009). The imagistic mode serves as an effective tool for bonding people tightly together in a manner that makes it difficult to change group membership. We would therefore expect imagistic rituals to dominate in low-relational-mobility societies. We have already discussed some of the archaeological evidence that points to a connection between imagistic rituals and smaller-scale communities, and it is also notable that the prototypical illustrations of imagistic rituals are derived from tribal societies (Whitehouse, 1995, 1996, 2000). Moreover, even within contemporary low mobility societies, such as Japan, where devotion to doctrinal religiosity is famously low (WIN-Gallup International, 2012), a wide variety of dramatic imagistic rituals abound and are often the central events within local communities (Kavanagh, 2016; Kavanagh & Jong, 2020; Kawano, 2005; Nelson, 1996; Reader & Tanabe, 1998). Conversely, doctrinal rituals, with their ability to generate large "imagined communities," are likely more suited to environments with higher relational mobility. Individuals raised in high-mobility societies are likely to extract more benefit from the greater numbers of in-group partners they are granted access to via their shared doctrinal ritual practices and the associated communities.

Though the relationships posited above imply that societal levels of social mobility are the antecedent factor that enables different kinds of ritual practices to become more or less adaptive, an alternative causal pathway may also function wherein certain ritual practices themselves generate high- and low-mobility environments. For instance, in contemporary societies there are many examples of tightly knit groups, including gangs and military fighting units, which utilize imagistic rituals, such as traumatic initiations or dramatic ritualized displays of commitment, to forge group bonds. In groups bonded by imagistic rituals, the penalty for leaving the group or violating group norms can often be severe, including the severing of appendages (Bosmia et al., 2014) or punishment beatings (Monaghan & McLaughlin, 2006; Nolan & McCoy, 1996). However, imagistic

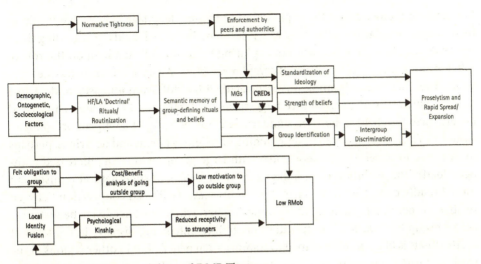

FIGURE 15.6 Relational mobility and DMR Theory.

rituals are also found in less extreme groups, including college fraternities (Campo et al., 2005; Cimino, 2013), splinter sects from mainstream religious traditions (Hood & Williamson, 2008), and various new religious movements (Lewis, 2008; McFarland, 1967). It may be that in all these cases, imagistic rituals help decrease relational mobility and prevent defection. Alternatively, doctrinal practices may serve as one method to *increase* relational mobility by enabling high-mobility social networks to grow within societies that are traditionally low in relational mobility. If this is correct, it could help to explain why new religions that prove effective at proselytizing and conversion are often diagnosed as representing an existential threat to traditional cultures and authority (Laver, 2011).

Although currently in need of empirical verification, the correspondence between low-mobility societies and the prevalence of imagistic rituals is striking. Efforts are now underway to examine these associations both by looking at the historical indicators of relational mobility and ritual practice in the Seshat database and examining contemporary groups and societies.

Conclusion

How do rituals bind communities together? The answer seems to be that different kinds of rituals bind together communities on different scales via distinct psychological processes. Specifically, imagistic practices, including imagistic rituals, are effective at binding smaller groups together through relationally focused local fusion. Large, imagined communities, alternatively, can be effectively bound together by doctrinal rituals producing group identification. In addition, perceptions of having shared life-defining moments and the exploitation of familial language may enable fusion to be projected onto larger collectives. Much still remains to be teased out regarding these processes and how they interact, but exploring them should shed light on the role of religion and ritual in the evolution of complex societies. We have evidence that the transition from foraging to farming was associated with a shift from imagistic to doctrinal modes, which helped to crystallize large-scale identities, based on shared rituals and beliefs, enabling these to become standardized. The policing of emergent orthodoxies would also have been assisted by a tightening of religious norms and doctrines, perhaps in response to novel dangers associated with large-group living (e.g., increased pathogen load). The evolution of moralizing gods, or beliefs in supernatural punishment more broadly conceived (e.g., karma), may also have facilitated cooperation between relative strangers, especially in multiethnic empires, where trust needed to be sustained across group boundaries. The spread of credibility-enhancing displays in the form of costly rituals is likely to have helped to stabilize such beliefs. But in other regions of the world, alternative ways of solving collective action problems in large-scale societies evolved. In East Asia, for example, low levels of relational mobility (arising partly from dependence on subsistence practices that required high levels of coordination and interdependence, such as the management of rice paddies) may have enabled cooperation to be maintained even in very large societies, without the need for moralizing high gods. More research is needed, however, to test and extend these hypotheses based on a continuous back-and-forth between the study of living populations (e.g., via field observation, surveys, and experiments) and quantitative analysis of human history and prehistory.

QUESTIONS FOR FUTURE RESEARCH

1. To what extent are a given community's collective rituals shaped by contemporary environmental factors versus historically entrenched traditions?
2. How long do the effects on group cohesion of participation in different kinds of collective rituals persist?
3. How and why did ritual behavior emerge in human evolution?

ACKNOWLEDGMENTS

This work was supported by an Advanced Grant ("Ritual Modes: Divergent Modes of Ritual, Social Cohesion, Prosociality, and Conflict," grant agreement no. 694986) from the European Research Council (ERC) under the European Union's Horizon 2020 Research and Innovation Programme and an award from the Templeton World Charity

Foundation, entitled "Cognitive and Cultural Foundations of Religion and Morality" (TWCF0164).

REFERENCES

Allen, M. R. (1967). *Male Cults and Secret Initiations in Melanesia*. Melbourne: Melbourne University Press.

Anderson, B. (1983). *Imagined communities: Reflections on the origin and spread of nationalism*. London: Verso.

Atkinson, Q. D., & Whitehouse, H. (2011). The cultural morphospace of ritual form: Examining modes of religiosity cross-culturally. *Evolution and Human Behavior*, 32(1), 50–62. https://doi.org/10.1016/j.evolhumbehav.2010.09.002

Bayly, S. (2004). Conceptualizing from Within: Divergent Religious Modes from Asian Modernist Perspectives. In H. Whitehouse & J. Laidlaw (Eds.) *Ritual and Memory: Towards a Comparative Anthropology of Religion*, pp. 111–134. Walnut Creek, CA: AltaMira Press.

Beck, R. (2004). Four men, two sticks, and a whip: Image and doctrine in a Mithraic ritual. In H. Whitehouse & L. H. Martin (Eds.), *Theorizing religions past: Archaeology, history, and cognition* (pp. 87–104). Walnut Creek, CA: AltaMira Press.

Berner, U. (2004). Modes of religiosity and types of conversion in medieval Europe and modern Africa. In H. Whitehouse & L. H. Martin (Eds.), *Theorizing religions past: Archaeology, history, and cognition* (pp. 157–172). Walnut Creek, CA: AltaMira Press.

Bosmia, A. N., Griessenauer, C. J., & Tubbs, R. S. (2014). Yubitsume: Ritualistic self-amputation of proximal digits among the Yakuza. *Journal of Injury and Violence Research*, 6(2), 54–56.

Boyer, P. (1994). *The naturalness of religious ideas: A cognitive theory of religion*. Berkeley: University of California Press.

Boyer, P. (2001). *Religion explained: The evolutionary origins of religious thought*. New York: Basic Books.

Boyer, P., & Liénard, P. (2006). Why ritualized behavior? Precaution systems and action parsing in developmental, pathological and cultural rituals. *Behavioral and Brain Sciences*, 29(6), 595–612. https://doi.org/10.1017/S0140525X06009332

Brown, S. D. (2006). Intergroup processes: Social identity theory. In D. Langdridge & S. Taylor (Eds.), *Critical reading in social psychology* (pp. 163–188). London, UK: Open University Press.

Buhrmester, M. D., Fraser, W. T., Lanman, J. A., Whitehouse, H., & Swann, W. B. (2014). When terror hits home: Fused Americans saw Boston bombing victims as "family" and rushed to their aid. *Self and Identity*, 14(3), 253–270. https://doi.org/10.1080/15298868.2014.992465

Campo, S., Poulos, G., & Sipple, J. W. (2005). Prevalence and profiling: Hazing among college students and points of intervention. *American Journal of Health Behavior*, 29(2), 137–149. https://doi.org/10.5993/AJHB.29.2.5

Cimino, A. (2013). Predictors of hazing motivation in a representative sample of the United States. *Evolution and Human Behavior*, 34(6), 446–452.

Clegg, J. M., & Legare, C. H. (2015). Instrumental and conventional interpretations of behavior are associated with distinct outcomes in early childhood. *Child Development*, 87, 527–542. https://doi.org/doi:10.1111/cdev.12472

Cohen, E., Mundry, R., & Kirschner, S. (2014). Religion, synchrony, and cooperation. *Religion, Brain & Behavior*, 4(1), 20–30.

Conway, M. A., Singer, J. A., & Tagini, A. (2004). The self and autobiographical memory: Correspondence and coherence. *Social Cognition, 22*(5), 491–529. https://doi.org/10.1521/soco.22.5.491.50768

Durkheim, É. (1965). *The elementary forms of the religious life* (J. M. Ward, Trans.). New York, USA: Free Press.

Fincher, C. L., Thornhill, R., Murray, D. R., & Schaller, M. (2008). Pathogen prevalence predicts human cross-cultural variability in individualism/collectivism. *Proceedings of the Royal Society B: Biological Sciences, 275*(1640), 1279–1285. https://doi.org/10.1098/rspb.2008.0094

Gantley, M., Whitehouse, H., & Bogaard, A. (2018). Material correlates analysis (MCA): An innovative way of examining questions in archaeology using ethnographic data. *Advances in Archaeological Practice, 6*(4), 328–341.

Good, A., Choma, B., & Russo, F. A. (2017). Movement synchrony influences intergroup relations in a minimal groups paradigm. *Basic and Applied Social Psychology, 39*(4), 231–238.

Gelfand, M. J., Raver, J. L., Nishii, L., Leslie, L. M., Lun, J., Lim, B. C., Duan, L., Almaliach, A., Ang, S., Arnadottir, J., Aycan, Z., Boehnke, K., Boski, P., Cabecinhas, R., Chan, D., Chhokar, J., D'Amato, A., Ferrer, M., Fischlmayr, I. C., . . . Yamaguchi, S. (2011). Differences between tight and loose cultures: A 33-nation study. *Science, 332*(6033), 1100–1104. https://doi.org/10.1126/science.1197754

Gragg, D. L. (2004). Old and new in Roman religion: A cognitive account. In H. Whitehouse & L. H. Martin (Eds.), *Theorizing religions past: Archaeology, history, and cognition* (pp. 69–86). Walnut Creek, CA: AltaMira Press.

Henrich, J. (2009). The evolution of costly displays, cooperation and religion: Credibility enhancing displays and their implications for cultural evolution. *Evolution and Human Behavior, 30*(4), 244–260. https://doi.org/10.1016/j.evolhumbehav.2009.03.005

Herrmann, P. A., Legare, C. H., Harris, P. L., & Whitehouse, H. (2013). Stick to the script: The effect of witnessing multiple actors on children's imitation. *Cognition, 129*(3), 536–543. https://doi.org/10.1016/j.cognition.2013.08.010

Hinde, R. A. (2005). Modes theory: Some theoretical considerations. In H. Whitehouse & R. N. McCauley (Eds.), *Mind and religion: Psychological and cognitive foundations of religiosity* (pp. 143–156). Walnut Creek, CA: AltaMira Press.

Hobson, N. M., Gino, F., Norton, M. I., & Inzlicht, M. (2017). When novel rituals lead to intergroup bias: Evidence from economic games and neurophysiology. *Psychological Science, 28*(6), 733–750. https://doi.org/10.1177/0956797617695099

Hogg, M. A. (2006). Social identity theory. In P. J. Burke (Ed.), *Contemporary social psychological theories* (pp. 111–136). Stanford, CA: Stanford University Press.

Hogg, M. A., & Turner, J. C. (1987). Intergroup behaviour, self-stereotyping and the salience of social categories. *British Journal of Social Psychology, 26*(4), 325–340. https://doi.org/10.1111/j.2044-8309.1987.tb00795.x

Højberg, C. (2004). Universalistic orientations of an imagistic mode of religiosity: The case of the West African Poro cult. In H. Whitehouse & J. Laidlaw (Eds.), *Ritual and memory: Toward a comparative anthropology of religion* (pp. 173–186). Walnut Creek, CA: AltaMira Press.

Hood, R., & Williamson, W. P. (2008). *Them that believe: The power and meaning of the Christian serpent-handling tradition*. Berkeley: University of California Press.

Hornsey, M. J. (2008). Social identity theory and self-categorization theory: A historical review. *Social and Personality Psychology Compass, 2*(1), 204–222. https://doi.org/10.1111/j.1751-9004.2007.00066.x

Hove, M. J., & Risen, J. L. (2009). It's all in the timing: Interpersonal synchrony increases affiliation. *Social Cognition, 27*(6), 949–960. https://doi.org/10.1521/soco.2009.27.6.949

Howe, L. (2004). Late Medieval Christianity, Balinese Hinduism, and the Doctrinal Mode of Religiosity. In H. Whitehouse & J. Laidlaw (Eds.), *Ritual and Memory: Towards a Comparative Anthropology of Religion*, pp. 135–154. Walnut Creek, CA: AltaMira Press.

Jackson, J. C., Jong, J., Bilkey, D., Whitehouse, H., Zollmann, S., McNaughton, C., & Halberstadt, J. (2018). Synchrony and physiological arousal increase cohesion and cooperation in large naturalistic groups. *Scientific Reports, 8*, 127. https://doi.org/10.1038/s41598-017-18023-4

Johnson, D. P. (2015). *God is watching you: How the fear of God makes us human.* Oxford, UK: Oxford University Press.

Jong, J., Whitehouse, H., Kavanagh, C. M., & Lane, J. (2015). Shared negative experiences lead to identity fusion via personal reflection. *PloS One, 10*(12), Article e0145611.

Kapitány, R., & Nielsen, M. (2015). Adopting the ritual stance: The role of opacity and context in ritual and everyday actions. *Cognition, 145*, 13–29. http://dx.doi.org/10.1016/j.cognition.2015.08.002

Kapitány, R., & Nielsen, M. (2016). The ritual stance and the precaution system: The role of goal-demotion and opacity in ritual and everyday actions. *Religion, Brain & Behavior, 7*(1), 27–42.

Kapitány, R., Kavanagh, C., & Whitehouse, H. (2020). Ritual morphospace revisited: the form, function and factor structure of ritual practice. *Philosophical Transactions of the Royal Society B, 375*(1805), 20190436

Kavanagh, C. M. (2016). Religion without belief. *Aeon Magazine.* https://aeon.co/essays/can-religion-be-based-on-ritual-practice-without-belief

Kavanagh, C. M., & Jong, J. (2020). Is Japan religious? *Journal for the Study of Religion, Nature, and Culture, 14*(1). https://doi.org/10.1558/jsrnc.39187

Kavanagh, C., & Yuki, M. (2017). Culture and group processes. *Online Readings in Psychology and Culture, 5*(4). https://doi.org/10.9707/2307-0919.1154

Kavanagh, C. M., Jong, J., McKay, R., & Whitehouse, H. (2019). Positive experiences of high arousal martial arts rituals are linked to identity fusion and costly pro-group actions. *European Journal of Social Psychology, 49*(4), 461–481. https://doi.org/10.1002/ejsp.2514

Kavanagh, C. M., Kapitány, R., Putra, I. E., & Whitehouse, H. (2020). Exploring the pathways between transformative group experiences and identity fusion. *Frontiers in Psychology, 11*:1172. doi: 10.3389/fpsyg.2020.01172

Kawano, S. (2005). *Ritual practice in modern Japan: Ordering place, people, and action.* Honolulu: University of Hawai'i Press.

Kertzer, D. I. (1989). *Ritual, politics, and power.* New Haven, CT: Yale University Press.

Khaldūn, I. (1958 [1377]). *The Muqaddimah: An Introduction to History.* Trans. Franz Rosenthal, from Arabic in 3 Vols. New York: Princeton University Press.

Laidlaw, J. (2004). Embedded Modes of Religiosity in Indic Renouncer Religions. In H. Whitehouse & J. Laidlaw (Eds.), *Ritual and Memory: Towards a Comparative Anthropology of Religion*, pp. 89–110. Walnut Creek, CA: AltaMira Press.

Lang, M., Bahna, V., Shaver, J. H., Reddish, P., & Xygalatas, D. (2017). Sync to link: Endorphin-mediated synchrony effects on cooperation. *Biological Psychology, 127*, 191–197.

Lang, M., Purzycki, B. G., Apicella, C. L., Atkinson, Q. D., Bolyanatz, A., Cohen, E., Handley, C., Kundtová Klocová, E., Lesorogol, C., Mathew, S., McNamara, R. A., Moya, C., Placek, C. D., Soler, M., Vardy, T., Weigel, J. L., Willard, A. K., Xygalatas, D., Norenzayan, A. & Henrich,

J. (2019). Moralizing gods, impartiality and religious parochialism across 15 societies. *Proceedings of the Royal Society B, 286*(1898), 20190202.

Laver, M. S. (2011). *The Sakoku edicts and the politics of Tokugawa hegemony*. New York, USA: Cambria Press.

Legare, C. H., & Wen, N. J. (2014). The effects of ritual on the development of social group cognition. *International Society for the Study of Behavioural Development, 66*(2), 9–12.

Lewis, J. R. (Ed.). (2008). *The Oxford handbook of new religious movements*. New York: Oxford University Press.

Lyons, D. E., Young, A. G., & Keil, F. C. (2007). The hidden structure of overimitation. *Proceedings of the National Academy of Sciences of the United States of America, 104*(50), 19751–19756. https://doi.org/10.1073/pnas.0704452104

McCauley, R. N., & Lawson, E. T. (2002). *Bringing ritual to mind: Psychological foundations of cultural forms*. Cambridge, UK: Cambridge University Press. https://doi.org/10.1017/CBO9780511606410

McFarland, H. N. (1967). *The rush hour of the gods: A study of new religious movements in Japan*. New York, USA: Macmillan.

McKay, R., & Whitehouse, H. (2015). Religion and morality. *Psychological Bulletin, 141*(2), 447–473. http://dx.doi.org/10.1037/a0038455

McKinnon, A. M. (2005). Reading Opium of the People: Expression, Protest and the Dialectics of Religion. *Critical Sociology, 31*(1-2), 15–38.

Monaghan, R., & McLaughlin, S. (2006). Informal justice in the city. *Space and Polity, 10*(2), 171–186.

Murdock, G. P., Ford, C., Hudson, A., Kennedy, R., Simmons, L., & Whiting, J. (2006). *Outline of cultural materials*. New Haven, CT: Human Relations Area Files.

Nelson, J. K. (1996). *A year in the life of a Shinto shrine*. Seattle: University of Washington Press.

Newson, M., Buhrmester, M. D., & Whitehouse, H. (2016). Explaining lifelong loyalty: The role of identity fusion and self-shaping group events. *PLoS One, 11*(8), Article e0160427.

Nolan, P., & McCoy, G. (1996). The changing pattern of paramilitary punishments in Northern Ireland. *Injury, 27*(6), 405–406.

Norenzayan, A. (2013). *Big Gods: How religion transformed cooperation and conflict*. Princeton, NJ: Princeton University Press.

Norenzayan, A., Shariff, A. F., Gervais, W. M., Willard, A. K., McNamara, R. A., Slingerland, E., & Henrich, J. (2016). The cultural evolution of prosocial religions. *Behavioral and Brain Sciences, 39*. https://doi.org/10.1017/S0140525X14001356

Páez, D., Rimé, B., Basabe, N., Wlodarczyk, A., & Zumeta, L. (2015). Psychosocial effects of perceived emotional synchrony in collective gatherings. *Journal of Personality and Social Psychology, 108*(5), 711–729.

Peel, J. (2004). Divergent modes of religiosity in West Africa. In H. Whitehouse & J. Laidlaw (Eds.), *Ritual and memory: Toward a comparative anthropology of religion* (pp. 11–30). Walnut Creek, CA: AltaMira Press.

Pronin, E., Wegner, D. M., McCarthy, K., & Rodriguez, S. (2006). Everyday magical powers: The role of apparent mental causation in the overestimation of personal influence. *Journal of Personality and Social Psychology, 91*(2), 218–231. https://doi.org/10.1037/0022-3514.91.2.218

Purzycki, B. G., & Sosis, R. (2013). The extended religious phenotype and the adaptive coupling of ritual and belief. *Israel Journal of Ecology & Evolution, 59*(2), 99–108. https://doi.org/10.1080/15659801.2013.825433

Purzycki, B. G., & Watts, J. (2018). Reinvigorating the cooperative, comparative ethnographic sciences of religion. *Free Inquiry, 38*(3), 26–29.

Purzycki, B. G., Willard, A., Klocová, E. K., Apicella, C. L., Atkinson, Q., Bolyanatz, A., Cohen, E., Handley, C., Henrich, J., Lang, M., Lesorogol, C., Mathew, S., McNamara, R., Moya, C., Norenzayan, A., Placek, C., Soler, M., Vardy, T., Weigel, J., Xygalatas, D., & Ross, C. T. (2020). The moralization bias of gods' minds: A cross-cultural test. [Preprint submitted to Religion, Brain and Behavior]. https://raw.githubusercontent.com/bgpurzycki/gods_moralization_bias/master/Moralization%20Bias.pdf

Pyysiäinen, I. (2004). Corrupt doctrine and doctrinal revival: On the nature and limits of the modes theory. In H. Whitehouse & L. H. Martin (Eds.), *Theorizing religions past: Archaeology, history, and cognition* (pp. 173–194). Walnut Creek, CA: AltaMira Press.

Rappaport, R. A. (1999). *Ritual and religion in the making of humanity*. Cambridge, UK: Cambridge University Press.

Reader, I., & Tanabe, G. J. (1998). *Practically religious: Worldly benefits and the common religion of Japan*. Honolulu: University of Hawai'i Press.

Reddish, P., Tong, E. M. W., Jong, J., Lanman, J. A., & Whitehouse, H. (2016). Collective synchrony increases prosociality towards non-performers and outgroup members. *British Journal of Social Psychology, 55*(4), 722–738. https://doi.org/10.1111/bjso.12165

Reese, E., & Whitehouse, H. (2021). The Development of Identity Fusion. *Perspectives on Psychological Science*. Advance online publication. doi.org/10.1177/1745691620968761

Richert, R. A., Whitehouse, H., & Stewart, E. (2005). Memory and analogical thinking in high arousal rituals. In H. Whitehouse & R. N. McCauley (Eds.), *Mind and religion: Psychological and cognitive foundations of religiosity* (pp. 127–145). Walnut Creek, CA: AltaMira Press.

Robertson-Smith, W. (1889). *Lectures on the religion of the Semites: First series*. London, UK: Adam and Charles Black.

Rose Addis, D., & Tippett, L. (2004). Memory of myself: Autobiographical memory and identity in Alzheimer's disease. *Memory, 12*(1), 56–74. https://doi.org/10.1080/09658210244000423

Rosenberg, M. (1987). Depersonalisation: The loss of personal identity. In T. Honess & K. M. Yardley (Eds.), *Self and identity: Perspectives across the lifespan* (pp. 193–206). London: Routledge & Kegan Paul.

Schug, J., Yuki, M., Horikawa, H., & Takemura, K. (2009). Similarity attraction and actually selecting similar others: How cross-societal differences in relational mobility affect interpersonal similarity in Japan and the USA. *Asian Journal of Social Psychology, 12*(2), 95–103.

Shankland, D. (2004). Modes of religiosity and the legacy of Ernest Gellner. In H. Whitehouse & J. Laidlaw (Eds.), *Ritual and memory: Toward a comparative anthropology of religion* (pp. 31–48). Walnut Creek, CA: AltaMira Press.

Sim, J. J., Goyle, A., McKedy, W., Eidelman, S., & Correll, J. (2014). How social identity shapes the working self-concept. *Journal of Experimental Social Psychology, 55*, 271–277.

Singh, M., Kaptchuk, T. J., & Henrich, J. (2021). Small gods, rituals, and cooperation: The Mentawai water spirit Sikameinan. *Evolution and Human Behavior, 42*(1), 61–72.

Slingerland, E., & Sullivan, B. (2017). Durkheim with data: The database of religious history. *Journal of the American Academy of Religion, 85*(2), 312–347.

Sosis, R., & Alcorta, C. S. (2003). Signalling, solidarity, and the sacred: The evolution of religious behavior. *Evolutionary Anthropology, 12*, 264–274.

Sosis, R., Kres, H. C., & Boster, J. S. (2007). Scars for war: Evaluating alternative signaling explanations for cross-cultural variance in ritual costs. *Evolution and Human Behavior, 28*(4), 234–247. https://doi.org/10.1016/j.evolhumbehav.2007.02.007

Swann, W. B., Buhrmester, M. D., Gómez, A., Jetten, J., Bastian, B., Vázquez, A., Ariyanto, A., Besta, T., Christ, O., Cui, L., Finchilescu, G. G., González, R., Goto, N., Hornsey, M. J., Sharma, S., Susianto, H., & Zhang, A. (2014). What makes a group worth dying for? Identity fusion fosters feelings of familial ties, promoting self-sacrifice. *Journal of Personality and Social Psychology, 106*(6), 912–926. https://doi.org/10.1037/a0036089

Swann, W. B., Gómez, A., Huici, C., Morales, J. F., & Hixon, J. G. (2010). Identity fusion and self-sacrifice: Arousal as a catalyst of pro-group fighting, dying, and helping behavior. *Journal of Personality and Social Psychology, 99*(5), 824–841. https://doi.org/10.1037/a0020014

Swann, W. B., Jetten, J., Gómez, A., Whitehouse, H., & Bastian, B., (2012). When group membership gets personal: A theory of identity fusion. *Psychological Review, 119*(3), 441–456. https://doi.org/10.1037/a0028589

Tajfel, H., & Turner, J. C. (1985). The social identity theory of intergroup behavior. In S. Worchel & W. G. Austin (Eds.), *Psychology of intergroup relations* (2nd ed., Vol. 2, pp. 7–24). Chicago: Nelson-Hall.

Thomson, R., Yuki, M., Talhelm, T., Schug, J., Kito, M., Ayanian, A. H., Becker, J. C., Becker, M., Chiu, C., Choi, H.-S., Ferreira, C. M., Fülöp, M., Gul, P., Houghton-Illera, A. M., Joasoo, M., Jong, J., Kavanagh, C. M., Khutkyy, D., Manzi, C., . . . Visserman, M. L. (2018). Relational mobility predicts social behaviors in 39 countries and is tied to historical farming and threat. *Proceedings of the National Academy of Sciences.* https://doi.org/10.1073/pnas.1713191115

Thorne, A., & McLean, K. C. (2003). Telling traumatic events in adolescence: A study of master narrative positioning. In R. Fivush & C. A. Haden (Eds.), *Connecting culture and memory: The development of an autobiographical self* (pp. 169–186). New Jersey, USA: Erlbaum.

Tulving, E. 1972. "Episodic and Semantic Memory." In E. Tulving and W. Donaldson(Eds.), *Organization of Memory* (pp. 590–600). New York: Academic Press.

Turchin, P., Brennan, R., Currie, T. E., Feeney, K. C., Francois, P., Hoyer, D., Manning, J. G., Marciniak, A., Mullins, D. A., & Palmisano, A. (2015). Seshat: The global history databank. *Cliodynamics: The Journal of Quantitative History and Cultural Evolution, 6*(1). https://doi.org/10.21237/C7clio6127917

Turchin, P., Currie, T. E., Whitehouse, H. François, P. Feeney, K. Mullins, D., Hoyer, D., Collins, C., Grohmann, S., & Savage, P. (2018). Quantitative historical analysis uncovers a single dimension of complexity that structures global variation in human social organization. *Proceedings of the National Academy of Sciences, 115*(2), E144–E151.

Turchin, P., Whitehouse, H., Larson, J., Cioni, E., Reddish, J., Hoyer, D., Savage, P. E., Covey, R. A., Baines, J., Altaweel, M., Anderson, E., Bol, P. K., Brandl, E., Carballo, D., Feinman, G., Korotayev, A., Kradin, N., Levine, J, Nugent, S., & François P. (2019, November 20). Explaining the rise of moralizing religions: A test of competing hypotheses using the Seshat databank. https://doi.org/10.31235/osf.io/2v59j

Turner, J. C., & Oakes, P. J. (1986). The significance of the social identity concept for social psychology with reference to individualism, interactionism and social influence. *British Journal of Social Psychology, 25*(3), 237–252.

Turpin, H., Andersen, M., & Lanman, J. A. (2018). CREDs, CRUDs, and Catholic scandals: Experimentally examining the effects of religious paragon behavior on co-religionist belief. *Religion, Brain & Behavior, 9*(2), 1–13.

Vial, T. (2004). Modes of religiosity and changes in popular religious practices at the time of the Reformation. In H. Whitehouse & L. H. Martin (Eds.), *Theorizing religions past: Archaeology, history, and cognition* (pp. 143–156). Walnut Creek, CA: AltaMira Press.

Watson-Jones, R. E., Legare, C. H., Whitehouse, H., & Clegg, J. M. (2014). Task-specific effects of ostracism on imitative fidelity in early childhood. *Evolution and Human Behavior, 35*(3), 204–210. https://doi.org/10.1016/j.evolhumbehav.2014.01.004

Watson-Jones, R. E., Whitehouse, H., & Legare, C. H. (2016). In-group ostracism increases high-fidelity imitation in early childhood. *Psychological Science, 27*(1), 34–42. https://doi.org/10.1177/0956797615607205

Watts, J. A., Greenhill, S. J., Atkinson, Q. D., Currie, T. E., Bulbulia, J. A., & Gray, R. D. (2015). Broad supernatural punishment but not moralizing high gods precede the evolution of political complexity in Austronesia. *Proceedings of the Royal Society B: Biological Sciences, 282*(1804). https://doi.org/10.1098/rspb.2014.2556

Wen, N. J., Herrmann, P. A., & Legare, C. H. (2016). Ritual increases children's affiliation with in-group members. *Evolution and Human Behavior, 37*(1), 54–60. https://doi.org/10.1016/j.evolhumbehav.2015.08.002

Whitehouse, H. (1992). Memorable religions: Transmission, codification, and change in divergent Melanesian contexts. *Man*, [n.s.] *27*, 777–797.

Whitehouse, H. (1995). *Inside the cult: Religious innovation and transmission in Papua New Guinea*. Oxford, UK: Oxford University Press.

Whitehouse, H. (1996). Rites of terror: Emotion, metaphor and memory in Melanesian initiation cults. *Journal of the Royal Anthropological Institute*, [n.s.] *2*(4), 703–715. https://doi.org/10.2307/3034304

Whitehouse, H. (2000). *Arguments and icons: Divergent modes of religiosity*. Oxford, UK: Oxford University Press.

Whitehouse, H. (2004). *Modes of religiosity: A cognitive theory of religious transmission*. Walnut Creek, CA: AltaMira Press.

Whitehouse, H. (2011). The Coexistence Problem in Psychology, Anthropology, and Evolutionary Theory. *Human Development, 54*: 191–9.

Whitehouse, H. (2018). Dying for the group: Towards a general theory of extreme self-sacrifice. *Behavioral and Brain Sciences, 41*(e192), 1–64. https://doi.org/10.1017/S0140525X18000249

Whitehouse, H., François, P., Savage, P. E., Hoyer, D., Feeney, K. C., Cioni, E., Turchin, P. (2021, April 3). Big Gods did not drive the rise of big societies throughout world history. https://doi.org/10.31219/osf.io/mbnvg

Whitehouse, H., François, P., & Turchin, P. (2015). The role of ritual in the evolution of social complexity: Five predictions and a drum roll. *Cliodynamics: The Journal of Quantitative History and Cultural Evolution, 6*(2). https://doi.org/10.21237/C7CLIO6229624

Whitehouse, H., & Hodder, I. (2010). Modes of religiosity at Çatalhöyük. In I. Hodder (Ed.), *Religion in the emergence of civilization: Çatalhöyük as a case study* (pp. 122–145). Cambridge, UK: Cambridge University Press.

Whitehouse, H., Jong, J., Buhrmester, M. D., Gómez, A., Bastian, B., Kavanagh, C. M., Newson, M., Matthews, M., Lanman, J. A., McKay, R., & Gavrilets, S. (2017). The evolution of extreme cooperation via shared dysphoric experiences. *Scientific Reports, 7*, Article 44292.

Whitehouse, H., & Lanman, J. A. (2014). The ties that bind us: Ritual, fusion and identification. *Current Anthropology, 55*(6), 674–695. https://doi.org/10.1086/678698

Whitehouse, H. & McQuinn, B. (2012). Ritual and violence: Divergent modes of religiosity and armed struggle. In M. Juergensmeyer, M. Kitts, & M. Jerryson (Eds.), *Oxford Handbook of Religion and Violence*, pp. 597–619. Oxford, UK: Oxford University Press.

Whitehouse, H., Mazzucato, C., Hodder, I., & Atkinson, Q. D. (2014). Modes of religiosity and the evolution of social complexity at Çatalhöyük. In I. Hodder (Ed.), *Religion at work in a Neolithic society* (pp. 134–158). New York: Cambridge University Press.

Whitehouse, H., McQuinn, B., Buhrmester, M. D., & Swann, W. B. (2014). Brothers in arms: Libyan revolutionaries bond like family. *Proceedings of the National Academy of Sciences of the United States of America, 111*(50), 17783–17785. https://doi.org/10.1073/pnas.1416284111

Wilson, A. E., & Ross, M. (2003). The identity function of autobiographical memory: Time is on our side. *Memory, 11*(2), 137–149. https://doi.org/10.1080/741938210

Wiltermuth, S. S., & Heath, C. (2009). Synchrony and cooperation. *Psychological Science, 20*(1), 1–5. https://doi.org/10.1111/j.1467-9280.2008.02253.x

WIN-Gallup International. (2012). Global index of religiosity and atheism. https://sidmennt. is/wp-content/uploads/Gallup-International-um-tr%C3%BA-og-tr%C3%BAleysi-2012.pdf

Worsley, P. (1957). *The Trumpet Shall Sound: A Study of Cargo Cults in Melanesia.* London: MacGibbon & Kee.

Yuki, M., & Schug, J. (2012). Relational mobility: A socioecological approach to personal relationships. In O. Gillath, G. Adams, & A. Kunkel (Eds.), *Decade of behavior 2000–2010. Relationship science: Integrating evolutionary, neuroscience, and sociocultural approaches* (pp. 137–151). Washington, DC, USA: American Psychological Association.

Yuki, M., Schug, J., Horikawa, H., Takemura, K., Sato, K., Yokota, K., & Kamaya, K. (2007). Development of a *scale to measure perceptions of relational mobility in society.* Working Paper Series no. 75, 12 December, Hokkaido University, Japan

CHAPTER 16

THE FAILURE OF RELIGIOUS SYSTEMS

HUGH TURPIN AND JONATHAN A. LANMAN

INTRODUCTION

FRACTIONATION, whereby socially constructed folk categories, including "religion," "belief," and "ritual," are broken down into more precise, scientifically tractable objects of analysis (such as "nonphysical agent beliefs" and "causally opaque social conventions") was key to the early success of the cognitive science of religion ([CSR]; Boyer, 2010; Whitehouse & Lanman, 2014). Nevertheless, some argue these distinct objects of analysis are connected in causally significant ways to each other, to social identities, and to material culture, thereby forming "religious systems" that can increase the cooperative success of social groups (Sosis, 2016; Wilson, 2002). They further argue that these systems deserve a place in our scientific ontology (Sosis, 2009).

Whether or not one agrees with this systemic perspective, the substantial increase in the numbers of atheists, religious "nones," and socially active antitheists presents a general challenge to the cognitive and evolutionary science of religion. This is because most cognitive scientists of religion accept some form of the naturalness of religion hypothesis (Barrett & Lanman, 2008; McCauley, 2011), which holds that religious beliefs and practices are cross-culturally recurrent because the operations of numerous pan-human, naturally developing cognitive mechanisms make them very likely to be produced and accepted. If such naturally developing cognitive systems are the most potent proximate causes of religious beliefs and practices, then how can we explain the decline of religious belief and affiliation in numerous countries, and the rise of antireligious sentiment and social action? Or, from the systemic perspective, how can we explain what clearly appears to be the failure of numerous religious systems?

This chapter aims to offer an account of how recent work across the social and cognitive sciences can address this question. First, we will discuss whether or not it makes scientific sense to talk about "religious systems" before outlining how the success or failure of such systems can be evaluated. After this, we examine the contributions of CSR to explaining the differential success of religious systems over time, such that some come to fail while others succeed. We then outline the relevance of CSR for explaining how and where religious systems lose influence altogether and various forms of nonreligion emerge, a process that has traditionally been called "secularization." The chapter closes with a case study outlining the applicability of the cognitive and evolutionary study of religion to the decline of Catholic belief, practice, and identification, as well as the rise in anti-Catholic social action, in the Republic of Ireland.

On the Nature and Failure of "Religious Systems"

Within the social sciences, the utility of the term "religion" has been endlessly debated and frequently dismissed as a western folk-concept with no universal purchase (Asad, 2003; Josephson, 2012). Such critiques have been accompanied by anthropological skepticism toward notions of hard group boundaries and cultural essences, and the labeling of any ideas of discrete social systems as reified snapshots of what, in reality, is a constantly shifting flux (e.g., Leach, 1954). If neither "religion" nor "sociocultural systems" are valid scientific concepts, how are we to proceed with developing a scientific account of the failure of religious systems? This would be the equivalent of "scientifically" explaining the failure of a constellation to exert astrological effects on human life.

Perhaps surprisingly, much work in CSR endorses the basic idea that "religion" is a socially constructed and historically contingent category rather than a natural kind, but in a way that may allow us to salvage some scientifically legitimate objects of analysis. CSR has frequently operated by "fractionating" the socially constructed umbrella "religion" into a number of more scientifically tractable phenomena and "building blocks" (e.g., Boyer, 2002, 2010; Taves, 2009; Whitehouse & Lanman, 2014). Although "religion" may not be a natural kind, beliefs in nonphysical agency (Barrett, 2004), natural teleology (Keleman et al., 2012), and magical causation (Rozin et al., 1986; Sørensen, 2000), as well as synchronous movement (Wiltermuth & Heath, 2009), dysphoric arousal (Xygalatas, 2012; Whitehouse, 2004), and sacred values (Atran, 2010), among others, may be. Clarifying these components allows us to subsequently examine not only their independent effects on human thought and action, but also their effects on each other and, potentially, how they combine to form "religious systems." Indeed, some see this as imperative: "Isolating particular features of religion for analysis without understanding their influence on the full religious system can be misleading and generate trivial results" (Purzycki et al., 2014, p. 75).

While there are still relevant scientific challenges to the idea of a "religious system" (e.g., given individual conceptual differences, how can one say that a belief or value is shared across a population?), we see the existence of what Boyd, Richerson, and other dual inheritance theorists have called "ethnic psychology" as offering a plausible cognitive foundation (Henrich & McElreath, 2007). Humans stand to benefit enormously both from the knowledge of those around them and by cooperating selectively with those who agree on basic social norms such as what is right, wrong, and fair. According to dual-inheritance theorists, this situation gave rise to stable intergroup differences in social norms, as well as evolved psychological mechanisms that lead individuals to preferentially learn from and interact with members of what they perceive to be *their* social group (McElreath et al., 2003; Henrich, 2015).

The implication of the existence of an evolved ethnic psychology is that humans have mental representations of their social group's identity and norms, including epistemic norms, credences (Van Leeuwen, 2014), and behaviors. Although these various concepts and norms are distinct, they are linked at a psychological level, as "symbolic identity markers." This linking leads to a number of downstream cognitive and behavioral outcomes, such as committing more to these individual markers in the face of both individual and normative threats (Navarette et al., 2004; Stenner, 2005).

If the dual-inheritance account of ethnic psychology is correct, then we might speak of religious systems in two senses. First, there are linked mental representations of social identities, including the elements CSR scholars have identified as fractionated components of religion. Second, there are the physical human beings who cooperate based on these mental representations to run economies, institutions and, more generally, social life itself. These two senses of the term "religious system" would be mutually reinforcing, because mental representations can produce behaviors that make human groups function more cohesively (e.g., refraining from cheating because of a fear of supernatural punishment) and vertically transmit the credences and norms of the group (e.g., costly rituals that can overcome the epistemic vigilance of cultural learners).

How, then, should we conceptualize the success and failure of religious systems? The answer is not straightforward because there are diverse metrics of success. We may choose, for instance, to view religious systems through a hedonistic or eudemonic lens, judging success and failure solely on the amount of subjective well-being enjoyed by bearers/members, regardless of their numbers. Further, we could follow the definitions of the religious systems themselves. For a Heaven's Gate member[1], for instance, success was the swift attainment of extraterrestrial evolution by a highly select few, a mission accomplished via mass suicide in 1997; for them, we who remain behind are the failures.

Placing emic and human flourishing sensitivities to one side, other dilemmas still present themselves. If the religious system contains several fractionated components

---

[1] Heaven's Gate, founded in 1974, was an American new religious movement syncretizing Christian millenarianism with Ufology. When one of the founders, Bonnie Nettles, died of cancer in 1985, the group developed a view of the body as a 'container' that must be abandoned to attain post-human apotheosis. In March 1997, the remaining 39 members of the group committed mass suicide at a house in San Diego. Their act was timed to coincide with the passage of the Hale-Bopp Comet.

of religion, some might fail while others succeed. For example, the failure to preserve and transmit particular representations or norms may not coincide with a decline in the number of those claiming allegiance to the religious group. The sociologist Christian Smith, for instance, believes that many Christian sects in the United States are failing from within because youthful adherents, though plentiful, are jettisoning the distinct representational content symbolic of their religious in-groups in favor of what he calls "moral therapeutic deism," a parasitic, interdenominationally homogeneous set of relativistic concepts revolving around a vague deity advocating self-help and tolerance (Smith, 2005). Others note that when copious adherents of a religious system begin to deviate from its norms, the result tends to be either reform, which preserves the coalition by readjusting standards, or schism, whereby purists form new coalitions (Wollschleger & Beach, 2011). Whether such transformations constitute adaptive successes or forms of failure via capitulation or fragmentation is difficult to answer. These concerns raise a Ship of Theseus–style question: What degree of change can a religious system undergo and still be described as a functioning religious system, or at least the same religious system that it was? When is something no longer a religious system at all?

Other contemporary sociologists have hypothesized new forms of "religiosity" that challenge the description of a religious system as a relatively stable nexus of interlocked beliefs, rituals, moral norms, and in-group identity. They have advanced concepts of "believing without belonging," whereby institutional and ritual participation declines but representations remain important in private form (Davie, 1994), or concepts of "belonging without believing," where a sense of tradition leads unbelievers to maintain participation in some forms of communal religious behavior (Mountford, 2011), or of "natal nominalism," where in-group identification is retained in the absence of doctrinal belief, moral agreement, participation, or even basic interest (Day, 2011). Should we consider all of these cases failures?

Our own position, following both Sperber's (1996) epidemiological approach to culture and evolution and the ethnic psychology account offered above, is to define the success of religious systems both according to their survivability in individual minds, and the survivability and expansion of the cooperative social groups employing religious components in their social identities. Consequently, a religious system that is forgotten or explicitly rejected would fail at the level of mental representations, and would fail at the level of cooperative social groups if those groups were to disintegrate (e.g., being physically wiped out through starvation or war, or breaking down through the cessation of cooperative interactions and shared identity among members). This distinction between cognitive and social failure helps account for some of the issues discussed above. Smith's moral therapeutic deism, for instance, would represent the failure of a particular type of religious system at an individual cognitive level but not necessarily at a social one, since the individuals concerned still cooperate with one another based on their linked representations of Christianity.

Cognitive Science and the Success or Failure of Religious Systems

Currently, CSR can be seen to offer two broad accounts that contribute to explanations of differential religious success, both based on the underlying concept of competitive selection. One strand concerns the varying competitiveness of supernatural representational content itself: some representational content is more epidemiologically catchy—more "viral" as it were—lending it greater power to supplant rivals (Sperber, 1996; Boyer, 2002). This corresponds to our *cognitive* understanding of success and failure. The other strand operates at a social level and suggests that "content catchiness" may be irrelevant in determining the success or failure of a given religious group in terms of survival and intergroup competition. These approaches adopt more sociofunctionalist arguments such that certain religious representations may endow certain social groups with the ability to outcompete others (e.g., Norenzayan, 2013; Wilson, 2002), or that differing social structures benefit from differing forms of ritual behavior (e.g., Whitehouse, 2004). This corresponds to our *social* understanding of success and failure.

The epidemiological, or byproduct, approach, emphasizes how certain conceptual content spreads through populations by appealing to cognitive mechanisms that evolved for other purposes (Boyer, 2002; Sperber, 1996). Candidates include an evolutionarily beneficial oversensitivity to cues of agency (Guthrie, 1993; Barrett, 2004); a cognitive default toward purpose-based explanations of natural phenomena (Kelemen et al., 2013); an innate dualism leading us to intuitively regard human beings as nonphysical minds harnessed to physical bodies (Bloom, 2004, 2007; Bering, 2006); and the possible mnemonic advantages of representations that minimally violate the boundaries of dedicated cognitive systems processing particular domains such as minds, artifacts, and natural kinds (Boyer & Ramble, 2001; Barrett & Nyhoff, 2001 Banerjee et al., 2013; Banerjee & Bloom, 2013), though the evidential basis and conceptual clarity of "minimal counterintuitiveness" and its relevance to religious transmission in actual social environments is currently a matter of some debate (Gervais & Henrich, 2010; Purzycki & Willard, 2016; but see also Barrett, 2016). The foregoing list is by no means exhaustive, and further examples can be easily hypothesized.

Over time then, concepts that are more in line with content biases are more successful in terms of memory and transmission. In the arena of epidemiological struggle, this yields advantages for religious representations that are cognitively optimal (i.e., catchy and easy to think with) rather than cognitively costly (i.e., ungraspable and laborious to process). It has been found, for instance, that people inadvertently default to reasoning in a "theologically incorrect" manner about incomprehensible deities (Barrett & Keil, 1996; Barrett, 1999; Slone, 2004). This can, in part, explain the notable failure of theologians' more abstruse formulations to gain popular purchase (e.g., why Paul Tillich's notion of a nonagentic God fails to become popular in Christianity, while the poem "Footprints,"[2] depicting a deity that can carry an individual and leave footprints on the beach, circulates widely). It may also have implications when maximally counterintuitive traditions encounter more cognitively optimized rivals; the theologian and religious historian Hans Kung, for instance, has argued that Islam overcame Christianity in North Africa in part due to the incomprehensibility of the doctrine of the Trinity as juxtaposed with the clarity of Allah (Kung, 1996).

These factors concern the success and failure of religious systems as linked mental representations of social identities involving fractionated religious components. Although each individual would retain linked mental representations of their social identities, the versions of those networks featuring more maximally counterintuitive components and other concepts that fail to appeal to content biases are replaced by those that do. One religious system fails and another is born within the same population. Such cognitive-epidemiological considerations, however, have little to do with the success or failure of physical human groups ordered around these networked concepts and faced with the challenges of intergroup competition. Other, more sociofunctionalist approaches in the cognitive and evolutionary study of religion examine this latter notion of success.

According to Whitehouse's theory of divergent modes of religiosity (DMR) (Whitehouse, 2004; Whitehouse & Kavanagh, this volume) ritual traditions cluster on two ends of a spectrum that runs from "doctrinal" to "imagistic" modes. The imagistic mode is characterized by intense, irregular, and frequently dysphoric rituals. Experiences of such rituals are encoded episodically as "flashbulb memories" and encourage an intense form of bonding (dubbed "identity fusion") with one's co-sufferers (Whitehouse & Lanman, 2014). Such traditions, for Whitehouse and his collaborators, are culturally evolved adaptations that allow small groups to flourish in situations presenting a high risk of defection, such as warfare and big-game hunting (Whitehouse et al., 2017). Imagistic systems explicitly eschew formulated doctrine, and individuals who have undergone the "rites of terror" together will often produce their own deeply personal and highly idiosyncratic exegeses on the meaning of what they have experienced (Whitehouse, 1995). Doctrinal traditions, by contrast, serve to overcome critical resistance and encode shared dogma in semantic memory via regularized repetition (weekly mass is, perhaps, the preeminent example). The doctrinal mode is thought to act as a gelling agent in large, geographically dispersed entities (such as ethnic-religious collectives) by generating a sense of shared identity with anonymous others. This sense of shared identity is facilitated by the widespread use of symbols and behaviors indicating

---

[2] "Footprints", also known as "Footprints in the Sand," is an allegorical poem that has transmitted widely across various Christian denominations and sects. The central motif is that of a believer walking on a beach, a stroll representing his journey through life. Behind him, he sees two sets of footprints (his own and the Lord's). Looking further back along the trail though, the believer notices that at the lowest moments of his life, there appear to have been only one set of footprints. He assumes from this that God tended to abandon him when he was at his lowest ebb. The poem culminates by revealing that these were in fact the times when God 'carried' the believer.

the acceptance of collective norms (Whitehouse, 2004; Whitehouse & Lanman, 2014). Evidence garnered thus far includes cross-cultural data sets demonstrating the existence of imagistic and doctrinal attractor positions in ritual systems (Atkinson & Whitehouse, 2011) and empirical studies demonstrating the power of shared dysphoric experiences to produce identity fusion (Whitehouse et al., 2017). DMR has implications for the question of why some cooperative religious-social systems may fail in the face of alternatives: over time, through conquest or imitation, ritual systems will tend to cleave closer to whichever of the two poles best produces the type of social cohesion most beneficial in the environment in question. Groups that do not change the content of their social identities to better match the more appropriate mode will be more likely to fail economically or militarily, a prediction supported by Brian McQuinn's analysis of the formation and success of civil-war armed groups (Whitehouse & McQuinn, 2013).

According to the "Big Gods" theory, effective social cooperation drives intergroup competitive fitness. While religious-representational candidates may well have originated via competitive catchiness, they were then subject to a process of cultural evolution whereby content enhancing the competitive potency of the groups in which it was instantiated prevailed (Norenzayan, 2013). Key here is that perceived supernatural monitoring encourages increased norm compliance, expanding cooperation beyond one's immediate circle of familiarity and allowing societies to grow beyond the numerical limits of face-to-face social networks solidified by direct reputational knowledge (e.g., Dunbar, 1996). The further innovation of Big Gods, that is, punitive, morally-interested deities whose interests extend beyond the tribal to the universal, further increases the power and size of groups by birthing large-scale civilizations composed of vast numbers of anonymous but norm-sharing and cooperative individuals. These societies were then capable of dominating rivals, and older religious systems built around parochial or morally-ambivalent supernatural agents found themselves outcompeted. Evidence garnered thus far includes large-scale historical analyses suggesting that group size correlates with the presence of moralizing supernatural-watcher beliefs (Roes & Raymond, 2003; Watts et al., 2015), and experiments suggesting that reminders of supernatural monitoring increase cooperation in economic games (Shariff & Norenzayan, 2007; Purzycki et al., 2016; Purzycki, Henrich, et al., 2018; Shariff et al., 2015).

Despite such evidence, Big Gods theory has been challenged on historical grounds, with some arguing that many large empires operated without morally interested deities (Baumard & Boyer, 2013). One current alternative is "life history" theory (Baumard & Chevallier, 2015): In late Antiquity, an increasingly safe and predictable environment in a number of key regions promoted a strategic shift to "slow" religious systems foregrounding the ethical over the immediately pragmatic, enabling the pursuit of larger but more long-term goals, especially by social elites. Over time, these soteriological and moralistic systems replaced older, transactional religious systems that were based on a "fast" strategy of trade with supernatural entities for immediate material benefits. As "the industrial revolution allowed more and more people to escape the vicissitudes of a Malthusian economy, slow strategies were adopted everywhere and world religions became truly popular" (Baumard & Chevallier, 2015, p. 5). Today, that popularity appears to be waning in certain environments.

COGNITIVE SCIENCE AND SECULARIZATION

We have just considered some reasons that certain religious systems win out over others. At the level of individual mental representations, cognitive biases can help explain why some beliefs (e.g. agentic deities versus nonagentic deities) are more likely to be retained and transmitted. At the level of cooperative social groups, particular types of ritual traditions (e.g., imagistic vs. doctrinal) and beliefs (e.g., moralistic vs. nonmoralistic deities) increase the potential to survive and expand. This brings us to the question of how religious systems may fail entirely, both in the sense of individuals' mental representations of their social groups that do not give credence to many of the fractionated components of religion and in the sense of social groups that are guided by religious components failing to maintain their numbers and social influence. Such failures appear to be occurring in many Western European societies (Bruce, 2002; Ribberink et al., 2013; Voas, 2009) but also more recently in the United States (Hout & Fischer, 2014), long considered a pious Western outlier (Stark & Iannaccone, 1994). In social scientific literature, this process is referred as *secularization*. Here, we discuss secularization primarily in terms of this Western European and now North American phenomenon of declining Christian theism and practice, alongside the waning social influence of the Christian churches. This transformation does not entail the extinction of all beliefs and behaviors that a cognitive scientist of religion might deem "religious" or "supernatural," but it does describe the breakdown of Christian religious systems in both of the senses just outlined. The exact nature and implications of these transformations are subject to much debate among social scientists. We will outline the secularization debate as a precursor to examining the potential for CSR to contribute to its resolution.

Sociologists once axiomatically assumed that religion was in inevitable decline everywhere (Comte, 2009; Durkheim, 1993); however, disagreement over this proliferated in the late twentieth century due to such factors as the robust religiosity of the United States, the rise of Islamic fundamentalism, and the emergence of the New Age movement. Far from an inevitability, secularization came to be portrayed as a Western cultural myth arising from a historically idiosyncratic quarantining of religion, by no means destined to be repeated elsewhere (Asad, 2003; Cannell, 2010). Even Western European secularization, seemingly so unquestionable, came to be doubted. This doubt hinged on Europe's combination of declining institutional attachment and practice with comparably low levels of outright, self-reported unbelief. For some anti-secularizationists, this was seen to herald a new and potentially stable form of privatized religiosity ("believing without belonging"; Davie, 1994, 2002). This privatized stance entails that secularization at the level of *belief* has failed to occur. Overall, religious change might be better described as institutional detachment (Davie, 1994; Inglis, 1998).

This trend is opposed by neo-secularizationists of various schools (e.g., Bruce, 2006; Brown, 2001, 2012), for whom innate religiosity is an optimistic illusion to which sociologists who are religiously inclined cling (Brown, 2012). Far from involving strong but autonomous belief arising from innate religious instincts, privatized theism and lingering affiliation may be little more than superficial socially desirable meta-representational habits encouraged by the structures of survey questionnaires (Demerath, 2000; Voas, 2009). For these scholars, what is of interest is the underanalyzed swathe who may or may not self-report as theistic and affiliated but do little to evince this orientation (Voas, 2009). Evidence from longitudinal datasets suggests that this pattern of attenuated religiosity shows signs of declining in most Western European societies (Bruce, 2002; Voas, 2009; Brown, 2012), and that residual religious identification tends to wane once committed secularists numerically outweigh the committedly religious (Voas, 2009; Ribberink et al., 2013). In tandem with these neosecularizationist developments, more nuanced historical work has sought to salvage secularization theory by disaggregating it into a number of interlocking components (Casanova, 1994; Taylor, 2007). Taylor (2007, 2011) for instance, describes "Secularization 1," the expulsion of religion from the public sphere; "Secularization 2," the decline of religious belief and practice; and "Secularization 3," the replacement of transcendent religious values with a long-gestating "secular humanist" moral ethic based on the maximization of earthly human flourishing.

The most robust empirical data currently available suggests the West is indeed becoming more secular across all three of Taylor's forms, but that, due to demographic patterns, the world as a whole is becoming more religious. Norris and Inglehart (2011) identify levels of existential security—freedom from or exposure to such factors as disease, high mortality, hunger, poverty, inequality, lack of social security, and natural disasters—as the critical determining factor. For example, the Scandinavian countries are exceptionally secular, while African and Middle Eastern nations are highly religious (Zuckermann, 2008). The main fault line between the secularizing West and the religious "rest" seems to be one of morality. The more-religious nations are cleaving to values that are religiously inflected and prioritize the group over the individual, because commitment is required for obtaining such goods as "communal mutual support, charitable services for those in need, and supernatural beliefs that help to 'explain' pain and suffering" (Zuckerman et al., 2017, p. 63). By contrast, data on US "nones" suggest that disaffiliation is primarily motivated by the rejection of baptismal denominations because their moral stances are seen to inhibit the freedom of the individual (Hout & Fischer, 2014).

CSR can advance the discussion on secularization by describing the proximate cognitive mechanisms behind the declining hold of orthodox religious beliefs and connected moral norms in existentially secure environments, thus paving the way for the emergence and proliferation of more individualized alternatives (Inglehart & Welzdel, 2005). Both Big Gods and life-history theories have addressed this question. For Norenzayan (2013), in contemporary secularized societies the monitoring function of a Big God has been usurped by highly effective state institutions. Societies such as Sweden and

Denmark have "climbed the ladder of religion, and then kicked it away" (Norenzayan, p. 172). Baumard and Chevallier (2015) suggest that secularization is related to slow strategies winning out so completely that the need to invoke divinely mandated disapproval of fast, materialistic strategies has become irrelevant (Baumard & Chevallier, 2015). Nevertheless, both accounts require further elaboration of the proximate factors behind such declines: how exactly do certain contemporary environments lead religious representations to become less tractable, and why for some people rather than others?

With respect to the second part of this question, a number of individual-level psychological factors likely contribute to the acceptance or rejection of religious belief, though the exact nature and extent of their influence is a matter of some debate. Ethnographic evidence suggests that lonely or isolated individuals may indeed gravitate toward religious groups, but that believing is a difficult, effort-intensive process, no matter how catchy the concept. In some contexts, such as Vineyard evangelical Christianity, belief cultivation requires elaborate practices analogous to "pretend-play" and is aided by certain cognitive traits, such as absorption-proneness (Luhrmann, 2012, 2018). More generally, autism has frequently been linked to a lack of interest in supernatural agents (e.g., Norenzayan et al., 2012), though this linkage has increasingly been challenged (e.g., Jack et al., 2016; Lindeman et al., 2015), and qualitative work further suggests that at least some fantasy-prone subsets of the autistic *prefer* to interact with imaginary beings (Visuri, 2018). Although analytic thinking styles may help to override religious intuitions (Gervais, 2012), meta-analyses show small effect sizes (Pennycook et al., 2016), some (but not all) influential studies have failed to replicate (Norenzayan & Gervais, 2012; Gervais et al., 2017; Sanchez et al., 2017), and new evidence suggests that the relationship pertains only to a handful of WEIRD (Western, educated, industrialized, rich, and democratic) societies and does not appear in other cultural contexts (Gervais et al., 2017). As this suggests, trait-focused accounts have limited applicability to the most salient feature of nontheism: its high level of intercultural variation. At both the individual and intercultural levels, upbringing remains the most reliable predictor of religiosity (e.g., Bengston, 2014); trait variables and vulnerability to content-features may, however, have greater influence on the acceptance of socially unendorsed content (e.g., paranormal beliefs; Willard & Cingl, 2017). Therefore the biggest question is what CSR can tell us about how intergenerational religious transmission declines within certain social contexts.

The answer may lie in how representations linked to religious social identities cease to benefit from cognitive adaptations that encourage the preferential adoption of information if it is linked to certain social cues (e.g., prestige or conformity; McElreath et al., 2003; Henrich, 2015). One particularly important sociocognitive factor that influences relative rates of theism and nontheism may be the environmental preponderance of theistic "credibility enhancing displays" ([CREDs]; Henrich, 2009). CRED theory assumes that the emergence of language made it far easier to manipulate others by deceiving them about one's actual beliefs (Henrich, 2009; Von Hippel & Trivers, 2011). Because of this, cultural learners have evolved the precautionary tendency to scrutinize cultural models for behavioral confirmation of a commitment to stated beliefs. Accordingly, belief transmission, particularly in the case of empirically unverifiable truth-propositions (such as religious beliefs) is strengthened when models "practice what they preach." Thus professed religious beliefs will appear more compelling and transmit more successfully when they are accompanied by actions that would be costly to undertake if the models did not believe what they said they did, actions such as painful or time-consuming rituals, charity, celibacy, martyrdom (Henrich, 2009; Sosis et al., 2007; Lanman & Burhmeister, 2017). Initial studies have been promising, establishing a strong correlational link between CRED exposure and religious belief, both between individuals (Lanman, 2012; Lanman & Buhrmeister, 2017; Turpin et al., 2018) and societies (Willard & Cingl, 2017).

Lanman (2012) has clarified the causal links between existential security and CRED performance. Much work has demonstrated that the contexts of threat, including mortality salience, feelings of uncertainty, a lack of control, and the normative threat of out-groups with contrasting worldviews, all serve to elevate ideological conformity and "worldview defense" (Stenner, 2005), likely as an index of coalitional commitment (Navarette et al., 2004). Such perceived threats, then, encourage individuals to behave in a way that telegraphs commitment to their in-groups, either inadvertently or deliberately. To the extent that religious beliefs are relevant components of a group's social identity, such dynamics would increase the level of religious CREDs being performed, increasing in turn the catchiness for cultural learners of mental representations linked to religious social identities. When environments become more existentially secure, threat declines, and with it, the need for costly action indexing commitment to in-group worldviews. For worldviews that include religious beliefs, this security would produce a decline in the effectiveness of intergenerational religious transmission. Potentially then, CRED theory can help to adjudicate the debate between sociological secularizationists and anti-secularizationists: If CREDs are indeed important to religious transmission, then the privatized belief posited by anti-secularizationists in secure Western European contexts may represent a stage on the way to widespread nontheism. However, we must still account for differences in the style of nonreligion in different social contexts. Why do some nontheistic people and social groups actively oppose religion, while others merely evince apathy to it?

The best evidence suggests that antitheism tends to proliferate where religious normativity is higher (Zuckermann, 2008; Lanman, 2012; Ribberink et al., 2013; Blankholm & Garcia, 2016), which can be accounted for in part by moral and coalitional psychology. Although a discussion of the strenuous disagreements over the fundamental cognitive substrates of human moral behavior cannot be entered into here (e.g., Baumard et al., 2013; Curry, 2016; Graham, 2015), most of the existing evolutionary literature argues that "moralities" are culturally evolved systems that secure social cooperation by building on underlying evolved intuitions that govern interpersonal behavior (Haidt & Kesebir, 2010). At least in Western contexts, religious and secular moral stances have been depicted as drawing on differing underlying moral intuitions. Current secular morality tends to be *individualizing*—that is, it prioritizes the rights of the individual within the group and emphasizes fairness and the prevention of harm; whereas the morality dominant religious traditions advocate tends to be *binding*—that is, it subordinates individual to in-group concerns by also drawing on intuitions around loyalty, subservience to authority, and the preservation of purity (Haidt & Graham, 2007). In social contexts where religious morality has significant social influence, it becomes a normative threat that drives up secular identity and worldview defense. As a result, explicit antitheism is far more common among nontheists in a religious environment such as the United States than in a largely secular one such as Denmark, where many nontheists are content to remain Lutherans on paper (Zuckerman, 2008; Lanman, 2012).

By way of further example, Ribberink et al. (2013) investigated "non-religion" (i.e., apathy) and "anti-religion" (i.e., overt antipathy) using 2008 European Value Survey data. Their results suggest that though the Republic of Ireland had the smallest unbelieving minority of the 14 Western European nations they analyzed, this minority harbored the strongest antireligious sentiment. Such antagonistic secular/religious situations are by no means static; they are examples of intense intercoalitional moral warfare as rivals committed to contrasting normative visions attempt to sway third-party bystanders with whatever moral affordances are at hand (e.g., Tooby & Cosmides, 2010; Mercier & Sperber 2017). Ribberink's data on the Irish Republic is now ten years out of date. Since then, the collapse of the Irish Catholic religious system has garnered international attention as a particularly prominent and rapid example of secularization. Therefore we now analyze the emergence and nature of Irish ex-Catholicism as a case study of the failure of a religious system, paying particular attention to the role mechanisms identified by cognitive and evolutionary scholars of religion played in this process.

COGNITIVE SCIENCE AND THE FAILURE OF CATHOLICISM IN THE REPUBLIC OF IRELAND

For much of the twentieth century, to be Irish was to be devoutly Catholic (Inglis, 1998; Fuller, 2002). In recent decades, this situation has unraveled. Irish self-reported weekly mass attendance declined from 85% in 1990 to 34% in 2012; priestly vocations are negligible; and legally encoded church dogma on divorce, same-sex marriage, and abortion has been publicly overturned. In 1979, more than one million people flocked to see Pope John Paul II in Dublin's Phoenix Park; in 2018, Pope Francis was greeted by a tenth this number. Protestors gathered in objection to the visit, bearing symbolic markers of their *rejection* of signature Catholic moral tenets, such as rainbow flags, pro-choice badges, and other accoutrements left over after recent referendum victories. By contrast, disappointed street vendors had to bin large quantities of unsold Vatican flags.

Some Irish sociologists have adopted variants of the anti-secularization thesis to explain the transformation (Ó Féich & O'Connell, 2015; Ganiel, 2016), and have concluded that deference to the Church has been replaced by privatized theism and a moral autonomy wedded to an ethnic Catholic identity, often glossed as "cultural Catholicism". This position has been increasingly challenged by the growth of outright religious rejection since the 2000s, so that the Republic now has the eighth-highest percentage of "convinced atheists" in the world (Win-Gallup International, 2012) and a "non-religious" population that increased from 14% in 2004 to 26.3% in 2016 (Bullivant, 2017), and the figures higher still among younger cohorts (Barna, 2017). The cognitive theories outlined in the previous section (see "Cognitive Science and Secularization")—including mental representations related to religious social identities, the role of CREDs in supporting such credences, and the role of moral intuitions and normative threat in the emergence of strong antireligious sentiment—can perhaps better explain this change.

First, we must clarify from a cognitive perspective what the Irish Catholic religious system was at its height, stretching roughly from the middle of the nineteenth century to the early 1960s (and in some accounts lingering on longer than this). During the nineteenth century, an expansion of religious infrastructure, personnel, and clerical discipline coincided with declines in existential security (notably, the Great Famine) and rising nationalism to create a new religious culture oriented around the consistent projection of an orthodox Catholic social identity (Inglis, 1998). From a DMR perspective, this was paradigmatically a doctrinal shift (Whitehouse, 2004) that gave birth to a rigorous, repetitive ritual system that reinforced a national ethnoreligious social identity (Connolly, 1985; Inglis, 1998; Miller, 1975). In the decades immediately following the Great Famine of 1845 to 1852, mass attendance rose from 40% to 95%. Confession became much more frequent, alongside "a whole series of devotional exercises" including "the rosary, forty hours, perpetual adoration, novenas, blessed altars, Via Crucis, benediction, vespers, devotion to the Sacred Heart and to the Immaculate Conception, jubilees, triduums, pilgrimages, shrines, processions, and retreats" (Larkin, 1976, p. 77). This public religious culture was reinforced domestically by the figure of the "Irish mother," "the living embodiment of Our Lady—humble, pious, celibate and yet fecund," who acted as "the Church's representative in the home" and "supervised the moral conduct of her husband and children" (Inglis, 1998, p. 249). This was a religious culture which was to persist deep into the twentieth century, if anything further reinforced by the policy of isolationist Catholic nationalism that characterized the State for decades after independence was won in 1922.

Daily interpersonal behavior, both public and domestic, was rich with symbolic identity markers indicating that that an individual was a good Catholic, and thus a true and trustworthy Irish person (Inglis, 1998). From a sociocognitive perspective, these signals constituted a canopy of religious CREDs. Signs of widespread adherence to orthodox religious credence frequently resulted, as evidenced, for instance, by queues of sinners outside confessionals, anxious to avoid damnation (Fuller, 2002; Whyte, 1980). Epidemiologically speaking, too, the representational content to which such sinners were committed was catchy, if harsh. God fully occupied the mind because he was exceptionally punitive and vigilant in the prosecution of norm violations (i.e., "sin";

Fuller, 2002). This was taking place amid some of the most impoverished conditions in Europe, favoring the kind of tight cleaving to and policing of God's binding moral norms, as is typical of existentially insecure societies today. Loyalty, authority, and purity foundations (Haidt & Kesebir, 2010) were recruited to form a moral culture defined by "duty, self-sacrifice and mortification, and fearfulness in relation to threats to sexual morality" (Fuller, 2002, p. 227), enhanced by hierarchical deference to a celibate elite preoccupied with "evil literature, indecent Hollywood movies, immodest dress, courting in public, excessive drinking, secularism, materialism," and the "the craze for pleasure" (Barr & Ó Corráin, 2017, p. 80).

This system began to decline in 1970s. Vatican II inadvertently reduced the catchiness of Catholic representational content, replacing the God who was a "stern taskmaster" with a "loving, understanding God," meaning that the "kind of dread that filled people's minds at the idea that they might have committed a mortal sin—and not be in a 'state of grace'—no longer had the same urgency" (Fuller, 2002, p.227). As anxious CREDs declined under the aegis of this vague new God of Love, social changes began to reduce CRED performance in other ways too. Notably, socioeconomic developments meant that women were afforded roles other than wife and mother, overturning the domestic pillar of CRED production (Inglis, 1998; Ganiel, 2016). Existential security began to increase, slowly at first, and then rapidly during the "Celtic Tiger" economic boom of the 1990s (McWilliams, 2005), leading to a shift toward a moral culture predicated on individualism (Fuller, 2002; Inglis, 1998). These factors, and others besides, precipitated a tacit compromise in which greater personal doxastic and moral autonomy, as well as reduced practice, were reconciled with the retention of ethnoreligious in-group bonds and Church influence on social institutions.

The trajectory described above marked the first stages in the failure of the Irish Catholic religious system: the failure of the established system of mental representations around what it meant to be an Irish Catholic at an individual cognitive level. An environment defined by growing existential security diminished incentives to project signature Catholic in-group markers. Doctrinal orthodoxy was displaced by idiosyncratic privatized representations and a decline in allegiance to strict Catholic moral norms. Behavioral corollaries ensued: attendance at mass declined steeply, public conduct deviating from religious standards became more acceptable, and the elaborate doctrinal-ritual scaffolding of jubilees, triduums, vespers, processions, and retreats atrophied, constituting a process of CRED depletion and undermining the sociocognitive dimensions of religious transmission. Consonant with this, correlational data indicates that Catholic CREDs have been declining intergenerationally, and that low CRED exposure is the best predictor of reduced Catholic belief and social identification among the baptized Catholic Irish population (Turpin, 2018).

To this must be added the exacerbating factor of Church moral scandals involving child abuse, cover-ups, and repressive institutions. These have accelerated CRED depletion through the activation by scandal of strong intuitions concerning unfairness, harm, and the violation of moral purity (e.g., Haidt & Kesebir, 2010; Hilliard, 2003; Orsi, 2017), inducing further withdrawal from public participation related to feelings of disgust, shame, and distrust. Increasingly, believers no longer wish to symbolically mark their affiliation to a contaminated institution (Egan, 2011). Perhaps more importantly, resistance to conformist practice was thoroughly legitimized. Church scandals empowered more distal cultural Catholics to reject the moral authority of the Church and set the costs of Catholic coalitional membership on an even lower bar, pushing CREDs down even further.

If things had stopped there, it could be possible to view the increasingly peripheral importance of official religious representational content and ritual participation alongside the retention of Catholic identity as a new, deinstitutionalized Catholic religious system that has grown out of the previous version. This is problematized by recent trends suggesting that this does not mark a new, harmonious homeostasis. The latest stage in the failure of the religious system operates at the second social level outlined earlier. It is marked by the disaggregation of previously tightly intertwined Irish and Catholic social identities, and the emergence of a rival coalitional ethic oriented around explicitly severing all ties with Catholicism. Newly emergent ex-Catholics tend toward strong atheism, and in particular, reject outright religious representations of a Catholic variety, often adopting this stance on moral grounds (Turpin, 2018). An associational free-list, a cognitive anthropological tool intended to elicit shared cultural models (Romney & D'Andrade, 1964), found that ex-Catholics' first association when presented with the term *Irish Catholic Church* is pedophilia, followed swiftly by authoritarianism, corruption, conservativism, and dishonesty (Turpin, 2018). Frequently, those who have adopted this stance also look askance at cultural Catholicism, viewing it as a form of inauthentic complicity with a harm-causing institution.

As noted, such strong antireligious stances tend to proliferate in circumstances where religion poses a normative threat to secular values. In the Irish case, the key factor is an increasingly existentially secure, CRED-depleted, liberalized populace for whom Catholic religious representations and norms have faded, coming into conflict with lingering Church-state entrenchment, particularly around the education system and (until recently) abortion laws. In this context, Church scandals re-enter the picture as a moral affordance in a scene of "offensive moral warfare" (Tooby & Cosmides, 2010) between secular and religious coalitional actors (Ruane, 1998), conditions defined by rival efforts to cause a "moral cascade" that will sway third-party bystanders by crafting and launching a "contagious representational bundle" using whatever moral affordances are at hand (Tooby & Cosmides, 2010, p. 225; Keane, 2015). In the Irish case, the secularist "representational bundle" is by far the catchiest, framed as it is within a compelling moral-historical narrative involving the obligation to break free from the Church, recast in a pitch-black light as a deceitful and abusive oppressor intent on retaining power and inhibiting secular liberal progress. As this moral narrative has flourished, explicit unbelief, while far from obligatory, has gone from something to be concealed to a marker of adherence to a new and growing normative stance.

CONCLUSION

While religion may not be a viable object of scientific enquiry, religious systems as linked representations of social identities involving fractionated "religious" content, and as networks of social cooperation based upon these representations, offer more tractable objects of scientific analysis. This chapter has attempted to show how CSR can help us to understand the failure of such systems at both mental-representational and social levels. Existing work on content transmission can explain why certain religious representations are likely to fail from the outset. Work on intergroup competition and cultural evolution explains why some cooperative religious groups are less likely to survive and spread than their rivals. Finally, CSR has enhanced our understanding of secularization by highlighting the importance of sociocognitive mechanisms to the transmission—and transmission failure—of religious representations. This account can help to provide a proximate, psychologically-plausible mechanism clarifying longstanding debates around secularization in the social sciences by describing how conditions of existential security drive down in-group focused signals of coalitional commitment, leading to an intergenerational decline in the transmission of associated religious representations due to a lack of supporting CREDs, allowing the emergence of new normative stances less oriented around binding moral foundations. When these normative stances find themselves frustrated by entrenched religious influence (such as in Ireland) or threatened by reactionary religious forces (such as in the United States), this sets the stage for anti-religious identities and social action to emerge.

QUESTIONS FOR FUTURE RESEARCH

1. Privatised, bespoke religious mental representations are said to be a growing norm in secularizing Western countries where the influence of religious institutions is in decline. What can CSR tell us about the potential intergenerational durability of privatized beliefs of this sort? Are these religious systems of one, and do they fail each time a person dies?

2. Demographics tell us that the nonreligious are growing numerically, but higher birth rates among the religious mean that they are shrinking as a proportion of the global population. Do these pronatalist demographic factors mean we will also see the failure of secular systems in time?

3. How can scholars from the cognitive science of religion apply their insights to the emergence and growth of new ideologies with religion-like features, such as transhumanism?

References

Asad, T. (2003). *Formations of the secular: Christianity, Islam, modernity*. Stanford, CA: Stanford University Press.

Atkinson, Q. D., & Whitehouse, H. (2011). The cultural morphospace of ritual form: Examining modes of religiosity cross-culturally. *Evolution and Human Behaviour, 32*, 50–62.

Atran, S. (2010). *Talking to the enemy: Violent extremism, sacred values, and what it means to be human*. London: Penguin.

Banerjee, K., & Bloom, P. (2013). Would Tarzan believe in God? Conditions for the emergence of religious belief. *Trends in Cognitive Sciences, 17*(1), 7–8.

Banerjee, K., Haque, O., & Spelke, E. (2013). Melting lizards and crying mailboxes: Children's preferential recall of minimally counterintuitive concepts. *Cognitive Science, 37*(7), 1251–1289.

Baumard, N., André, J. B., & Sperber, D. (2013). A mutualistic approach to morality. *Behavioral and Brain Sciences, 36*(1), 59–122.

Baumard, N., & Boyer, P. (2013). Explaining moral religions. *Trends in Cognitive Sciences, 17*(6), 172–180.

Baumard, N., & Chevallier, C. (2015). The nature and dynamics of world religions: A life-history approach. *Proceedings of the Royal Academy B: Biological Sciences, 282*, 1818.

Barna Group. (2017). *The faith crisis of today's Irish youth*. [Research report].Retrieved 12/10/2017 (https://www.barna.com/research/faith-crisis-todays-irish-youth/)

Barr, C., & Ó Corráin, D. (2017). Catholic Ireland, 1740–2016. In E. F. Biagini & M. Daley (Eds.), *The Cambridge social history of modern Ireland*. (pp.68–87) Cambridge: Cambridge University Press.

Barrett, J. L. (1999). Theological correctness: Cognitive constraint and the study of religion. *Method & Theory in the Study of Religion, 11*, 325–339.

Barrett, J. L. (2004). *Why would anyone believe in God?* Walnut Creek, CA: AltaMira Press.

Barrett, J. L. (2016). The (modest) utility of MCI theory. *Religion, Brain & Behavior, 6*(3), 249–251. doi:10.1080/2153599X.2015.1015049

Barrett, J. L., & Keil, F. (1996). Conceptualizing a nonnatural entity: Anthropomorphism in God concepts. *Cognitive Psychology, 31*, 219–247.

Barrett, J., & Lanman, J. (2008). The science of religious beliefs. *Religion, 38*(2), 109–124.

Barrett, J., & Nyhof, M. (2001). Spreading non-natural concepts: The role of intuitive conceptual structures in memory and transmission of cultural materials. *Journal of Cognition and Culture, 1*(1), 69–100.

Bengston, V. L. (with Putney, N. M., & Harris, S). (2013). *Families and faith: How religion is passed down across generations*. New York: Oxford University Press.

Bering, J. M. (2006). The folk psychology of souls. *Behavioral and Brain Sciences, 29*, 1–46.

Blankholm, J., & Garcia, A. (2016) The social context of organized nonbelief: County-level predictors of nonbeliever organizations in the United States. *Journal for the Scientific Study of Religion, 55*(1), 70–90.

Bloom, P. (2004). *Descartes' baby: How child development explains what makes us human*. London: Arrow Books.

Bloom, P. (2007). Religion is natural. *Developmental Science, 10*(1), 147–151.

Boyer, P. (2002). *Religion explained: The evolutionary origins of religious thought*. New York: Basic Books.

Boyer, P. (2010). *The fracture of an illusion: Science and the dissolution of religion.* Götingen: Vandenhoeck & Ruprecht.

Boyer, P., & Ramble, C. (2001). Cognitive templates for religious concepts: Cross-cultural evidence for recall of counter-intuitive representations. *Cognitive Science, 25,* 535–564

Brown, C. G. (2001). *The death of Christian Britain.* London: Routledge.

Brown, C. G. (2012). *Religion and the demographic revolution: Women and secularisation in Canada, Ireland, UK and USA since the 1960s.* Woodbridge, UK: Boydell Press.

Bruce, S. (2002). *God is dead: Secularization in the West.* Oxford: Blackwell.

Bruce, S. (2006). Secularization and the impotence of individualized religion. *Hedgehog Review, 8*(1–2), 35–46.

Bullivant, S. (2017, August 24). *Religion in Ireland: Recent trends and possible futures.* [Presentation]. Iona Institute, Dublin.

Cannell, F. (2010). Anthropology of secularism. *Annual Review of Anthropology, 39,* 85–100.

Casanova, J. (1994). *Public religions in the modern world.* Chicago: University of Chicago Press.

Comte, A. (2009). *A general theory of positivism.* Cambridge University Press. (Original work published in 1865).

Connolly, S. J. (1985). *Priests and people in pre-famine Ireland, 1780–1845.* Dublin: Gill and MacMillan

Curry, O. S. (2016). Morality as cooperation: A problem-centred approach. In T. K. Shackelford & R. D. Hansen (Eds), *The evolution of morality.* (pp. 27–52). New York: Springer International.

Davie, G. (1994). *Religion in Britain since 1945: Believing without belonging.* Blackwell.

Davie, G. (2002). *Europe: The exceptional case. parameters of faith in the modern world.* London: Darton Longman & Todd.

Day, A. (2011). *Believing in belonging: Belief and social identity in the modern world.* Oxford: Oxford University Press.

Demerath, N.J., III. (2000). The rise of cultural religion in European Christianity: Learning from Poland, Northern Ireland, and Sweden. *Social Compass, 47*(1), 127–139.

Dunbar, R. (1996). *Grooming, gossip and the evolution of language.* London: Faber and Faber.

Durkheim, É. (1993). *The division of labor in society.* New York: Free Press.

Egan, K. (2011). *Remaining a Catholic after the Murphy Report.* Dublin: Columba Press.

Fuller, L. (2002). *Irish Catholicism since 1950: The undoing of a culture.* Dublin: Gill & MacMillan.

Ganiel, G. (2016). *Transforming post-Catholic Ireland: Religious practice in late modernity.* Oxford: Oxford University Press.

Gervais, W. M., & Henrich, J. (2010). The Zeus problem: Why representational content biases cannot explain faith in gods. *Journal of Cognition and Culture, 10,* 383–389.

Gervais, W. M., van Elk, M., Xygalatas, D., McKay, R., Aveyard, M., Buchtel, E. E. K., Dar-Nimrod, I., Klocová, E. K., Ramsay, J.E., Riekki, T. , Svedholm-Häkkinen, A. M., Bulbulia, J. (2017). Analytic atheism: A cross-culturally weak and fickle phenomenon? *Judgement and Decision Making, 13*(3), 268–274.

Graham, J. (2015). Explaining away differences in moral judgment: Comment on Gray & Keeney. *Social Psychological and Personality Science, 6,* 869–873.

Guthrie, S. (1993). *Faces in the clouds: A new theory of religion.* Oxford: Oxford University Press.

Haidt, J., & Graham, J. (2007). When morality opposes justice: Conservatives have moral intuitions that liberals may not recognize. *Social Justice Research, 20,* 98–116.

Haidt, J., & Kesebir, S. (2010). Morality. In S. T. Fiske, D. T. Gilbert & G. Lindzey (Eds.), *Handbook of Social Psychology* (5th ed.). (pp. 797–832). Hoboken, NJ: John Wiley & Sons.

Henrich, J. (2009). The evolution of costly displays, cooperation, and religion: Credibility enhancing displays and their implications for cultural evolution. *Evolution and Human Behaviour, 30*, 244–260.

Henrich, J. (2015). *The secret of our success: How culture is driving human evolution, domesticating our species, and making us smarter.* Princeton, NJ: Princeton University Press.

Henrich, J., & McElreath, R. (2007). Dual inheritance theory: The evolution of human cultural capabilities and cultural evolution. In R.I. M. Dunbar & L. Barrett (Eds.), *The Oxford handbook of evolutionary psychology* (pp. 555–570). Oxford: Oxford University Press.

Hilliard, B. (2003). The Catholic Church and married women's sexuality: Habitus change in late 20th century Ireland. *Irish Journal of Sociology, 12*(2), 28–49.

Hout, M., & Fischer, C. (2014). Explaining why more Americans have no religious preference: Political backlash and generational succession, 1987–2012. *Sociological Science, 1*(4), 423.

Inglehart, R., & Welzel, C. (2005). *Modernization, cultural change, and democracy: The human development sequence.* Cambridge, UK: Cambridge University Press.

Inglis, T. (1998). *Moral monopoly: The rise and fall of the Catholic Church in modern Ireland.* Dublin: University College Dublin.

Jack, A. L., Friedman, J. P., Boyatzis, R. E., & Taylor, S. N. (2016). Why do you believe in God? Relationships between religious belief, analytic thinking, mentalizing and moral concern. *PLoS One, 11*(3), Article e0149989.

Josephson, J. A. (2012). *The invention of religion in Japan.* Chicago: University of Chicago Press.

Keane, W. (2015). *Ethical life: Its natural and social histories.* Princeton, NJ: Princeton University Press.

Kelemen, D., Rottman, J., & Seston, R. (2013). Professional physical scientists display tenacious teleological tendencies: Purpose-based reasoning as a cognitive default. *Journal of Experimental Psychology: General, 142*(4), 1074–1083

Kung, H. (1996). *Christianity: Essence, history and future.* New York: Continuum.

Lanman, J. (2008). In defence of "belief": A cognitive response to behaviourism, eliminativism and social constructivism. *Issues in Ethnology and Anthropology, 3*(3), 49–62.

Lanman, J. (2012). The importance of religious displays for belief acquisition and secularisation. *Journal of Contemporary Religion, 27*(1), 49–65.

Lanman, J. A., & Buhrmeister, M. (2017). Religious actions speak louder than words: Exposure to CREDs predicts theism. *Religion, Brain & Behavior, 7*(1), 3–16.

Larkin, E. J. (1976). *The historical dimensions of Irish Catholicism.* New York: Arno Press.

Leach, E. (1954). *Political systems of highland Burma: A study of Kachin social structure.* Cambridge, MA: Harvard University Press.

Lindeman, M., Svedholm-Hakkinen, A. M., & Lipsanen, J. (2015). Ontological confusions but not mentalizing abilities predict religious belief, paranormal belief, and belief in supernatural purpose. *Cognition, 134*, 63–76.

Luhrmann, T. (2012). *When God talks back: Understanding the American evangelical relationship with God.* New York: Vintage Books.

Luhrmann, T. (2018). The faith frame: Or, belief is easy, faith is hard. *Contemporary Pragmatism, 15*, 302–318.

McCauley, R. N. (2011). *Why religion is natural, and science is not.* New York: Oxford University Press.

McElreath, R., Richerson, T. J., & Boyd, R. (2003). Shared norms and the evolution of ethnic markers. *Current Anthropology, 44*(1), 122–130.

McWilliams, D. (2005). *The Pope's Children: Ireland's New Elite.* Dublin: Gill & MacMillan.

Mercier, H., & Sperber, D. (2017). *The enigma of reason: A new theory of human understanding.* New York: Penguin Books.

Miller, D. W. (1975). Irish Catholicism and the Great Famine. *Journal of Social History, 9*(1), 81–98.

Mountford, B. (2011). *Christian atheist: Belonging without believing.* Winchester: O-Books.

Navarratte, C., Kurzban, R., Fessler, D., & Kirkpatrick, L. (2004). Anxiety and intergroup bias: Terror management or coalitional psychology. *Group Processes and Intergroup Relations, 7*, 370–397.

Norenzayan, A. (2013). *Big Gods: How religion transformed cooperation and conflict.* Princeton, NJ: Princeton University Press.

Norenzayan, A., & Gervais, W. M. (2012). Analytic thinking promotes religious disbelief. *Science, 336*, 493–496.

Norenzayan, A., & Gervais, W. M. (2013). The origins of religious disbelief. *Trends in Cognitive Sciences, 17*, 20–25.

Norenzayan, A., Gervais, W. M., & Trzesniewski, K. H. (2012). Mentalizing deficits constrain belief in a personal god. *PLoS One, 7*, e36880.

Norris, P., & Inglehart, R. (2011). *Sacred and secular: Religion and politics worldwide* (2nd ed.). New York: Cambridge University Press.

Ó Féich, P., & O'Connell, M. (2015). Changes in Roman Catholic beliefs and practices in Ireland between 1981 and 2008 and the emergence of the liberal Catholic. *Journal of Contemporary Religion, 30*, 38–54.

Orsi, R. (2017). What is Catholic about the clergy sex abuse crisis? In K. Norget, V. Napolitano, & M. Mayblin (Eds.), *The anthropology of Catholicism: A reader.* Berkeley: University of California Press.

Pennycook, G., Ross, R. M., Koehler, D. J., & Fugelsang, J. A. (2016). Atheists and agnostics are more reflective than religious believers: Four empirical studies and a meta-analysis. *PloS One, 11*(4), e0153039.

Purzycki, B. G., Haque, O., & Sosis, R. (2014). Extending evolutionary accounts of religion beyond the mind: Religions as adaptive systems. In F. Watts & L. Turner (Eds.), *Evolution, religion, and cognitive science: Critical and constructive essays* (pp. 74–91). New York: Oxford University Press.

Purzycki, B. G., & Willard, A. K. (2016). MCI theory: A critical discussion. *Religion, Brain & Behavior, 6*, 207–248.

Purzycki, B. G., Apicella, C., Atkinson, Q., Cohen, E., McNamara, R. A., Willard, A. K., Xygalatas, D., Norenzayan, A., & Henrich, J. (2016). Moralistic Gods, supernatural punishment and the expansion of human sociality. *Nature, 530*(7590), 327–330.

Purzycki, B. G., Henrich, J., Apicella, C., Atkinson, Q., Baimel, A., Cohen, E., McNamara, R. A., Willard, A. K., Xygalatas, D., & Norenzayan, A. (2018). The evolution of religion and morality: A synthesis of ethnographic and experimental evidence from eight societies. *Religion, Brain & Behavior, 8*(2), 101–132.

Ribberink, E., Achterberg, P., & Houtman, D. (2013). Deprivatization of disbelief? Non-religiosity and anti-religiosity in 14 Western European countries. *Politics and Religion, 6*(1), 101–120.

Roes, F. L., & Raymond, M. (2003). Belief in moralizing gods. *Evolution and Human Behavior, 24*, 126–135.

Romney, A. K., & D'Andrade, R. G. (1964). Cognitive aspects of English kin terms. *American Anthropologist, 68*(3), 146–170.

Rozin, P., Millman, L., & Nemeroff, C. J. (1986). Operation of the laws of sympathetic magic in disgust and other domains. *Journal of Personality and Social Psychology, 50*(4), 703–712.

Ruane, J. (1998). Secularisation and ideology in the Republic of Ireland. In P. Brennan (Ed.), *La Secularisation en Irlande* (pp. 239–253). Caen: Presses de Universitaire de Caen.

Sanchez, C., Sundermeier, B., Gray, K., & Calin-Jageman, R. J. (2017). Direct replication of Gervais and Norenzayan (2012): No evidence that analytic thinking decreases religious belief. *PloS One, 12*(2), e0172636.

Shariff, A. F., & Norenzayan, A. (2007). God is watching you: Priming God concepts increases prosocial behavior in an anonymous economic game. *Psychological Science, 18*(9), 803–809.

Shariff, A. F., Willard, A. K., Andersen, T., & Noranzayan, A. (2015). Religious priming: A meta-analysis with a focus on prosociality. *Personality and Social Psychology Review, 20*(1), 27–48.

Slone, J. D. (2004). *Theological incorrectness: Why religious people believe what they shouldn't.* New York: Oxford University Press.

Smith, C. (2005). *Soul searching: The religious and spiritual lives of American teenagers.* New York: Oxford University Press.

Sperber, D. (1996). *Explaining culture: A naturalistic approach.* Oxford: Blackwell.

Stenner, K. (2005). *The authoritarian dynamic.* Cambridge, UK: Cambridge University Press.

Sørensen, J. (2006). *A cognitive theory of magic.* Lanham, MD: AltaMira Press.

Sosis, R. (2009). The adaptationist-byproduct debate on the evolution of religion: Five misunderstandings of the adaptationist program. *Journal of Cognition and Culture, 9,* 315–332.

Sosis, R. (2016). Religions as complex adaptive systems. In N. Clements (Ed.), *Mental religion: The brain, cognition, and culture* (pp. 219–236). MacMillan Interdisciplinary Handbooks on Religion. Farmington Hills, MI: Macmillan.

Sosis, R., Kress, H. C., & Boster, J. S. (2007). Scars for war: Evaluating alternative signaling explanations for cross-cultural variance in ritual costs. *Evolution and Human Behavior, 28*(4), 234–247.

Stark R., & Iannaccone, L. R. (1994). A supply-side reinterpretation of the secularization of Europe. *Journal for the Scientific Study of Religion, 33*(3), 230–252.

Taves, A. (2009). *Religious experience reconsidered: A building block approach to the study of religion and other special things.* Princeton, NJ: Princeton University Press.

Taylor, C. (2007). *A secular age.* Cambridge, MA: Belknap Press of Harvard University Press.

Taylor, C. (2011). Western secularity. In Calhoun, C., Juergensmeyer, M, & VanAntwerpen, J. (Eds.), *Rethinking Secularism.* (pp.31–53). Oxford: Oxford University Press.

Tooby, J., & Cosmides, L. (2010). Groups in mind: The coalitional roots of war and morality. In H. Høgh-Olesen (Ed.), *Human Morality and Sociality: Evolutionary and Comparative Perspectives* (pp. 91–234). New York: Palgrave MacMillan.

Turpin, H. (2018). *Failing God? A cognitive anthropological examination of the relationship between Catholic scandals and Irish secularization* [Doctoral thesis]. Queen's University Belfast and Aarhus University.

Turpin, H., Andersen, M., & Lanman, J. A. (2018). CREDs, CRUDs, and Catholic scandals: Experimentally examining the effects of religious paragon behavior on co-religionist belief. *Religion, Brain & Behavior, 87,* 1–13.

Van Leeuwen, N. (2014). Religious credence is not factual belief. *Cognition, 1*(33), 698–715.

Visuri, I. (2018). Rethinking autism, theism and atheism: Bodiless agents and imaginary realities. *Archive for the Psychology of Religion, 40*(1), 1–31.

Voas, D. (2009). The rise and fall of fuzzy fidelity in Europe. *European Sociological Review*, 25(2), 155–168.

Von Hippel, W., & Trivers, R. (2011). The evolution and psychology of self-deception. *Behavioural and Brain Sciences*, 34, 1–56.

Watts, J., Greenhill, S. J., Atkinson, Q. D., Currie, T. E., Bulbulia, J., & Gray, R. D. (2015). Broad supernatural punishment but not moralizing high gods precede the evolution of political complexity in Austronesia. *Proceedings of the Royal Society B: Biological Sciences*, 282(1804), 20142556.

Whitehouse, H. (1995). *Inside the cult: Religious innovation and transmission in Papua New Guinea*. Oxford: Oxford University Press.

Whitehouse, H. (2004). *Modes of religiosity: A cognitive theory of religious transmission*. Walnut Creek, CA: AltaMira Press.

Whitehouse, H., Jong, J., Buhrmester, M.D., Gómez, Á., Bastian, B., Kavanagh, C., Newson, M., Matthews, M., Lanman, J. A., McKay, R., & Gavrilets, S. (2017). The evolution of extreme cooperation via shared dysphoric experiences. *Scientific Reports*, 7, Article p.srep44292.

Whitehouse, H., & Lanman, J. A. (2014). The ties that bind us: Ritual, fusion and identification. *Current Anthropology*, 55(6), 674–695.

Whitehouse, H., & McQuinn, B. (2013). Divergent modes of religiosity and armed struggle. In M. Kitts, M. Juergensmeyer, & M. Jerryson (Eds.), *The Oxford Handbook of religion and violence* (pp. 597–619). Oxford: Oxford University Press.

Whyte, J. H. (1980). *Church and state in modern Ireland 1923–1979*. Dublin: Gill and MacMillan.

Willard, A. K., & Cingl, L. (2017). Testing theories of secularization and religious belief in the Czech Republic and Slovakia. *Evolution and Human Behavior*, 38(5), 604–615.

Wilson, D. S. (2002). *Darwin's cathedral: Evolution, religion and the nature of society*. Chicago: University of Chicago Press.

Wiltermuth, S. S., & Heath, C. (2009). Synchrony and cooperation. *Psychological Science*, 20, 1–5.

Win-Gallup International. (2012). International Index of Religiosity and Atheism. Retrieved 4/10/2015 from https://sidmennt.is/wp-content/uploads/Gallup-International-um-tr%C3%BA-og-tr%C3%BAleysi-2012.pdf.

Wollschleger, J., & Beach, L. (2011). A cucumber for a cow: A theoretical explanation of the causes and consequences of religious hypocrisy. *Rationality and Society*, 23(2), 155–174.

Xygalatas, D. (2012). *The burning saints: Cognition and culture in the fire-walking rituals of the Anastenaria*. Equinox.

Zuckerman, P. (2008). *Society without God: What the least religious nations can tell us about contentment*. New York: New York University Press.

Zuckerman, P., Galen, L., & Pasquale, F. (2017). *The Nonreligious: Understanding secular people and societies*. Oxford University Press.

PART VII

CSR'S RELATIONS AND IMPLICATIONS

CHAPTER 17

NEUROSCIENCE
OF RELIGION

UFFE SCHJOEDT AND MICHIEL VAN ELK

INTRODUCTION

NEUROSCIENCE *of religion* is the attempt to describe and explain religious thought and behavior at the level of the brain. Unlike the cognitive science of religion (CSR), which mainly seeks to model the cognitive mechanisms involved in religious thought and behavior, and the evolutionary psychology of religion (EPR), which attempts to uncover the selection pressures that may have led to those mechanisms, neuroscience of religion aims to identify the neurobiological substrates of such mechanisms.

Neuroscience, however, is sometimes used inappropriately by nonexperts who wish to increase the credibility of particular cognitive or evolutionary accounts of religion by suggesting a link to the physical brain. To avoid speculative uses of neuroscience in other religion disciplines, we suggest that neuroscience of religion be more narrowly defined as scientific research on religion that is primarily based on the methods and theories used in the brain sciences. We use an attributional definition of religion, which means that experiences, behaviors, cognitions, beliefs, and attitudes that people "deem" religious qualify as the research object of the neuroscience of religion (akin to other attributional definitions of religion, e.g., Taves, 2009).

As such, neuroscience of religion is an umbrella term for widely different topics and approaches. Empirically, it includes studies that use brain-imaging technologies such as magnetic resonance imaging (MRI), magnetoencephalography (MEG), and electroencephalography (EEG) and stimulation devices such as transcranial magnetic stimulation (TMS) or transcranial direct-current stimulation (tDCS). Theoretically, it includes work that centers around neuroscientific models of the functional brain, its anatomical regions, neural signals, and principles of encoding to understand and explain various religious phenomena, for example, religious attitudes, supernatural beliefs, ritualized behaviors, and mystical states.

Neuroscience versus Neurotheology

Many believers experience religious cognition as fundamentally different from ordinary cognition. Neuroscientists who share this feeling have spent decades searching for specialized neural substrates of religious cognition. The attempts to map the uniqueness of religious experience in terms of brain function has been termed "neurotheology" (d'Aquili & Newberg, 1999, p. 176). Instead of applying conventional insights to the human brain, d'Aquili and Newberg and like-minded researchers propose new brain models for understanding the distinct aspects of religious experience. Such theories are intriguing and popular in the media, but evidence for their core assumptions about the brain is often lacking. Examples include d'Aquili's and Newberg's (1999) fascinating work on the experience of Absolute Unitary Being as a consequence of the deafferentiation of the posterior superior parietal lobe. Other examples include Persinger's (1983) innovative theory that mystical experience is the result of quasi-epileptic activity in the temporal lobe, and McNamara's (2009) insightful attempt to explain the transformative power of religious experience by an overlap between a self-processing network and a religion circuitry (for critical reviews, see Schjoedt, 2009, 2011).

A potential danger in neurotheology is inventing "new theories" based on studies that have used small sample sizes by modern neuroscience standards. By adopting theories that are too liberal, the field incurs the risk of becoming marginalized and not taken seriously by mainstream neuroscience. Another potential concern is the temptation of nonprofessionals to seek nonnaturalistic explanations for religious experiences based on uncertain interpretations. For instance, the link between electromagnetic stimulation and the feeling of a presence in Persinger's work may lead people to explain unusual experiences by referring to external and weak electromagnetic fields, for example, because of changes in the earth's magnetic field or variation in solar activity (Spottiswoode, 1997; Spottiswoode & May, 1997).

Most neuroscientists of religion, however, examine religious cognition from a conventional neuroscience perspective in which religious thought and behavior are assumed to recruit known neurocognitive networks and processes. Religious experience is conceived of neither as a uniform category nor as a function of dedicated neural circuitry. It is simply a label for any experience deemed religious by believers (Taves & Asprem, 2017). Religious cognition and experience are therefore as diverse as any other kind of cognition and experience with corresponding language, reward, emotion, and executive processes depending on its specific content.

A Fragmented Field

The field's empirical findings are published in widely different subfields, such as religious studies, cognitive science, social psychology, psychiatry, neurology, neuroscience, medicine, and pain research. Although the results are often cited selectively in popular-science books to promote specific ideas, the proper academic integration of empirical evidence across disciplines is largely missing. The field's fragmented landscape reflects the fact that most contributors to it come from disciplines in which religion is secondary, for example, medical doctors, psychiatrists, and cognitive neuroscientists. The research is often motivated by an individual researcher's interest in the topic. Very few researchers are committed full time to the neuroscience of religion.

This "secondary" nature of the field means that state-of-the-art developments in the frontier neuroscience disciplines are only slowly integrated. It also means that the issue of scanning time and cost leads to relatively small sample sizes in comparison to the contemporary standards in neuroscience.

We will present five distinguishable neuroscientific approaches to religion. The first approach (Approach 1), which is the most common, examines the neural correlates of religion using adapted versions of standard paradigms of experimental psychology. The second line of research (Approach 2) examines religion and spirituality in relation to structural differences in brain anatomy, for example, cases of brain lesions and atrophy in neuropsychological patients. A third line of research (Approach 3) examines the religion-brain link by analogy, using hypnosis and illusion paradigms, for instance. A fourth approach (Approach 4) attempts to directly examine the neurocognitive processes in authentic religious practices and experiences in the laboratory. Finally, as a fifth approach (Approach 5), we discuss the curious case of neuroenchantment, by which researchers seem capable of eliciting religious experiences in participants by exploiting their belief in neuroscience.

In practice, the different research approaches are not as separate and delineated as presented here, but the typology should help clarify the strengths and weaknesses researchers need to consider when evaluating and designing neuroscientific research on religion. The chapter thus presents the complex and heterogeneous field of neuroscience of religion, but it does not provide a systematic review of the field's studies (for recent reviews of the field, see McNamara, 2019; Grafman et al., 2020).

Methodological Problems and Trade-offs

The neuroscience of religion is generally challenged by three major methodological problems pertaining to *experimental control*, *authenticity*, and *reverse inference*. Experimental research generally strives to reach full experimental control in order to make causal inferences. When studying complex cultural phenomena like religion, however, too much attention to experimental control runs the risk of ruining the authenticity and ecological validity of a given phenomenon. Brain scanners and scalp electrodes make for highly artificial environments. Exposure to abstract cognitive tasks and meaningless control conditions challenges researchers' ability to elicit and measure authentic religious cognition and behavior. To maintain authenticity, it is often necessary to compromise on the amount of experimental control.

Sacrificing experimental control to obtain a more authentic experience and behaviors, however, hampers efforts to isolate the unique effect of the independent variable of interest. Confounding variables in social psychology such as demand characteristics (cues in the experiment that reveal the study purpose to the participants) and the social-desirability effect (participants' tendency to respond in socially desirable ways) are especially problematic in studies measuring explicit religious behavior. A lack of experimental control may leave researchers with observed patterns of neural activity that are difficult to interpret because they cannot be linked to well-defined cognitive constructs and functions. If prayer, for instance, elicits activity in several areas of the brain, how can we make sense of the cognitive functions subserved by these regions during prayer? Typically, researchers then look at other studies to find similar brain activations in order to make meaningful interpretations. This approach is called *reverse inference*, and it is considered a controversial method in neuroscience because each brain region subserves many different functions and is functionally connected to many other regions. Surely, any inference about cognition based on overlapping brain activity alone will be speculative at best; in some instances, however, informed speculation based on reversed inference is the only viable approach.

Hence we see an inverse relationship between experimental control and authenticity, as well as a tendency to make reverse inferences in studies that emphasize authenticity over experimental control (Figure 17.1). Solving all three issues in a single study seems impossible, so researchers typically make trade-offs when they design their study.

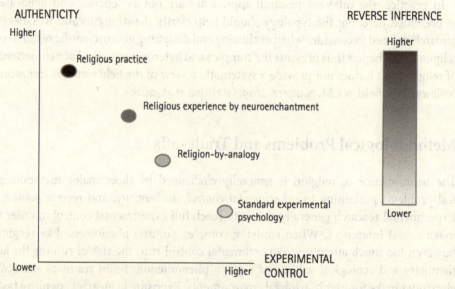

FIGURE 17.1 Four approaches in the neuroscience of religion varying on the critical dimensions of experimental control, authenticity, and degree of reverse inference. Note that structural brain research is not represented in the figure because no experimental conditions are used in this approach.

Five Approaches in Neuroscience of Religion

In this section, we introduce the various approaches in neuroscience of religion. For each approach, several studies are presented to illustrate its strengths and weaknesses, focusing on varying degrees of experimental control, authenticity, and reverse inference.

Standard Experimental Psychology

The most widely used approach in the neuroscience of religion involves recording a time series of brain activity (e.g., with a fMRI or an EEG) under various experimental and control conditions that are relevant to a particular aspect of religion. In this line of research, religion may be treated as a continuous independent variable (*what does religion do to some other variable?*), the dependent variable (*what does some other variable do to religion?*), or a differentiator of groups (*how do religious participants compare to nonreligious participants on a given task?*)

Because research questions are often social-psychological in scope, experiments tend to use generic religious stimuli (images, statements, and words like "God," "Heaven," "Divine") that are of relevance to a broad population in society (e.g., Christians, supernatural believers). The experiments are designed to isolate the effect of a psychological construct relevant to a particular aspect of religion (e.g., God beliefs). In order to reach a high degree of experimental control and generalizability, religious stimuli are typically presented repeatedly in adapted versions of standard experimental paradigms.

Inzlicht and Tullett (2009), for example, recorded EEG during a cognitive control task (Stroop task; $n = 41$) to examine the modulation of error processing as a function of participants' religiosity and religious priming. In the Stroop task, participants tend to commit errors when they attempt to categorize incongruent stimuli. Inzlicht and Tullett found that stronger religious beliefs were associated with a reduced error-related negativity (ERN) signal from the anterior cingulate cortex (ACC), which is known to correlate with a negative affective response to committing an error. The results are used by the authors as evidence of an affective function of religion as a palliative worldview (Inzlicht et al., 2011), but this interpretation appears somewhat speculative since the results could just as well support a purely cognitive interpretation (Schjoedt & Bulbulia, 2011). The affective interpretation holds that religion has the capacity to act as a buffer against the distress that comes from committing errors; a cognitive interpretation proposes that religion can somehow decrease the cognitive processing in ACC in response to committing such errors. However, in a recent conceptual replication fMRI study we found no evidence for the hypothesized relationship between religiosity and ACC activity (Hoogeveen et al., 2020), casting doubt on both theoretical accounts.

Kapogiannis, Barbey, Su, Krueger et al. (2009) recorded the blood oxygen level dependent (BOLD) signal in 40 participants. The BOLD signal is used in most fMRI studies as a correlate of brain metabolism and blood flow. In this study, the signal was used to measure the neural responses to statements about God of religious and nonreligious participants. The researchers found that reflecting on particular dimensions of God beliefs (God's emotional states, God's involvement with the world, etc.) was associated with different neural networks corresponding to the content of specific beliefs. For instance, reflecting on God's level of involvement with the world was associated with the activation of the medial prefrontal cortex and the precuneus—areas that have been associated with self-referential processing and mind-wandering. According to Kapogiannis et al., this may indicate that reflecting on God's level of involvement engages deliberate reflection on how their view of God relates to themselves. Although this interpretation is based on reverse inference, the authors' findings support the idea that religious cognition recruits ordinary neural circuitry, which is involved in other cognitive tasks as well, rather than a dedicated circuitry for religion.

In another study examining misattributions of intentionality in paranormal believers (beliefs in telepathy, mindreading, clairvoyance, etc.), Riekki et al. (2014) recorded brain activity (fMRI) while 12 paranormal believers watched geometrical shapes that were moving intentionally and arbitrarily. Compared with skeptics, the paranormal believers were more likely to attribute intentionality to arbitrary movements, an observation that correlated with stronger activation of the medial prefrontal cortex (mPFC). This finding is in line with the interpretation that at least one class of paranormal believers may be more prone to processing arbitrary events as intentional and perhaps even to engage in "hypermentalizing," that is, overattributing intentions to nonintentional objects.

Other studies of this kind include Wiech et al. (2008), in which Christian ($n = 12$) and nonreligious ($n = 12$) participants received a painful stimulus while looking at images of the Virgin Mary. Observed analgesic effects of such images were reflected in activation of the right ventrolateral prefrontal cortex (VLPFC), an area that has been associated with higher-order pain modulation. Epley et al. (2009) reported convergence of neural activity (fMRI) in the medial prefrontal cortex (mPFC) in 17 participants who estimated their own attitudes and God's attitudes on topics like euthanasia; this activation of the mPFC was not found when participants estimated other people's attitudes. Harris et al. (2009) used fMRI to examine the neural correlates of participants (15 believers and 15 nonbelievers), who evaluated the truth and falsity of religious and nonreligious propositions. They found similar neural activation in response to both categories across participants, which is taken to indicate that evaluating religious statements recruits the same neural systems used in comparable evaluations of general semantic knowledge. Han et al. (2008, 2009) examined Chinese participants with different cultural backgrounds (14 Christians and 14 nonreligious). They found that Christians (Han et al., 2008) recruited the dorsomedial prefrontal cortex (DMPFC)

> **Box 17.1 Standard experimental psychology in neuroscience of religion**
>
> | Strengths: | Weaknesses: |
> | --- | --- |
> | - High experimental control | - Lack of authenticity |
> | - Generalizable to target population | - Lack of meaningful experience |
> | - Few demand characteristics | - Lack of cultural specificity |
> | - Few social desirability effects | |

during a self-evaluation task, which was interpreted to suggest that Christian beliefs result in more evaluative processing in response to self-referential stimuli. Lindeman et al. (2013) recorded brain activity (fMRI) while 12 supernatural believers and 11 skeptics watched pictures suggestive of a dramatic ending to a fictive story and found that the supernatural believers rated the pictures as more indicative of what was about to happen than did skeptics, which was reflected in activation of the right inferior frontal gyrus (IFG).

Standardized experimental psychology offers a relatively high degree of experimental control because it uses implicit priming and examines well-documented neural responses to standardized cognitive tasks. If they are properly controlled, studies like Inzlicht and Tullett's (2009) allow for advanced analyses of the unconscious effects of religion on neural processing. Using standardized stimuli and measures, however, comes at a cost. Exposure to abstract and standardized stimuli unavoidably leads to decreased ecological validity. Indeed, participants in such studies rarely feel that they are engaging in religious activities because the conscious experience of being religious is deliberately removed in order to increase the internal validity of the experimental findings. In fact, if participants consciously perceived the conditions as religious, the researchers' ability to make causal inferences would be compromised because of the potential effects of demand characteristics and social desirability. Removing conscious experience effectively rules out noise from such confounding factors. Alas, it also detracts from the ability to study authentic religious thought and behavior. Box 17.1 summarizes the strengths and weakness of standard experimental psychology in neuroscience of religion.

Structural Brain Research

Not all studies use recordings of brain activity to examine the neural correlates of religious cognition. Another approach is to correlate various religious traits, beliefs, and behaviors with differences in brain anatomy. This approach is very different from the first approach because it measures structural differences in the physical brain (brain anatomy), rather than the dynamic measures of the brain's metabolism or electrical charges (brain activity). Researchers have used both cross-sectional and longitudinal brain imaging data to study the neuroanatomical correlates of religiosity and spirituality in relation to brain lesions and cases of atrophy, as well as in normal healthy subjects.

Kapogiannis et al. (2009) performed structural MRI on participants who reported different patterns of religiosity (n = 40). Distinct aspects of religiosity were associated with different regional cortical volumes as measured by voxel-based morphometry. For example, experiencing an intimate relationship with God and engaging in religious behavior was associated with an increased volume of the right middle temporal cortex, and experiencing fear of God was associated with a decreased volume of the left precuneus and left orbitofrontal cortex. These findings were used as evidence that variation in religiosity is associated with cortical-volume differences.

Owen et al. (2011) found that hippocampal atrophy in late life (n = 268) was predicted by affiliation with religious minorities and by whether participants had reported a life-changing religious experience. This finding is interpreted as reflecting the detrimental effects of stress caused by being a member of a minority or undergoing a dramatic life-changing event. Miller et al. (2014) measured cortical thickness in high- and low-risk groups for depression (n = 103) to see if individual religiosity or spirituality could provide a buffer against the detrimental effects of depression. In line with their predictions, self-reported importance of religion and spirituality was indeed associated with thicker cortices in several areas of the brain. Blanke et al. (2014) analyzed felt-presence experiences caused by brain lesions in 12 neurological patients. Three distinct brain regions, which were involved in patients' sensorimotor loss, the temporoparietal cortex, the insular cortex, and especially the frontoparietal cortex, appeared to underlie these reported experiences. Cristofori et al. (2016) examined the link between mystical experience and executive brain functions in a sample of veterans who had suffered penetrating traumatic brain injury (n = 116). As predicted, lesions to the dorsolateral prefrontal cortex, which are strongly associated with impaired executive processing, were linked with more self-reported mystical-type experiences.

Other studies include Johnstone et al. (2009), who studied the relationship between spirituality/religiousness and health in patients with traumatic brain injury (n = 61). Johnstone found that aspects of spirituality/religiousness, for example, meaning making and forgiveness, correlated with both physical and mental health in this group. Butler et al. (2010) examined a sample of patients with Parkinson's disease (n = 25), which is a neurodegenerative disease that causes cell death in the dopaminergic system and found that this group did not respond to priming of religious words to the same extent that control participants did. Finally, Urgesi et al. (2010) examined the responses of neuropathological patients (n = 88) on the Self-Transcendence Scale before and after neurosurgery. The ability to take measures before and after an intervention is rare and makes this approach highly attractive because it allows for stronger causal inferences. Urgesi et al. found that selective damage to the left and right inferior posterior parietal regions increased participants' scores on the scale. This finding supports the idea that religious and spiritual cognition recruits the temporoparietal junction, which has previously been observed only in exploratory neuroimaging studies on religious practice and experiences (see Approach 4).

Structural imaging studies on religious cognition currently rely on diagnostic scans of predefined groups of patients with brain lesions or atrophy, and a few large datasets with high-resolution structural brain images of the general population. Most studies simply correlate structural brain differences with a battery of self-reported data and/or simple cognitive tests, including background data on participants' religious beliefs and practices. Still, the approach has some notable advantages over functional brain studies. First, structural changes to the brain are more robust than the more volatile functional activations. Second, structural brain studies avoid issues of social desirability and demand characteristics affecting the neural signals (though social desirability could still affect participants' self-reported religiosity). Third, the large-population datasets have a much higher numbers of participants, which further increases the robustness of findings.

To associate self-report variables on religion with structural changes in the brain, however, represents a purely correlational approach. There is no way to establish causality between brain differences and religiosity measures because no variables are experimentally manipulated. The uniqueness of Urgesi et al.'s (2010) study is precisely that they use neurosurgery as experimental manipulation to test whether damage to specific brain areas affects transcendent thoughts and feelings. However, even in this study, it is impossible to know how the spirituality measure is connected to the structural damage. Brain lesions and atrophy often result in general cognitive degradation, which makes models beyond such general effects difficult or speculative.

Another concern with structural brain research is that the interpretations of existing findings are often ambiguous (see van Elk & Aleman, 2017, for review). There is no one-to-one correspondence between changes in structural brain volume and functional brain data. Brain-behavior correlations are notoriously difficult to replicate. In fact, only very obvious characteristics, such as gender, appear to be consistently related to structural brain differences (Snoek et al. 2021). In a recent high-powered replication attempt, we failed to find any evidence for the hypothesized relation between religiosity and grey-matter differences in three key brain regions that had been identified in the literature (van Elk & Snoek, 2019), casting further doubt on the robustness of the relationships between religiosity and brain areas described above. Box 17.2 summarizes the strengths and weakness of structural brain research in neuroscience of religion.

Religiosity is a complex construct, and it remains to be seen whether it is reliably associated with any neuroanatomical markers at all. Future research, may instead use the network analyses of anatomically distinct neural circuitry (e.g., DTI) to capture the cognitive processes underlying religiosity and mystical experience—as they tap more directly into the efficiency with which neural networks process information (Bullmore & Sporns, 2009). In other words, these techniques allow researchers to determine the flow of information throughout the brain (akin to the traffic on a highway) instead of focusing only on the structure of the brain (akin to the infrastructure).

> **BOX 17.2 Structural brain research in neuroscience of religion**
>
> Strengths:
> - Anatomical differences more robust than neural activations
> - High number of participants
> - Brain damage is convincing for causal inferences
>
> Weaknesses:
> - Lack of theoretical precision (due to secondary nature of datasets, e.g., on lesion patients)
> - A poor link between structural differences and behavior in healthy subjects

Religion by Analogy

A third line of research attempts to study religion indirectly by eliciting cognitions, behaviors, and experiences in the lab that somehow resemble phenomena reported by religious practitioners (e.g., trance, possession, felt presence, and out-of-body experiences). Because religion draws on almost every aspect of human cognition, we narrow our description of this approach to cover studies that explicitly use experimental manipulations to examine religious phenomena by analogy.

Unlike standard experimental psychology in which conscious experience is often deliberately removed from the equation, this line of research tends to focus on experience. Hypnosis and illusion paradigms are popular tools for examining experience and have several strengths from the perspective of religion research. First, they enable researchers to examine aspects of conscious experience that may be relevant to religious experiences without the risk of proreligious response biases in participants. Second, focusing on specific cognitive aspects of religious experience rather than full-blown authentic religious experience reduces the problem of authenticity in the lab. To report visual illusions or hypnotically induced hallucinations is perfectly compatible with the laboratory context. Third, rather than customizing experimental designs to elicit authentic religious experience in particular groups of believers (as in Approach 4), illusion and hypnosis studies use standardized paradigms that can also be used with nonreligious participants.

Many examples could be given of the religion-by-analogy approach, ranging from research on the induction of delusional beliefs and conditioned hallucinations to psychedelic experiences. Especially the growing field of psychedelic research and the neuroscientific study of psychedelics offer great opportunity for studying the effects of set and setting on mystical-like experiences and its neural correlates (Carhart-Harris et al., 2014). An exhaustive review of this topic would be beyond the scope of this chapter. Here, we selectively focus on other examples of the neuroscience-based research on extraordinary experiences that are relevant for the study of religion.

Blanke et al. (2005) studied out-of-body experiences by asking participants ($n = 11$) to imagine taking visual perspectives associated with a visual avatar in different orientations. They found selective activation of the temporoparietal junction (TPJ). Transcranial magnetic stimulation (TMS) was then used to interfere with the TPJ, which impaired this mental task. Remarkably, the TMS interference had no effect on similar mental tasks involving external objects, which indicates that the TPJ may be selectively implicated in mental imagery of one's own body, including out-of-body experiences. Relatedly, several labs have used virtual- reality technology to experimentally induce out-of-body-like experiences—that is, by manipulating the observed and felt location of one's body (Lenggenhager et al., 2007; Ehrsson, 2007). This experimental induction of out-of-body experiences has also been used in a neuroimaging study, showing that the felt perspective of one's body is associated with a selective activation of the TPJ (Ionta et al., 2011). In another study by the Blanke lab (Blanke et al., 2014), which was based on insights from the structural brain study of neurological patients, a sensorimotor robot was used to experimentally induce a feeling of a presence in healthy subjects ($n = 21$). Blanke et al. showed that the illusion of feeling another person nearby appears to be caused by misperceiving the source and identity of sensorimotor (tactile, proprioceptive, and motor) signals of one's own body.

Inspired by cultural possession phenomena, Deeley et al. (2013) used hypnotic suggestion in an fMRI study to induce a felt loss of control and awareness of movements of the right hand in highly hypnotizable subjects ($n = 15$). The loss of perceived control of movements was associated with reduced connectivity between the supplementary motor area (SMA), associated with planning movement sequences, and the motor regions, suggesting that the reduced functional coupling of SMA with motor systems may underlie similar experiences reported in various cultures. Deeley et al. (2014) continued to investigate this phenomenon in a follow-up study with 15 highly hypnotically susceptible volunteers in which different experiences of a loss of movement control were modeled over distinct cultural phenomena, such as delusions of control and spirit possession. Differential modulation of activity in brain networks supporting error detection, object imagery, and representation of self and others were found to characterize these different types of experiences, suggesting that no common neural substrates could be identified for cultural possession phenomena.

The religion-by-analogy approach has lower experimental control compared with standard experimental psychology due to its use of suggestion and its focus on experience, which may both introduce effects of demand characteristics, compliance, and social desirability. Another weakness from the perspective of religion research is the possibility that examining religion by analogy may reveal limited insights into authentic religious experiences reported by believers. Even at the cognitive level, there may be fundamental differences between imagining that someone is controlling your arm and believing that your arm is being controlled by a spirit. The extent to which such beliefs affect the cognitive processing in possession phenomena is unknown, but we know that cognition is influenced by context and framing, and that religion offers a powerful interpretative framework. As such there may be a fundamental difference between authentic religious experiences and lab-based inductions of similar experiences. Box 17.3 summarizes the strengths and weakness of religion-by-analogy research in neuroscience of religion.

Box 17.3 Religion by analogy research in neuroscience of religion

Strengths:
- Standardized experimental procedures
- Possibility to study experience
- Avoids issues associated with scrutiny of participants' religion

Weaknesses:
- Lack of religiously meaningful manipulations
- Relatively weak experimental control

Authentic Religious Practice

A fourth approach attempts to directly examine authentic religious practice and experience in a laboratory setting. Contrary to the standardized designs of Approach 1, this approach uses customized experimental designs to accommodate the participants' beliefs and practices. The primary virtue is maintaining authenticity while at the same time collecting data for meaningful analyses. In neuroimaging studies, such analyses usually require contrast conditions that control for aspects of a practice that are irrelevant to the aspect of interest. For instance, verbalized prayer will almost by definition activate language-related regions in the brain. To control for this, one needs to come up with an experimental condition that uses linguistic utterances as well, but without the religious content.

Often, if it is done properly, this approach is slower than the other approaches because it takes time to recruit a specific group of practitioners and to customize the experimental design to study authentic experiences. Recruitment requires an inside collaborator with connections into a specific group, or sufficient fieldwork in which rapport with participants can be established. Neuroimaging technology and experimental procedures are often combined with qualitative research, including focus-group interviews and participant observations. The research questions are usually similar to those asked in qualitative research in the humanities. Typically, the aim is not to examine a cognitive mechanism but to understand a specific practice or experience.

For instance, in a pioneering study Azari et al. (2001) examined religious recitation in Christian ($n = 6$) and non-Christian ($n = 6$) participants. They found activation in the dorsolateral and medial prefrontal cortex when contrasting religious recitation with a secular recitation. This finding was used as evidence suggesting that religious experience may reflect an attributional process of conscious thought evaluation rather than being preconceptual in nature.

Newberg et al. conducted a series of pioneering and influential neurotheological studies, which are characterized by the use of very few participants and highly exploratory analyses. In one study by Newberg et al. (2001) using single-photon emission computed tomography (SPECT), Tibetan Buddhist meditators ($n = 8$) showed increased activity in the dorsolateral prefrontal areas and decreased activity in the superior parietal cortex (SPL), which was interpreted as evidence that meditators may experience a suspension of the self-other dichotomy. In another study, Newberg et al. (2003)

instructed Franciscan nuns ($n = 3$) to recite prayers in the scanner and found a negative correlation between prefrontal activity and SPL activations. In a third study, Pentecostal participants ($n = 5$) were scanned during glossolalia (Newberg et al., 2006) and showed decreased activity in the prefrontal cortex but increased activity in the SPL, an opposite pattern to the Buddhist meditation study. This decrease of prefrontal activity was interpreted as a correlate of the lack of control during glossolalia, as opposed to the focused attention of Tibetan meditation.

Beauregard and Paquette (2006) attempted to study mystical experience in Carmelite nuns (fMRI) ($n = 15$). The nuns, however, rejected the idea of having a spontaneous experience in the scanner, so instead they were instructed to recall their most intimate divine encounter. An assumption of the study was that this recall task would reactivate the neural patterns of the original mystical experience. This type of design, of course, seriously compromises ecological validity. Using a similar logic, Miller et al. (2018) asked participants to think about a spiritual experience and found reduced activity in the left inferior parietal lobule (IPL) compared with a neutral-relaxed condition. This finding was then interpreted as a correlate of perceptual processing and self-other representations during spiritual experiences.

Schjoedt et al. (2008) showed that both formalized and improvised prayers in Danish Christians ($n = 20$) activated the striatal reward system compared with secular control conditions, suggesting that praying may stimulate the dopaminergic system. In a related study, Schjoedt et al. (2009) showed that personal prayer recruits areas associated with social cognition, suggesting that praying to God may be comparable to normal interpersonal interaction. Schjoedt et al.'s finding was later replicated in a study ($n = 14$) by Neubauer (2014) who used fMRI to examine similar prayers and control conditions in an American Christian sample.

In another fMRI study, Schjoedt et al. (2011) examined the effect of charismatic authority on Pentecostal ($n = 18$) and nonreligious ($n = 18$) recipients of intercessory prayer. When the believers received prayers of healing from a charismatic healer (compared with prayers by a peer Christian or a nonbeliever), they showed a decreased activity of the frontal executive network and other areas of the brain. This down-regulation in the brain predicted participants' subsequent ratings of the speakers' charisma, as well as the felt presence of God during the prayers, which was interpreted to suggest a link between frontal down-regulation and vividness of the prayer experience.

Ferguson et al. (2016) used fMRI with a sample of Mormons ($n = 19$) and found that subjective ratings of "feeling the spirit" during various tasks with religious content were associated with activity in the striatal reward system, among other regions of the brain. Galanter et al. (2017) used fMRI to study prayer among members of Alcoholics Anonymous ($n = 20$), which is sometimes considered a religious organization (see Taves, 2016), and found activation in areas associated with social cognition and self-referential processing, which was interpreted to reflect the participants' deliberate control of attention and emotion.

Unlike Approach 1, where meaningful experiences are deliberately removed to avoid confounding variables, and unlike Approach 3, where the experiences are religious only

> ### Box 17.4 Authentic religious practice in neuroscience of religion
>
> | Strengths: | Weaknesses: |
> |---|---|
> | - Authentic practice | - Lack of experimental control |
> | - Religiously meaningful experience | - Low generalizability |
> | - High cultural specificity | - Lack of theoretical precision |
> | | - Reliance on reverse inference |

by analogy, this approach examines experiences deemed religious by the participants themselves. If done properly, participants engage in authentic religious practices and report meaningful religious experiences.

Alas, as fascinating as this may sound, studying religious practice directly in the laboratory setting introduces serious methodological problems. First, the issue of whether the neuroscience-lab setting and being inside a brain scanner can provide a context for having authentic religious experience remains controversial (Ladd et al., 2015). Beauregard and Paquette's (2006) study of mystical experience in Carmelite nuns illustrates this problem. Second, the degree to which the design was customized to the specific phenomenon reduces the generalizability of the study to populations beyond the study participants. Third, the lack of experimental control introduces a lack of theoretical precision. Which cognitive process are we actually measuring in the brain? The problem extends to the overreliance on reverse inference. Again, the Beauregard and Paquette study serves as an extreme example, in which the functional correlates of multiple brain activations are interpreted by reference to previous underpowered studies within neurotheology, for example, the work of Andrew Newberg and Michael Persinger. Box 17.4 summarizes the strengths and weakness of examining authentic religious practice in neuroscience of religion.

Neuroenchantment

The approaches presented so far use neuroscience technology to study brain structure and function in different groups and under different circumstances. Recently, however, researchers have begun to use neuroscience technology, not only as a device for measuring brain activity, but as a powerful and suggestive framing tool. This line of research exploits people's fascination with and belief in neuroscience to induce extraordinary experiences by means of placebo brain stimulation.

People in Western countries generally show a remarkable belief in neuroscience and a high degree of uncertainty about its limitations. Ali et al. (2014), for example, demonstrated how easily even psychology students could be tricked into believing that a mock scanner could read their exact thoughts. The authors termed this effect "neuroenchantment." Neuroenchantment research lies somewhere between Approaches 3 and 4 because it can be used to elicit experiences that are analogical to religious experiences, as well as proper religious experiences deemed religious or spiritual by the participants.

Much of the recent neuroenchantment research has been inspired by Michael Persinger's so-called God helmet, which is supposed to induce mystical experiences in normal healthy subjects by weak transcranial magnetic stimulation. Granqvist et al. (2005) did an independent double-blind replication study ($n = 89$) and found that participants did indeed report having mystical-type experiences when they were using the God helmet. However, it did not matter whether the helmet was active or inactive. Evidence like this has made most conventional neuroscientists of religion skeptical of Persinger's claims, but sham versions of the God helmet are now being used as an effective experimental manipulation for eliciting extraordinary experiences by suggestion. Andersen et al. (2014) demonstrated that intense mystical experiences could be induced with a placebo God helmet, and that these had lasting effects on the participants ($n = 23$). Similar observations have been made in other samples and settings (Maij et al., 2019; Simmonds-Moore et al., 2019, but none of these studies recorded brain activity during the reported experiences. In an EEG study, van Elk (2015) failed to experimentally induce extraordinary experiences in a sample of psychology students, although differences in Theta/Alpha power were observed between those who believed in the efficacy of the helmet and those who did not. Thus, despite the God helmet's ability to induce mystical-type experiences, the neural correlates of those experiences are currently understudied.

Another instance of neuroenchantment, which is more akin to Approach 3, uses placebo brain stimulation to study religious phenomena by analogy. Hoogeveen et al. (2018) used placebo brain stimulation to induce expected cognitive enhancement and impairment in participants ($n = 23$). Expected enhancement was found to increase participants' error-related negativity (ERN) in response to personal errors on a cognitive task (Flanker's task), and decreased ERN predicted attributions of personal errors to the brain stimulation device when the participants expected impairment. However, this neural finding was not replicated in a high-powered study, even though the subjective effects of neuroenchantment were replicated (van Elk et al., 2020). By analogy, then, when believers commit errors and blame voodoo or witchcraft, their claims may indeed be more than simply bad excuses; they may reflect a fundamental attribution error to outsource agency to an external power.

Similarly, Slama et al. (2013) used neuroenchantment to convince participants that a transformed EEG cap was capable of affecting their color perception. When they measured participants performance on a color-word Stroop task they found that suggestions of enhanced color perception resulted in stronger interference effects, whereas suggestions of impaired color perception were associated with a reduced interference effect. Another study found that suggestions related to binaural beats as enhancing or decreasing performance were, indeed, associated with strong changes in subjective performance, though objective performance was unaffected (Schwarz & Büchel, 2015). These studies show that expectancy manipulations that capitalize on people's trust in neuroscience and brain stimulation techniques can exert powerful effects on subjective experience and influence even basic cognitive processing.

Neuroenchantment is a curious phenomenon. Modern Western beliefs in neuroscience appear to express something in secular people that resembles traditional magic beliefs in other parts of the world. As such, evidence on neuroenchantment may indeed reveal something deeper about supernatural and external attributions, rather than simply being an analogue to religion.

To summarize, each of the approaches presented above have contributed insights to our current understanding of how, when, and why religious thought, behavior, and experience result from human brain function. No approach is superior because the relative strength of all of them depends on the questions asked. They all suffer from issues of varying degrees of experimental control, ecological validity, generalizability, authenticity, demand characteristics, social desirability, and interpretability, but each approach tends to solve the issues of the other. They are, in fact, complementary.

THEORETICAL INTEGRATION

Many of the studies reviewed here appear to support particular models of the brain and functions of specific brain areas, as interpreted by the authors. Although some of these models are highly controversial, most build on specific theories from other, more established neuroscience fields, including research on sensory-motor processing, memory, attention, executive functions, the resting brain, and social cognition. Observations on religious cognition are often linked to contemporary neuroscience research by means of reverse inference to infer the functionality of individual brain areas and networks. How can we understand such specialized knowledge of the brain and its involvement in religion in a wider context? Is there a model of the brain that spans all these functions, including beliefs, attitudes, emotions, practices and experiences, by which insights from different experimental paradigms and cognitive models can be integrated?

The Predictive Processing Framework

Brain scientists across disciplines have recently embraced a unifying model of brain function, the so-called *predictive processing framework*, in which the brain is assumed to use Bayesian inference to optimize perception and cognition. Mental representations are conceptualized as consisting of top-down models based on prior experience (generative models and predictions), which are constantly compared with bottom-up information from the senses. If prediction errors are detected, the brain corrects and updates its models in order to minimize prediction error in the future (Frith, 2007; Friston & Kiebel, 2009; Friston, 2010).

The predictive processing framework has already impacted the field of the cognitive science of religion (Schjoedt et al., 2013a; 2013b; Hermans, 2015; van Elk & Aleman, 2017; Taves & Asprem, 2017; Andersen, 2019). For instance, predictive processing has been used to analyze how features in rituals seem to modulate the relative weight of prior models (predictions) and incoming sensory models in order to increase the probability of people reporting religious experiences and interpretations (Schjoedt et al., 2013a). In the neuroscience of religion, Schjoedt et al. (2013a) interpret neuroimaging findings on intercessory prayer as evidence that charismatic authority decreases believers' error monitoring in charismatic interactions to elicit experiences that correspond with religious teachings. Taking this idea one step further, van Elk and Aleman (2017) use the predictive processing framework to account for the involvement of the default mode network in self-transcendent experiences, the social cognitive network in prayer experiences and attributions of supernatural intentionality, the temporal cortex in religious visions and ecstatic experiences, and the anterior cingulate cortex and the medial prefrontal cortex in processing supernatural beliefs.

At present however, the predictive processing framework leaves CSR with more questions than answers (Schjoedt & Andersen, 2017; van Elk & Wagenmakers, 2017). How should we understand religious experience in a framework where minimizing prediction error constitutes the core function of cognition and perception? One of the major challenges for future research will be to design experimental paradigms in which predictive processes in religious experience and practice can be studied. Early attempts that use eye-tracking, EEG, and fMRI to this end seem promising, but the ambitious goal of explaining religious experience in predictive minds has not yet been achieved.

CONCLUDING REMARKS

CSR and Neuroscience of Religion

We began this chapter by setting the neuroscience of religion apart from mainstream CSR. In CSR, models and simulations, which explain a given cognitive bias or behavior, have explanatory power, but ultimately, such models need to comply with knowledge about the human brain. Human brains are organized in ways that constrain cognition and behavior. It is necessary to translate CSR models into testable hypotheses about the brain if the ambition is to understand human cognition (e.g., models of supernatural-agency representations, ritualized behavior, and religious experience). Neuroscience, at the same time, needs cognitive science to bring testable hypotheses about the brain to the table. Beyond basic neurophysiology, the human brain is still a mystery. Understanding the link between the brain and religion is impossible without the intermediate level of cognitive science to constrain predictions and interpretations.

The implicit physiological measures in neuroscience present researchers with a unique opportunity to explore human cognition, including its religious dimension. They allow cognitive scientists to test their models directly on the object they attempt to describe. This obvious advantage may be why neuroscience seems almost magical to nonprofessionals, who easily become enchanted by brain images composed of brightly colored dots and captions suggesting what they mean. Indeed, neuroscience is heavily popularized, not only by the media, but also by researchers in other fields. The only solution to this public misunderstanding of neuroscience is to propose more concise cognitive models and preregistered hypotheses, and to refrain from speculation and sensationalism.

In summary, the neuroscience of religion in its present form is fraught with problems. Studies that aim for experimental control compromise the authenticity of their study object, while studies that sacrifice control for authenticity fail to link neural activity with well-documented cognitive theories. Instead, they rely on reverse inference despite the incredible complexity of the human brain. Even the theoretical assumptions made in the image analysis of brain data make observations uncertain, from the raw signal extraction to pre-processing adjustment and normalization of data to the final statistical parametric maps of brain activity. On top of that, most studies in the study of religion use old-fashioned methods and low sample sizes that make the detection of true effects unreliable. Taken together, then, one might ask if we should pursue this research at all.

To answer such a question, we might remind ourselves of the role experimentation has played throughout science history. Experimenting with new technologies and applying measures on new subject matter has driven science and technology for centuries. Bad studies are usually followed by better ones. In psychology, experiments have a long history of suboptimal methods and wrong interpretations, but even flawed studies have led to important new understandings. For us, the answer to this question is a resounding yes! We absolutely need to do this kind of research, and we eagerly anticipate groundbreaking new research in the decade to come.

QUESTIONS FOR FUTURE RESEARCH

1. How does religious cognition work in predictive brains?
2. Do the empirical findings from different neuroscience approaches converge on religious cognition?
3. Does neuroscience provide measures that avoid the biases inherent to self-report measures?
4. Are the neural effects of religious cognition similar to or different from the effects of other worldviews such as atheism or political conservatism?

REFERENCES

Ali, S. S., Lifshitz, M., & Raz, A. (2014). Empirical neuroenchantment: From reading minds to thinking critically. *Frontiers in Human Neuroscience, 8*, 357.

Andersen, M. (2019). Predictive coding in agency detection. *Religion, Brain & Behavior, 9* (1), 65–84.

Andersen, M., Schjoedt, U., Nielbo, K. L., & Sørensen, J. (2014). Mystical experience in the lab. *Method & Theory in the Study of Religion, 26*(3), 217–245.

Azari, N. P., Nickel, J., Wunderlich, G., Niedeggen, M., Hefter, H., Tellmann, L., Herzog, H., Stoerig, P., Birnbacher, D. & Seitz, R. J. (2001). Neural correlates of religious experience. *European Journal of Neuroscience, 13*(8), 1649–1652.

Beauregard, M., & Paquette, V. (2006). Neural correlates of a mystical experience in Carmelite nuns. *Neuroscience Letters, 405*(3), 186–190.

Blanke, O., Mohr, C., Michel, C. M., Pascual-Leone, A., Brugger, P., Seeck, M., Landis, T.& Thut, G. (2005). Linking out-of-body experience and self processing to mental own-body imagery at the temporoparietal junction. *Journal of Neuroscience, 25*(3), 550–557.

Blanke, O., Pozeg, P., Hara, M., Heydrich, L., Serino, A., Yamamoto, A., Higuchi, T., Salomon, R., Seeck, M., Landis, T., Arzy, S., Herbelin, B., Bleuler, H., & Rognini, G. (2014). Neurological and robot-controlled induction of an apparition. *Current Biology, 24*(22), 2681–2686.

Bullmore, E., & Sporns, O. (2009). Complex brain networks: Graph theoretical analysis of structural and functional systems. *Nature Reviews Neuroscience, 10*(3), 186–198.

Butler, P. M., McNamara, P., & Durso, R. (2010). Deficits in the automatic activation of religious concepts in patients with Parkinson's disease. *Journal of the International Neuropsychological Society, 16*(2), 252–261.

Carhart-Harris, R. L., Leech, R., Hellyer, P. J., Shanahan, M., Feilding, A., Tagliazucchi, E., Chialvo, D. R.& Nutt, D. (2014). The entropic brain: A theory of conscious states informed by neuroimaging research with psychedelic drugs. *Frontiers in Human Neuroscience, 8*, 20.

Cristofori, I., Bulbulia, J., Shaver, J. H., Wilson, M., Krueger, F., & Grafman, J. (2016). Neural correlates of mystical experience. *Neuropsychologia, 80*, 212–220.

d'Aquili, E. G., & Newberg, A. B. (1999). *The mystical mind: Probing the biology of religious experience*. Minneapolis, MN. Fortress Press.

Deeley, Q., Oakley, D. A., Walsh, E., Bell, V., Mehta, M. A., & Halligan, P. W. (2014). Modelling psychiatric and cultural possession phenomena with suggestion and fMRI. *Cortex, 53*, 107–119.

Deeley, Q., Walsh, E., Oakley, D. A., Bell, V., Koppel, C., Mehta, M. A., & Halligan, P. W. (2013). Using hypnotic suggestion to model loss of control and awareness of movements: An exploratory fMRI study. *PloS One, 8*(10), Article e78324.

Epley, N., Converse, B. A., Delbosc, A., Monteleone, G. A., & Cacioppo, J. T. (2009). Believers' estimates of God's beliefs are more egocentric than estimates of other people's beliefs. *PNAS, 106*(51), 21533–21538.

Ehrsson, H. H. (2007). The experimental induction of out-of-body experiences. *Science, 317*(5841), 1048.

Friston, K. (2010). The free-energy principle: A unified brain theory? *Nature Reviews Neuroscience, 11*(2), 127–138.

Friston, K., & Kiebel, S. (2009). Predictive coding under the free-energy principle. *Philosophical Transactions of the Royal Society of London B: Biological Sciences, 364*(1521), 1211–1221.

Frith, C. D. (2007). *Making up the mind: How the brain creates our mental world*. Malden, MA: Blackwell.

Ferguson, M. A., Nielsen, J. A., King, J. B., Dai, L., Giangrasso, D. M., Holman, R., Korenberg, J. R., & Anderson, J. S. (2016). Reward, salience, and attentional networks are activated by religious experience in devout Mormons, *Social Neuroscience, 13*(1), 104–116.

Galanter, M., Josipovic, Z., Dermatis, H., Weber, J., & Millard, M. A. (2017). An initial fMRI study on neural correlates of prayer in members of Alcoholics Anonymous. *American Journal of Drug and Alcohol Abuse, 43*(1), 44–54.

Grafman, J., Cristofori, I., Zhong, W., & Bulbulia, J. (2020). The neural basis of religious cognition. *Current Directions in Psychological Science, 29*(2), 126–133.

Granqvist, P., Fredrikson, M., Unge, P., Hagenfeldt, A., Valind, S., Larhammar, D., & Larsson, M. (2005). Sensed presence and mystical experiences are predicted by suggestibility, not by the application of transcranial weak complex magnetic fields. *Neuroscience Letters, 379*(1), 1–6.

Han S., Mao, L., Gu, X., Zhu, Y., Ge, J., & Ma, Y. (2008). Neural consequences of religious belief on self-referential processing. *Social Neuroscience, 3*, 1–15.

Han, S., Gu, X., Mao, L., Ge, J., Wang, G., & Ma, Y. (2009). Neural substrates of self-referential processing in Chinese Buddhists. Social Cognitive and Affective *Neuroscience, 5*(2–3), 332–339.

Harris, S., Kaplan, J. T., Curiel, A., Bookheimer, S. Y., Iacoboni, M., & Cohen, M. S. (2009). The neural correlates of religious and nonreligious belief. *PLoS One, 4*(10), Article e7272.

Hermans, C. A. (2015). Towards a theory of spiritual and religious experiences. *Archive for the Psychology of Religion, 37*(2), 141–167.

Hoogeveen, S., Schjoedt, U., & van Elk, M. (2018). Did I do that? Expectancy effects of brain stimulation on error-related negativity and sense of agency. *Journal of Cognitive Neuroscience, 30*(11), 1720–1733.

Hoogeveen, S., Snoek, L., & van Elk, M. (2020). Religious belief and cognitive conflict sensitivity: A preregistered fMRI study. *Cortex, 129*, 247–265.

Inzlicht, M., & Tullett, A. M. (2009). Reflecting on God: Religious primes can reduce neurophysiological response to errors. *Psychological Science, 21*(8), 1184–1190.

Inzlicht, M., Tullett, A. M., & Good, M. (2011). The need to believe: a neuroscience account of religion as a motivated process. *Religion, Brain & Behavior, 1*(3), 192–212.

Ionta, S., Heydrich, L., Lenggenhager, B., Mouthon, M., Fornar, E., Chapuis, D., Gassert, R. & Blanke, O. (2011). Multisensory mechanisms in temporo-parietal cortex support self-location and first-person perspective. *Neuron, 70*(2), 363–374.

Johnstone, B., Yoon, D. P., Rupright, J., & Reid-Arndt, S. (2009). Relationships among spiritual beliefs, religious practises, congregational support and health for individuals with traumatic brain injury. *Brain Injury, 23*(5), 411–419.

Kapogiannis, D., Barbey, A. K., Su, M., Zamboni, G., Krueger, F., & Grafman, J. (2009). Cognitive and neural foundations of religious belief. *PNAS, 106*(12), 4876–4881.

Kapogiannis, D., Barbey, A. K., Su, M., Krueger, F., & Grafman, J. (2009). Neuroanatomical variability of religiosity. *PloS One, 4*(9), Article e7180.

Ladd, K. L., Cook, C. A., Foreman, K. M., & Ritter, E. A. (2015). Neuroimaging of prayer: Questions of validity. *Psychology of Religion and Spirituality, 7*(2), 100–108.

Lenggenhager, B., Tadi, T., Metzinger, T., & Blanke, O. (2007). Video ergo sum: Manipulating bodily self-consciousness. *Science, 317*(5841), 1096–1099.

Lindeman, M., Svedholm, A. M., Riekki, T., Raij, T., & Hari, R. (2013). Is it just a brick wall or a sign from the universe? An fMRI study of supernatural believers and skeptics. *Social Cognitive and Affective Neuroscience, 8*(8), 943–949.

McNamara, P. (2009). *The neuroscience of religious experience.* Cambridge, UK: Cambridge University Press.

McNamara, P. (2019). *Religion, neuroscience and the self: A new personalism.* New York: Routledge.

Miller, L., Balodis, I. M., McClintock, C. H., Xu, J., Lacadie, C. M., Sinha, R., & Potenza, M. N. (2018). Neural correlates of personalized spiritual experiences. *Cerebral Cortex, 29*(6), 2331–2338.

Miller, L., Bansal, R., Wickramaratne, P., Hao, X., Tenke, C. E., Weissman, M. M., & Peterson, B. S. (2014). Neuroanatomical correlates of religiosity and spirituality: A study in adults at high and low familial risk for depression. *JAMA Psychiatry, 71*(2), 128–135.

Newberg, A. B., Alavi, A., Baime, M., Pourdehnad, M., Santanna, J., & d'Aquili, E. (2001). The measurement of regional cerebral blood flow during the complex cognitive task of meditation: A preliminary SPECT study. *Psychiatric Research: Neuroimaging, 106*, 113–122.

Newberg, A. B., Pourdehnad, M., Alavi, A., & d'Aquili, E. G. (2003): Cerebral blood flow during meditative prayer: Preliminary findings and methodological issues. *Perceptual and Motor Skills, 97*(2), 625–630.

Newberg, A. B., Wintering, N, Morgan, D., & Waldman, M. R. (2006) The measurement of regional blood flow during glossolalia: A preliminary SPECT study. *Psychiatry Research: Neuroimaging,.148*, 67–71.

Neubauer, R. L. (2014). Prayer as an interpersonal relationship: A neuroimaging study. *Religion, Brain & Behavior, 4*(2), 92–103.

Owen, A. D., Hayward, R. D., Koenig, H. G., Steffens, D. C., & Payne, M. E. (2011). Religious factors and hippocampal atrophy in late life. *PloS One, 6*(3), Article e17006.

Persinger, M. A. (1983): Religious and mystical experiences as artifacts of temporal lobe function: A general hypothesis. *Perceptual and Motor Skills, 57*, 1255–1262.

Riekki, T., Lindeman, M., & Raij, T. T. (2014). Supernatural believers attribute more intentions to random movement than skeptics: An fMRI study. *Social Neuroscience, 9*(4), 400–411.

Schjoedt, U. (2009). The religious brain: A general introduction to the experimental neuroscience of religion. *Method & Theory in the Study of Religion, 21*(3), 310–339.

Schjoedt, U. (2011). The neural correlates of religious experience. *Religion, 41*(1), 91–95.

Schjoedt, U., & Andersen, M. (2017). How does religious experience work in predictive minds? *Religion, Brain & Behavior, 7*(4), 320–323.

Schjoedt, U., & Bulbulia, J. (2011) The need to believe in conflicting propositions. *Religion, Brain & Behavior, 1*(3), 236–239.

Schjoedt, U., Stødkilde-Jørgensen, H., Geertz, A. W., Lund, T. E., & Roepstorff, A. (2011). The power of charisma: Perceived charisma inhibits the frontal executive network of believers in intercessory prayer. *Social Cognitive and Affective Neuroscience, 6*(1), 119–127.

Schjoedt, U., Stødkilde-Jørgensen, H., Geertz, A. W., & Roepstorff, A. (2008). Rewarding prayers. *Neuroscience Letters, 443*(3), 165–168.

Schjoedt, U., Stødkilde-Jørgensen, H., Geertz, A. W., & Roepstorff, A. (2009). Highly religious participants recruit areas of social cognition in personal prayer. *Social Cognitive and Affective Neuroscience, 4*(2), 199–207.

Schjoedt, U., Sørensen, J., Nielbo, K. L., Xygalatas, D., Mitkidis, P., & Bulbulia, J. (2013a). Cognitive resource depletion in religious interactions. *Religion, Brain & Behavior, 3*(1), 39–55.

Schjoedt, U., Sørensen, J., Nielbo, K. L., Xygalatas, D., Mitkidis, P., & Bulbulia, J. (2013b). The resource model and the principle of predictive coding: A framework for analyzing proximate effects of ritual. *Religion, Brain & Behavior, 3*(1), 79–86.

Schwarz, K. A., & Büchel, C. (2015). Cognition and the placebo effect–dissociating subjective perception and actual performance. *PloS One, 10*(7), Article e0130492.

Simmonds-Moore, C., Rice, D. L., O'Gwin, C., & Hopkins, R. (2019). Exceptional experiences following exposure to a sham "God Helmet": Evidence for placebo, individual difference, and time of day influences. *Imagination, Cognition and Personality, 39*(1), 44–87.

Slama, H., Caspar, E. A., Gevers, W., & Cleeremans, A. (2013). Placebo-suggestion modulates conflict resolution in the Stroop task. *PloS One, 8*(10), Article e75701.

Snoek, L., Miletić, S., & Scholte, H. S. (2019). How to control for confounds in decoding analyses of neuroimaging data. *NeuroImage, 184,* 741–760.

Snoek, L., van der Miesen, M. M., Beemsterboer, T., Van Der Leij, A., Eigenhuis, A., & Scholte, H. S. (2021). The Amsterdam Open MRI Collection, a set of multimodal MRI datasets for individual difference analyses. *Scientific Data, 8*(1), 1–23.

Spottiswoode, S. J. P. (1997). Geomagnetic fluctuations and free response anomalous cognition: A new understanding. *Journal of Parapsychology, 61*(1), 3–12.

Spottiswoode, S. J. P., & May, E. C. (1997). Anomalous cognition effect size: Dependence on sidereal time and solar wind parameters. *The Parapsychological Association 40th Annual Convention* [Conference publication]. Brighton, England.

Taves, A. (2009). *Religious experience reconsidered: A building-block approach to the study of religion and other special things.* Princeton, NJ: Princeton University Press.

Taves, A., & Asprem, E. (2017). Experience as event: event cognition and the study of (religious) experiences. *Religion, Brain & Behavior, 7*(1), 43–62.

Urgesi, C., Aglioti, S. M., Skrap, M., & Fabbro, F. (2010). The spiritual brain: selective cortical lesions modulate human self-transcendence. *Neuron, 65*(3), 309–319.

van Elk, M., (2015. An EEG study on the effects of induced spiritual experiences on somatosensory processing and sensory suppression. *Journal for the Cognitive Science of Religion, 2*(2), 121–157.

van Elk, M., & Aleman, A. (2017). Brain mechanisms in religion and spirituality: An integrative predictive processing framework. *Neuroscience & Biobehavioral Reviews, 73,* 359–378.

van Elk, M., Groenendijk, E., & Hoogeveen, S. (2020). Placebo brain stimulation affects subjective but not neurocognitive measures of error processing. *Journal of Cognitive Enhancement, 4,* 389–400.

van Elk, M., & Snoek, L. (2019). The relationship between individual differences in gray matter volume and religiosity and mystical experiences: A preregistered voxel-based morphometry study. *European Journal of Neuroscience, 51*(3): 850–865.

van Elk, M., & Wagenmakers, E. J. (2017). Can the experimental study of religion be advanced using a Bayesian predictive framework? *Religion, Brain & Behavior, 7*(4), 331–334.

Wiech, K., Farias, M., Kahane, G., Shackel, N., Tiede, W., & Tracey, I. (2008). An fMRI study measuring analgesia enhanced by religion as a belief system. *Pain, 139*(2), 467–476.

CHAPTER 18

SOUL MATES? CONFLICTS AND COMPLEMENTARITIES IN THE EVOLUTIONARY AND COGNITIVE SCIENCES OF RELIGION

RICHARD SOSIS, JOHN SHAVER,
BENJAMIN GRANT PURZYCKI, AND
JORDAN KIPER

INTRODUCTION

THE cross-cultural prevalence and persistence of religious expression demands evolutionary investigation and explanation. It is thus unsurprising that evolutionary approaches to the study of religion have flourished in recent years. Although evolutionary theory has informed some work in the cognitive science of religion (CSR), the field in general has not fully embraced selectionist analyses.

We aim to (a) provide a brief overview of the evolutionary study of religion, (b) examine how the evolutionary and cognitive sciences of religion differ, and (c) explore areas of potential integration between these two scientific fields of inquiry. We conclude that although the evolutionary and cognitive sciences of religion could continue as quasi-independent fields, both would benefit from theoretical and methodological integration.

THE EVOLUTIONARY STUDY OF RELIGION:
A BRIEF HISTORY

The evolutionary study of religion begins with Charles Darwin. Darwin, after all, offered a mechanism to explain evolutionary change—namely, natural selection. Yet, despite an illustrious founder, the beginnings of the evolutionary study of religion were not auspicious. Remarkably, Darwin thought the solution to the problem of the origin of religion was self-evident. In *Descent of Man, and Selection in Relation to Sex* (1871), he wrote: "As soon as the important faculties of the imagination, wonder, and curiosity, together with some power of reasoning, had become partially developed, man would naturally crave to understand what was passing around him, and would have vaguely speculated on his own existence" (Darwin, 2005; p. 678). In other words, once the human mind evolved, people needed answers to existential problems; religions, Darwin suggested, evolved to provide those answers.

Reading Darwin's comments on religion is a mildly disturbing experience for those of us who hold him as one of our intellectual heroes. How could Darwin, who was so careful in his analyses of the hundreds of species he discussed throughout his writings, completely miss that the structure and form of religion cry out for explanation? Simply contemplating one's existence does not lead one to build ornate cathedrals, undergo circumcision, forgo sex, or turn one's dinner into charcoal for immaterial beings. And as anthropologists have long noted, unlike typical explanations of events, which seek to clarify and simplify, religious explanations make things more complicated (Evans-Pritchard, 1937). Religions, as Sperber (1985, p. 85) observes, "create relevant mysteries." Darwin was correct that humans gravitate toward religious explanations, but he apparently did not appreciate the complexity of this process. As Hume famously commented, "explanation is where the mind rests"; but Darwin took us no further in understanding why the human mind so often rests on religious explanations.

Following Darwin, the evolutionary study of religion proceeded, by all measures, rather slowly. It was nearly a full century after Darwin's initial thoughts before another biologist would seriously engage the study of religion. It was marine biologist and Oxford professor Sir Alister Hardy, who is most famous or, more accurately, infamous for his aquatic ape hypothesis—but he also had a deep interest in religion. He was invited to give the Gifford Lectures at Aberdeen University in 1963–1964 and 1964–1965, and he used them to offer an evolutionary explanation of religion. Hardy was impressed by the universality of religious experience and proposed that religion evolved because it was favored by natural selection. Hardy's lectures were published in two volumes, regrettably entitled *The Living Stream* (Hardy, 1965) and *The Divine Flame* (Hardy, 1966). With these titles, these works were probably shelved next to books on new age spirituality and, not surprisingly, they have largely been forgotten. Although Hardy founded the Religious Experience Research Centre, for which he was awarded the Templeton Prize in 1985, his work did not jumpstart the still embryonic evolutionary study of religion.

A decade later, however, the evolutionary study of religion began showing signs of life. The eminent Harvard entomologist, E. O. Wilson, included a chapter on religion in his award-winning *On Human Nature* (1978). Wilson proposed that successful religions were those that enhanced the survivorship and reproduction of populations. Motivated by Wilson's writings, biological anthropologist Vernon Reynolds and sociologist Ralph Tanner (1983) collaborated on an innovative study entitled *The Biology of Religion*, in which they argued that religion was a "handbook of parental investment." They showed that in economically poor environments, whose populations experienced high mortality rates, religions were generally pronatalist; whereas in areas of greater health and wealth religions were antinatalist. Their findings were important because they suggested that religion was not irrational or impervious to external forces such as economics and the environment; rather, religions adapted to their local ecologies. Indeed, Reynolds and Tanner (1995) retitled the revised version of their book *The Social Ecology of Religion*.

The rest of the 1980s and most of the 1990s remained notably stagnant for the evolutionary study of religion. But by the mid- to late 1990s, an avalanche had begun, and suddenly a spate of books and articles by well-known academics applied evolutionary theory to the study of religion. For example, the renowned scholar of Greek religion and myth Walter Burkert (1996), examined Greek religion through a Darwinian lens in *The Creation of the Sacred*. And another prominent scholar, Cambridge zoologist Robert Hinde (1999), published *Why Gods Persist*.

It is not until biologist David Sloan Wilson published *Darwin's Cathedral* (2002), however, that the evolutionary study of religion appears to have crossed the Rubicon. Wilson argued that religion had evolved because it benefits groups. In other words, religion is a group-level adaptation. Despite Wilson's reliance on group selection as an explanatory mechanism, an approach that elicited great skepticism among evolutionary researchers who were studying human behavior at the time, the book did catalyze the evolutionary study of religion. It would probably be overstating the impact of *Darwin's Cathedral* to say that Wilson was the founder of the contemporary evolutionary study of religion, but his work is surely one of the major influences in the field. Although evolutionary anthropologists Lee Cronk (1994) and William Irons (1996) had pursued pioneering adaptationist analyses of religion in the 1990s, it was Wilson's work, and subsequent collaborations, that gave the adaptationist approach to religion visibility, and introduced the evolutionary study of religion to religious studies and other humanities-based scholars.

It is worth noting that prior to *Darwin's Cathedral*, research in the cognitive science of religion was not completely devoid of evolutionary thinking. Several landmark studies by scholars who focused on religious cognition, such as Guthrie's (1980, 1993) work on anthropomorphism, relied on evolutionary frameworks to support their theories. But it was not until the early 2000s that the evolutionary and cognitive sciences of religion began to cross-pollinate. The early 2000s saw the publication of seminal books in the cognitive science of religion by two cognitive anthropologists: *Religion Explained* by Pascal Boyer (2001), and *In Gods We Trust* by Scott Atran (2002). Both volumes, whose impact on the cognitive science of religion can hardly be overstated, drew from evolutionary psychology and treated religion as an evolutionary byproduct. However, as we will see, by defining religion as a byproduct, an analytical dead end, they were not well positioned to contribute to subsequent evolutionary analyses of religion.

EVOLUTIONARY APPROACHES TO RELIGION

The efforts to apply evolutionary theory to the study of religion do not represent a single unified endeavor or research program. Some of the differences, as we discuss below, are disciplinary and methodological in nature. Other differences, however, have deep theoretical roots. Among evolutionary scholars of religion, two of the most salient areas of disagreement concern (a) whether religion is a cognitive byproduct or a manifestation of adaptive behavioral plasticity, and (b) whether individual- or group-level selection processes have been a more potent evolutionary force in shaping the significant features of religion. The first of these disagreements has also been a topic of considerable debate between adaptationists and cognitive scientists of religion.

Researchers' focus of study strongly influences how they interpret the effects of natural selection on religion. When, for instance, researchers concentrate on the cognitive requirements of religious thought, they typically conclude that religious beliefs are merely byproducts of psychological adaptations that were designed for other purposes (e.g., Boyer, 2001; Guthrie, 1993). But when researchers examine the social consequences of ritual behavior, the adaptive benefits of religion become salient (e.g., Alcorta & Sosis, 2005). When research emphasizes individual variation in religious behavior, it is obvious that these adaptive benefits are not equally achieved; some benefit more than others (Cronk, 1994; Shaver, 2015; Shaver & Sosis, 2014). However, research that has focused on group-level dynamics reveals that some religious groups are more successful than others. Scholars who are study these dynamics argue that religious groups function as adaptive units that are subject to cultural group selection (Norenzayan, 2013; Wilson, 2002).

These differences in research foci roughly correspond to three relatively distinct evolutionary approaches to the study of human behavior: *evolutionary psychology*, *human behavioral ecology*, and *dual inheritance theory* (Smith, 2000). We will describe how each of these evolutionary subfields has approached the study of religion.

Before proceeding, and by way of disclosure, we mention that the first author's background and training is primarily, but not exclusively, in human behavioral ecology. The coauthors, however, have broader training in all the evolutionary subfields. Moreover, we have collectively pursued research in all three subfields (e.g., Kiper & Sosis, 2016; Shaver, 2015; Shaver & Sosis, 2014; Wildman & Sosis, 2011) and in the cognitive sciences (e.g., Purzycki et al., 2012). Elsewhere, we have argued that viewing these evolutionary approaches as complementary, rather than contradictory, offers the greatest potential to explain the complex phenomenon of religion (Shaver et al., 2016). Since evolved cognitive faculties, memory and its organization, behavioral expression, interpersonal social psychological responses, and the social and natural environments are all at play in the formation of religious systems, diverse approaches are necessary if we wish to uncover the evolutionary origins and development of religion.

Evolutionary Psychology of Religion

Evolutionary psychologists use the theory of natural selection to generate hypotheses about pan-human psychological design; they contend that the human mind consists of several cognitive systems that were designed to solve specific adaptive problems that ancestral human populations faced (Tooby & Cosmides, 1992). Because the human brain consists of cognitive adaptations that are designed to solve ancestral problems, and because modern environments often differ substantially from ancestral ones, cognitive adaptations can produce thoughts and behaviors that are neutral, maladaptive, or even unrelated to the problems they arose to solve. Indeed, the majority of evolutionary psychologists of religion hold that the human tendency toward supernatural belief is an evolutionary byproduct of cognitive systems that were originally meant to solve adaptive problems unrelated to religion (Kirkpatrick, 2006, 2008). That is, the human proclivity to believe in the supernatural is the result of an evolved pan-human psychological design; but the cognitive architecture that supports supernatural belief did not arise because belief in supernatural agents was itself adaptive.

The theoretical stance of evolutionary psychologists motivates their research questions, which include questions about the developmental trajectories of the cognitive abilities that are assumed to contribute to supernatural belief, their presence in adults, and their cross-cultural prevalence. Evolutionary psychologists generally test their assumptions in laboratory and field experiments, as well as survey research. Cognitive scientists of religion who rely on evolutionary thinking have primarily allied themselves with evolutionary psychology. Indeed, the cognitive science of religion considers many of the researchers employing evolutionary psychology in the study of religion, such as Guthrie, Boyer, and Bering, as part of their intellectual community.

Evolutionary psychologists of religion assume that several cognitive systems contribute to our propensity to believe in the supernatural. Notably, Guthrie (1993) argues that the human tendency to anthropomorphize arose as a result of selection pressures that favored the ability to perceive agents and agency in the environment, and that these abilities contribute to the human propensity to interpret events in terms of supernatural agency. He suggests that perceiving agents, even when there are none, is advantageous because *not* detecting harmful agents that are present would be deleterious. Although this promiscuous agency detection did not emerge for purposes relating to religion, and though the evolutionary roots of this capacity run deep, it is nonetheless the ability to perceive unseen agents that gives rise to religious perceptions and explanations of the mysterious (Barrett, 2004; cf. Andersen, 2019; Van Leeuwen & van Elk, 2018). Furthermore, perceptions of spirits, demons, gods, and other supernatural agents are the natural byproduct of such a sensitive system. Humans explain the world in terms of agency, and frequently believe that events are caused by supernatural agents.

Human social interactions require the ability to understand and appreciate what others are thinking and feeling. Indeed, human sociality is built on the cognitive ability to interpret other individuals as having their own distinct perceptions, desires, and beliefs. This capacity, known as theory of mind ([ToM]; Premack & Woodruff, 1978), arose for reasons unrelated to religion, but it now contributes to the human propensity to believe that supernatural agents have minds and their own wishes and desires. But perceiving and thinking about such entities would contribute little to human sociality unless it tapped into moral cognition as well (Gray et al., 2012). Some evidence suggests that it does (Purzycki et al., 2012), even when the gods are not thought of as concerned with moral behavior (Purzycki, 2013, 2016).

Other work suggests that humans are primed from an early age to accept teleological explanations. Deborah Kelemen, for example, has suggested that children are "intuitive theists," who believe that things in the natural world have been purposefully designed (Kelemen, 2004). Her studies have shown that children readily assert that both natural objects and artifacts exist for a reason. Moreover, this bias is not limited to children; lesser educated adults show the same tendency (Casler & Kelemen, 2007), and under conditions of high cognitive load, even scientifically trained adults exhibit the same biases (Kelemen & Rossett, 2009). Although "promiscuous teleology" is thought to be the result of cognitive modules that evolved to reason about the biological world (e.g., Atran, 1995), it also renders belief in a creator intuitive, and leads to interpretations that events happen for a purpose—an interpretive framework that many religions share.

Although the mainstream view among evolutionary psychologists is that religious representations are evolutionary byproducts, a few scholars have proposed that selection processes have resulted in specific psychological adaptations for religion. For example, Bering (2006) has provided evidence in support of the contention that humans are intuitive dualists, and unless formally taught otherwise, they exhibit a tendency to conceptually separate minds from bodies. This propensity leads to the belief that minds and/or souls can continue to exist after death (Bering, 2006). Additionally, Johnson and Bering (2006) argue that the human tendency to fear supernatural punishment is an adaptation that arose because individuals who feared supernatural punishment were able to inhibit self-interested behaviors and social transgressions that would have been punished by other group members. Because god-fearing individuals were more successful at reaping the benefits of cooperation in ancestral environments, selection favored these propensities. Others argue that religions evolved, at least in part, to support mate discrimination or finding other individuals who prefer monogamous long-term relationships and high fertility (Slone, 2008; Weede et al., 2008). Indeed, several authors interpret the lower promiscuity and higher fertility levels of religious people as an outcome of such strategies (Blume, 2010; Bulbulia et al., 2015; Kaufmann, 2010).

Human Behavioral Ecology of Religion

The majority of evolutionary psychologists of religion speculate that religious beliefs and behaviors are a byproduct of cognitive systems that evolved to respond to selection pressures in ancestral environments (and that these selection pressures were unrelated to those that now motivate religious beliefs and behaviors). However, behavioral ecologists assume that selection has produced behavior-generating mechanisms that enable individuals to respond optimally to diverse environmental conditions, and that cross-cultural variation in behavior represents a manifestation of this behavioral plasticity. Contrary to the majority of cognitive approaches, behavioral ecologists begin their analyses by assessing how behaviors are adapted to current socioecologies. For the behavioral ecologist, determining adaptiveness means measuring the costs and benefits of a behavior, given available alternatives, in an effort to understand the selection pressures at work in any given environment. In general, behavioral ecologists of religion start by testing hypotheses derived from models that assume an individual's behavior is adaptive in its current environment. Human behavioral ecologists are typically anthropologists, who engage in long-term ethnographic research and use data derived from field experiments and systematic behavioral observation to test hypotheses. They attempt to address research questions about the adaptiveness of individuals' religious behavior in a particular environment. While the behavioral ecology of religion is still in its infancy (Sosis & Bulbulia, 2011), research to date has been both diverse and fruitful. Here we focus on just a few of these research programs.

At first glance, religious behavior appears maladaptive; it is often materially, energetically, and temporally expensive and thus superficially appears to be detrimental to individuals' immediate somatic and reproductive self-interest. However, behavioral ecologists interpret these costs as investments that return material benefits that positively impact fitness. To explain the adaptive benefits of ritual behavior, behavioral ecologists borrow two key insights from social theorists. First, Durkheim (2001) speculated that the effervescent nature of collective rituals binds group members together and increases within-group cohesion. Second, Rappaport's (1999) definition of ritual as "the performance of more or less invariant sequences of formal acts and utterances not entirely encoded by the performer" (Rappaport, p. 24). has been widely employed by behavioral ecologists. He argued that rituals are able to increase social solidarity because they communicate adherence to a moral code and commitment to a social order, which in turn promotes trust, and hence cooperation.

Like all collectivities, religious groups are susceptible to exploitation by free-riders, who reap the benefits of group cooperation without cooperating themselves. Irons (2001) argued that the costliness of religious obligations functions as commitment devices and serves to minimize the free-rider problem, because only those who are truly committed to the group would be willing to incur the costs of these obligations. In other words, individuals who observe religious taboos and perform religious rituals communicate (or "signal") their commitment to the group and, in turn, benefit from increased cooperation; these material benefits are ultimately translated into reproductive success.

This theoretical framework, known as the *costly signaling theory of religion*, suggests that religious groups that require costly behaviors of their members will exhibit high levels of cooperation. For example, Sosis and Bressler (2003) found that nineteenth-century religious communes in United States that demanded more costly behaviors of group members out-survived those with fewer costly obligations. Moreover, the ritual costs associated with group membership vary across environments and increase as a function of the risks of exploiting these resources via free-riding. Perhaps the greatest risks of freer-riding occur among groups engaged in warfare, where shirking on one's commitment to the group might mean death to other group members. Indeed, Sosis et al. (2007) found that cultures engaged in endemic warfare have the most taxing religious rites. Research has also shown that religious communities are able to stabilize at larger group sizes (Dunbar & Sosis, 2018), presumably affording them greater defense and resource exploitation capacities. In general, a significant body of empirical research now provides support for the premise that costs paid in ritual performance return high levels of cooperation (e.g., Power, 2017a, 2017b; Ruffle & Sosis, 2007; Soler, 2012; Sosis & Ruffle, 2003).

Behavioral ecologists have also explored the socioecological conditions that have favored specific religious behavioral patterns. For example, Strassmann's (1992, 1996) work with the Dogon of Mali examined the manner in which religious taboos and rituals surrounding sexual activity, such as attending menstrual huts, reduce the risks of cuckoldry. And Strassmann et al. (2012) specifically showed how the various religions practiced by the Dogon differentially impact cuckoldry rates.

In other studies, behavioral ecologists have begun to address the "paradox of religious fertility" (Shaver, 2017). Many religious families globally have large families, and because resources are finite, there is typically a negative relationship between family size and child success on education and health measures. But large family size does not seem to negatively impact religious children. Shaver and his colleagues have suggested that religious families receive help raising their children from coreligionists, known as *allocare*, which offsets the costs of their large families. Shaver et al. (2019), for example, found that religious New Zealanders were more likely to engage in allocare than their secular counterparts. Moreover, Shaver et al. (2020) showed that religious women in the United Kingdom receive more social support than secular women and that this support is positively associated with fertility and children's cognitive development.

Dual Inheritance Theories of Religion

The aforementioned evolutionary approaches to the study of religion focus on the individual-level evolutionary forces that led to the emergence of religious belief and behavior. But there is a third group of scholars who emphasize that selection operating at the group level might explain the origins and proliferation of religions. Dual inheritance theory (DIT) posits that genes and culture provide separate but interacting forms of inheritance. DIT theorists suggest that cultures, like genes, exhibit the three necessary conditions for evolution by natural selection: variation, inheritance, and fitness consequences. Because people acquire a significant amounts of information from other group members and cultures differ, the information some groups accumulate allows them to overcome adaptive problems better, and thus they spread at the expense of less successful groups (Boyd & Richerson, 1985).

Proponents of DIT are, typically, evolutionary biologists, anthropologists, and economists, who rely upon computer simulations and field and laboratory experiments to test mathematical models of cultural evolutionary processes. Many DIT scholars have suggested that religious groups are subject to these cultural evolutionary processes.

Notably, D. S. Wilson (2002) argues that because religious groups limit self-interested behavior but provide secular utility to their members, they function as adaptive units. When communities function as units, they are subject to the forces of cultural group selection, and better adapted religions spread at the expense of those less equipped to overcome socioenvironmental challenges. Wilson shows how religions, such as Calvinist Christianity and Jainism, provide material benefits for their members, while limiting self-interested behaviors and encouraging altruism toward other group members.

Other dual inheritance theorists share with evolutionary psychologists the assumption that supernatural beliefs are byproducts of cognitive systems and processing tendencies, such as an agency detection device, theory of mind mechanisms, and teleological reasoning. But the dual inheritance theorists also argue that variants of supernatural belief and religious groups are subject to cultural selection (e.g., Atran & Henrich, 2010; Norenzayan, 2013). These theorists note that groups committed to omniscient high gods who they believed intervene in human affairs and punish noncooperators were more successful than groups whose belief systems did not promote cooperation as effectively. In this way, cultural evolutionary processes led to the current global pattern of limited religious diversity—more than half the world's population practices Christianity or Islam, which affirm belief in an omniscient high god that can punish uncooperative behavior. To support these assertions, DIT theorists cite the results of experimental studies showing that people are more cooperative under perceived social monitoring (e.g., Bering et al., 2005); that religious primes decrease cheating behavior and increase generosity, fairness, cooperation, and the punishment of noncooperators (Norenzayan & Shariff, 2008), and that religious individuals are trusted more than nonreligious individuals (Purzycki & Arakchaa, 2013).

Norenzayan (2013), who has developed this argument extensively, recognizes that the widespread cooperation among non-kin in large-scale human societies is a significant evolutionary puzzle. He speculates that powerful, morally interested "Big Gods," with their ability to promote prosocial behavior, enabled large-scale societies to emerge. Specifically, he posits that through coevolutionary processes, the groups that embraced watchful and omniscient gods were able to cooperate and outcompete groups that were unable to extend cooperation beyond kin and reciprocal relations.

Dual inheritance theorists also assume that humans are endowed with psychological adaptations for general-purpose learning, which allow for the rapid gathering of fitness-relevant information from other group members. These evolved abilities bias attention and learning toward successful group members, which contributes to the cultural accumulation of solutions to significant fitness concerns, such as techniques for tool construction or methods of agricultural production (Boyd & Richerson, 1985; Richerson & Boyd, 2005). One of these biases is the *frequency bias*, which increases the probability of learning information that is copious in a social environment. In terms of religious beliefs, the more people believe something and express that belief, the more likely an individual is to learn that belief and act on it as well (Henrich, 2016). Another such bias is the *prestige bias*, which concerns specific sources of informational transfers. Like parents and successful hunters, priests, rabbis, shamans, lamas, mullahs, and other religious leaders are likely to transfer information with high fidelity, because it is assumed that selection has favored learning mechanisms that encourage us to copy the behavior of successful individuals.

Differences between the Evolutionary and Cognitive Sciences of Religion

Scholars have identified various key events, conferences, or milestone publications—spanning decades—that allegedly mark the founding of cognitive science of religion (CSR) (Sosis, 2017). Here is not the place to debate these alternative narratives. What is relevant here is that regardless of when the field was actually founded, by the 2000s, when cognitive scientists of religion began to regularly engage with scholars trained in evolution, CSR was already a well-established field of study. Again, this is not to say that some of the founding CSR researchers did not consider evolutionary perspectives or attempt to explain the evolution of religious cognition. They did. However, adaptationist approaches were absent from early discourse in cognitive science of religion. Consequently, two key areas of disagreement emerged once evolutionary and cognitive scientists began to seriously engage each other's work: whether religious expressions should be understood as adaptations or byproducts, and whether religion should be characterized by maturational or practiced naturalness.

Adaptationist versus Byproduct Debate

The pioneering work of early CSR researchers, including E. Thomas Lawson, Robert McCauley, Justin Barrett, Harvey Whitehouse, and Pascal Boyer, uniformly maintained that the psychological mechanisms involved in the production of religious beliefs and behaviors were not designed to produce these beliefs and behaviors. This position has become axiomatic among cognitive scientists of religion.

In the early 2000s, when evolutionary scholars finally began to engage with the burgeoning CSR literature, they were puzzled by what they encountered. Biologists argue for high standards before a trait can be accepted as an adaptation, but they caution that nonadaptive explanations should be offered as a last resort because they stifle further scientific enquiry (Krebs & Davies, 1993, p. 31). Yet the cognitivists embraced religion as a byproduct even though adaptationist hypotheses had never been evaluated. As noted, not until the publication of D. S. Wilson's (2002) *Darwin's Cathedral* was there a significant challenge to the byproduct position; and Wilson did not tackle the byproduct position of the cognitivists but the byproduct views of the prominent sociologists Rodney Stark, William Bainbridge, and Roger Finke. Wilson offered an adaptationist account of religion based on cultural group selection models that focused on the secular utility of religion at the group level. Although Wilson demonstrated that religion can confer great benefits on its constituents, he did not address the underlying psychology of religious beliefs that were of interest to the cognitive scientists, and thus did little to sway them from their anti-adaptationist stance (e.g., Boyer, 2004).

The burden of evidence required to demonstrate an adaptation is considerable and unfortunately there is no agreed-upon protocol for accepting or rejecting what counts as an adaptation. Andrews et al. (2002) reviewed six evidentiary standards that have been employed by biologists to identify adaptations, including phylogenetic comparisons, fitness maximization, and beneficial effects in ancestral environments, but their thorough review also highlights the limitations of each of the approaches they discuss. Williams (1966), the recognized father of the adaptationist program, cautioned that alternative explanations for the emergence of trait characteristics had to be eliminated, but he also recognized that there is no universal list of evidentiary standards that can be applied to all traits. He argued that adaptations should exhibit evidence of "special design"; they should efficiently solve the adaptive problem they are purported to solve and demonstrate reliability, economy, and precision.

Despite the adaptationists' inability to conclusively eliminate all alternative explanations of a trait's emergence in a particular round of hypothesis testing, the cumulative output of sustained, rigorous hypothesis testing can reasonably support the existence of an adaptation. What is often unappreciated is that meeting the standards of evidence necessary to support the position that a trait is a byproduct is no less burdensome than establishing that a trait is an adaptation. Indeed, adaptationist hypotheses must be tested as alternative explanations (Andrews et al., 2002). In other words, hypotheses about functionless byproducts must meet rigorous scientific standards. These standards include a functional analysis of the original adaptations responsible for producing the functionless byproducts, and an analysis of the existing human cognitive and motivational mechanisms responsible for the co-opting. Needless to say, such standards of evidence are rarely met, especially by those claiming that religion is a byproduct (see Buss et al., 1998).

One reason for the communication impasse between evolutionists and cognitivists over the adaptive nature of religion is that they appear to be engaging different levels of analysis. Evolutionary analyses often begin with Niko Tinbergen's four questions, or four levels of analysis (Tinbergen, 1963). Importantly, these four types of explanations are not mutually exclusive but complementary. Ontogenetic analyses ask questions about the development of a trait over the life course of an organism. Mechanistic analyses ask questions about how underlying physiological and psychological mechanisms produce the observed behaviors. Ontogenetic and mechanistic explanations are more broadly understood as proximate explanations. They address how behaviors become manifest; in other words, how they are produced and develop. Proximate explanations contrast with ultimate explanations, which aim to understand why certain traits evolved. One ultimate explanation concerns phylogeny—that is, analyses that focus on the evolutionary history of a trait. The other ultimate explanation concerns the functional value of a trait. Specifically, functional analyses are concerned with how a trait helps an organism survive and reproduce.

Most evolutionary studies of religion focus on ultimate-level explanations, aiming to determine whether there are selective advantages that could explain the patterns of religious expression in our species. Initial evolutionary forays sought to explain the costs of religious behavior. Such work turned toward behavioral ecological models of signaling, discussed above (Bulbulia, 2004; Bulbulia & Sosis, 2011; Irons, 2001; Sosis, 2003; Sosis & Alcorta, 2003). These models broadly showed that religious behaviors could serve as commitment devices that limit freeriding in communal endeavors; the collective gains from successful cooperation could outweigh the costs of religious performance. Other evolutionary researchers, also recognizing the cooperative nature of many religious groups, argued that adherence to supernatural agents helped resolve the inherent freeriding problems that plague collective endeavors (Schloss & Murray, 2011). This class of models includes supernatural punishment theory (Johnson, 2016, 2017), *supernatural monitoring theory* (Shariff & Norenzayan, 2007), and *Big Gods theory* (Norenzayan, 2013, 2015). These theories have generated an impressive body of empirical studies that have sought to assess and distinguish between these competing theories (e.g., Hartberg et al., 2016; McNamara et al., 2016).

Some of the most exciting recent advances in the evolutionary study of religion have been the use of phylogenetic analyses. Watts et al. (2015), for example, were able to evaluate between two leading theories that aim to explain the role of religion in the rise of complex societies. Using phylogenetic methods, Watts and colleagues showed that commitments to supernatural punishing agents preceded political complexity, whereas contrary to predictions from Big Gods theory, beliefs in moralizing high gods did not. In subsequent phylogenetic work, Watts et al. (2016) demonstrated that human sacrifice emerged before strict class systems, and these rituals were used to develop and sustain systems of inequality. Phylogenetic tools offer a powerful way to evaluate hypotheses about the evolutionary origins, function, and trajectory of religious practices and beliefs.

At a fundamental level, cognitivists and evolutionists differ in their approach to religious beliefs. Evolutionists, in general, treat religious beliefs as proximate mechanisms.

CONFLICTS AND COMPLEMENTARITIES   361

Beliefs, it is argued, are simply one of the underlying mechanisms capable of motivating behavior. Consequently, the psychological underpinnings of supernatural beliefs are typically not the focus of adaptationist analyses. Evolutionists have been more concerned with how such beliefs inspire religious behaviors that can impact aspects of fitness, such as survivorship, resource accrual, and mating opportunities. Cognitive scientists of religion, on the other hand, have been deeply interested in explaining the psychological mechanisms that enable and foster supernatural beliefs. Cognitivists and evolutionists, thus, are often operating at different levels of analysis. This does not fully explain their disagreement over the adaptive nature of religion (we will return to this debate below), but it does help to explain some instances where researchers from each field are talking past each other (see Sosis, 2009).

Maturational versus Practiced Naturalness Debate

Many cognitive scientists of religion argue that human cognitive systems inevitably yield religious beliefs and commitments. This view is known as the *naturalness of religion thesis*. Some scholars take a strong position on the naturalness thesis, denying the relevance of much environmental input in the development of the cognitive systems that produce religion, whereas others support a weaker form of the thesis that recognizes environmental contributions to the developmental timing and manifestation of these systems, seeking to incorporate the role of cultural factors in religious expression. The naturalness of religion thesis has generated significant academic interest and discussion (see McCauley, 2013); however, its implications extend well beyond purely academic concerns. Whether or not religion is "natural" is relevant for understanding issues concerning the legal protection of religious expression, basic human rights, and conflict resolution between religious and secular values (Barrett, 2018; Sosis & Kiper, 2018). It is also central to understanding what it means to be human.

McCauley (2011) advanced the most thorough articulation of the naturalness thesis in his seminal book *Why Religion Is Natural and Science Is Not*. McCauley describes *naturalness* as thought processes or behaviors characterized by ease, automaticity, and fluency. He distinguishes between two basic types of naturalness that should be considered as existing along a continuum. On one side of the continuum, maturational naturalness arises as a consequence of normal development and requires relatively less socioecological input. Behaviors such as learning to walk, learning to speak, and recognizing faces, for example, are "maturationally natural." On the other side, practiced naturalness arises not through the normal course of physical and psychological development, but rather through repeated practice and training, such as learning to play a musical instrument.

McCauley places religious cognition (but not theological reflection) on the maturational side of the continuum. His argument relies on a growing body of research demonstrating that core elements of religious expression—such as supernatural agent beliefs, teleological reasoning, and afterlife beliefs—are the natural outcome of normal cognitive development. Evolutionary scholars generally have not contested these studies, however, they have argued that religion falls more toward the practiced end of the religious continuum (e.g., Sosis & Kiper, 2018).

From an evolutionary perspective, the underlying cognitive structures of religion represent only the seeds of the potential development of religious systems (Sosis & Kiper, 2014). After all, theory of mind, mind-body dualism, and other cognitive features are necessary but not sufficient to produce religious traditions. To be sustained throughout the life course and across generations, religious beliefs require reinforcement, and religious behaviors require practice. Therefore, without further qualification, most evolutionists doubt that religious behaviors are nearly inevitable, as the naturalness of religion thesis suggests. Religious expression requires cultural inputs and cultivation, not just cognitive potential. Whether one believes in Zeus, Vishnu, or Allah will depend on the cultural environment in which one is raised. But mere exposure to teachings about these figures is not enough to generate commitments. Rather, adherents throughout the world believe in their gods, and the gods of other people, regardless of exposure, because adherents perform rituals for their particular deities (Alcorta & Sosis, 2005). In other words, though humans possess the cognitive machinery to believe in gods, the commitment to a particular god must be cultivated. In this way, belief is not automatic but achieved through ritual behaviors, such as supplications to a particular god, ritual presentations of myth, ascetic practices, and healing ceremonies, all of which instill sacred experiences.

In terms of cultivating religious experience, religious ritual is universally used to identify the sacred, and in so doing, separate it from the profane. As Durkheim (2001) argued, the sacred emerges through ritual and reflects issues concerning the social order, which take on a seemingly cosmic significance in light of religious discourse. Additionally, Rappaport (1999) noted, ritual does not merely identify that which is sacred—it *creates* the sacred. This is because rituals collectively alter participants' cognitive schema, giving them a template for differentiating sacred objects and activities from profane ones. Most importantly, from a behavioral perspective, the emotional significance of sacred and profane activities is quite distinct; it is not only inappropriate to traffic in the profane, it is emotionally repugnant to do so. Thus, while religious adherents differentiate sacred and profane things, their cognitive discrimination would be empty without an emotional reaction to the sacred, for it is the emotional significance of the sacred that underlies "faith," and it is ritual participation that invests the sacred with emotional meaning. This emotional valancing of the sacred and profane is learned.

The debate over where religious cognition falls along the naturalness continuum may partially be a consequence of disciplinary and methodological differences. Cognitive scientists are interested in uncovering the universal cognitive architecture that produces religious concepts. They are therefore more likely to emphasize the maturational character of religion because they study the cognitive mechanisms that produce religious beliefs and behavior; it is indeed the case that human cognition naturally produces religious expression. But evolutionary scientists—particularly evolutionary anthropologists—are often struck by the extraordinary plasticity of human behavior in contrast to other organisms. They generally perceive religion as lying toward the practiced end of the naturalness continuum because their attention is on the diversity of religious expression and how religious behaviors are critical for forming and sustaining belief and commitment.

Toward Integration: Religions as Complex Systems

Cognitive scientists of religion focus on how cognitive systems produce, retain, and transmit religious thought. Conversely, adaptationist approaches to religion emphasize variation in the costs and benefits of religious behavior. Thus these two perspectives differentially emphasize some features of religions while neglecting others. However, religions are made up of both features—and a host of others—including emotionally evocative symbols, myths, and taboos. Some recent evolutionary approaches recognize that these core elements of religion constitute an adaptive system designed for promoting cooperation (Alcorta & Sosis, 2005; Purzycki & Sosis, 2009, 2010; Sosis, 2009, 2016). This approach incorporates the insights from all three evolutionary perspectives, as well as CSR research, and aims to explain the central elements of religion taking into consideration the local environment in which people operate.

Religious systems typically maintain eight core elements: authority, meaning, moral obligation, myth, ritual, the sacred, supernatural agents, and taboo (Sosis, 2016, 2019). They are the building blocks of religious systems (Sosis, 2019; cf. Taves, 2009). Each element is most usefully conceived of as a unique category, which may have an independent phylogenetic history but which within a religious system is inherently interconnected with the other elements in that system. The core structure of religious systems consists of interactions between the eight core elements we have identified. Ritual is at the center of religious systems, and though all the elements may not interact with each other directly, they do all interact with and through ritual.

Our understanding of these interactions is rudimentary, but various cognitive theories shed light on these interactions, and it is here where integration between the evolutionary and cognitive sciences of religion is most promising. For example, Whitehouse's (2004) modes theory of religion provides a useful framework for understanding the mechanisms that enable rituals to create meaning, and significantly, how variation in the frequency of ritual performance is related to variation in the formation of meaning. Modes theory also captures how ritual intensity is related to religious authority; religious leaders are more likely to emerge under the doctrinal mode (low intensity rituals) than the imagistic mode (high intensity rituals) of religion. Other cognitivist theories, such as minimally counterintuitive or MCI theory (Purzycki & Willard, 2016), hazard precaution system theory (Liénard & Boyer, 2006), and ritual form theory (McCauley & Lawson, 2002), offer further insights about how the core elements of religious systems interrelate. These theories, alongside evolutionary theories, including supernatural punishment and signaling theories, are laying the groundwork for a more holistic analysis of religions (Sosis, 2020; Wood & Sosis, 2019). The patterns by which the core elements of religion interact likely constitute a grammar (Bulbulia, 2012); it is the ongoing task of evolutionary and cognitive researchers studying religion to uncover these grammatical rules.

The systemic approach to religion can also help resolve the adaptationist-byproduct debate discussed above. Adaptationists have been accused of not specifying "what it is that evolved or is evolving" (Wiebe, 2008, p. 344). The systemic approach clarifies what selection has operated on—a coalescence of cognitive, emotional, and behavioral elements—and directs us to the appropriate questions for an adaptationist analysis. Even if the category of religion is simply a Western construct as some contend (Klass, 1995), it *is* a collection of cognitive processes and behaviors that form an appropriate unit of evolutionary analysis. To clarify, we are not arguing that we should abandon the study of individual core elements of the religious system, such as supernatural agent beliefs, ritual, or religious authority. Quite the contrary; studying these core elements is essential. The point here is that the religious system—the coalescence of these elements—must be the focus of adaptationist analyses. To claim that the cognitive systems that produce supernatural agent belief have not evolved to produce such beliefs and therefore "religion" is not adaptive is misleading. It is the religious system that produces functional effects, not the constituent parts. A proper byproduct account of religion, which has yet to be offered, must explain why the religious system's constituent parts recurrently coalesce across cultures.

CONCLUSION

The title of our chapter questions the nature of the relationship between the evolutionary and cognitive sciences of religion. On the one hand, these fields have independent academic histories. One draws inspiration from Darwin and the modern evolutionary sciences; the other sees it roots in the cognitive revolution inspired by Chomsky and others. On the other hand, the contemporary cognitive sciences have widely incorporated evolutionary perspectives. Moreover, the intellectual promiscuity of CSR, welcoming nearly all nonsociological scientific research into the fold, has meant that evolutionists and cognitivists have been bedfellows for nearly two decades. Admittedly, sharing the same bed has not always been comfortable. The tensions between the evolutionary and cognitive sciences of religion in some ways mirror those between evolutionary psychology, on which much CSR thinking is based, and behavioral ecology and dual inheritance theory. Although competition between fields of study can advance understanding, the history of collaboration between these evolutionary subfields also suggests that complementarity can foster progress and provide a more complete picture of the human condition (Sosis, 2017). We think an integration of the cognitive and evolutionary sciences of religion holds similar promise.

Questions for Future Research

1. What data are needed to evaluate byproduct theories of religion?
2. Can behavioral ecological and cultural evolutionary models inform cognitive science approaches to religion?
3. How can the cognitive and evolutionary sciences of religion become better integrated?

References

Alcorta, C., & Sosis, R. (2005). Ritual, emotion, and sacred symbols: The evolution of religion as an adaptive complex. *Human Nature, 16*, 323–359.

Andersen, M. (2019). Predictive coding in agency detection. *Religion, Brain & Behavior, 9*. 65–84. doi:10.1080/2153599X.2017.1387170

Andrews, P. W., Gangestad, S. W., & Matthews, D. (2002). Adaptationism: How to carry out an exaptationist program. *Behavioral and Brain Sciences, 25*(4), 489–553.

Atran, S. (1995). Causal constraints on categories. In D. Sperber, D. Premack, & A. J. Premack (Eds.), *Causal cognition: A multi-disciplinary debate* (pp. 263–265). Oxford: Clarendon Press.

Atran, S. (2002). *In Gods we trust: The evolutionary landscape of religion.* Oxford: Oxford University Press.

Atran, S., & Henrich, J. (2010). The evolution of religion: How cognitive by-products, adaptive learning heuristics, ritual displays, and group competition generate deep commitments to prosocial religions. *Biological Theory, 5*(1), 18–30.

Barrett, J. (2004). *Why would anyone believe in God?* Walnut Creek, CA: AltaMira Press.

Barrett, J. (2018). On the naturalness of religion and religious freedom. In T. S. Shah & J. Friedman (Eds.), *Homo religiosus? Exploring the roots of religion and religious freedom in human experience* (pp. 67–88). Cambridge: Cambridge University Press.

Bering, J. (2006). The folk psychology of souls. *Behavioral and Brain Sciences, 29*, 453–498.

Bering, J., McLeod, K., & Shackelford, T. (2005). Reasoning about dead agents reveals possible adaptive trends. *Human Nature, 16*(4), 360–381.

Blume, M. (2010). Von Hayek and the Amish fertility: How religious communities manage to be fruitful and multiply; a case study. In U. Frey (Ed.), *The nature of God: Evolution and religion* (pp. 159–175). Marburg, Germany: Tectum Verlag.

Boyd, R., & Richerson, P. J. (1985). *Culture and the evolutionary process.* Chicago: University of Chicago Press.

Boyer, P. (2001). *Religion explained: The evolutionary origins of religious thought.* New York: Basic Books.

Boyer, P. (2004). Religion, evolution, and cognition. *Current Anthropology, 45*(3), 430–433.

Bulbulia, J. (2004). Religious costs as adaptations that signal altruistic intention. *Evolution and Cognition, 10*, 19–38.

Bulbulia, J. (2012). Spreading order: Religion, cooperative niche construction, and risky coordination problems. *Biology & Philosophy, 27*(1), 1–27.

Bulbulia, J., Shaver, J. H., Greaves, L., Sosis, R., & Sibley, C. (2015), Religion and parental cooperation: An empirical test of Slone's sexual signaling model. In D. J. Slone & J.

Van Slyke (Eds.), *The attraction of religion: A sexual selectionist account* (pp. 29–62) Bloomsbury Press.

Bulbulia, J., & Sosis, R. (2011). Signalling theory and the evolution of religious cooperation. *Religion, 41*(3), 363–388.

Burkert, W. (1996). *Creation of the sacred: Tracks of biology in early religions.* Cambridge, MA: Harvard University Press.

Buss, D. M., Haselton, M. G., Shackelford, T. K., Bleske, A. L., & Wakefield, J. C. (1998). Adaptations, exaptations, and spandrels. *American Psychologist, 53*(5), 533–548.

Casler, K., & Kelemen, D. (2007). Reasoning about artifacts at 24 months: The developing teleo-functional stance. *Cognition, 103*(1), 120–130.

Cronk, L. (1994). Evolutionary theories of morality and the manipulative use of signals. *Zygon, 29*(1) , 81–101.

Darwin, C. (2005). The descent of man, and selection in relation to sex. In J. D. Watson (Ed.), *Darwin: The indelible stamp* (pp. 607–1059). Philadelphia, PA: Running Press. (Original work published in 1871).

Dunbar, R. I. M., & Sosis, R. (2018). Optimising human community sizes. *Evolution and Human Behavior, 39*(1), 106–111.

Durkheim, É. (2001). *The elementary forms of religious life.* Oxford University Press. (Original work published in 1915).

Evans-Pritchard, E. E. (1937). *Witchcraft, oracles and magic among the Azande.* London: Clarendon Press.

Gray, K., Young, L., & Waytz, A. (2012). Mind perception is the essence of morality. *Psychological Inquiry, 23*(2), 101–124.

Guthrie, S. E. (1980). A cognitive theory of religion. *Current Anthropology, 21*(2), 181–203.

Guthrie, S. .E. (1993). *Faces in the clouds: A new theory of religion.* New York: Oxford University Press.

Hardy, A. C. (1965). *The living stream: Evolution and man.* London: Harper & Row.

Hardy, A. C. (1966). *The divine flame: An essay towards a natural history of religion; the second of two series of Gifford lectures in science, natural history and religion delivered in the University of Aberdeen, during the session 1964–5.* London: Collins.

Hartberg, Y., Cox, M., & Villamayor-Tomas, S. (2016). Supernatural monitoring and sanctioning in community-based resource management. *Religion, Brain & Behavior, 6*(2), 95–111.

Henrich, J. (2016). *The secret of our success.* Princeton University Press.

Hinde, R. A. (1999). *Why gods persist: A scientific approach to religion.* London: Routledge.

Irons, W. (1996). In our own self-image: The evolution of morality, deception, and religion. *Skeptic, 4*(2), 50–61.

Irons, W. (2001). Religion as a hard-to-fake sign of commitment. In R. Nesse (Ed.), *Evolution and the capacity for commitment* (pp. 292–309). New York: Russell Sage Foundation.

Johnson, D. (2016). *God is watching you: How the fear of God makes us human.* Oxford: Oxford University Press.

Johnson, D. (2017). Book symposium: Dominic Johnson's God Is Watching You. *Religion, Brain and Behavior, 8*(3), 279–350.

Johnson, D., & Bering, J. (2006). Hand of God, mind of man: Punishment and cognition in the evolution of cooperation. *Evolutionary Psychology, 4*, 219–233.

Kaufmann, E. (2010). *Shall the religion inherit the earth?* London: Profile Books.

Kelemen, D. (2004). Are children "intuitive theists"? Reasoning about purpose and design in nature. *Psychological Science, 15*(5), 295–301.

Kelemen, D., & Rosset, E. (2009). The human function compunction: Teleological explanation in adults. *Cognition, 111*(1), 138–143.

Kiper, J., & Sosis, R. (2016). Shaking the tyrant's bloody robe: An evolutionary perspective on ethnoreligious violence. *Politics and the Life Sciences, 35*(1), 27–47.

Kirkpatrick, L. A. (2006). Religion is not an adaptation. In P. McNamara (Ed.), *Where God and science meet: How brain and evolutionary studies alter our understanding of religion; evolution, genes, and the religious brain* (Vol. 1, pp. 159–179). Westport, CT: Praeger.

Kirkpatrick, L. A. (2008). Religion is not an adaptation: Some fundamental issues and arguments. In J. Bulbulia, R. Sosis, E. Harris, C. Genet, R. Genet, & K. Wyman (Eds.), *The evolution of religion: Studies, theories, and critiques* (pp. 61–65). Santa Margarita, CA: Collins Foundation Press.

Klass, M. (1995). *Ordered universes: Approaches to the anthropology of religion.* Boulder, CO: Westview Press.

Krebs, J. R., & Davies, N. B. (1993). *An introduction to behavioral ecology.* London: Blackwell Science.

Liénard, P., & Boyer, P. (2006). Whence collective rituals? A cultural selection model of ritualized behavior. *American Anthropologist, 108*(4), 814–827.

McCauley, R. N., & Lawson, E. T. (2002). *Bringing ritual to mind: Psychological foundations of cultural forms.* Cambridge, UK: Cambridge University Press.

McCauley, R. N. (2011). *Why religion is natural, and science is not.* New York: Oxford University Press.

McCauley, R. N. (2013). Book symposium: Robert McCauley's "Why religion is natural and science is not." *Religion, Brain & Behavior, 3*(2), 119–182.

McNamara, R. A., Norenzayan, A., & Henrich, J. (2016). Supernatural punishment, in-group biases, and material insecurity: experiments and ethnography from Yasawa, Fiji. *Religion, Brain & Behavior, 6*(1), 34–55.

Norenzayan, A. (2013). *Big Gods: How religion transformed cooperation and conflict.* Princeton, NJ: Princeton University Press.

Norenzayan, A. (2015). Book symposium on Big Gods by Ara Norenzayan. *Religion, Brain & Behavior, 5*(4), 266–342.

Norenzayan, A., & Shariff, A. F. (2008). The origin and evolution of religious prosociality. *Science, 322*(5898), 58–62.

Premack, D., & Woodruff, G. (1978). Does the chimpanzee have a theory of mind? *Behavioral and Brain Sciences, 1*(4), 515–526.

Power, E. A. (2017a). Discerning devotion: Testing the signaling theory of religion. *Evolution and Human Behavior, 38*(1), 82–91.

Power, E. A. (2017b). Social support networks and religiosity in rural South India. *Nature Human Behaviour, 1*(3), Article 0057.

Purzycki, B. G. (2013). The minds of Gods: A comparative study of supernatural agency. *Cognition, 129*(1), 163–179.

Purzycki, B. G. (2016). The evolution of Gods' minds in the Tyva Republic. *Current Anthropology, 57*(S13), S88–S104.

Purzycki, B. G., & Arakchaa, T. (2013). Ritual behavior and trust in the Tyva Republic. *Current Anthropology, 54*(3), 381–388.

Purzycki, B. G., Finkel, D. N., Shaver, J., Wales, N., Cohen, A. B., & Sosis, R. (2012). What does God know? Supernatural agents' access to socially strategic and non-strategic information. *Cognitive Science*, *36*(5), 846–869.

Purzycki, B. G., & Sosis, R. (2009). The religious system as adaptive: Cognitive Flexibility, Public Displays, and Acceptance. In E. Voland & W. Schiefenhövel (Eds.), *The biological evolution of religious mind and behavior* (pp. 243–256). Dordrecht: Springer

Purzycki, B. G., & Sosis, R. (2010). Religious concepts as necessary components of the adaptive religious system. In U. Frey (Ed.), *The nature of God: Evolution and religion* (pp. 37–59). Marburg: Tectum.

Purzycki, B. G., & Sosis, R. (2013). The extended religious phenotype and the adaptive coupling of ritual and belief. *Israel Journal for Ecology and Evolution*, *59*(2): 99–108.

Purzycki, B. G., & Willard, A. K. (2016). MCI theory: A critical discussion. *Religion, Brain & Behavior*, *6*(3), 207–248.

Rappaport, R. A. (1999). *Ritual and religion in the making of humanity*. Cambridge, UK: Cambridge University Press.

Reynolds, V., & Tanner, R. E. (1983). *The biology of religion*. London: Longman.

Reynolds, V., & Tanner, R. E. (1995). *The social ecology of religion*. Oxford: Oxford University Press.

Richerson, P., & Boyd, R. (2005). *Not by genes alone*. Chicago: University of Chicago Press.

Ruffle, B. J., & Sosis, R. (2007). Does it pay to pray? Costly rituals and cooperation. *B.E. Press of Economic Policy and Analysis*, *7*(1), 1–35.

Schloss, J. P., & Murray, M. J. (2011). Evolutionary accounts of belief in supernatural punishment: A critical review. *Religion, Brain & Behavior*, *1*(1), 46–99.

Shariff, A., & Norenzayan, A. (2007). God is watching you: Priming God concepts increases prosocial behavior in an anonymous economic game. *Psychological Science*, *,18*(9), 803–809.

Shaver, J. H. (2015). The evolution of stratification in Fijian ritual participation. *Religion, Brain & Behavior*, *2*, 101–117.

Shaver, J. H. (2017). Why and how do some religious individuals, and some religious groups, achieve higher relative fertility? *Religion, Brain & Behavior*, *7*(4), 324–327.

Shaver, J. H., Power, E., Purzycki, B., Watts, J., Sear, R., Shenk, M., Sosis, R., Bulbulia, J. (2020). Church attendance and alloparenting: An analysis of fertility, social support, and child development among English mothers. *Philosophical Transactions of the Royal Society B*, *375*, Article 20190428.

Shaver, J. H., Purzycki, B. G., & Sosis, R. (2016). Evolutionary theory in the study of religion. In M. Stausberg and S. Engler (Eds.), *The Oxford handbook of the study of religion* (pp. 124–136). Oxford: Oxford University Press.

Shaver, J. H., Sibley, C., Sosis, R., Galbraith, D., & Bulbulia, J. (2019). Alloparenting and religious fertility: A test of the religious alloparenting hypothesis. *Evolution and Human Behavior*, *40*, 315–324.

Shaver, J. H., & Sosis, R. (2014). How does male ritual behavior vary across the lifespan? *Human Nature*, *25*(1), 136–160.

Slone, D. J. (2008). The attraction of religion: A sexual selectionist account. In J. Bulbulia, R. Sosis, E. Harris, C. Genet, R. Genet, & K. Wyman (Eds.), *The evolution of religion: Studies, theories, and critiques* (pp. 181–187). Santa Margarita, CA: Collins Foundation.

Smith, E. A. (2000). Three styles in the evolutionary study of human behavior. In L. Cronk, W. Irons, & N. Chagnon (Eds.), *Human behavior and adaptation: An anthropological perspective* (pp. 27–46). Hawthorne, NY: Aldine de Gruyter.

Soler, M. (2012). Costly signaling, ritual and cooperation: Evidence from Candomblé, an Afro-Brazilian religion. *Evolution and Human Behavior, 33*(4), 346–356.

Sosis, R. (2003). Why aren't we all Hutterites? Costly signaling theory and religion. *Human Nature, 14,* 91–127.

Sosis, R. (2009). The adaptationist-byproduct debate on the evolution of religion: Five misunderstandings of the adaptationist program. *Journal of Cognition and Culture, 9*(3), 315–332.

Sosis, R. (2016). Religions as complex adaptive systems. In N. Clements (Ed.) *Mental religion: The brain, cognition, and culture* (pp. 219–236). Farmington Hills, MI: Macmillan..

Sosis, R. (2017). The road not taken: Possible paths for the cognitive science of religion. In L. Martin & D. Wiebe (Eds.), *Religion explained? The cognitive science of religion after 25 years* (pp. 155–167). London: Bloomsbury Press.

Sosis, R. (2019). The building blocks of religious systems: Approaching religion as a complex system. In G. Y. Georgiev, J. M. Smart, C. L. Flores Martinez, & M. Price (Eds.), *Evolution, development and complexity: Multiscale models of complex adaptive systems* (pp. 421–449). New York: Springer.

Sosis, R. (2020). Four advantages of a systemic approach to religion. *Archive for the Psychology of Religion, 42,* 142–157.

Sosis, R., & Alcorta, C. (2003). Signaling, solidarity and the sacred: The evolution of religious behavior. *Evolutionary Anthropology, 12,* 264–274.

Sosis, R., & Bressler, E. (2003). Cooperation and commune longevity: A test of the costly signaling theory of religion. *Cross-Cultural Research, 37,* 211–239.

Sosis, R., & Bulbulia, J. (2011). The behavioral ecology of religion: The benefits and costs of one evolutionary approach. *Religion, 41*(3), 341–362.

Sosis, R., & Kiper, J. (2014). Religion is more than belief: What evolutionary theories of religion tell us about religious commitment. In M. Bergmann and P. Kain (Eds.) *Challenges to Religion and Morality: Disagreements and Evolution,* (pp. 256–276). New York: Oxford University.

Sosis, R., & Kiper, J. (2018). Sacred versus secular values: Cognitive and evolutionary sciences of religion and religious freedom. In T. S. Shah & J. Friedman (Eds.), *Homo religiosus? Exploring the roots of religion and religious freedom in human experience* (pp. 89–119). Cambridge, UK: Cambridge University Press.

Sosis, R., Kress, H., & Boster, J. (2007). Scars for war: Evaluating alternative signaling explanations for cross-cultural variance in ritual costs. *Evolution and Human Behavior, 28*(4), 234–247.

Sosis, R., & Ruffle, B. (2003). Religious ritual and cooperation: Testing for a relationship on Israeli religious and secular kibbutzim. *Current Anthropology, 44,* 713–722.

Sperber, D. (1985). Anthropology and psychology: Towards an epidemiology of representations. *Man, 25,* 73–89.

Strassmann, B. I. (1992). The function of menstrual taboos among the Dogon: Defense against cuckoldry? *Human Nature, 3*(2), 89–131.

Strassmann, B. I. (1996). Menstrual hut visits by Dogon women: A hormonal test distinguishes deceit from honest signaling. *Behavioral Ecology, 7*(3), 304–315.

Strassmann, B. I., Kurapati, N. T., Hug, B. F., Burke, E. E., Gillespie, B. W., Karafet, T. M., & Hammer, M. F. (2012). Religion as a means to assure paternity. *Proceedings of the National Academy of Sciences, 109*(25), 9781–9785.

Taves, A. (2009). *Religious experience reconsidered: A building-block approach to the study of religion and other special things.* Princeton, NJ: Princeton University Press.

Tinbergen, N. (1963). On aims and methods of ethology. *Zeitschrift für Tierpsychologie*, 20(4), 410–433.

Tooby, J., & Cosmides, L. (1992). The psychological foundations of culture. In J. Barkow, L. Cosmides, & J. Tooby (Eds.), *The adapted mind: Evolutionary psychology and the generation of culture* (pp. 19–136). New York: Oxford University Press.

Van Leeuwen, N., & van Elk, M. (2018). Seeking the supernatural: The interactive religious experience model. *Religion, Brain & Behavior*, 9(3), 221–251.

Watts, J., Greenhill, S. J., Atkinson, Q. D., Currie, T. E., Bulbulia, J., & Gray, R. D. (2015). Broad supernatural punishment but not moralizing high gods precede the evolution of political complexity in Austronesia. *Proceedings of the Royal Society B: Biological Sciences*, 282(1804), Article 20142556.

Watts, J., Sheehan, O., Atkinson, Q. D., Bulbulia, J., & Gray, R. D. (2016). Ritual human sacrifice promoted and sustained the evolution of stratified societies. *Nature*, 532(7598), 228.

Weeden, J., Cohen, A. B., & Kenrick, D. T. (2008). Religious attendance as reproductive support. *Evolution and Human Behavior*, 29(5), 327–334.

Whitehouse, H. (2004). *Modes of religiosity: A cognitive theory of religious transmission*. Walnut Creek, CA: Alta Mira Press.

Wiebe, D. (2008). Does talk about the evolution of religion make sense? In J. Bulbulia, R. Sosis, E. Harris, C. Genet, R. Genet, & K. Wyman (Eds.), *The evolution of religion: Studies, theories, and critiques* (pp. 339–346). Santa Margarita, CA: Collins Foundation Press.

Wildman, W. J., & Sosis, R. (2011). Stability of groups with costly beliefs and practices. *Journal of Artificial Societies and Social Simulation*, 14(3), 6.

Williams, G. (1966). *Adaptation and natural selection*. Princeton, NJ: Princeton University Press.

Wilson, D. S. (2002). *Darwin's cathedral: Evolution, religion, and the nature of society*. Chicago: University of Chicago Press.

Wilson, E. O. (1978). *On human nature*. Cambridge, MA: Harvard University Press.

Wood, C., & Sosis, R. (2019). *Simulating religions as adaptive systems*. In S. Diallo, W. J. Wildman, F. L. Shults, & A. Tolk (Eds.), *Human simulation: Perspectives, insights, and applications* (pp. 209–232). New York: Springer.

CHAPTER 19

CSR AND RELIGIOUS BELIEF: EPISTEMIC FRIENDS OR FOES?

HANS VAN EYGHEN

INTRODUCTION

FROM early on in its young history, cognitive science of religion (CSR) has attracted the attention of epistemologists. Some argue that CSR theories raise a negative epistemic verdict for religious beliefs. Others argue for the opposite, a positive verdict.[1] In this chapter, I discuss what I believe to be the main arguments based on CSR theories for and against the rationality of religious beliefs.[2]

In the next section ("CSR and the Genealogy of Belief"), I make some preliminary remarks on the relationship between CSR theories and the genealogy of individual religious beliefs. I argue that the relationship is not as obvious as some defenders of arguments involving CSR theories assume.

In the third section ("CSR as Epistemic Foe"), I discuss two arguments *against* the rationality of religious beliefs. One argument claims that CSR theories show that religious beliefs were a product of natural selection and are therefore suspect. While the suspicion can be removed for some beliefs shaped by evolution, no such redemption is available for religious beliefs. A second argument claims religious beliefs are the result of misattributions according to CSR theories. If CSR theories are true, people form religious beliefs by wrongfully attributing super natural input to something natural. After

---

[1] For various arguments in this area, see Schloss and Murray (2009); Trigg and Barrett (2014), Braddock (2018).
[2] Other arguments against religious belief were raised by Matthew Braddock (2016) and Liz Goodnick (2016).

discussing both arguments, I will argue that both fail to show that religious beliefs are not rationally held.

In the fourth section ("CSR as Epistemic Friend"), I look at the opposing side of the debate—that is, arguments *for* the rationality of religious beliefs. Here, the main argument claims that CSR theories show that religious beliefs are formed naturally, or intuitively. Because naturally or intuitively formed religious beliefs can be prima facie rationally held, CSR theories therefore support religious beliefs. Against this argument, I will argue that CSR theories show only that some religious beliefs, which stand in contradiction to most of the supernatural beliefs people hold nowadays, are naturally formed. Therefore, CSR theories do not support most of the supernatural beliefs that are dominant in most major religions today.

CSR and the Genealogy of Belief

All arguments I discuss below look at the epistemic implications for religious beliefs held by individual subjects. CSR theories do not directly explain religious beliefs at the level of the individual. Instead, they rather aim to explain why beliefs (or ideas, rituals, etc.) are common in a population. For example, Justin Barrett (2004) points to the operations of the hypersensitive agency-detection device (HADD) to (partly) explain why religious belief is widely prevalent. The theory draws on work by Stewart Guthrie (1993) and argues that the cognitive mechanism, by means of which humans detect agents, attributes agency based on very limited evidence. Since HADD is hypersensitive, people are prone to easily form beliefs that agents are around. This hypersensitivity, in turn, makes them prone to believe in invisible agents.

If Barrett's theory is true, the operations of HADD make populations of people prone to form religious beliefs. In this way, HADD explains why many people hold religious belief, but it does not necessarily explain why any given individual does so. Even if HADD is instrumental in generating a case of agency detection, the impetus to doubt that attribution or act on it or the degree to which it is shared with others or woven into one's cultural practices, and so forth are all causal contributors to an individual's belief. Likewise, an individual can have many reasons for holding religious beliefs beyond a single detection of agency. She can hold religious beliefs because she has heard a persuasive philosophical argument or testimony by trusted kin, for instance. In these cases, her religious beliefs do not appear to be caused simply by the operations of HADD.

The arguments I discuss here do not take these additional complexities into account. Instead, they assess the impact of CSR theories for religious believers who came to hold their beliefs because of the isolated operations of the various cognitive mechanisms discussed by CSR theories, independently of additional causes or reasons that may support them. Since the cognitive mechanisms discussed by CSR theories often operate at the subpersonal or unconscious level, people are often not aware of how their religious beliefs are formed. For how many people this is the case remains an open question.[3] For all arguments, the caveat must therefore be that the epistemic status of religious beliefs can also be affected by other reasons in the subject's evidence base. This holds for both kinds of arguments. If negative arguments are true, the negative status of religious beliefs can be overturned by the reasons I have mentioned. If positive arguments are true, their positive status could be overturned if arguments for atheism are true, or for other reasons, to deny religious beliefs. Often, defenders of CSR-based arguments do not make this explicit.

There is another aspect of individual religious belief that CSR theories does not explain. HADD can explain how cognitive mechanisms may lead to the detection of invisible agents. It does not explain why an individual believes the invisible agent is "God" or a "god" or "spirit." To use these concepts, cultural input is needed. Other CSR theories do explain why people believe in gods rather than spirits (e.g., see Barrett, 2012; Norenzayan, 2013; and Scott & Barrett, this volume), but these still allow for a great variety in God concepts. It is not clear how much cultural input is needed to form specific beliefs in God or gods or to what extent cognitive mechanisms contribute aside from these inputs. The more religious beliefs are shaped by cognitive mechanisms alone, the greater the effects of the arguments that I discuss will be, if these arguments are successful. For the purposes of this chapter, I have assumed that religious beliefs are significantly shaped by cognitive mechanisms working relatively independently within individual believers.

CSR as Epistemic Foe

Most participants in the discussion about CSR's epistemic implications wonder if CSR has negative epistemic implications for religious belief.[4] Opinions diverge on what the negative epistemic implications are. CSR could render religious belief undermined, *unjustified, not rational,* or *unwarranted.* These epistemic qualifications have different meanings, and their exact definitions are hotly contested. For the purposes of this chapter, I will consider CSR's implications for the *rationality* of religious belief. In the next sections I consider whether CSR renders holding religious beliefs *not rational.*

I will use the terms *rational* and *not rational* in line with how they are used in rational choice theory.[5] On this account, a belief can be rationally held if the content of the belief

---

[3] Elsewhere, I argue that the scope of debunking arguments is likely rather large. See Van Eyghen (2020).

[4] Not all of these authors argue that CSR theories in fact have negative epistemic implications. Interestingly, arguments for negative implications are of later date than rebuttals against similar arguments. See, for example, Leech and Visala (2011b); Murray and Goldberg (2009).

[5] I will not use the term *irrational* in this chapter. Being irrational is often considered a greater epistemic bad than being not rational. Arguments that conclude to the irrationality of holding religious beliefs are therefore also arguments for their nonrationality.

is more probably true than false given the evidence a subject has. Applying this definition to CSR, I consider whether a subject can judge her religious beliefs to be true after she has learned about various CSR theories. In other words, I consider what changes when a subject adds CSR theories to her evidence base. Does it force her to give up her religious beliefs? Does it add evidence? Or does nothing change?

With this in mind, I first discuss whether CSR theories force people without additional reasons for their religious belief to give them up, beginning with the best-known argument of this kind.

Not Rational Because Evolved

A popular reason CSR theories could render holding religious beliefs not rational is that CSR theories show that the propensity to form religious beliefs evolved by means of natural selection.[6] The argument goes as follows:

1. CSR theories show that propensities to form religious beliefs (PFRBs) evolved by means of natural selection.
2. Religious beliefs that result from PFRBs, which evolved by means of natural selection, are not rational in the absence of additional reasons to judge that PFRBs are reliable.
3. There are no additional reasons to judge that PFRBs are reliable.
4. Therefore, religious beliefs are not rational.

A similar argument was raised by John Wilkins and Paul Griffiths (2013). Though their argument is more refined, my statement resembles their core claim as well as similar, less elaborate arguments. I will discuss all premises in greater detail and show why I find the argument unconvincing.

Premise 1 is clearly true. Though CSR theories disagree about many things, they all claim that PFRBs evolved by means of natural selection. Whether the theory claims that religious belief evolved as an adaptation in its own right or as a byproduct makes little difference. In both cases, the force driving the evolution of religious beliefs was survival or increased odds of reproduction. On theories wherein religious belief is an adaptation in its own right, religious beliefs themselves provide a benefit for survival or reproduction. For example, on Dominic Johnson's (2015) *supernatural punishment theory* belief in a punishing God or gods evolved because it fostered cooperation and cooperation benefits for human survival. On theories wherein religious beliefs are a byproduct, religious beliefs co-evolved—or piggybacked—with other adaptive traits. Here, the evolution of PFRBs is still driven by survival or reproduction, for example, in Justin

---

[6] Evolutionary arguments were raised by Liz Goodnick (2016) and John Wilkins and Paul Griffiths (2013).

Barrett's (2004) HADD *theory*, religious beliefs co-evolved with the human proneness to overdetect agency. The overdetection of agency yielded better chances of survival. On HADD, overdetection of agency and religious belief are a package deal. If subjects have one, they very likely have the other. The mechanisms of natural selection therefore also explain how byproducts evolved.

Premise 2 takes the claim that evolution by means of natural selection is (mainly)[7] driven by survival and reproduction to be a reason to look with suspicion toward these evolved propensities. It notes that belief propensities evolved because of their adaptive function and not because they yielded true or approximately true beliefs. On Johnson's theory, belief in a punishing god arose because it fostered cooperation; and on Barrett's theory, religions have become common because hypersensitivity in detecting agents helped survival. PFRBs did not evolve because the beliefs they produce were true under either theory.

The second premise does not claim that everyone who holds beliefs that have arisen because of evolved propensities is not rational or that all the resulting beliefs are false. Many propensities for other beliefs we rationally hold have also arisen through natural selection. Our perceptual faculties, which produce perceptual beliefs, were subject to evolutionary pressures, yet claiming that all perceptual beliefs are therefore not rational or false is surely absurd. For this reason, premise 2 is weaker and leaves open the possibility that beliefs of this sort can be rational if there are additional reasons to believe that the propensities that produce them are reliable. The premise merely claims that beliefs that arise from evolved propensities are initially suspect because the process by which humans came to have these beliefs (i.e., evolution by natural selection) is driven not by truth considerations but by fitness considerations.

Note here that the argument relies on a naturalistic reading of evolution. On theistic accounts of evolution, evolution by naturalistic selection aims—or can be aimed—at truth. Some philosophers argue that God could have set up the initial conditions for evolution or that God can intervene in the evolutionary process. If either is the case, God could easily have made sure that evolution led to true beliefs, at least much of the time. On theistic accounts, survival and reproduction would still be important drivers of evolution. They are not the only main drivers though. On theistic evolution, truth is also an important driver.[8] Although a response in terms of theistic evolution is valid, I will not further pursue this line of argument here, and will proceed with a naturalistic account of evolution in mind.

Premise 2 also states that the initial suspicion toward beliefs arising from evolved propensities can be overcome. As with all suspect propensities or cognitive mechanisms, their resulting beliefs can be rationally held if there is sufficient evidence to judge that they are reliable. Wilkins and Griffiths (2013) give a reason to let perceptual beliefs off the hook. They argue that perceptual systems would likely not have evolved to produce

---

[7] According to many biologists, evolution by means of natural selection can also be driven by genetic drift or mutation (Lynch, 2007).

[8] See, for example, Plantinga (2011).

the kinds of beliefs they commonly do if the beliefs they produce were not true. Having false perceptual beliefs about one's environment would have made survival more difficult. If evolution had fostered in our ancestors the belief that tigers are lambs or that water is solid, for example, our forebears likely would have been unable to transmit their DNA due to premature death. Since perceptual beliefs need to be true—or approximately true—in order to be adaptive, subjects have a good reason to trust their perceptual propensities. For this reason, perceptual beliefs can be rationally held.[9]

Premise 3 states that no reason is available to overcome the initial suspicion for PFRBs. Wilkins and Griffiths (2013) argue that CSR theories show that truth made no difference for the adaptive value of religious beliefs. A similar defense to the one they offered for perceptual beliefs is therefore not available. They do leave open the possibility that religious beliefs can be salvaged by natural theology but don't discuss this in detail.

In my response, I will accept a naturalistic account of evolution by natural selection and will contest premise 3. Wilkins and Griffiths (2013) note that natural theology can help overcome the suspicion toward PFRBs. If famous arguments such as the cosmological or teleological argument are convincing to a person, such a person could rationally hold that God exists.[10] Nevertheless, the vast majority of religious believers have never heard of these arguments. Thus, even if they are convincing, they will help only a limited number of believers, and perhaps with only a narrow range of religious beliefs, such as the belief that God exists.[11]

A better additional reason for religious belief is a more pragmatic one.[12] Wilkins and Griffiths (2013), in their defense of evolved perceptual propensities, make an appeal to their pragmatic success. Because of this pragmatic success, our evolved perceptual propensities can be regarded as good guides to reality and their outputs can be rationally held, without any need for additional reasons or evidence. Religious beliefs do not have the same pragmatic success. Some do, however, allow for spiritual pragmatic success. William Alston (1991, p. 251) argued that religious belief could yield spiritual fruit, such as growth in sanctity, serenity, peace, joy, fortitude, and love. Alston discusses the epistemic value of spiritual fruits in his defense of the reliability of mystical experiences. He compares mystical experience to sense perception and claims the two are similar in significant ways. One of way in which they are similar is that they both receive self-support.[13] Sense perception receives self-support because it allows us to make

---

[9] One could respond that having true perceptual beliefs is not needed for evolutionary success. Animals that arguably do not have anything close to mental states like "beliefs" also successfully navigate their environments. It therefore seems that other "pre-belief states," such as subdoxastic states or aliefs, could suffice in successfully navigating one's environment. I thank Justin Barrett for this suggestion.

[10] Wilkins and Griffiths also argue that scientific beliefs can be rationally held because of the evidence and reasons scientists provide. By responding in this way, they suggest that all initial suspicion of evolved propensities to form beliefs can be overcome by additional reasons for those beliefs.

[11] A response along these lines could also help a religious believer who hears about CSR theories and wants a response.

[12] This argument and counterarguments are discussed at length in (Van Eyghen & Bennett, 2020).

[13] Alston's main goal is defending the reliability of mystical perceptions. Although he claims that both receive self-support, he does not argue that sensory perception and mystical perception are reliable

predictions that turn out to be correct by allowing us to anticipate events and to control events. The self-support mystical experiences receive does not lie in prediction or control but in other fruits that are more appropriate to its aims. Since one of the aims of mystical experiences is spiritual development, growth in spiritual development can yield self-support for mystical experiences. Alston argues that the spiritual development that follows from mystical experiences are best explained by the reliability of the belief-forming process behind religious beliefs (Alston, 1991, pp. 173–175).

If reasons are required to regard a PFRB as reliable, as Wilkins and Griffiths do, self-support can fulfill that role. If PFRBs can be regarded as reliable, the beliefs they produce can be regarded as rational. The self-support of our perceptual propensities gives a reason to overcome the initial evolutionary suspicion and regard their outputs (perceptual beliefs) as rational. Similarly, our ability to grow spiritually supports both the practice of seeking mystical experiences and religious beliefs. Applied to our discussion, spiritual growth and spiritual fruits also constitute a reason to regard PFRBs as reliable. Leading a life of greater sanctity goes well beyond the evolutionary function of religious beliefs that CSR theories lay out. It gives the subject the additional reason she needs to rationally hold religious beliefs.

One could respond that the self-support of spiritual fruits is not nearly as direct or immediate as the self-support of perceptual propensities. False perceptual beliefs are immediately checked when a subject acts on them to navigate her environment. A belief that "water is solid" will be checked when the subject touches water for the first time. Spiritual fruits can also be a check on religious beliefs, but the check is far less direct. People can also lead their lives without spiritual fruits, whereas they can't lead their lives without navigating their environments. My response is that weaker self-support is still self-support. Demanding the same self-support as for perceptual propensities is too much to ask of PFRBs.

The third premise of the argument is therefore not established. Hence, the argument does not show that CSR is an epistemic foe of religious belief. While the argument (and similar arguments) could cast some initial doubt about beliefs that evolved for reasons of fitness, it cannot cast doubt on additional evolutionary reasons to hold religious beliefs, such as the greater spiritual fruits they yield. Tackling these additional reasons, however, is beyond the scope of what CSR theories can currently show.

Not Rational Because of Misattribution

A second argument for concluding that religious beliefs are not rationally held looks closer at the proximate causes[14] of religious beliefs. Defenders of the argument argue

---

because they receive self-support. Instead, Alston argues that the reliability of sense perception cannot be proven conclusively by means of evidence or argument. We are, however, still entitled to regard sense perception as reliable. Since mystical perception is sufficiently similar, it can be regarded as reliable as well.

[14] The proximate causes of religious beliefs are the cognitive mechanisms or propensities that produce religious beliefs. These are different than its distant causes, i.e. natural selection and (according to theists) God. For a discussion of the distinction, see (Szocik and Van Eyghen 2021).

that CSR theories show that religious beliefs result from a misattribution.[15] The argument is more straightforward than the previous one and goes as follows:

1. CSR theories show that religious beliefs result from a misattribution.
2. Beliefs that result from a misattribution are not rational.
3. Therefore, religious beliefs are not rational.

Although the argument is straightforward, one key term, *misattribution*, stands in need of clarification. A misattribution occurs when a subject forms a false belief by misreading the world or events. This is best explained with an example. A well-documented case of a misattribution is the Rubber Hand Illusion. Multiple studies have show that people can easily be convinced that a fake rubber hand is their own. In experiments participants were asked to take a seat and to put their real hands out of sight A fake rubber hand was put in sight and an experimenter touched one of the participant's real hands and the fake rubber hand using similar movements. After a short while—sometimes only 10 seconds—participants began to have the feeling that the fake rubber hand was their own (Ehrsson et al., 2005).

The Rubber Hand Illusion is a clear example of a misattribution. Subjects falsely come to believe that the rubber hand is theirs because their minds misidentify sensory input. In this case, they wrongfully identify sensory input of a fake hand as input from their own hand. The misattribution resulted in a false belief—namely, "the rubber hand is mine." The experiment does not show that humans often or usually misidentify bodily sensations. It also does not show that humans are bad at forming beliefs about themselves. It does show that the human cognitive apparatus can lead people astray and produce false beliefs in situations that are similar to those of the experimental setup.

Keeping the rubber-hand example in mind, it is clear that beliefs resulting from a misattribution can no longer be rationally held once the misattribution has been discovered. When a subject learns that her cognitive apparatus is prone to false identifications, such as thinking a rubber hand is her own, she should not judge the beliefs she forms in a situation similar to the experimental setting as true. Premise 2, that beliefs based on a misattribution are not rational, is therefore rather obvious.

Premise 1 is more difficult to establish. Most CSR theories do not straightforwardly argue that religious beliefs result from misattributions. Many merely claim that religious beliefs resulted from the operations of some cognitive mechanism, or that religious beliefs gave our ancestors an evolutionary advantage. Sometimes, however, defenders of CSR theories do claim that cognitive mechanisms go astray when they produce religious beliefs. Guthrie made one such claim when he defended a theory that is

---

[15] The term "misattribution" is drawn from Luke Galen (2017), who makes an argument that closely resembles this one. Another similar argument was raised by Robert Nola (2013, 2018) and Stephen Law (2018).

similar to Barrett's HADD theory, arguing that religious beliefs are produced by a tendency to anthropomorphize. For our ancestors, it was important to be on guard against predators or malevolent humans. It was important to spot agents in their environment quickly, and it was safer to spot too many agents rather than too few. Spotting too many agents, at worst, could lead to the waste of energy and time, whereas spotting one agent too few could lead to instant death. This favored hyperactivity in detecting agents or anthropomorphizing nature. Because of hyperactivity, humans easily *erroneously* conclude that agents are all around based on very limited evidence, such as the rustling of leaves or vague pattern-like forms. Guthrie argues that this tendency can easily lead to a belief in spirits and gods. The sense of agency humans perceive when their cognitive systems are triggered by vague inputs can lead them to believe that an invisible agent caused it. Belief in invisible agents can easily lead to belief in gods according to Guthrie (1993).

Guthrie has unambiguously claimed that religious beliefs result from "false positives."[16] He claims that the human cognitive system often misidentifies input for an agent. Importantly, he claims that these misidentifications foster the belief in invisible agents, which, in turn, leads to belief in gods. A misattribution thus lies at the root of religious beliefs, according to Guthrie (2002).

Other CSR theorists make similar suggestions. Gray and Wegner (2010) argue that religious beliefs result from the way people intuitively characterize moral situations. People intuitively distinguish moral agents and moral patients when they encounter morally significant events. Moral agents are those that do the moral harm or good, and moral patients are those who suffer or benefit from those actions. Although the dichotomy works well in most moral situations, problems arise in situations where there is no apparent moral agent. Natural disasters are a good example. Disasters are very often judged as morally significant. In almost every disaster there are moral patients—that is, those who lost their lives or whose homes were destroyed. There is, however, no apparent moral agent.[17] Here, humans are prone to seek an ultimate moral agent with the power to bring such an enormous event about; in other words, humans intuitively conclude to a god who is responsible. Though Gray and Wegner are not as outspoken as Guthrie, they also suggest that people—or rather their cognitive systems—are making a mistake when they attribute large, morally significant events to God.[18]

---

[16] See, for example: "In scanning for such agents, we encounter *false positives*: we think we see agents where none exist" (Guthrie, 2002, p. 1, emphasis added).

[17] In recent years, some natural disasters have been attributed to global warming. A case can be made that humans, whose activities release too much carbon dioxide into the atmosphere, are the moral agents in these disasters. Such considerations are, however, usually not on the radar of people who have experienced a natural disaster and thus human actions are not intuitively seen as the culprit.

[18] They write: "[W]e have reviewed evidence suggesting that people believe in God . . . because they need to *find* a moral agent to account for their suffering." They also write: "The research reviewed in this article suggests that God may be more accurately characterized as 'God of the Moral Gaps,'

We have seen the case some CSR theorists make for premise 1. I will now argue that their case is not well supported. First, Guthrie does not give a good reason to believe that religious beliefs result from misattributions. His claim that humans are promiscuous in detecting agents is plausible, but the additional claim that belief in invisible agents results from misattributing agency is far less plausible. If humans are indeed prone to jump to agency conclusions, they will soon learn that they often make mistakes. Usually, they will check their hunches and have a closer look. When they do not find any agent around, they will correct their initial hunch and not form a stable belief that an agent is or was around. This idea is shared by a number of prominent CSR-scholars. Pascal Boyer claims that beliefs triggered by hyperactive agency detection will be easily overridden (Boyer, 2002). Barrett, agrees with Boyer. He argues that hunches of agency *must be* easily overridden. If they are not, hyperactive detection would lead to survival difficulties, not advantages. He also notes that detecting invisible agents does not give rise to religious beliefs as we know them because other cultural factors that contribute to religious beliefs must be taken into account (Barrett, 2004, pp. 40–41).

Gray and Wegner (2010) also do not make sufficiently clear how moral typecasting leads to religious belief. They do cite evidence that societies with harsher conditions—and thus more suffering—have a higher prevalence of belief in God. This, however, does not establish that the moral typecasting of moral agents and moral patients produces religious belief. It could very well be that causation goes in the opposite direction, and that people first believe in a God who can cause natural disasters before they explain large morally significant events in terms of God's agency. If this is the case, people do not infer God's existence in order to account for disasters, but merely infer God's agency.

Apart from the question of whether these misattribution-claims provide a detailed explanation of how religious belief is formed, they do not show that religious beliefs cannot result from a correct attribution. Though agent detection could be hyperactive and thus prone to error, Guthrie does not show how beliefs in invisible agents and gods result from misattributions. Believers in most religious traditions believe that God or other supernatural beings can make themselves known to humans. The fact that human detection of physical agents is hyperactive does not rule out the possibility that humans can correctly pick up signals from supernatural beings in their environments. To show that religious beliefs result from misattributions, Guthrie would need to show that the sensory input that leads to religious beliefs is in fact natural and not the action of a god or spirit. He does not do this. In fact, Guthrie gives few details about the input that triggers HADD. A strong case for misattribution requires a strong case for exclusively natural input. Guthrie assumes there are no gods and, hence, all attributions to gods are misattributions.

The same holds for Gray and Daniel Wegner's (2010) theory. They do not show that people cannot correctly infer a divine cause of morally significant events. Looking for

a supernatural mind *introduced* into our perception of the world because of the underlying dyadic structure of morality" (Gray & Wegner, 2010, pp. 13–14, emphasis added).

moral agents is appropriate in many situations. In many, if not most, morally significant situations one or more agents did in fact cause the moral harm or good. To argue that moral typecasting goes astray in a given situation, one needs to show—or at least make plausible—that there is no moral agent in that situation or that God could not have caused the event. Some religious traditions hold that God does in fact cause natural disasters.[19] God is often also held responsible for situations that are regarded as morally good, for instance, if someone escapes death or has a child. Gray and Wegner's theory does not show that inferring to God's activity in these cases is a mistake. Like Guthrie, they appear to assume that there is no ultimate moral agent and therefore that concluding to one is a misattribution.

My last point hints to a inherent feature of CSR-theories and of scientific theories in general. Scientific theories do not refer to supernatural entities in explaining phenomena. This practice is known as *methodological naturalism*. Methodological naturalism is the thesis that scientific theories ought not refer to nonnatural entities to explain phenomena. With respect to CSR, methodological naturalism prevents CSR theories from appealing to anything supernatural to explain how religious beliefs came about (see Visala, this volume). If explanations of religious beliefs cannot refer to anything supernatural, the theories cannot refer to supernatural input. Concluding that supernatural belief results from a misattribution in this way is question-begging.

Methodological naturalism does appear to explain why some CSR theorists claim that religious beliefs result from a misattribution. Methodological naturalism casts doubt on existing misattribution claims, but it does not make them impossible nor does it show that all misattribution claims presuppose atheism. For example, if studies could be conducted that demonstrate how subjects attribute supernatural agency to natural agency (e.g., a human or animal) in ecologically valid conditions, such demonstrations would support the ideas that misattributions may generate some religious beliefs.[20] To support this claim, the defender need not explicitly check whether religious beliefs are caused by supernatural input (if doing so would even be possible). If they can document enough examples of people forming religious beliefs after misidentifying natural input, we will have a strong case for premise 1. At the moment, premise 1 is not sufficiently supported and the misattribution argument fails.

Another response against misattribution arguments claims that God is indirectly involved in the genealogy of religious belief. A friend of this response could cede that PFRBs produce religious beliefs when triggered by natural input. She could add that

---

[19] Many contemporary Christians are reluctant to attribute natural disasters directly to God's activity; however, there are passages in the Bible where God clearly causes disasters. The most famous is the great flood in Genesis 6–9.

[20] Some scholars made several attempts to test Guthrie's and related theories, but most of the results did not support the claim that religious belief is formed after misidentifying natural input. See Van Leeuwen & van Elk, (2018, sec. 3.2) for a summary of the studies. These studies, however, mainly tested whether hyperactivity in agency detection co-varies with religious commitment (a claim that neither Guthrie's nor Barrett's predicts), and not whether religious belief is caused by misattributing natural input.

God set everything up to be this way. God could have directed evolution to have people with PFRBs that often produce religious beliefs prompted by natural input.

David Leech and Aku Visala (2011a) argue that this *indirect response* would make God resemble a *deus deceptor*. By setting up the evolutionary process God is only an ultimate cause in the genealogy of religious beliefs, he is not a proximate cause. Yet phenomenologically, it seems to people that God is a proximate cause. On HADD, people believe they are witnessing God's agency. If that belief results from a misattribution, they are not actually witnessing God's agency. Their PFRB's are therefore still making a misattribution and the beliefs they form remain suspect.

CSR AS EPISTEMIC FRIEND

Some authors argue in the opposite direction and claim that CSR theories show that religious beliefs are prima facie rationally held.[21] CSR theories allegedly show that in the absence of defeaters, religious beliefs are natural and therefore rationally held. The argument goes as follows:

1. CSR theories show that religious beliefs are formed naturally.
2. Beliefs that are formed naturally can be prima facie rationally held.
3. Therefore, religious beliefs can be prima facie rationally held.

The argument is straightforward. Both premises are, however, controversial. Before I discuss them, it is necessary to clarify the conclusion. The argument does not conclude that religious beliefs can be rationally held. Its conclusion is less firm. Like Clark and Barrett (2010), I use the term *prima facie* in the sense of "innocent until proven guilty". A belief can be proven "guilty" when a defeater is available. The burden of proof is on the challenger to argue for the existence of a defeater. For a belief, a defeater is, roughly, a reason to accept the negation of that belief or that makes it less likely to be true.[22] Therefore, even if both premises 1 and 2 are true, it does not necessarily follow that all religious beliefs can be rationally held. If the subject has a defeater,[23] her religious beliefs will still be rendered not rational.

Premise 1 states that religious beliefs are naturally formed according to CSR theories.[24] The qualifier "natural" does not refer to the distinction between natural and

---

[21] Arguments of this kind were defended by Kelly Clark and Justin Barrett (2010) and by Barrett and Ian Church, (2013).

[22] The first kind of defeater is often called a *rebutting* defeater; and the second, an *undercutting* defeater. The distinction was first introduced by John Pollock (1986).

[23] Arguments like the problem of evil or divine hiddenness (see Schellenberg, 2006; Rowe, 1979), if sound, could provide such a defeater. I lack the space to discuss these arguments in more detail.

[24] CSR theories don't pretend to apply to all beliefs that someone might deem religious. Some authors, Barrett (2012) for example, are explicit. Barrett argues that belief in the Trinitarian God is not natural.

supernatural to which I referred to in section "CSR as Epistemic Friend". Instead, natural beliefs are beliefs that are easily formed by the human mind because of the way the human mind is constituted or structured.[25] Nonnatural beliefs are harder to form, and explicit instruction is required. Many CSR theorists argue that some religious beliefs are formed without the need for explicit instruction and that human minds operate in such a way that religious beliefs are easily formed. For example, the above-mentioned HADD theory states that people form beliefs in invisible agents because their agency-detection devices are easily triggered. Although the beliefs HADD produces can be molded by instruction, they were initially produced without it.

Premise 2 is in line with an influential tradition in contemporary epistemology.[26] It hinges on the claim that most of the human belief-forming faculties are reliable. Sometimes defenders argue that not relying on naturally formed beliefs implies that most people do not rationally hold moral beliefs or other common-sense beliefs, such as belief that other people have minds or that there is an external world. A full assessment of premise 2 lies beyond the scope of this paper. Therefore, I will assume its truth in the remainder of this section.

I will contest premise 1. Although I will not contest that CSR theories make a good case for the naturalness of some beliefs, these beliefs are not the religious beliefs that most contemporary religious believers affirm. According to many CSR theories, belief in anthropomorphic gods or spirits comes naturally, but not belief in a transcendent God, let alone belief in the Trinitarian God. These beliefs are the result of learning or socialization and are therefore not natural.

Jonathan Jong, Christopher Kavanaugh, and Aku Visala, make a similar objection. They argue that CSR theories are largely irrelevant to classical theism (Jong et al., 2015, p. 253). They note that, on most CSR theories, gods are things in the world. Most theories also suggest that people naturally believe in supernatural beings that live in and are bound by the spatiotemporal realm. CSR theories have little to say about belief in the God of classical theism, who stands above the spatiotemporal realm and is not a thing in the world but its creator and sustainer (Jong et al., 2015).[27]

An additional mismatch between theism and the beliefs produced by CSR mechanisms is anthropomorphism. Many CSR theorists argue that human subjects naturally form beliefs in supernatural beings who are much like humans. Like humans, they are conceived as being limited. The Trinitarian God is not subject to human

---

[25] See Visala and Barrett (2019), McCauley (2011).

[26] For well-known, elaborate defenses, see Reid (1872); Plantinga (1993); Huemer, (2007). The accounts diverge to some extent. Michael Huemer argues that justification of beliefs is grounded in how things appear or seem to the subject who believes. Thomas Reid defends the validity of common-sense judgments. Alvin Plantinga argues that beliefs formed by a properly functioning apparatus that functions according to a design plan and in a suitable environment have warrant. On all three accounts, many naturally formed beliefs have a positive epistemic status.

[27] Deborah Kelemen and Cara DiYanni (2005) did argue that belief in a creator comes naturally. They conducted experiments, which showed that young children are prone to see teleology in nature. This propensity would foster belief in a creator

limitations and is conceived as vastly different than humans. The same holds for how God is conceived in Judaism and Islam.

Jong et al. (2015) conclude that CSR theories, at best, suggest that a flawed religious belief is formed naturally. Their objection to premise 1 is, however, vulnerable. A defender could argue that detailed beliefs about God's nature do not come naturally, but that a vague belief that supernatural beings exist or that a supernatural realm exists does. The argument goes as follows:

1. Belief in anthropomorphic, time-bound gods is formed naturally.
2. Beliefs that are formed naturally are prima facie rational.
3. Therefore, belief in anthropomorphic time-bound gods is prima facie *rational*.
4. If belief in anthropomorphic, time-bound supernatural beings is prima facie rational, belief that some supernatural being exists is prima facie rational as well.
5. Therefore, belief that some supernatural being exists is prima facie rational.

Belief in anthropomorphic, time-bound supernatural beings logically implies the more general belief that at least one supernatural being exists.[28] Therefore, if one is rational in believing the former, one is also rational in believing the latter. This obviously does not work in the opposite direction, but that is not necessary for our purposes.

The revised argument does not conclude to prima facie rational belief in classical theism. If we look closer at what defenders of naturalness arguments argue, we see that they do *not* conclude that CSR theories support classical theism as defined by Jong et al. (2015). Clark and Barrett (2010) argue that the operations of the cognitive mechanisms CSR theories laid bare resemble those of the *sensus divinitatis*. The *sensus divinitatis* is usually regarded as a cognitive mechanism that produces vague supernatural beliefs or a vague sense of the divine.[29] Theistic belief is way more qualified than the vague sense of the divine Clark and Barrett argue for.

If CSR theories support the rationality of belief that some supernatural being exists— as most defenders of naturalness arguments contend—they also provide some support for more substantial religious beliefs, like belief in the Trinitarian God. How much support is transferred to more detailed religious beliefs is not clear.

Although defenders of naturalness arguments can avoid the problem Jong et al. (2015) raised, this solution comes at a cost. I argue that CSR theories only support rational belief in a limited number of religious beliefs. As Jong et al. rightly point out, most CSR theories show that people naturally believe in supernatural beings that are anthropomorphic and live in and are bound by the spatiotemporal world. If this belief is natural, it prima facie supports the belief that something supernatural exists. It, however,

---

[28] It also implies that a supernatural realm exists. For reasons of brevity, I focus on the belief that some supernatural being exists.

[29] Clark and Barrett (2010, p. 176) do, however, refer to Alvin Plantinga, who argues that the *sensus divinitatis* produces belief in the Abrahamic God.

does not support beliefs that *contradict* the natural belief. Therefore, it does not aid the rationality of belief in supernatural beings that are non-anthropomorphic, live outside the spatiotemporal world, and are unbound by it. Although many members of most religious traditions believe in supernatural beings who are bound by the spatiotemporal world, like angels and demons, they also usually believe that at least one supernatural being that is not anthropomorphic exists or can exist outside the spatiotemporal world. This belief is not only unsupported by CSR theories, it is directly contradicted by naturally formed beliefs.

A successful naturalness argument could be made if CSR theories were to show that belief in supernatural beings comes naturally but remained silent on further attributes of those supernatural beings. If they show that humans naturally form religious beliefs that are not anthropomorphic or bound by the spatiotemporal realm, a naturalness argument can support theism. For now, it seems that most CSR theories do suggest that humans naturally conceive supernatural beings in a limited, anthropomorphic way.[30] Future developments can change this. On current CSR theories, however, a naturalness argument at best supports anthropomorphic religious beliefs, and not theism or belief in any nonanthropomorphic God.

I conclude that, although a good case can be made that some religious beliefs are formed naturally, these naturally formed beliefs contradict religious beliefs, such as belief in a nonanthropomorphic, transcendent God that is not bound by the spatiotemporal realm. Premise 1, though valid for some beliefs, can therefore not support the rationality of theism or the religious belief that most Christians, Jews, and Muslims affirm. The argument therefore does not support the rationality of most of the religious beliefs that contemporary people affirm.

CONCLUSION: CSR AS NEUTRAL

In this chapter, I reviewed three arguments based on CSR theories. I argued that none of them are convincing. Although other arguments can be raised, the failure of these three arguments suggests that CSR theories are neutral with regard to the epistemic status of religious belief.

[30] One could argue that adaptationist theories like the Big Gods theory (Norenzayan, 2013) are largely silent about the specific content of religious beliefs. Big Gods theory argues that belief in a powerful, morally concerned supernatural being gave certain groups an advantage because it allowed for large-scale cooperation. To be adaptive in this way, religious belief need not involve details about anthropomorphism. However, adaptationist theories primarily aim to explain why religious belief persisted and was transmitted. They don't primarily address the more proximate causes of religious beliefs such as cognitive mechanisms or biases. Four notable defenders of the Big Gods theory state clearly that their adaptationist theory fits well with other cognitive explanations of the proximate causes of religious beliefs (Gervais et al., 2011). It therefore seems that defenders of adaptationist theories like the Big Gods theory will also argue that anthropomorphic religious beliefs come naturally.

My assessment of the arguments was based on the current status of CSR. It seems that new CSR theories can only make a difference for the second and third arguments.[31] I argued that the role evolutionary pressures play in the genesis of religious beliefs does not allow for negative epistemic conclusions. Future CSR theories that support the evolved nature of religious belief will therefore not undermine the rationality of religious belief either. Future CSR theories could make a stronger case that religious belief results from a misattribution. Before they can do so, they will need to make a stronger case that religious belief is based on natural input. Future CSR theories could also show that religious beliefs which come naturally do not contradict religious beliefs which are affirmed in some of the largest religious traditions (Christianity, Islam and Judaism).

For now, I merely conclude that current CSR theories are epistemically neutral. Future theories might not be. This will depend on what the theories claim and cannot be decided a priori.

QUESTIONS FOR FUTURE RESEARCH

1. How could theories show that religious belief is (often) not rationally held?
2. How could theories show that religious belief is (often) rationally held?
3. How much do atheistic or theistic presuppositions guide arguments in favor of or against religious belief?

REFERENCES

Alston, W.. P. (1991). *Perceiving God: The epistemology of religious experience.* Ithaca NY: Cornell University Press.

Barrett, J. L. (2004). *Why would anyone believe in God?* Cognitive Science of Religion Series. Walnut Creek, CA: Altamira Press.

Barrett, J. L. (2012). Towards a cognitive science of Christianity. In J. B. Stump & A. G. Padgett (Eds.), *The Blackwell companion to science and Christianity*, p. 319–334. Oxford: Blackwell.

Barrett, J. L., & Church, I. M. (2013). Should CSR give atheists epistemic assurance? On beer-goggles, BFFs, and skepticism regarding religious belief. *The Monist*, 96, 311–324.

Boyer, P. (2002). *Religion explained: The human instincts that fashion gods, spirits and ancestors.* London: Vintage.

Braddock, Matthew. 2016. Debunking Arguments and the Cognitive Science of Religion. *Theology and Science* 14: 268–87.

Braddock, M. (2018). An evidential argument for theism from the cognitive science of religion. In H. Van Eyghen, R. Peels, & G. Van den Brink (Eds.), *New developments in cognitive science of religion: The rationality of religious belief*, pp. 171–198. Dordrecht: Springer.

---

[31] I thus part ways with the idea that CSR theories cannot or do not make a difference in debunking arguments (e.g., Launonen, 2021). The question of whether religious beliefs result from a misattribution or are natural is an empirical question that can be answered by CSR theories.

Clark, K. J., & Barrett, J. L. (2010). Reformed epistemology and the cognitive science of religion. *Faith and Philosophy, 27*(2), 174–189.

Ehrsson, H. H., Holmes, N. P., & Passingham, R. E. (2005). Touching a rubber hand: Feeling of body ownership is associated with activity in multisensory brain areas. *Journal of Neuroscience: The Official Journal of the Society for Neuroscience, 25*(45), 10564–10573. https://doi.org/10.1523/JNEUROSCI.0800-05.2005

Galen, L. (2017). Overlapping mental magisteria: Implications of experimental psychology for a theory of religious belief as misattribution. *Method & Theory in the Study of Religion, 29*, 221–267.

Gervais, W., Willard, A. K., Norenzayan, A., & Henrich, J. (2011). The cultural transmission of faith: Why innate intuitions are necessary, but insufficient, to explain religious belief. *Religion, 41*, 389–410.

Goodnick, L. (2016). A de jure criticism of theism. *Open Theology, 2*(1), 23–33.

Gray, K., & Wegner, D. M. (2010). Blaming God for our pain: Human suffering and the divine mind. *Personality and Social Psychology Review, 14*, 7–16.

Guthrie, S. E. (1993). *Faces in the clouds: A new theory of religion*. New York: Oxford University Press.

Guthrie, S. (2002). Animal animism: Evolutionary roots of religious cognition. In I. Pyysiainen and V. Anttonen (Eds.) *Current Approaches in the Cognitive Science of Religion*, pp. 38-67. London: Continuum.

Huemer, M. (2007). Compassionate phenomenal conservatism. *Philosophy and Phenomenological Research, 74*, 30–55.

Johnson, D. P. (2015). *God is watching you: How the fear of God makes us human*. New York: Oxford University Press.

Jong, J., Kavanagh, C., & Visala, A. (2015). Born idolaters: The limits of the philosophical implications of the cognitive science of religion. *Neue Zeitschrift Für Systematische Theologie Und Religionsphilosophie, 57*, 244–266.

Kelemen, D., & DiYanni, C. (2005). Intuitions about origins: Purpose and intelligent design in children's reasoning about nature. *Journal of Cognition and Development 6*, 3–31.

Law, S. (2018). The X-claim argument against religious belief. *Religious Studies, 54*(1), 15–35.

Launonen, L. (2021). Debunking arguments gain little from cognitive science of religion. *Zygon, 56*(2), 416–433.

Leech, D., & Visala, A. (2011a). The cognitive science of religion: A modified theist response. *Religious Studies, 47*, 301–316.

Leech, D., & Visala, A. (2011b). The cognitive science of religion: Implications for theism? *Zygon, 46*, 47–65.

Lynch, M. (2007). The frailty of adaptive hypotheses for the origins of organismal complexity. *Proceedings of the National Academy of Sciences, 104*, 8597–8604.

McCauley, R. N. (2011). *Why religion is natural and science is not*. New York: Oxford University Press.

Murray, M., & Goldberg, A. (2009). Evolutionary accounts of religion: Explaining and explaining away. In J. Schloss & M. Murray (Eds.), *The believing primate: Scientific, philosophical, and theological reflections on the origin of religion* (pp. 179–199). Oxford: Oxford University Press.

Nola, R. (2013). Do naturalistic explanations of religious beliefs debunk religion? In G. W. Dawes & J. Maclaurin (Eds.), *A new science of religion*, pp. 162–188. Routledge Studies in Religion. New York: Routledge.

Nola, R. (2018). Demystifying religious belief. In H. Van Eyghen, R. Peels, & G. van den Brink (Eds.), *New developments in the cognitive science of religion: The rationality of religious belief* (pp. 71–92). Heidelberg: Springer.

Norenzayan, A. (2013). *Big Gods: How religion transformed cooperation and conflict.* Princeton NJ: Princeton University Press.

Plantinga, A. (1993). *Warrant and proper function.* New York: Oxford University Press.

Plantinga, A. (2011). *Where the conflict really lies: Science, religion, and naturalism.* Oxford: Oxford University Press.

Pollock, J. L. (1986). *Contemporary theories of knowledge.* Rowman & Littlefield Texts in Philosophy. Totowa, NJ: Rowman & Littlefield.

Reid, T. (1872). *Inquiry into the human mind* (7th ed., Vol. 1). The Works of Thomas Reid. Edinburgh: Maclachlan & Stewart.

Rowe, W. L. (1979). The problem of evil and some varieties of atheism. *American Philosophical Quarterly, 16*(4), 335–341.

Schellenberg, J. L. (2006). *Divine hiddenness and human reason.* Ithaca, NY: Cornell University Press.

Schloss, J., & Murray, M. (Eds.). (2009). *The believing primate: Scientific, philosophical, and theological reflections on the origin of religion.* New York: Oxford University Press.

Szocik, K., & Hans Van E. (2021). *Revising cognitive and evolutionary science of religion: Religion as an adaptation.* Vol. 8. London: Springer Nature.

Trigg, R. & Barrett, J. L. (2014). The roots of religion: Exploring the cognitive science of religion (Ashgate Science and Religion Series). Farnham, UK: Ashgate Publishing Group, 2014.

Van Eyghen, H. (2020). *Arguing from cognitive science of religion: Is religious belief debunked?* London: Bloomsbury Academic.

Van Eyghen, H., & Bennett, C. T. (2020). Did natural selection select for true religious beliefs? *Religious Studies.* https://doi.org/10.1017/S0034412520000141

Van Leeuwen, N., & van Elk, M. (2018). Seeking the supernatural: The interactive religious experience model. *Religion, Brain & Behavior, 9*(3), 221–225.

Visala, A., and Barrett, J. L. (2019). In what senses might religion be natural? In P. Copan and C. Taliaferro (eds.), *The Naturalness of Belief: New Essays on Theism's Rationality*, pp. 67–84. Lanham, MD: Lexington Books.

Wilkins, J. S., & Griffiths, P. E. (2013). Evolutionary debunking arguments in three domains: Fact, value, and religion. In G. Dawes & J. Maclaurin (Eds.), *A new science of religion* (pp. 133–146). New York: Routledge.

CHAPTER 20

THE CULTURAL AND DEVELOPMENTAL NICHE OF RELIGIOUS COGNITIONS

Educational Implications of the Cognitive Science of Religion

REBEKAH A. RICHERT

INTRODUCTION

MUCH of the research into the cognitive science of religion (CSR) delineates the nature of intuitive belief systems that provide fundamental cognitive foundations (e.g., causal reasoning, essentialism, folk psychology) for the evolution, transmission, and development of religious thinking. This chapter considers how two primary theories of cognitive development contribute to an understanding of the role cultural and educational practices play in the development of religious cognitions. First, cultural approaches to the study of cognitive development indicate that cultural and social processes support the development of the intuitive systems that provide the foundation for religious cognitions. Information-processing approaches to cognitive development highlight how cognitions come to be intuitive and the potential for critical periods in the development of religious cognitions. The chapter begins with a description of information-processing and theory-theory approaches to cognitive development. It then outlines sociocultural approaches to cognitive development and considers how they highlight the role of education in the development of religious cognitions.

Information-Processing and Theory-Theory Approaches to Cognitive Development

Much research and theory in the field of CSR are based on assumptions and arguments that religious cognitions arise as byproducts of cognitive systems or from propensities that evolved to solve nonreligious problems in human ancestry (Atran, 2002; Bering, 2006; Boyer, 2001). According to the evolutionary accounts commonly drawn upon in the CSR field, humans have default, intuitive cognitive patterns that structure thinking and learning. McCauley (2011) refers to these as "maturationally natural" cognitions. Allegedly, many types of religious cognition are widespread (and perhaps ubiquitous) in part because the cognitions map closely onto these default patterns for reasoning about the world. These postulated patterns of thinking have included assumptions about psychological immortality (i.e., minds do not die with bodies) and the symbolic meaning of natural events (Bering, 2006); that there is purposeful design in natural objects (Kelemen & DiYanni, 2005); and about agency/mind detection (Atran & Norenzyan, 2004; Barrett et al., 2001; Guthrie, 1993). In order to consider the role education plays in developing religious cognitions, it is critical to unpack how different theoretical approaches explain the mechanisms through which concepts are (or become) intuitive.

Automatic and Effortful Cognitions

A primary assumption of information-processing approaches to cognitive development is that all cognitions exist on a continuum from effortful to automatic (Bjorklund & Causey. 2018). Developing human cognition can be characterized as refining both intuitive and explicit processing systems (e.g., Bjorklund & Causey, 2018). Purely effortful cognitions (and explicit processing systems) are available to consciousness, and they may interfere with other processes, improve with practice, and are influenced by individual differences in intelligence, motivation, or education. In contrast, purely automatic cognitions (and intuitive processing systems) occur without intention or awareness, do not interfere with other processes, do not improve with practice, and are not influenced by individual differences in general intelligence, motivation, or education (Bjorklund & Causey, 2018).

From information-processing perspectives, the presence of intuitive cognitive processes can be accounted for in two ways. On the one hand, cognitions develop from being effortful to being automatic through experience and via mechanisms of neural development, such as the complementary processes of the synaptic pruning of unused synaptic connections and the myelination of regularly used synaptic connections (Bjorklund & Causey, 2018). On the other hand, some cognitive processes may be automatic at or shortly after birth. Neurological development accounts for the early presence of intuitive cognitions through characterizations of experience-expectant plasticity (Greenough et al., 1987). In this case, the brain has evolved to expect to receive the kinds of environmental stimuli that generally characterize all human environments (e.g., all humans live on a planet that abides by laws of nature; all humans are exist in social environments that include other members of their species).

Intuitive Theories

As Richert and Lesage (this volume), outline more explicitly, cognitive development also can be characterized as the active acquisition and construction of folk or naive theories about how the world works (Gopnik & Wellman, 1994; ojalehto & Medin, 2015). Folk theories are similar to scientific theories in that they involve theory generation, theory testing, and theory (or conceptual) change; however, folk theories differ from scientific theories in that they result from individuals' natural experiences in the world rather than explicit instruction (Bjorklund & Causey, 2018). Cultural differences in folk theories appear to reflect differences in how the concepts are organized, as opposed to reflecting stable differences in the concepts themselves (ojalehto & Medin, 2015).

Decades of research have documented evidence of early and intuitive folk theories about agents and objects. For example, infants appear to intuitively associate rational, motivational, and epistemic mental states in predicting the actions of intentional agents (Baillargeon et al., 2016) and expect objects to conform to principles of continuity, cohesion, and persistence (Baillargeon, 2008). This definition of "intuitive" is qualitatively different from the definition of "implicit" used in information-processing approaches in that the cognitive processes are considered innate, or processing biases that are present at birth rather than developing from more effortful processes into automatic processes (Bjorklund & Ellis, 2014).

The Cognitive Niche

The documentation of early intuitive concepts and theories by developmental psychologists is consistent with a cognitive-niche hypothesis for the evolution of human cognition, according to which humans evolved into a "cognitive niche," which has allowed the species to overtake others' defenses by cause-and-effect reasoning and through cooperative action (Pinker, 2010; Tooby & DeVore, 1987). Pinker's (2010) version of the argument goes something like this: Given that all animals are potentially other animals' food sources and therefore evolve mechanisms to avoid being eaten, the human species has also evolved such mechanisms. Over the course of evolving predation and defense mechanisms, each species evolves into a niche, which can be considered as the role an organism fills in an ecosystem. In response to selection pressures, most species develop fixed action patterns that protect them from some predators, sometimes make them predators, and sometimes make them prey, resulting in that particular species' evolutionary niche (Pinker, 2010).

In theory, however, in any ecosystem, it is possible for an organism to overtake others' defenses by cause-and-effect reasoning and cooperative action (Pinker, 2010). The evolution of these cognitive capacities characterizes the cognitive niche into which humans have evolved (Pinker, 2010), a niche characterized by the evolution of domain-specific mechanisms designed by natural selection to specialize in processing specific aspects of the physical or social environment (Bjorklund & Ellis, 2014). Regarding the development of religious cognitions, these intuitive (or potentially innate) cognitive predispositions (e.g., agency attribution, assumptions of causality) also allow for the relatively easy transmission of supernatural and religious concepts, across both ontogeny and phylogeny (Bering, 2006).

Summary

To sum up: the term *intuitive* as applied to cognitive development could imply either cognitive biases for processing environmental information that is present from early in development or even birth, or automatic cognitive processes that started as effortful in development and became (more) automatic through repeated use and practice. Of particular note in a developmental context is that intuitive reasoning does not negate or supplant the potential for explicit reasoning (Baillargeon et al., 2016); however, both adults and children will generally default to intuitive and automatic reasoning unless the context or other motivational factors cue them to reason more explicitly or effortfully (Bjorklund & Causey, 2018).

Much research in CSR has focused on arguments that the ubiquity of religious cognitions in human cultures can be explained by the fact that humans have innate, intuitive, domain-specific cognitive mechanisms for processing physical and social environmental stimuli. Findings from young children, educated adults under cognitive load, or adults who have not had formal schooling, have suggested humans may have default cognitive mechanisms that lead to the overattribution of (superknowing) agency (Jarnefelt et al., 2015), teleological reasoning concerning natural phenomena (Kelemen, 2004), and essentialism (or the belief that species members have a shared inner nature that determines the outward appearance; Evans, 2000; Shtulman & Schulz, 2008). These cognitive mechanisms enable us to reason about varieties of agents (supernatural, alive, dead) and natural phenomena without any need to invoke a set of dedicated, input-restricted mechanisms for religion (Pyysiäinen & Hauser, 2010).

In many of these accounts, cultural practices or religious instruction "fill in" these default cognitive assumptions with specific religious content (Kelemen, 2004). Rather than thoroughly review these arguments (presented elsewhere in this handbook), this chapter unpacks the developmental processes through which religious cognitions that begin as effortful can develop through cultural construction to become default intuitive assumptions on which young children and adults rely.

SOCIOCULTURAL APPROACHES TO COGNITIVE DEVELOPMENT

Consistent with experience-expectant neurological plasticity, the ubiquity of religious cognitions in human minds could be explained by unpacking the shared nature of species-typical exposure (Gottlieb, 2007) to religious concepts and ritualized actions (Richert & Smith, 2010). From this developmental perspective, social interaction plays a fundamental role in shaping not only the content, but also the *structure* of children's cognition (Bandura, 1989; Bruner, 1990; Gauvain, 2001; Tomasello, 1999; Vygotsky, 1978). This characterization of cognitive development is outlined in three theoretical approaches: the general genetic law of cultural development (Vygotsky, 1981), the developmental niche (e.g., Super & Harkness, 1986, 2002), and social learning (Bjorklund & Causey, 2018).

The General Genetic Law of Cultural Development

The *general genetic law of cultural development* (Vygotsky, 1981) is the principle that any cognitive function developing in a cultural environment begins first on the social plane, between the child and a social partner, before becoming internalized as a cognitive process in an individual child's mind. This approach allows researchers to actively consider how elementary-level cognitions that are present at birth (i.e., attention, sensation, perception, memory) are transformed as "socially-constituted cognitive activities" (Gauvain, 2001) into higher-order cognitions. Additionally, children are actively involved in re-evaluating and reshaping the socially constructed concepts ("scientific"; see Vygotsky, 1986) into their own spontaneous cognitions.

Cultural Construction of Concepts

According to a Vygotskian (1986) approach to concept development, children's development of concepts progresses through three basic phases: unorganized categories, thinking in complexes, and abstraction. In the first steps toward concept formation (unorganized categories), children's categories exist primarily as a "heap" (Vygotsky, 1986, p. 110) of objects or ideas that share some form of vague, syncretic organization in the child's mind. At this phase, concepts are highly unstable, and the features incorporated into a given concept change regularly based on children's subjective perceptions of the relations between things.

In the *unorganized categories* phase, children progress through three stages of concept development (Vygotsky, 1986). The first stage involves trial and error, when children randomly add features to concepts and try out the revised concepts in social interactions. When a feature of the concept is shown to be inconsistent with the conventional use of that concept, children revise the concept. In the second stage, children rely on the organization of the visual field. In this stage, they incorporate features into concepts based on the continuity in space or time between the feature and the concept. During the third stage, children swap elements from separate categories that have already been formed; however, the newly combined elements still result in incoherent concepts.

According to Vygotsky's (1986) outline of concept development, the second major phase is *thinking in complexes.* In this stage, the features incorporated into a child's concept are not only subjective, but concepts also begin to incorporate the objective bonds that actually exist between features and concepts. In this stage, complexes serve as the "functional equivalence" (Vygotsky, p. 112) of adult concepts; however, Vygotsky argues that concepts in this stage are still profoundly different from the adult forms of concepts, and that complexes form by different rules than real concepts do, specifically through concrete and factual bonds rather than abstract and logical bonds. In practice, this means that when children are developing an abstract concept (like that of God), they primarily rely on the observable actions, objects, people, and words that co-occur with the use of the concept, rather than coming to an understanding of the meaning of the concept through logical or abstract thinking.

The preschool years are an important transition stage in concept development generally. According to Vygotsky (1986), in the preschool years children's concepts are pseudo-concepts, or "shadows" of adult concepts. Preschoolers' pseudo-concepts are initially formed through an associative relationship between the word for the concept and concrete components that are associated with the concept, such as the actions performed while learning the concept or the environment in which the concept was learned. According to Vygotsky, children "practice" with a concept before it is fully formed; and thus early religious concepts are fundamentally "concepts-for-others" before they are "concepts-for-myself."

The implications of this characterization of concept development are far-reaching for understanding the role of education in religious concept development. First, when children use a religious term such as "God" or "prayer," we cannot assume they mean the same thing that an adult member of the religious group would mean. Second, the context in which children are first exposed to a word (or concept) provides the preliminary structure of that concept. In relation to the development of religious concepts, therefore, the contexts in which children are exposed to and learn about religious concepts are themselves a fundamental feature of those concepts.

Third, there may be a critical period for the development of intuitive religious concepts that occurs during early childhood as pseudo-concepts develop into abstracted concepts. Importantly, once cognitive intuitions have become more automatic they are difficult to overwrite with explicit reasoning or education (Shtulman, 2017).

Social and Cultural Learning

Social learning, or learning from others, is typically characterized as taking five basic forms: local enhancement, mimicry, emulation, imitative learning, and teaching (Bjorklund & Causey, 2018). Local enhancement is learning that happens simply because a child notices an activity that another child is doing and goes to the same location and discovers a useful new behavior through trial-and-error learning (e.g., seeing a child playing in the sandbox and going over to the sand box to play as well). In the case of local enhancement, the child does not repeat a modeled behavior or understand the goal of the behavior. In mimicry, children reproduce a modeled behavior without understanding the goal of that behavior (e.g., stepping on a scale after seeing dad step on a scale). In emulation, children understand the goal of a modeled behavior, but do not directly copy the modeled behavior to achieve the same goal (e.g., a child has seen a sibling filling up a pail with sand using a scoop, then the child uses a different item to scoop up the sand). In imitative learning, children reproduce the same action that was modeled while also understanding the goal of performing the action that way. In teaching, children acquire a new skill through the direct instruction of a knowledgeable and experienced social partner (Bjorklund & Causey, 2018).

Developmentally, mimicry begins to emerge around the age of 6 months, and rational imitation begins to emerge around 14 months (Bjorklund & Causey, 2018). In rational imitation, infants will directly mimic an action sequence if they do not know why an actor is performing the action sequence that way, but will emulate the goal of an action sequence they understand by eliminating unnecessary actions (Buttelman et al., 2007; Gergely et al., 2002). For example, a common paradigm for testing infants' imitation involves a person demonstrating how to turn on a light box using their head; of note, the light box can just as easily be turned on using one's hands (Gergely et al., 2002). In this paradigm, if an infant sees a person turning on the box with their head while their hands are clearly available to turn on the box, the infants will mimic the action sequence by also using their head to turn on the box. In contrast, if the hands of the model turning on the box with their head are clearly unavailable for use (e.g., wrapped up in a blanket), the infants will emulate the goal by turning on the box with their hands, not their head (Gergely et al., 2002).

The mimicry of unnecessary actions in an action sequence appears to be present in young children but not chimpanzees (Horner & Whiten, 2005; Lyons et al., 2007). This tendency has been termed "overimitation" (Lyons et al., 2007) and has been documented in children cross-culturally (Neilsen & Tomaselli, 2010). Overimitation appears to reflect children's assumption that certain actions must serve a broader (likely social) function if the mature members of the cultural group are performing them, but the children are unsure why (Legare & Nielsen, 2015).

Cultural learning can be considered a form of social learning. According to Tomasello et al. (1993), cultural learning is uniquely human and is a type of social learning that other species do not share. What distinguishes cultural learning from other forms of social learning is the importance of social cognition in cultural learning. According to Tomasello et al., general social learning can be explained by multiple processes that do not require activating social cognitive processes. For example, general social learning can occur through mere exposure to new ways of doing things, by drawing children's attention to an object or location, and through local enhancement. In contrast, "the cognitive representation resulting from cultural learning includes something of the perspective of the interactional partner, and this perspective continues to guide the learner even after the original learning experience is over" (Tomasello et al., p. 496). The idea of cumulative cultural evolution suggests that human ontogeny occurs in an environment of new artifacts and social practices that carry the collective wisdom of the social group, accumulated throughout the course of cultural history (Dewey, 1963; Durkheim, 1947; Luria, 1928; Tomasello, 1999; Vygotsky, 1929).

Major tasks of development include learning the behavior and activities of the culture and internalizing the tools that support thinking (Gauvain, 1998; Rogoff, 1998). For example, in Vygotskian (1978) theory, children begin to internalize the actions they conduct in the presence of more experienced partners. In cultural learning theory, imitation plays a key role because it constitutes the internalization of communicative intent (Tomasello, 1999). In addition, children develop in the context of structured social activities that provide them with opportunities to discern the process and function of the activities, as well as the function of the social roles within the activities. Overimitation plays a critical role in cumulative cultural evolution, facilitates the rapid acquisition of cultural skills and social skills, and maintains social interaction and group membership (Legare & Nielsen, 2015).

The Developmental Niche

The theory of the developmental niche is echoed in the *cultural niche hypothesis* (Boyd et al., 2011) proposed as an extension of the cognitive niche hypothesis summarized above (see "The Cognitive Niche"). The cultural niche hypothesis specifically addresses the role of cultural processes in human evolution and considers why humans are better than other species at adapting to novel environments. The focus of this account is primarily on the human ability to learn from others, particularly in a cumulative fashion. Thus understanding the mechanisms of cultural and social learning is critical for understanding the development of religious cognitions.

The *developmental niche* (e.g., Super & Harkness, 1986, 2002) is a framework for considering how cultural practices and contexts structure development, with a particular focus on *processes* of human development as opposed to the adult-like final product of development. The developmental niche approach provides valuable insights into the role of education in the development of religious cognitions. In particular, it delineates three operational subsystems along which the cultural construction of religious thinking may systematically differ from the cultural construction of other kinds of thinking (e.g., scientific): the physical and social settings in which development occurs, child-care practices and customs, and parent ethnotheories.

The dimension of *physical and social settings* highlights the ways in which cultural values structure the places in which, and people around whom, a child's development occurs. As Bronfenbrenner and Morris (2006) highlighted, the varying levels at which the environment can impact development (chronosystem, macrosystem, microsystem) filter into direct influences on development via proximal processes and interactions in the child's most immediate environments (most commonly, parents, other caregivers, objects, and symbols. Researchers should consider the unique physical settings (e.g., inside vs. outside the home, school, sacred space, times of the day devoted to engaging these cognitions) and social settings (e.g., parents, religious experts, special agents, academic educators, tutors, peers, siblings) in which children interact with religious cognitions.

The dimension of *child-care practices and customs* highlights the historically constituted customs and practices of child care and childrearing. One useful way of concretizing and operationalizing this dimension is through Rogoff et al.'s (2015) description of repertoires of cultural practice. Rogoff et al. have outlined various ways in which children can be involved in cultural practices, and they particularly highlight that many of the means of support provided for development are "invisible," or not made explicit by members of a particular cultural group or community. This approach has identified three traditions of learning: learning by observing and pitching in (children observe the activities of other community members and actively contribute to these activities), assembly-line instruction (experts coordinate teaching outside the context of the actual productive use of that skill within the community until the child has achieved expertise), and guided repetition of text (children learn specific cultural texts through observation, imitation, and repetition).

The dimension of *parent ethnotheories* generally relates to the psychology of the caretakers. As Super and Harkness (1986) outlined, ethnotheories on parenting typically incorporate "beliefs concerning the nature and needs of children, parental and community goals for rearing, and caretaker beliefs about effective rearing techniques" (Super & Harkness, p. 556). Regarding the development of religious thinking, parents' ethnotheories may incorporate views about the appropriate age at which children should be engaged in religious and ritual practices, parents' beliefs about their own role and efficacy in engaging their children in religious practices and discourse, and about whether and when children should question or accept religious teachings, etc.

The Cultural and Developmental Niche of Religious Cognitions

Understanding the developmental niche of religious cognitions involves unpacking the nature of the practices and contexts that structure this development. According to cultural learning theories, it is also critical to trace children's understandings of these contexts (Tomasello et al., 1993). The remainder of this chapter focuses on three aspects of the developmental context of religious cognitions: parents' own intuitive religious cognitions, explicit testimony about religious concepts and beliefs, and the involvement of children in shared religious activities (e.g., prayer, rituals).

Parents' Intuitive Religious Cognitions

Given that children's development of religious concepts depends on the testimony of those around them rather than direct observation (Harris & Richert, 2008), it is critical to consider the ways in which adults' language structures the transmission of religious concepts. As noted, adults hold varieties of intuitive religious cognitions, including the overattribution of (omniscient) agency (Atran & Norenzayan, 2004), teleological causes of natural phenomena (Kelemen, 2004), and essentialism (Evans, 2000; Shtulman & Schulz, 2008). To understand how these intuitions may structure children's developing religious concepts, it is critical to take a child-oriented view to understanding the influence of language input on children's development (see Nelson & Kessler-Shaw, 2002). Instead of considering language input as having a top-down effect on development, through which parents' explicit transmission of concepts is unidirectional, a child-oriented approach highlights that children develop in a shared communicative environment in which they use social learning skills, such as joint attention and fast mapping, to gather the meaning of concepts through the environmental, syntactical, and grammatical context in which they are embedded.

As a thought exercise, consider the context in which children hear the word "God." Certainly, young children are exposed to the word "God" in the context of explicit religious instruction or in communication with God (e.g., in prayer), whether at home or at a religious institution. However, children also commonly hear the word "God" in nonreligious and unrelated linguistic contexts, such as, "Oh my God!" Because there is no concrete object in the child's environment to which this term "God" refers, the child must piece together the varying contexts in which this term is used, distill the key defining features of the concept, and learn the appropriate contexts in which to use the term. Considering the Vygotskian approach to concept development, young children's concepts of God should be expected to reflect the features to which children have the most frequent exposure.

This is where it becomes critical to unpack the anthropomorphic biases that structure adults' concepts of God (Barrett & Keil, 1996; Heiphetz et al., 2016; Lane & Harris, 2014). The (presumed) ubiquity of these anthropomorphic biases in adults' concepts of supernatural agents may be considered a species-typical experience in cognitive development, which leads early in development to strong anthropomorphic intuitions about God. However, a cultural approach to concept development would suggest that the strength of the anthropomorphic bias may be expected to vary with the strength of parent's own anthropomorphic biases in their concepts of God.

Richert et al. (2017) tested this hypothesis by interviewing parents and their 4- to 7-year-old children from four religious traditions: Protestant, Catholic, Muslim, and Non-Affiliated. The parents completed a checklist indicating their level of certainty that God has a set of humanlike properties (e.g., can get wet in the rain, eats food, forgets things). Although the parents from all the religious traditions indicated generally that they did not believe God had humanlike properties, there were significant differences in parents' certainty in their judgments. The Muslim parents had significantly greater certainty than the Protestant, Catholic, and Non-Affiliated parents that God was not humanlike. The children in the study indicated their belief that God and humans would have omniscience. Like their parents, Muslim children were more likely than the children from the other religious groups to indicate that God would have omniscience but humans would not.

In predictive models, children's differentiation of God's mind from human minds was not predicted by general frequency of participation in formal religious activities (e.g., going to religious services, attending a religious school). Children's differentiation was, however, significantly predicted by parents' certainty about God's anthropomorphic properties. Specifically, children whose parents were more certain that God did not have anthropomorphic properties had greater differentiation between God's mind and human minds. Richert et al. (2017) hypothesized that these anthropomorphic biases likely emerge in the language parents use when they talk with their children about God. Support for this hypothesis comes from research by Lane et al. (2012), who found that children who were tested using anthropomorphic depictions of or language about God were more likely than children tested without such anthropomorphic depictions to attribute ignorance to God

In summary, if adults' intuitive anthropomorphic concepts of God are reflected in the anthropomorphic language they use to describe God, it follows that children's early concepts will reflect these propensities in adults' language use. Within a developmental niche approach, then, it becomes critical to unpack the function of an anthropomorphic concept of God for adults and the resulting ethnotheories about the function of God concepts in development. Some evidence for the functional utility of God concepts can be found in a study examining parents' beliefs about the role of ritualized actions in prayer (Richert et al., 2016). Protestant and Catholic parents were more likely than Muslim parents to indicate that the actions of prayer facilitated direct communication with God, whereas Muslim parents were most likely to focus on the role of prayer actions in facilitating internalized reflection about God. These findings suggest that different foundations in a concept of God can facilitate different kinds of relationships with God.

Explicit Religious Teaching

Children regularly evaluate whom they can trust to teach them new information or skills, a tendency described as "selective trust" (Harris et al., 2018) or "naive skepticism" (Woolley & Ghossainy, 2013). Children's learning about religious concepts such as supernatural agents and the afterlife reflects their reliance on the explicit testimony of those around them (Harris & Richert, 2008). Research has suggested that preschool-aged children are sensitive to the characteristics of potential informants when determining whether they can trust those informants to teach them new information (Harris et al., 2018).

Most of the research on children's trust of informants has evaluated children's selective trust by asking them to identify unreliable informants and to endorse novel claims made by reliable informants (Koenig & Harris, 2005). In this method, both 3- and 4-year-olds exposed to reliable informants (e.g., always gives the correct word label for a common object, like a ball) and unreliable informants (e.g., gives the incorrect word label for common objects, like calling a ball a shoe) can identify which informant is the unreliable one (Koenig & Harris, 2005). However, 4-year-olds tend to be significantly more likely than 3-year-olds to indicate that the reliable informant will provide accurate information in the future and to endorse the reliable informant. Based on this and similar methodologies, studies have found that 4-year-old children selectively learn grammar morphology and object functions from reliable informants (Corriveau et al., 2011) and that children's memory for which informants are reliable persists for four to seven days (Corriveau & Harris, 2009).

Despite the persistence of children's memory for informant reliability, children can easily take into account new information about a previously reliable informant and then update their perspective on that informant as unreliable. This capability has been demonstrated in studies in which a previously reliable informant was shown to be incorrect (Jaswal et al., 2008) or was blindfolded and incapable of providing accurate information (Nurmsoo & Robinson, 2009). In contrast, children do not as easily switch from perceiving a previously unreliable informant as reliable (Nurmsoo & Robinson, 2009).

Beyond providing accurate information (e.g., correct object labels), children's selective trust of informants is related to a variety of other informant characteristics. Children will consistently endorse an informant with unknown expertise over an informant who has demonstrated incompetence in a domain (Koenig & Jaswal, 2011). For example, when children were presented with an informant with a good reason for having information and an informant with a poor reason for knowing information, children were more likely than chance to choose the informant with a good reason (Koenig, 2012). In studies examining whether children can attribute knowledge to the relevant expert (doctor vs. mechanic, eagle vs. car), 3-year-olds assigned stereotypical roles to relevant experts, and 4- and 5-year-olds associated stereotypical roles, relevant knowledge, and underlying principles with relevant experts at above chance levels (Landrum et al., 2013; Lutz & Keil, 2002). Finally, children also consider personality characteristics when determining which informants to trust for information. Children are more likely to endorse a nice but ignorant informant over a mean expert (Landrum et al., 2013) and significantly more likely to endorse a confident informant (Tenney et al., 2011).

Related to the developmental niche of intuitive religious cognitions, it is relevant to consider who presents children with religious testimony in early childhood, in particular parents, religious leaders, and religious instructors. Studies suggest that children's endorsement of the reality status of fictional and supernatural entities relates to parents' explicit encouragement of children's beliefs in those entities (Canfield & Ganea, 2014; Luce et al., 2013; Tenenbaum & Hohenstein, 2016; Woolley et al., 2004). One example of the role of explicit parent testimony in children's development of supernatural concepts comes from a study of parent-child conversations about impossible and improbable events (Nolan-Reyes et al., 2016). Children were more likely to indicate that improbable events were impossible if their parents had provided an explanation for why an impossible event could not occur. Additionally, Rosengren and Hickling (2000) found that children's use of the term "magic" to explain physical causes only emerges in response to parents' use of the term.

The degree of broad cultural endorsement of the existence of unobservable entities also influences children's belief in those entities. For example, Harris et al. (2006) found that 4- to 6-year-old children were more certain of the existence of unobservable entities for which there was collective endorsement (e.g., germs) than of unobservable entities for which there was familial variation in endorsement (e.g., Santa Claus). This pattern is evident even in communities with collective cultural support for both scientific and religious phenomena (Davoodi et al., 2016). For example, in a study conducted with Iranian parents and children, the parents collectively endorsed the existence of religious phenomena (e.g., God), but were more certain of the existence of scientific phenomena (e.g., germs). The 5- to 10-year-old children of these parents reflected the same pattern of greater certainty in the existence of scientific phenomena than of religious phenomena.

Additionally, children's emotional attachment to an information source will influence the likelihood that they will trust information from that informant (Corriveau et al., 2009). The role of emotional bonds is especially illuminated in studies examining children's preferences for their mother or a stranger as a source of information when the information that the mother gives conflicts with that of the stranger. In one study, 4- to 5-year-old children who had been categorized as having a secure attachment at 15 months of age were more likely to rely on a stranger than their mother for information in a task if that stranger had previously been shown to know more than the mother about the specific task (Corriveau et al., 2009). In contrast, children who had an insecure-avoidant attachment style relied less on their mothers' claims in general; and children who had an insecure-resistant attachment style relied more on their mothers' claims in general (Corriveau et al., 2009).

Shared Religious Activities

According to Tomasello et al. (1993), imitation involves the internalization of communicative intent and the model's perspective. As such, religious concepts may be internalized forms of ritual actions or of the intentions and perspectives underlying ritual actions (Richert & Smith, 2010). Religious rituals incorporate actions that are causally opaque (Legare & Souza, 2012; Watson-Jones & Legare, this volume). As Legare and Souza (2012) have noted:

> Rituals are irretrievably causally opaque because they (1) are not bound by the same kinds of intuitive physical-causal constraints that characterize nonritualistic actions and (2) lack an intuitive causal connection between the specific action performed (e.g., rubbing a ceramic pot) and the desired outcome or effect (e.g., making it rain). (p. 1)

Evidence from research with adults has suggested that adults are sensitive to variations in ritual practices that may communicate efficacy, if not the causal mechanisms of the efficacy. Specifically, adults were more likely to judge an unfamiliar ritual effective if the ritual practice contained more procedural steps, incorporated repetition, and was performed in the presence of religious icons (Legare & Souza, 2012).

In addition to these factors, theorists have discussed the social-cognitive and procedural factors involved in intuitions about ritual efficacy (Lawson & McCauley, 1990; McCauley & Lawson, 2002). Lawson and McCauley (1990) proposed a Ritual Action Representation System built on Fodor's (1987) Action Representation System. From this perspective, rituals can be broken into their constituent aspects: a ritual actor (who performs the ritual) and the ritual elements, including a ritual action; a ritual instrument used in performing the ritual action; and a ritual object (or person) toward which the ritual is directed (Lawson & McCauley, 1990). According to this theoretical approach, religious rituals are defined as "acts in which someone does something to someone or something in order to bring about some nonnatural consequence by virtue of appeal to superhuman agency" (Barrett & Lawson, 2001, p. 184). Key to this definition is the role of supernatural agency as the causal mechanism of ritual efficacy and the implication that ritual actions and sequences are a form of communication with a supernatural agent.

A child's imitation of rituals and religious practices involves internalizing the intentions, of not only the actor, but all the actors who have performed those actions over the course of evolutionary history (Richert & Smith, 2010). If we consider rituals to be culturally symbolic action forms, it is important to consider the role rituals play in children's religious concept development. In a strict application of cultural learning theory, religious concepts may be internalized forms of ritual actions or of the intentions and perspectives underlying the actions. If this is the case, participation in religious rituals may have been a primary factor in structuring religious concepts over the course of evolutionary history. The particular forms of these practices for our ancestors and in modernity would be expected to vary as a function of the specific cultural context, as they would reflect an accumulation of cultural changes and practices.

Factors related to overimitation would be expected to relate specifically to children's imitation of (and subsequent internalization of the intentions of) religious rituals. Studies have suggested that children are more likely to overimitate the actions of people who have the same accent as the child (Kinzler et al., 2011), are considered to be in a high-status group (McGuigan, 2013), and appear to be knowledgeable (Bucshbaum et al., 2011).

Few studies have specifically examined children's intuitions about *how* religious rituals work and *what* makes them work. In one study, 4- to 12-year-old Catholic children were told a vignette about an infant being baptized. The children were then asked what about the infant would be different after the baptism. Across all ages, the children indicated that the baptism changed something internal about the baby, specifically, the baby's mind or soul but not the baby's physical brain (Richert & Harris, 2006). These findings suggest that children view rituals as having an invisible effect on the person on whom a ritual is performed, perhaps reflecting an assumption that these "causally opaque" actions (Legare & Souza, 2012) will affect aspects of a person that cannot be observed directly.

An additional set of studies specifically examined children's understanding of the efficacy of ritual actions (Richert, 2006). In three experiments, Richert (2006) interviewed 4- to 12-year-old children about whether altering a ritual's actions would affect the outcome of the ritual. In the first experiment, children were interviewed about novel ritual actions (e.g., standing on one foot while singing) that were given either a ritual (i.e., social group history) explanation (e.g., they don't know why people stand on one leg, that's just how it's always been done) or a functional explanation (e.g., people sing better when they stand on one leg). Children were then asked how bad it would be if the protagonist did not perform the ritual action. By the age of 9, children differentiated the ritual actions from the functional actions and claimed it would be "a little" bad if a person did not perform the ritual actions but not the functional actions (Richert, 2006).

In follow-up experiments, children were asked about the actions involved in a familiar religious ritual (baptism) and a familiar routine (the nighttime bath; Richert, 2006). Instead of the question how bad would it be not to perform the actions, the children were asked whether people had to perform the sequence of actions in a particular way (Experiment 2) and whether a ritual would still work if changes to the actions were made while the ritual was being performed (Experiment 3). Children at all ages were more likely to say that the sequence of actions in a baptism had to be performed a specific way than the sequence of actions in a bath; however, the 4- to 6-year-old children were more likely than the 7- to 12-year-old children to claim that a ritual would not work if the actions were altered (Richert, 2006).

Two recent studies have examined the factors related to differences in whether children have a ritualistic view of prayer (Richert et al., 2016) and how children's developing social cognition relates to their understanding of the ritualized aspects of prayer (Shaman et al., 2016). Richert et al. (2016) found that 3.5- to 6-year-old children from a variety of religious traditions (Protestant, Catholic, and Muslim) were more likely than their parents to view the actions of prayer as serving a ritualistic function (e.g., helped the person praying to communicate with God) as opposed to an instrumental-internal function (e.g., helped the person praying to think about God). Children with a ritualistic view of prayer also had more anthropomorphic views of God (e.g., viewed God as embodied and with limited knowledge).

Shaman et al. (2016) found that preschoolers had generally inflexible views of prayer actions, claiming that prayers had to incorporate conventional actions of their own religious tradition. However, the view that prayer actions have to be conventional was related to their view of their mother's mind, not God's mind. More specifically, children who believed that their mothers had fallible access to their own intentions (i.e., false beliefs) had more inflexible views about how prayers had to be performed, even after controlling for age. These findings indicate that children have some sense that ritualistic practices, such as prayer, involve a supernatural agent's influence and psychological aspects of the people engaging in the practice.

In summary, one area related to religious concept development in early childhood that is ripe for research is in the nature of the relationship between engaging in shared religious activities (e.g., prayer) and the development of intuitive and explicit religious cognitions (Richert & Granqvist, 2013). One hypothesis is that in observing the people around them participating in rituals, and overimitating the actions of rituals, children may be internalizing the intentions of the people they are imitating (e.g., Tomasello et al., 1993). These intentions often include communication with an unseen supernatural agent and assumptions of supernatural causality. As such, participation in shared religious activities plays a critical role in laying the foundation for the development and education of religious cognitions.

Conclusion

Critical questions remain about the ways in which complex religious cognitions that exist at the cultural level become internalized as personal cognitions and beliefs in the course of development. Theories of cognitive development that highlight the cultural context suggest that it is critical to unpack how the development of religious thinking occurs in unique physical and social spaces; engages the body in different ways; and is guided by parental ethnotheories about developmental timing, goals for religious thinking, and children's active participation in this domain of thought at different ages.

Despite these remaining questions, the theories and research that have been described here indicate that religious education can occur in multiple ways. Certainly, religious education can occur through direct instruction; however, for young children, religious education is more likely to occur through informal interactions with their parents, observations of their parents' language and behaviors, and participation in ritual. As early-occurring cognitions become more automatic over time and with use, the nature of religious experiences in early childhood will form the conceptual foundation for children's future learning about and interaction with their religious beliefs.

Questions for Future Research

1. What is the nature of the physical and social spaces in which religious thinking develops? How does the nature of these spaces shape religious and spiritual development?
2. What are similarities and variations in parental ethnotheories about goals for religious thinking, developmental timing for achieving these goals, and children's active participation in this domain of thought at different ages?
3. How do children process and internalize different kinds of testimony received from different "experts" in their religious lives (e.g., parents, religious teachers, religious leaders, siblings, peers, texts, etc.)?
4. What is the role of action and embodiment in children's developing religious thinking?

Acknowledgments

The writing of this chapter was supported by a grant to the author from the John Templeton Foundation (#JTF61062).

References

Atran, S. (2002). *In gods we trust: The evolutionary landscape of religion*. Oxford: Oxford University Press.

Atran, S., & Norenzyan, A. (2004). Religions evolutionary landscape: Counterintuition, commitment, compassion, communion. *Brain and Behavioral Sciences, 27*(6), 713–730. doi:10.1017/S0140525X04000172

Baillargeon, R. (2008). Innate ideas revisited: For a principle of persistence in infants' physical reasoning. *Perspectives on Psychological Science, 3*(1), 2–13. doi:10.1111/j.1745-6916.2008.00056.x

Baillergeon, R., Scott, R. M., & Bian, L. (2016). Psychological reasoning in infancy. *Annual Review of Psychology, 67*, 159–186. doi:10.1146/annurev-psych-010213-115033

Bandura, A. (1989). Social cognitive theory. In R. Vasta (Ed.), *Annals of child development. Vol. 6: Six theories of child development*, pp. 1–60. Greenwich, CT: JAI Press.

Barrett, J. L., & Keil, F. C. (1996). Conceptualizing a non-natural entity: Anthropomorphism in God concepts. *Cognitive Psychology, 31*, 219–247. doi:10.1006/cogp.1996.0017

Barrett, J. L., & Lawson, E. T. (2001). Ritual intuitions: Cognitive contributions to judgments of ritual efficacy. *Journal of Cognition & Culture, 1*(2), 183–201. doi:10.1163/156853701316931407

Barrett, J. L., Richert, R. A., & Driesenga, A. (2001). God's beliefs versus mother's: The development of nonhuman agent concepts. *Child Development, 72,* 50–65. doi:10.1111/1467-8624.00265

Bering, J. M. (2006). The folk psychology of souls. *Behavioral and Brain Sciences, 29,* 453–462. doi:10.1017/S0140525X06009101

Bjorklund, D. F., & Causey, K. B. (2018). *Children's thinking: Cognitive development and individual differences* (6th ed.). Thousand Oaks, CA: Sage.

Bjorklund, D. F., & Ellis, B. J. (2014). Children, childhood, and development in evolutionary perspective. *Developmental Review, 34,* 225–264. doi:10.1016/j.dr.2014.05.005

Boyd, R., Richerson, P. J., & Heinrich, J. (2011). The cultural niche: Why social learning is essential for human adaptation. *PNAS, 108*(2), 10918–10925. doi:10.1073/pnas.1100290108

Boyer, P. (2001). *Religion explained.* London: Vintage.

Bronfenbrenner, U., & Morris, P.A. (2006). The ecology of developmental processes. In W. Damon & R. M. Lerner (Eds.), *Handbook of child psychology* (5th ed., Vol. 1). New York: Wiley.

Bruner, J. S. (1990). *Acts of meaning.* Cambridge, MA: Harvard University Press.

Bucshbaum, D., Gopnik, A., Griffiths, T. L., & Shafto, P. (2011). Children's imitation of causal action sequences is influenced by statistical and pedagogical evidence. *Cognition, 120*(3), 331–340. doi:10.1016/j.cognition.2010.12.001

Buttelmann D., Carpenter, M., Call, J., & Tomasello, M. (2007). Enculturated chimpanzees imitate rationally. *Developmental Science, 10*(4), F31–38. doi:10.1111/j.1467-7687.2007.00630

Canfield, C. F., & Ganea, P. A. (2014). "You could call it magic": What parents and siblings tell children about unobservable entities. *Journal of Cognition and Development, 15*(2), 269–286. doi:10.1080/15248372.2013.777841

Corriveau, K. H. & Harris, P. L. (2009). Preschoolers continue to trust a more accurate informant 1 week after exposure to accuracy information. *Developmental Science, 12,* 188–193. doi:10.1111/j.1467-7687.2008.00763.x

Corriveau, K. H., Harris, P. L., Meins, E., Femyhough, C., Arnott, B., Elliot, L., Liddle, B., Hearn, A., Vittorini, L., & de Rosnay, M. (2009). Young children's trust in their mother's claims: Longitudinal links with attachment security in infancy. *Child Development, 80*(3), 750–761. doi:10.1111/j.1467-8624.2009.01295.x

Corriveau, K. H., Pickard, K, & Harris, P. L. (2011). Young children's selective trust in informants. *Philosophical Transactions of the Royal Society, Series B: Biological Sciences, 366,* 1179–1187. doi:10.1098/rstb.2010.0321

Davoodi, T., Corriveau, K. H., & Harris, P. L. (2016). Distinguishing between realistic and fantastical figures in Iran. *Developmental Psychology, 52*(2), 222–231. doi:10.1037/dev0000079

Dewey, J. (1963). *Experience and education.* New York: Simon and Schuster. (Original work published in 1938).

Durkheim, É. (1947). *The elementary forms of religious life.* London: George Allen & Unwin. (Original work published in 1912).

Evans, E. M. (2000). The emergence of beliefs about the origins of species in school-age children. *Merrill-Palmer Quarterly, 46,* 221–254.

Fodor, J. A. (1987). *Psychosemantics: The problem of meaning in the philosophy of mind.* Cambridge, MA: MIT Press.

Gauvain, M. (1998). Cognitive development in social and cultural context. *Current Directions in Psychological Science, 7*(6), 188–192. doi:10.1111/1467-8721.ep10836917

Gauvain, M. (2001). *The social context of cognitive development.* New York: Guilford Press.

Gergely, G., Bekkering, H., & Kiraly, I. (2002). Rational imitation in preverbal infants. *Nature*, *415*(6873), 755. doi:10.1038/415755a

Gopnik, A., & Wellman, H. M. (1994). The theory theory. In L. A. Hirschfeld & S. A. Gelman (Eds.), *Mapping the mind: Domain specificity in cognition and culture*, pp. 257–293. New York: Cambridge University Press. http://dx.doi.org/10.1017/CBO9780511752902.011

Gottlieb, G. (2007). Probabilistic epigenesis. *Developmental Science*, *10*(1), 1–11. doi:10.1111/j.1467-7687.2007.00556.x

Greenough, W. T., Black, J. E., & Wallace, C. S. (1987). Experience and brain development. *Child Development*, *58*, 539–559.

Guthrie, S. (1993). *Faces in the clouds: A new theory of religion*. Oxford: Oxford University Press.

Harris, P. L., Koenig, M. A., Corriveau, K. H., & Jaswal, V. K. (2018). Cognitive foundations of learning from testimony. *Annual Review of Psychology*, *69*, 251–273. doi:10.1146/annurev-psych-122216-011710

Harris, P. L., Pasquini, E. S., Duke, S., Asscher, J. J., & Pons, F. (2006). Germs and angels: The role of testimony in young children's ontology. *Developmental Science*, *9*(1), 76–96. doi:10.1111/j.1467-7687.2005.00465.x

Harris, P. L., & Richert, R. A. (2008). William James, "The World of Sense" and trust in testimony. *Mind & Language*, *23*(5), 536–551. doi:10.1111/j.1468-0017.2008.00354.x

Heiphetz, L., Lane, J. D., Waytz, A., & Young, L. L. (2016). How children and adults represent God's mind. *Cognitive Science*, *40*(1), 1–24. doi:10.1111/cogs.12232

Horner, V., & Whiten, A. (2005). Causal knowledge and imitation/emulation switching in chimpanzees (*Pan troglodytes*) and children (*Homo sapiens*). *Animal Cognition*, *8*(3), 164–181. doi:10.1007/s10071-004-0239-6

Jarnefelt, E., Cantfield, C. F., & Kelemen, D. (2015). The divided mind of a disbeliever: Intuitive beliefs about nature as purposefully created among different groups of non-religious adults. *Cognition*, *140*, 72–88. doi:10.1016/j.cognition.2015.02.005

Jaswal, V. K., McKercher, D. A., & VanderBorght, M. (2008). Limitations on reliability: Regularity rules in the English plural and past tense. Child Development, *79*(3), 750–760. doi:10.1111/j.1467-8624.2008.01155.x

Kelemen, D. (2004). Are children "intuitive theists"? Reasoning about purpose and design in nature. *Psychological Science*, *15*(5), 295–301. doi:10.1111/j.0956-7976.2004.00672.x

Kelemen, D., & DiYanni, C. (2005). Intuitions about origins: Purpose and intelligent design in children's reasoning about nature. *Journal of Cognition and Development*, *6*(1), 3–31. doi:10.1207/s15327647jcd0601_2

Kinzler, K. D., Corriveau, K. H., & Harris, P. L. (2011). Children's selective trust in native-accented speakers. *Developmental Science*, *14*(1), 106–111. doi:10.1111/j.1467-7687.2010.00965.x

Koenig, M. A. (2012). Beyond semantic accuracy: Preschoolers evaluate a speaker's reasons. *Child Development*, *83*(3), 1051–1063. doi:10.1111/j.1467-8624.2012.01742.x

Koenig, M. A., & Harris, P. L. (2005). Preschoolers mistrust ignorant and inaccurate speakers. *Child Development*, *76*, 1261–1277. doi:10.1111/j.1467-8624.2005.00849.x

Koenig, M. A., & Jaswal, V. K. (2011). Characterizing children's expectations about expertise and incompetence: Halo or pitchfork effects? *Child Development*, *82*(5), 1634–1647. doi:10.1111/j.1467-8624.2011.01618.x

Landrum, A., Mills, C. M., & Johnston, A. (2013). When do children trust the expert? Benevolence information influences children's trust more than expertise. *Developmental Science*, *16*(4), 622–638. doi:10.1111/desc.12059

Lane, J. D., & Harris, P. L. (2014). Confronting, representing, and believing counterintuitive concepts: Navigating the natural and supernatural. *Perspectives on Psychological Science*, 9(2), 144–160. doi:10.1177/1745691613518078

Lane, J. D., Wellman, H. M., & Evans, E. M. (2012). Socio-cultural input facilitates children's developing understanding of extraordinary minds. *Child Development*, 83(3), 1007–1021. doi:10.1111/j.1467-8624.2012.01741.x

Lawson, T. E., & McCauley, R. N. (1990). *Rethinking religion*. Cambridge, UK: Cambridge University Press.

Legare, C. H., & Nielsen, M. (2015). Imitation and innovation: The dual engines of cultural learning. *Trends in Cognitive Science*, 19(11), 68–699. doi:10.1016/j.tics.2015.08.005

Legare, C. H., & Souza, A. L. (2012). Evaluating ritual efficacy: Evidence from the supernatural. *Cognition*, 124(1), 1–15. doi:10.1016/j.cognition.2012.03.004

Luce, M. R., Callanan, M. A., & Smilovic, S. (2013). Links between parents' epistemological stance and children's evidence talk. *Developmental Psychology*, 49(3), 454–461. doi:10.1037/a0031249

Luria, A. R. (1928). The problem of the cultural behavior of the child. *Journal of Genetic Psychology*, 35, 493–506. Retrieved from https://www.marxists.org/archive/luria/works/1928/cultural-behaviour-child.htm

Lutz, D. J., & Keil, F. C. (2002). Early understanding of the division of cognitive labor. *Child Development*, 73, 1073–1084. doi:10.1111/1467-8624.00458

Lyons, D. E., Young, A. G., & Keil, F. C. (2007). The hidden structure of overimitation. *PNAS*, 104(50), 19751–19756. doi:10.1073/pnas.0704452104

McCauley, R. N. 2011). *Why religion is natural, and science is not*. New York Oxford University Press.

McCauley, R. N., & Lawson, E. T. (2002). *Bringing ritual to mind: Psychological foundations of cultural forms*. New York: Cambridge University Press.

McGuigan, N. (2013). The influence of model status on the tendency of young children to over-imitate. *Journal of Experimental Child Psychology*, 116(4), 962–969. doi:10.1016/j.jecp.2013.05.004

Nelson, K., & Kessler Shaw, L. (2002). Developing a socially shared symbolic system, in language, literacy and cognitive development. In E. Amsel & J. P. Byrnes (Eds), *Language, literacy, and cognitive development: The development and consequences of symbolic communication*, pp. 27–62. Mahwah, NJ: Erlbaum.

Nielsen, M., & Tomaselli, K. (2010). Over-imitation in Kalahari bushman children and the origins of human cultural cognition. *Psychological Science*, 21(5), 729–736. doi:10.1177/0956797610368808

Nolan-Reyes, C., Callanan, M. A., & Haigh, K. A. (2016). Practicing possibilities: Parents' explanations of unusual events and children's possibility thinking. *Journal of Cognition and Development*, 17(3), 378–395. doi:10.1080/15248372.2014.963224

Nurmsoo, E., & Robinson, E. J. (2009). Children's trust in previously inaccurate informants who were well or poorly informed: When past errors can be excused. *Child Development*, 80(1), 23–27. doi:10.1111/j.1467-8624.2008.01243.x

ojalehto, b. l., & Medin, D. L. (2015). Perspectives on culture and concepts. *Annual Review of Psychology*, 66, 249–275. doi:10.1146/annurev-psych-010814-015120

Pinker, S. (2010). The cognitive niche: Coevolution of intelligence, sociality, and language. *Proceedings of the National Academy of Sciences*, 107(2), 8893–8999. doi:10.1073/pnas.0914630107

Pyysiäinen, I., & Hauser, M. (2010). The origins of religion: Evolved adaptation or by-product? *Trends in Cognitive Science, 14*(3), 104–109. doi:10.1016/j.tics.2009.12.007

Richert, R. A. (2006). The ability to distinguish ritual actions in children. *Method & Theory in the Study of Religion, 18,* 144–165. doi:10.1163/157006806777832850

Richert, R. A., & Granqvist, P. (2013). Religious and spiritual development in childhood. In R. F. Paloutzian & C. L. Park (Eds.), *Handbook of the psychology of religion and spirituality* (2nd ed.), pp. 165–192. New York: Guilford Press.

Richert, R. A., Saide, A. R., Lesage, K. A., & Shaman, N. J. (2017). The role of religious context in children's differentiation between God's mind and human minds. *British Journal of Developmental Psychology, 35*(1), 37–59. doi:10.1111/bjdp.12160

Richert, R. A., Shaman, N. J., Saide, A. R., & Lesage, K. A. (2016). Folding your hands helps god hear you: Prayer and anthropomorphism in parents and children. *Research in the Social Scientific Study of Religion, 27,* 140–157. doi:10.1163/9789004322035_010

Richert, R. A., & Smith, E. I. (2010).The role of religious concepts in the evolution of human cognition. In U. Frey (Ed), *The nature of God: Evolution and religion,* pp. 93–110. Antwerp, Belgium: Tectum.

Rogoff, B. (1998). Cognition as a collaborative process. In W. Damon (Ed.), *Handbook of child psychology. Vol. 2: Cognition, perception, and language,* pp. 679–744. Hoboken, NJ: John Wiley & Sons.

Rogoff, B., Moore, L. C., Correa-Chavez, & Dexter, A. L. (2015). Children develop cultural repertoires through engaging in everyday routines and practices. In J. E. Grusec & P. D. Hastings (Eds.), *Handbook of socialization: Theory and research* (2nd ed.), pp. 472–498. New York: Guilford.

Rosengren, K. S., & Hickling, A. K. (2000). Metamorphosis and magic: The development of children's thinking about possible events and plausible mechanisms. In K. S. Rosengren, C. N. Johnson, & P. L. Harris (Eds.), *Imagining the impossible: Magical, scientific, and religious thinking in children,* pp. 75–98. New York: Cambridge University Press.

Shaman, N. J., Saide, A. R., Lesage, K. A., & Richert, R. A. (2016). Who cares if I stand on my head when I pray? Social cognition and ritual inflexibility in preschoolers. *Research in the Social Scientific Study of Religion, 27,* 122–139. doi:10.1163/9789004322035_009

Shtulman, A. (2017). *Scienceblind: Why our intuitive theories about the world are so often wrong.* New York: Basic Books.

Shtulman, A., & Schulz, L. (2008). The relation between essentialist beliefs and evolutionary reasoning. *Cognitive Science, 32*(6), 1049–1062. doi:10.1080/03640210801897864.

Super, C. M., & Harkness, S. (1986). The developmental niche: A conceptualization at the interface of child and culture. *International Journal of Behavioral Development, 9*(4), 545–569. doi:10.1177/016502548600900409

Super, C. M., & Harkness, S. (2002). Culture structures the environment for development. *Human Development, 45*(4), 270–274. doi:10.1159/000064988

Tenenbaum, H. R., & Hohenstein, J. M. (2016). Parent-child talk about the origins of living things. *Journal of Experimental Child Psychology, 150,* 314–329. doi:10.1016/j.jecp.2016.06.007

Tenney, E. R., Small, J. B., Kondrad, R. L., Jaswal, V. K., & Spellman, B. A. (2011). Accuracy, confidence, and calibration: How young children and adults assess credibility. *Developmental Psychology, 47*(4), 1065–1077. doi:10.1037/a0023273

Tomasello, M. (1999). *The cultural origins of human cognition.* Cambridge, MA: Harvard University Press.

Tomasello, M., Kruger, A. C., & Ratner, H. H. (1993). Cultural learning. *Behavioral and Brain Sciences*, *16*(3), 495–552. doi:10.1017/S0140525X0003123X

Tooby, J., & DeVore, I. (1987). The reconstruction of hominid behavioral evolution through strategic modeling. In W. G. Kinzey (Ed.), *Primate models for the origin of human behavior*, pp. 183–237. Albany: State University of New York Press.

Vygotsky, L. S. (1929). The problem of the cultural development of the child. *Journal of Genetic Psychology*, *36*, 415–434.

Vygotsky, L. S. (1978). *Mind in society: The development of higher psychological processes* (M. Cole, V. John-Steiner, S. Scribner, & E. Souberman, Trans.). Cambridge, MA: Harvard University Press.

Vygotsky, L. S. (1981). The genesis of higher mental function. In J. V. Wertsch (Ed.), *The concept of activity in Soviet psychology*, pp.144–188. Armonk, NY: Sharp.

Vygotsky, L. S. (1986). *Thought and language*. Cambridge, MA: MIT Press. (Original work published in 1934).

Woolley, J. D., Boerger, E. A., & Markman, A. B. (2004). A visit from the candy witch: Factors influencing young children's belief in a novel fantastical being. *Developmental Science*, *7*(4), 456–468. doi:10.1111/j.1467–7687.2004.00366.x

Woolley, J. D., & Ghossainy, E. M. (2013). Revisiting the fantasy-reality distinction: Children as naïve skeptics. *Child Development*, *84*, 1496–1510. doi:10.1111/cdev.12081

CHAPTER 21

LIVED FAITH AND COGNITIVE INTUITIONS

Some Theological Implications of Cognitive Science of Religion

LAIRD R. O. EDMAN AND MYRON A. PENNER

INTRODUCTION

OUR task in this chapter is to examine the ways in which data and theories from the cognitive science of religion (CSR) can and should impact theology. Suppose that the model of religious cognition emerging from CSR is reasonably accurate, as far as it goes. What difference should that make to theology's content and method? Answering that question is the focus of this chapter. We set out to answer it in the following outline. First, we do a bit of conceptual ground clearing by making explicit what we mean by both "CSR" and "theology." After describing what theology is, we present a general model for how theology can be done, using a model for theological method that we hope will be both recognizable to professionals and intelligible to those outside the guild of professional theologians. Second, we look at how findings from CSR can inform theology in two key areas: attributions of divine purpose and understanding ritual and worship. While we will write specifically about how CSR should affect the task of Christian theologizing, much of what we say here will work (with minor adjustment) for other theological paradigms, whether they be the conceptual and lived framework of another established religious tradition or, more broadly, any type of personal reflection on supernatural agency and meaning one could reasonably dub "religious" or "spiritual" in nature.

What Is CSR?

We understand CSR to be a pan-disciplinary endeavor that examines the ways ordinary human cognition informs and influences those cultural expressions most people deem "religious" (Barrett, 2013). These cognitive foundations or common mental tools make it easy for humans to develop and maintain religious beliefs. Core to the cognitive architecture involved in these processes is our dual-system thinking, often characterized as "system 1" and "system 2" thinking (Kahneman, 2003, 2011; Stanovich & West, 2000). Our unreflective, automatic, nonconscious cognition (system 1) serves as a foundation for our more analytic, reflective thinking (system 2), which can recursively influence our nonreflective intuitions to develop in new directions, which in turn influence our reflective cognition. This circular process creates the mental conditions that "smooth the cognitive path" for people to interpret events and generate ideas that today we deem religious.

The central research areas of CSR reveal a complex interaction of cognitive functions and propensities that appear to be foundational to religious beliefs, behaviors, and social arrangements. In brief, the story CSR tells about the generation of religious beliefs and behaviors includes the way dual-system thinking interacts with the human tendency to easily detect agents, our use of theory of mind to consider what others might be thinking, our tendency to impute purpose as the reason for the existence of objects and events, and our easy default to dualistic thinking about mind and body. Since our dual-system thinking relies on our nonconscious intuitions as the foundation for our reflective beliefs, our hypersensitive agency-detection device (HADD) makes it easy to sense agents even when we don't see anything, and our theory of mind then imputes thoughts, intentions, and desires to those invisible agents. Our overactive teleological thinking makes it seem reasonable and logical that something made all that we see and that everything that happens must happen for a reason, conclusions that support what our HADD and theory of mind have been telling us. Our intuitive dualism encourages us to assume that life continues in some form after death. Finally, the concepts generated by these intuitions that are most easily remembered and passed on to others, are those that give the believer some advantage and which violate only one or two folk intuitions. Minimally counterintuitive concepts with inferential advantage, generated at least in part by nonreflective intuitions, tend to make up the core of human religious beliefs.

The operations of this cognitive architecture are not independent of social or cultural influence, no more than learning a language is independent of the cultural and social context into which someone is born. We speak not of "innate" predispositions or propensities, but rather of the ways in which normal human cognitive functioning (operating within and interacting with the environments typical for humans) leads to the development of particular sorts of "religious" beliefs and behaviors that may or may not be specifically adaptive. Because of the interaction of how our minds work with the circumstances in which we find ourselves, beliefs in the existence and abilities of invisible supernatural agents, in an afterlife and mind-body dualism, in an agentic creator, and in the efficacy of causally opaque rituals are developed and transmitted easily. Some forms of religious belief and behavior are "natural," and others are much less so (McCauley, 2000, 2011). This has deep implications for theological inquiry and the work of religious leaders and teachers.

What Is Theology?

One feature of CSR that has led to its productivity as a research program in the scientific study of religion, is its focus on mapping the cognitive processes involved in specific activities that form part of the human experience of religion. This has allowed CSR to make substantial progress in offering explanations of, for example, the near-universal, cross-cultural, recurrent experience of belief in supernatural agents, without getting bogged down in definitional debates about what constitutes "religion" (Barrett, 2013; Barrett & Trigg, 2014) or whether religion itself is something that can be studied. Thus, though "religion" might be too wide a thing to be studied scientifically with confidence, one has a better chance at giving scientific explanation for narrower objects of study: for example, the ease with which children form beliefs about mind-body dualism (Barrett, 2012; Bloom, 2004, 2007; Boyer, 2001) or the role of mentalizing cognitive processes in prayer to gods (Barrett, 2012; Edman, 2018). The piecemeal approach then generates data that can be synthesized to form more comprehensive theories that are wider in scope.[1]

Theology, like religion, is challenging to define but recognizable when one sees it, and no definition of theology is going to be without detractors. At its most general level of analysis, theology can be understood as an attempt to organize one's thoughts about the divine.[2] Some are happy to equate thinking about the divine with thinking about whatever one has in view as being the source of life's meaning, or happiness, or ultimate value. Casting the net so widely means that one is doing something akin to theology whenever one articulates one's views about what constitutes meaning and value.

For now, we're going to narrow our description of theology to organized thinking about the divine, and in short order we're going to narrow down our description even further. What our discussion thus far shows, however, is that on one level of definition, it makes sense to think about "theology" as a legitimate activity for participants of any and every type of religion, and perhaps even for those who follow Socrates's injunction to live the examined life and ask what, if anything, constitutes a meaningful life. Nonetheless, taking a cue from CSR researchers, who tend to focus on the cognitive processes involved in specific aspects of religious life, we will use Christian theology as a specific aspect of the theological life; we will present ways in which CSR specifically impacts Christian theologizing.

---

[1] Ara Noranzayan's *Big Gods* (2013) is an example; it synthesizes data from related fields into a comprehensive theory with wider scope.

[2] Describing the *logos* (systematic, organizing rational principle) that maps on to *theos* (god, God, the divine).

THEOLOGY AND OTHER DISCIPLINES

Theology, like philosophy, is something done both by professionals and nonexperts. For example, the person who lacks formal training in philosophy might still reflect on philosophical questions, employ reason in constructing and evaluating arguments, and so forth. Similarly, the Christian who lacks formal training in theology might still reflect on theological questions, drawing on various resources to articulate who God is, what God's purposes might be, and how creaturely experience in all its forms relates to God. Explicitly, Christian theology looks to articulate God's nature and purposes from a Christian perspective, the central shaping event being the life and work of Jesus of Nazareth. This means that the texts, traditions, influencers, and communities that reflect Christian experience—including the Hebrew Bible and the Jewish communities out of which early Christianity emerged—shape the contours of Christian theology.

One feature that distinguishes the flavor of academic theology from the layperson's practice of theology is that academic theology reflects a sustained, scholarly research program that draws on and synthesizes a variety of academic disciplines. These disciplines include, but are not limited to, biblical studies, historical theology, systematic theology, biblical languages, and philosophical theology. Because theology is an integrative discipline whose ultimate goal is articulating how all things relate to God, it is proper for theologians to look at our best data across academic disciplines to see what impact, if any, our best information about the world has on our understanding of God and God's purposes. Properly incorporated, information from other disciplines should influence theology in two main ways.

The first way is *corrective*, when it turns out that a theological claim needs revision because new and better information has come to light from another (i.e., nontheological) domain of inquiry. An easy example of this is the way in which theological models of creation, which held the universe to be less than 10,000 years old, required revision in light of data from geology, physics, chemistry, and cosmology, each of which, and in different ways, demonstrated that the universe is much, much older.

The second way information from other disciplines influences theology is *generative*, where insights from one nontheological domain generate new areas of theological inquiry, or new ways of conceiving and addressing perennial theological questions. An example of this is how models of species development stemming from evolutionary biology generate new ways of thinking through doctrines of the fall of humanity and the nature and scope of original sin (Cavanaugh & Smith, 2017; Enns, 2012; Venema & McKnight, 2017).[3] Similarly, CSR can serve both as a corrective and generative source for theology.

---

[3] Consider a standard claim of Christian theology that the human condition includes sin and a kind of structural moral shortcoming often described as a fall from a prior state where that shortcoming was not manifested in, say, a first human couple. Models of human origins from evolutionary biology and genomic science indicate that *Homo sapiens* descended from other hominin species, and at no point

Teleological Reasoning and Theology

A central part of the human endeavor to understand and make sense of the world is to explain observations in terms of other events or processes. Using the language of dual-processing models of cognition mentioned earlier, explanatory narratives can arise from slow, reflective, system 2–type processes, or from quick, automatic system 1–type processes. Scientific explanation is a paradigm of a type of explanation arising from system 2 processes, where often, an observation is explained by describing its causes and interpreted by being embedded in a wider theoretical framework. Scientific explanation engages system 2 because the type of cognition involved in articulating and grasping scientific descriptions, explanations, and theoretical context (often involving the language of mathematical formalism), is slower, reflective, and requires concerted attention and heavier cognitive load.

But not all explanations that we seek or provide are scientific, and not all putative explanations are causal in this sense: sometimes we explain observations by appealing to the purposes or goals that agents have in view in bringing something about. These types of explanations are called *teleological* explanations, stemming from the Greek word *telos*, which can be translated as *goal, end,* or *purpose* (Keleman, 1999). Much of the work in cognitive psychology in general and CSR in particular suggests that teleological reasoning—the propensity to explain observations in terms of some intended purpose or function—is an intuitive part of human cognition and manifested in quick and automatic pre-reflective system 1 cognitive processes (e.g., see Scott & Barrett, this volume).

Children, for example, seem naturally inclined to favor purposive explanations for physical features of both living and inanimate objects. Mountains or dogs are viewed as being *made for* something (Kundert & Edman, 2017; Keleman, 1999). Rocks are pointy *so that* animals will not sit on them. As Kundert and Edman (2017) state, "It appears likely that children are naturally inclined to engage in teleological reasoning without being taught to do so" (p. 81). Interestingly, these results were replicated among atheist and secular adults, such that "even highly motivated atheists and committed nonbelievers display a heightened tendency to judge natural phenomena as purposefully created by a supernatural agent(s) when time constraints inhibit reflective censorship" (Kundert & Edman, p. 85; see also Järnefelt et al. 2015; Canfield, & Kelemen, 2015). This demonstrates that the human cognitive propensity to attribute purpose to events and actions is manifested in religious and nonreligious contexts.[4] The tendency to seek purposive explanations stays with humans across their life span, even for people who say they don't believe in God or divine purpose but still tend to see their lives as having a narrative plot,

---

in evolutionary history did the *Homo sapiens* population dip below approximately 10,000. Thus, the scientific data give theologians an impetus to develop theological accounts of origins and structural shortcomings of the human condition that are consistent with our best science.

[4] Routledge, Abeyta, & Roylance (2017) make a similar claim with respect to extraterrestrial intelligence (ETI) beliefs—our cognitive propensity for religious beliefs needs to be exercised even when religiosity is low—hence, the rise in ETI beliefs in low religious belief contexts.

determined by purposive forces. And for religious believers, this cognitive disposition makes it easy to see divine purpose in human history, as well as in the past, present, and future trajectories of their own lives (Luhrmann, 2012). Understanding this cognitive tendency can enrich theological accounts of human experience by supplementing theological accounts of human experience with an understanding of the mechanisms that structure that experience.

Corrective Application

Recall our earlier distinctions between the corrective and generative applications of information from other disciplines to theology (see "Theology and Other Disciplines"). We stated that theology can incorporate data from other disciplines as a corrective to certain theological claims that conflict with well-supported claims from other modes of inquiry. Now, we can expand this to note that data from other disciplines can be utilized as a corrective—or at the very least, sound a cautionary note—for certain types of practices, even when, possibly, those practices are sanctioned by one's theology.

For example, consider the practice, common in many, many Christian contexts, of attributing divine purpose to specific events, large or small, tragic or fortuitous. Natural disasters, wars, the outcomes of political elections, rainbows, sunsets, job offers, scraped knees, and even finding prime parking spots are seen as evidence of divine action. For millennia, Christians have attempted to explain events like these in terms of some wider narrative of purposive agency. However, what the CSR research on teleological reasoning suggests is that the practice of seeking out explanations—and for Christians, the practice of seeking out explanations that describe God's purposes with respect to natural occurrences—is motivated by deep and pervasive intuitive cognitive processes that may have little to do with the motive of discovering truth. And because the proclivity to seek purposive explanations is entrenched in our cognitive architecture, it is easy to screen off evidence that complicates or doesn't easily fit with our initial preferred explanation. The danger in this practice is being satisfied with an explanatory account primarily because adopting it requires little cognitive effort, and not because it is plausibly true.

To illustrate, recall the devastating earthquake that struck Haiti in January 2010 in which over 200,000 people were killed (DesRoches et al., 2011). Massive mudslides followed and added to the loss of life. A tent city that was put up outside Port-au-Prince housed several thousand Haitians who had lost their homes in the earthquake. The day after the earthquake a massive mudslide narrowly missed the camp, resulting (in this case) in no more deaths. The argument was made to one of the present authors (and published in the local newspaper) that the mudslide missed the camp as a result of God's protective hand. What the CSR literature on teleological reasoning shows is that this kind of explanation is natural—that is, it is cognitively natural to jump to quick explanations that attribute good outcomes to God and to screen off other data that don't fit the explanatory narrative—in this case, the data point that is screened off is the question of God's role, if any, in causing the earthquake and devastation in virtue of which the tent city was required in the first place. But just because such explanations are cognitively natural does not mean that they are accurate or even plausible. Nor does it mean these intuitions are false. The central issue is that simply unreflectively trusting the intuitions can be problematic. It is important to note as well, that many theologians from different Christian traditions have written treatises outlining positions on, for example, divine action, the relationship between divine sovereignty and human agency, the degree to or sense in which human agents are free to act contrary to God's purposes, and the ways in which events in nature are related to divine decree. Thus, mitigating the potential cognitive bias that is the result of natural teleological reasoning has applications to the lived experience of Christians and Christian leaders who seek to minister to the faithful in times of suffering, as well as for theologians who reflect on what it all means for theology.

In a word, the corrective that CSR suggests for all these areas of application is *caution*: namely, caution concerning the intuitive inferences one makes based on observation to conclusions about divine purpose. Quick and easy inferences to conclusions about divine purpose can lead to inappropriate levels of certainty when epistemic humility is more appropriate. The potential negative effect of intuitive teleological reasoning is compounded in that a high degree of certainty that some quick explanation is true cuts off the search for other explanations; and the longer one considers only one possible explanation for some phenomenon, the more likely it seems to be true—not on its merits, but simply because it is the only one being considered.[5]

But note also that merely checking system 1 intuitions with system 2 processes is no guarantee that one is closer to a better explanation for a phenomenon. Suppose that one decides, after engaging with slower, more effortful system 2 processes, that the mind should be trained in a certain way. As a result, one tries to "tune the mind" to engage experience in ways that shape one's intuitive interaction with the world. But just being able to train the mind to experience the world a certain way is not sufficient; it is also important, theologically and philosophically, to ask, "why *those* ways?" and "to what end?"

Tanya Luhrmann's (2012) excellent book *When God Talks Back: Understanding the American Evangelical Relationship with God* documents how reflectively supported cultural scaffolding in two Vineyard[6] congregations helps participants quickly and intuitively form beliefs about God's immediate presence in their lives. Lurhmann spent two years embedded in two different Vineyard congregations, and her anthropological research is supplemented with theory and data from cognitive psychology and historical theology. Luhrmann explores how members of Vineyard congregations—typically adult, well-functioning, educated people—come to believe that God is immediately and tangibly present, and available for ongoing, interactive conversation. Luhrmann reserves judgment about whether these habits of mind are truth-conducive and is unwilling to assert that these congregants are irrational. However, it is clear from Luhrmann's analysis that second-order reflective practices shape first-order experiences

---

[5] Elliot Sober (2020) identifies "the only game in town fallacy" as the mistake in reasoning where one concludes that an explanation is correct because it is the only explanation one can think of.

[6] Vineyard congregations are Pentecostal churches in the Evangelical tradition.

in ways that shape what members of the Vineyard congregations intuitively see, hear, and feel as they navigate the world of everyday experience.

To review: teleological reasoning—the quick and easy tendency of the mind to form purposive explanations for one's experiences—is part of human cognitive architecture. As such, a corrective theological implication is for caution in two senses. First, one should be careful about immediately adopting some explanation of a particular event in terms of God's purposes. Humans are primed to see purpose everywhere, even when there is none or when myriad competing purposive explanations are available. Second, even if one is able to train the mind to structure experience in certain ways, including some that constrain and shape one's propensity for purposive explanations, that by itself is no guarantor of acquiring truth-conducive explanations.

Generative Application

It would be a mistake, however, to infer that because it is cognitively easy to attribute a purpose behind events, that there are therefore *no* reasons or purposes behind events. Consider actions involving human agents. Sometimes people do act out of a cognitive base that includes reflective consideration of reasons. And though the causally efficacious reasons in a particular case might be difficult to discern, either from the outside by observers of the action or from the inside by the actor herself, it does seem that, in some cases, a causally significant reason that someone performed an action is, in fact, that they had a particular purpose in view. And the same principle applies to attempts to discern what purpose, if any, God may have had in view in allowing some event to happen. Epistemological humility about the accuracy of attributions of divine purpose is not the same thing as pervasive epistemological skepticism that there is any purpose whatsoever.

We think that a more productive application of the CSR literature on teleological reasoning to theology is not to abandon the attempt to discern divine purpose, but rather, to do so with a sustained commitment to seek out, consider, and engage with multiple narratives of what God's purposes may be. Considering multiple possible divine reasons that may be behind some event opens up a space for mystery and humility. We are cognitively primed to see purpose. Understanding the intuitive tendency to see purpose not only serves as a caution, but also helps us understand, perhaps even more deeply, the ways scripture, reason, and experience endorse *and* caution against this intuition.

The book of Job, for example, is, partly, an exposition against the unreflective causal interpretation of events. Job's friends insist that his troubles must have been brought on by his actions, that they had a purpose and an identifiable cause, and that it is Job's sin that is at the root of his suffering. Although the book of Job does not undermine the notion of teleological thinking itself, its conclusion could be interpreted as a repudiation of easy "blame the victim" intuitions. The story of Joseph in Genesis includes an assertion that Joseph's abduction and slavery in Egypt had teleological purpose (Genesis 50:20). Both the book of Romans and Jesus as he is portrayed in the gospels endorse teleological explanations of events and creation (Romans 1:19–20; John 9:3; John 11:4) but also caution against such interpretations (Matthew 5:45). The seeming contradictions in these texts and others can be informed by research on intuitive teleological thinking. The intuition to see purpose can both make it easier to see the hand of God in the world and lead people to overinterpret events in ways that undermine the mystery of God-in-the-world. Defaulting to quick and easy explanations can cut off further inquiry and make things simpler than they are in a way that undermines an appreciation for the complexity of creation and God's nature.

In terms of applied theology, this speaks to the ways in which system 2 processes should be used to constrain and train the intuitions. Scripture, theology, and church teaching in spiritual formation include many examples of the need to discipline the mind and train the imagination. The implication is that there are times when discerning teleological purpose is good and appropriate, and times when it is not. Understanding how cognitive defaults and heuristics inform thinking about religious topics and lead to intuitive teleological beliefs can be useful in developing ways to test the approaches to spiritual formation that currently exist *and* ways to help people overcome what Pascal Boyer calls "the tragedy of the theologian" (Boyer, 2001), the tendency of believers to default to intuitions that are actually theologically incorrect.

RITUALS AND WORSHIP

CSR and the Scientific Study of Ritual

CSR has much to say about how corporate worship, ritual, and liturgy are effective in religious contexts. Dimitris Xygalatas's work on extreme rituals (Xygalatas, 2019, and this volume), Lawson and McCauley's work on the ritual form hypothesis (Lawson & McCauley, 2002; Lawson, this volume), and Christine Legare's work on ritual efficacy (Legare & Souza, 2012; Watson-Jones & Legare, 2016), as well as theories about costly signaling and religious ritual (Atran & Henrich, 2010; Bulbulia & Sosis, 2011; Sosis et al., this volume; Wood, 2016) generate important implications for how theologians and religionists think about and engage in ritual and liturgy.

The cognitive study of ritual participation reveals a consistent effect of religious rituals on social cohesion and prosociality for in-group members. Research among members of religious and secular Israeli kibbutzim (Sosis & Ruffle, 2003) and participants in fire-walking ceremonies in Spain (Konvalinka et al., 2011), and the extreme rituals practiced by Tamil Hindus in Mauritius (Xygalatas et al., 2013) all support the connection between religious ritual and social cohesion. Although many secular rituals promote social cohesion (e.g., fraternity pledging, military training rituals), religious rituals, in particular, appear to create powerful social bonds—people who worship together, at least in a ritualistic way, do stick together (Whitehouse & Kavanagh, this volume). The mechanisms of this ritual-cohesion effect are complex and embedded in the social context (Sosis, 2019; Xygalatas, 2019), but they include synchronized action (movement, singing, and speaking), social signaling, and, perhaps, even the transformation of beliefs from nonintuitive to intuitive via repetition within the social group.

The ritual form hypothesis (RFH), proposed by E. Thomas Lawson and Robert N. McCauley, explores the cognitive logic of ritual action, how the very structure of many rituals makes an essential difference in how they are experienced and understood by participants and observers (Lawson, this volume; Lawson & McCauley, 2002; Malley, 2019). The starting premise of RFH theory is that when people engage in many religious rituals, they mentally represent the action of the ritual using the same categories as are used in everyday social interactions. For example, in everyday actions of social exchange, an agent does something to, for, or with someone in actions that can be described in a subject–verb–direct object format (e.g., Laird thanked Myron for the gift). The RFH applies the same template to the social exchanges involved in religious rituals (e.g., The congregation confessed their sins to God). Common human interactions are cognitively coded by locating the agent and the object of the action. We understand many human events in terms of who is doing what to whom, and we assess these relationships almost instantaneously and intuitively.

Recognizing these relationships allows researchers to make predictions about how participants understand and experience particular kinds of rituals: which rituals are repeatable, which are reversible, how much sensory pageantry should be involved, and how emotionally powerful and engaging the ritual is or should be. The key role in a ritual, according to the RFH, is the one played by the "culturally postulated super-human agent" (the god). To simplify, the foundational question in a Christian context would be: Is God the agent, doing the action of the ritual, or is God the object, receiving the action of the ritual? The answer to this question is essential for how people experience and understand religious rituals. The theory stipulates that, at least for certain classes of rituals, if there is a disconnect between how the ritual is carried out and what it is supposed to represent (e.g., if an "everyday" ritual such as the congregant makes an offering or confesses something to God is performed with high level of sensory stimuli and pageantry), the ritual participants will, in the long run, not sustain the ritual behavior. Only rituals in which God is the acting agent require such sensory pageantry (e.g., a wedding, when God "creates" a new family of two people who belonged to different families prior to the ritual). Another feature of rituals in which God is the agent is that they can only be performed by someone who was previously irrevocably changed in a ritual in which God was the agent (e.g., only ordained priests or pastors can perform weddings).

The mechanisms involved in perceived ritual efficacy appear to include the intensity and cost of the ritual. The more intense or painful the ritual—that is, the higher its "costs"—the greater the sense of social inclusivity it fosters among the participants. The higher the cost of participation in terms of time, resources, or comfort, the more the ritual serves to create a tighter community and increases trust among the community members (Xygalatas, 2019; Sosis, 2019). This "costly signaling" may be one of the ways people identify those who are part of the accepted social "in-group" as an authentic, trustworthy, true believers. Rituals and nonverbal signals communicate shared religious identity, and they do so better than verbal assent (Atran & Henrich, 2010; Bulbulia & Sosis, 2011).

Related to this signaling is the way rituals allow participants to develop a shared identity. It has been noted across many contexts that synchronous action builds social connection and community (Hobson et al., 2018; Lang et al., 2017; Morgan et al., 2017; Whitehouse & Kavanagh, this volume). This is true in contexts ranging from shared cheering and other actions of sports fans to the rigid synchronous marching of military units. Even social dancing has this effect—couples who dance together develop a stronger shared bond than those who dance separately (which is a point in favor of ballroom dancing; Tarr et al., 2016). Christine Legare's work with children and ritual expands upon this "shared action" effect to note that ritualistic action not only creates tighter social bonds among children, but ritualized directions are remembered better than nonritualized directions. Children use ritual to help them develop and maintain social groups, identify who is in and who is out, and to remember how to do complicated tasks (Legare & Nielsen, 2015; Watson-Jones & Legare, 2016). Children who have been ostracized use rigorous adherence to the group's unstated rituals as a way to gain acceptance back into the group (Watson-Jones et al., 2016). Ritual is a powerful way for groups to gain coherence and tight bonds and for group members to learn and remember complicated tasks and principles that are associated with group membership.

Corrective Application

Group bonds, a sense of shared community, and adherence to social norms are important, even essential components of a religious community. Using what we know about the ways rituals and shared worship experiences enhance group identification and commitment can be very useful in helping religiously bonded groups grow and develop. However, the potential downside of developing a strong sense of shared identity and commitment is that the increased group affiliation is associated with increased in outgroup derogation and rejection (Hobson, et al., 2018; Johnson et al., 2012). It may be this aspect of ritualized worship that the "seeker sensitive" development in evangelical protestant worship[7] is designed to address (Redman, 2001).

This issue, of identifying the insiders and outsiders to solidify group social bonds and, perhaps, to protect and enhance the individual's ego strength, as well as the strength of the religious organization, is an interesting lens through which one can interpret Jesus's interactions and conflict with the religious leaders of his day. One corrective that understanding this aspect of ritual provides is recognizing how rituals can serve to separate and draw lines between those who are part of the group and those who are not. This recognition itself can help church liturgists develop strategies to overcome the problem. There are many instances in church practice of very tightly bound, ritual-infused groups

---

[7] "Seeker Sensitive" worship is that which demands little "insider knowledge" of participants about church life, liturgy, or worship and tends to mimic common public gatherings such as concerts or sporting events. The purpose is to create fewer barriers to participation for those who are not already a part of the worshipping community, to help put "seekers" at ease in the worship setting.

who have also been focused on welcoming and serving outsiders (the Franciscans or Benedictines in Roman Catholicism, for example). If one of the central tasks of the church is to offer winsome invitation to those who are not part of the church body, then finding a way to engage in rituals that build group cohesion while at the same time welcoming and extending hospitality to outsiders should be the goal. More research about how this can be accomplished is needed.

Ritual is necessary, however. For a church group to endure, it must engage in worship and ritual to build community and transmit core commitments and practices across generations. The quandary is to design worship that includes rituals that speak to congregants' intuitive understanding of and desires for ritual, on the one hand, but to develop and practice rituals that also create space for invitation to outsiders rather than serving to identify and exclude them. Worship services that take place in auditoriums and coffee shops and that forgo formalized liturgies and rituals are more invitational to outsiders. They rank low on the need for specialized "insider" information to decode their architecture and rituals. Most people know how to attend and what to expect at a concert or sporting event, and these worship spaces and services resemble common public events more than they resemble traditional liturgical worship services.

And yet one of the common complaints of those who lead churches that eschew traditional liturgies and worship styles is that those that resemble large-scale concerts do not seem to engender commitment to a specific worship community among parishioners. If leaders or music styles change, or someone feels insulted or ignored in one church, they find it easy to move on and engage in "church shopping." This lack of deep commitment to a local worship community is undoubtedly related to many other aspects of modern life, such as the individualization of contemporary society and the erosion of local social connections (see Putnam, 2000). But it may also be that dispensing with specialized liturgies and church rituals in order to draw outsiders in has led to the weaker commitment and social bonds among those who are already in the group.[8]

Lawson and McCauley, in their RFH, indicate (and have case studies in support) that for a worshipping community to be stable and pass on the faith across generations, the types of rituals and the way they are performed need to be intuitively congruent. The community needs to have high sensory pageantry *special agent rituals* in which God is the actor (weddings, ordinations, and some approaches to baptism and communion) balanced with low sensory pageantry *special patient rituals* in which the congregants are the actors offering something to God (confession, participation in worship, offering time and resources). If a worshipping community has too many special agent rituals— if every service is a highly emotional sensory experience related to intense personal

---

[8] Research is needed on the difference in the kinds of affiliative bonds created by different types of worship rituals and liturgies. It may be that some "seeker sensitive" approaches to worship lead to shallow commitments among those already there. For example, Willow Creek Church, the American mega-church often associated with founding the "seeker sensitive" movement, has moved away from this approach to worship in order to "deepen" the commitment of current members (Branaugh, 2008).

transformations directly by God—it will lose its power and meaning. The community will need to seek ever more intense emotional engagement and experiences, a trajectory that is not sustainable over time. As a result, the community itself will have little staying power over the years. There is a sense here that, perhaps, the evangelical megachurch with its fog machines, light shows, and rock bands is sowing the seeds of its own destruction by forgoing the mundane common rituals that are necessary for building deep commitments and cross-generational transference of the faith. If rituals that are intuitively special patient rituals are performed with the sensory pageantry of special agent rituals, congregants will sense a disconnect between the meaning of the ritual and the structure of what is happening. Moreover, this approach to worship may be unsustainable, since this cognitive disconnect will eventually lead people to become cynical or even bored with spectacle that is not tied to its intuitive meaning.

By the same token, if rituals that should be highly emotionally charged are treated casually or do not occur at all in the life of a church, then the church will also have difficulty with cross-generational continuity and deep commitment on the part of congregants. The RFH, and the research that supports it across many different religious contexts, makes it clear that intuitions about the structure and meaning of religious rituals are deeply held. Emotion-laden special agent rituals create powerful memories around which meaning is made and community is formed. Common ritual actions that seem almost mundane serve to rehearse and encode the more counterintuitive and abstract aspects of theology into the memory and daily life of the worshipper and help the worshipper identify with the worshipping community (Whitehouse, 2004). A worshipping body needs both types of ritual in the right balance to survive and thrive.

Generative Application

The CSR work on ritual has made clear the importance of ritual to successful group cohesion and commitment, the formation of religious identity across generations, and both group and individual memory for theological concepts. Religious groups with established, balanced participatory rituals are more resilient than those without such practices. A CSR analysis of ritual not only can help explicate what people intuitively experience when they engage in religious rituals, but it can also help religionists and theologians critique and design rituals that more effectively accomplish the mission of the church.

The use of sacrifices for sin is an example of how CSR can help explicate the intuitive meaning in rituals. The regular depictions of sacrifices and offerings depicted in the Hebrew Bible are examples of special patient rituals (Edman, 2015). The human participants are the agents, making sacrifices to God, who receives their sacrifices. These special patient rituals were repeated daily among the ancient Hebrews, were not reversible, did not necessarily require the intervention of the priest, and were relatively low in sensory pageantry. The crucifixion of Christ, however, transforms what was a special patient ritual (making ritual sacrifices for sin) into a special agent ritual (the ultimate ritual sacrifice for sin). Now God is the actor, who is sacrificed on the cross, and who, simultaneously, receives the sacrifice for the sin of humanity. The ritual does not need to be repeated; it is the climax of the drama of salvation and the effect is permanent. The way the church expresses, celebrates, and retells this central event of the faith has deep implications for how people understand and remember the crucifixion, and the transformation of the relationship of humanity and God it suggests is undergirded and supported by our intuitions about the meaning of such rituals.

This profound theological concept maps onto our intuitions about how rituals work in a powerful way. The connection between ritual intuitions and theology should be explored more fully by theologians and by cognitive scientists. Research questions arise here regarding other intuitions about rituals and their theological underpinnings. It may be that Christians' tendency to believe the wrong things (e.g., confusing grace with social exchange, misinterpreting the incarnation to mean that Jesus is half-god half-man, defaulting to inappropriately anthropomorphic notions about God, Barrett, 1999; Barrett, 2002; Slone, 2004) has to do with the misuse, or rejection, of church rituals. Rituals that appropriately reflect theology while being intuitively congruent are those that will most effectively help religious groups pursue their aims.

Moreover, given this analysis, we can imagine CSR scholars advising churches and religious communities to consider the following:

- Communal rituals are powerful means by which groups can create strong social bonds, provided they are participatory in the right ways: synchronized, with a proscribed order and vocabulary, and make it possible for participants to see and hear each other participating in a shared experience.[9]
- But ritual power to strengthen in-group bonds may also alienate strangers and new members of religious groups; it is therefore important for those designing rituals to purposefully involve newcomers or the formerly excluded or ignored in performing and leading the rituals.
- The rituals of the church should also be carefully designed to engage the appropriate amount of emotion-laden sensory pageantry. Rituals that are part of life-transformation (weddings, ordinations, and in some traditions, baptisms) should be the most spectacular rituals in which the church engages.[10]

---

[9] These rituals not only serve to help people feel that they are a part of a community, but also to reconnect people with a community from which they have been alienated. For example, Vern Bengtson Bengtson et al. 2013) in his excellent longitudinal study of how faith is passed down across generations, delineates the importance of shared religious rituals and activities in both the church and the home. The sharing of these rituals (and especially if they are part of the fabric of family life as well) help to explain why some religious traditions have higher rates of transgenerational faith transfer.

[10] What is unclear and should be examined more fully is how the RFH maps onto rituals that do not fit the forms delineated by Lawson and McCauley. Do rituals that do not seem to fall into the categories specified by the RFH still generate intuitive expectations and interpretations? In what ways can rituals deepen social connection but also be invitational, broaden the social group rather than create boundaries that identify insiders versus outsiders? The difficulty is that ritual appears to be a practice the church needs to thrive, but ritual can also create the very conditions churches must avoid if they are to be vibrant, welcoming communities that grow and thrive.

Conclusion

Cognitive science of religion provides important information for understanding and even predicting the types of beliefs and behaviors people tend to develop with respect to God, angels, demons, spirits, life after death, and design and origins (Barrett, 2011, 2012, 2013; Bloom, 2004; Boyer, 2001; De Cruz, 2014; Kelemen, 2004; Lawson & McCauley, 2002; Slone, 2004). These conceptions are usually developed in childhood but often persist into adulthood. The purpose of this chapter is both to lay out a framework for how this information can be profitably used by theologians and to provide several examples of that framework in action.

The two areas we focus on in the chapter, teleological thinking and ritual, provide examples of ways in which theologians can and should engage CSR. However, these two areas are not the only areas of CSR research and theory that can provide fertile ground for theologians. For example, the operation of our default notions about the minds of agents and our ability to imagine what emotions and thoughts another agent is having are essential intuitive components for how we understand God and God's "mind." Our "theory of mind" has important implications for the ways we experience prayer, intimacy with God, and God's purposes and desires (Edman, 2018; Gervais, 2013; Luhrmann, 2012; Norenzayan et al., 2012; Willard & Norenzayan, 2013).

The impact of individual differences in theory of mind could help explain part of the differences not just in belief in God, but in the ways people experience God in prayer and worship, as well as differences in individual theologies of God's will and purposes. It has been shown that particular religious expressions (e.g., conservative fundamentalism, liberal Protestantism) are related to the values, moral codes, and politics of adherents (Brown & Brown, 2015; Rowatt et al., 2013). The implications of this research are that people tend to attribute to God values, politics, and moral codes that are consistent with and even reflect their own values and preferences. The process of discerning the "mind of God" implicates the working of theory of mind. It may be that individual differences in theory of mind are, in part, responsible for differences in how much people believe God's values are the same as their own (an issue calling for more research). This has implications for how one approaches teaching about God and what one's goals should be in spiritual and religious identity formation.

Theory of mind, teleological thinking, ritual forms, along with our intuitive beliefs about the afterlife and the memory and transmission advantages of some minimally counterintuitive theological concepts, all provide important corrective and generative applications for theology. The challenge moving forward is to develop useful responses to what CSR tells us about human religious cognition. One prominent CSR scholar, who is also a priest in the Church of England, has called CSR the "cognitive science of idolatry" (Jong et al., 2015), because CSR helps us understand why Christians tend to default to beliefs and behaviors that are incongruent with what they have been taught in the church and through biblical texts for years. CSR can help us understand the persistence of "bad religion," wherein the people's religious faith serves to create an exclusivist tribal identity, enhance superstitious thinking and beliefs, and generate an image of God that is really a reflection of the believer's values and not of the divine being presented in scripture and church teaching. Framed in this way, a goal for churches may be overcoming these intuitions and generating church practices that enhance spiritual formation as well as the cross-generational transmission of the faith. However, doing so also requires an understanding of how human cognitive processes generate the way we are religious. CSR can help us to understand both where and why religious belief and practice goes awry, and what one can do to guide effective, theologically informed practice. The marriage of CSR and theology is both a necessary and fruitful one for those involved in thinking about and guiding the life of faith. Those wishing to do so effectively cannot afford to ignore cognitive science of religion.

QUESTIONS FOR FUTURE RESEARCH

1. What are the primary differences in how CSR concepts interact with and are expressed in the practices and theologies of different religions?
2. What are the structural differences in ritual practices that invite strangers into a community versus those that set up barriers to strangers?
3. In what ways do differences in mentalizing and theory of mind influence differences in divine experiences?

ACKNOWLEDGMENTS

We gratefully acknowledge that this work was supported by a grant from the Templeton Religion Trust.

REFERENCES

Atran, S., & Henrich, J. (2010). The evolution of religion: How cognitive by-products, adaptive learning heuristics, ritual displays, and group competition generate deep commitments to Prosocial religion. *Biological Theory*, 5, 18–30.

Barrett, J. L. (1999). Theological correctness: Cognitive constraint and the study of religion. *Method & Theory in the Study of Religion*, 11, 325–339.

Barrett, J. L. (2002). Smart gods, dumb gods, and the role of social cognition in structuring ritual intuitions. *Journal of Cognition and Culture*, 2, 183–193.

Barrett, J. L. (2012). *Born believers: The science of children's religious belief*. New York: Free Press.

Barrett, J. L. (2011). *Cognitive science of religion and theology: From human minds to divine minds*. Conshohocken, PA: Templeton Press.

Barrett, J. L. (2013). Exploring religion's basement: The cognitive science of religion. In R. F. Paloutzian & C. L. Park (Eds.), *Handbook of the psychology of religion and spirituality* (2nd ed.), pp. 234–255. New York: Guilford Press.

Barrett, J. L., & Trigg, R. (2014). Cognitive and evolutionary studies of religion. In J. L. Barrett and R. Trigg (Eds.), *The roots of religion: Exploring the cognitive science of religion*, pp. 1–15. Farnham, UK: Ashgate.

Bengtson, V. L., Putney, N. M., & Harris, S. (2013). *Families and faith: How religion is passed down across generations.* New York: Oxford University Press.

Bloom, P. (2004). *Descartes' baby: How child development explains what makes us human.* London: William Heinemann.

Bloom, P. (2007). Religion is natural. *Developmental Science, 10*(1), 147–151.

Boyer, P. (2001). *Religion explained: The evolutionary origins of religious thought.* New York: Basic Books.

Branaugh, M. (2008). Willow creek's "huge shift": Influential megachurch moves away from seeker-sensitive services. *Christianity Today, 52*(6), 13.

Brown, K. B., & Brown, R. E. (2015). Race/ethnicity, religion, and partisan leanings. *Review of Religious Research, 57*(4), 469–505.

Bulbulia, J., & Sosis, R. (2011). Signalling theory and the evolution of religious cooperation. *Religion, 41,* 363–388.

Cavanaugh, W. T., & Smith, J. K. A. (Eds.). (2017*). Evolution and the fall.* Grand Rapids, MI: Eerdmans.

De Cruz, H. (2014). Cognitive science of religion and the study of theological concepts. *Topoi, 33,* 487–497.

DesRoches, R., Comerio, M., Eberhard, M., Mooney, W., & Rix, G. J. (2011). Overview of the 2010 Haiti earthquake. *Earthquake Spectra, 27,* S1–S21.

Edman, L. (2015). Applying the science of faith: The cognitive science of religion and Christian practice. *Journal of Psychology and Christianity, 34,* 238–249.

Edman, L. (August 12-16, 2018). *Theory of mind, imagination, and the experience of God* (paper presentation). The 7th bi-annual Conference of the International Association for the Cognitive Science of Religion, Boston, MA.

Enns, P. (2012). *The evolution of Adam: What the Bible does and does not say about human origins.* Grand Rapids, MI: Brazos Press.

Gervais, W. M. (2013). Perceiving minds and gods: How mind perception enables, constrains and is triggered by beliefs in gods. *Perspectives in Psychological Science, 8*(4), 380–394.

Hobson, N. M., Scheroeder, J., Risen, J. L., Xygalatas, D., & Inzlicht, M. (2018). The psychology of rituals: An integrative review and process-based framework. *Personality and Social Psychology Review, 22*(3), 260–284.

Järnefelt, E., Canfield, C. F., & Kelemen, D. (2015). The divided mind of a disbeliever: Intuitive beliefs about nature as purposefully created among different groups of non-religious adults. *Cognition, 140,* 72–88.

Johnson, M. K., Rowatt, W. C., & LeBouff, J. P. (2012). Religiosity and prejudice revisited: In-group favoritism, out-group derogation, or both? *Psychology of Religion and Spirituality, 4*(2), 154–168.

Jong, J., Kavanagh, C., & Visala, A. (2015). Born idolaters: The limits of the philosophical implications of the cognitive science of religion. *Neue Zeitschrift für systematische Theologie und Religionphilosophie, 57*(2), 244–266.

Kahneman, D. (2003). A perspective on judgment and choice: Mapping bounded rationality. *American Psychologist, 58*(9), 697–720.

Kahneman, D. (2011). *Thinking fast and slow.* New York: Farrar, Straus and Giroux.

Kelemen, D. (1999). The scope of teleological thinking in preschool children. *Cognition, 70,* 241–272.

Kelemen, D. (2004). Are children "intuitive theists"? Reasoning about purpose and design in nature. *Psychological Science, 15,* 295–301.

Konvalinka, I., Xygalatas, D., Bulbulia, J., Schjoedt, U., Jegindø, E.-M. E., Wallot, S., Van Orden, G., & Roepstorff, A. (2011). Synchronized arousal between performers and related spectators in a fire-walking ritual. *Proceedings of the National Academy of Sciences of the United States of America, 108*(20), 8514–19.

Kundert, C., & Edman, L. R. O. (2017). Promiscuous teleology: From childhood through adulthood and from east to west. In R. G. Hornbeck, J. L. Barrett, & M. Kang (Eds.), *Religious cognition in China: "Homo Religiosus" and the dragon,* pp. 79–96. Cham, Switzerland: Springer.

Lang, M., Bahana, V., Shaver, J., Reddish, P., & Xygalatas, D. (2017). Endorphin-mediated synchrony effects on cooperation. *Biological Psychology, 127,* 191–197.

Lawson, E. T., & McCauley, R. N. (2002). *Bringing ritual to mind: Psychological foundations of cognitive forms.* New York: Cambridge University Press.

Legare, C. H., & Nielsen, M. (2015). Imitation and innovation: The dual engines of cultural learning. *Trends in Cognitive Sciences, 19,* 688–699.

Legare, C. H. & Souza, A. L. (2012). Evaluating ritual efficacy: Evidence from the supernatural. *Cognition, 124,* 1–15.

Luhrmann, T. M. (2012). *When God talks back: Understanding the American evangelical relationship with God.* New York: Alfred A. Knopf.

Mally, B. (2019). How are rituals thought to work? In D. Jason Slone & W. W. McCorkle Jr. (Eds), *The cognitive science of religion: A methodological introduction to key empirical studies,* pp. 211–227. London: Bloomsbury Academic Press.

McCauley, R. N. (2000). The naturalness of religion and unnaturalness of science. In F. C. Keil & R. A. Wilson (Eds.), *Explanation and cognition,* pp. 61–85. Cambridge, MA: MIT Press.

McCauley, R. N. (2011). *Why religion is natural, and science is not.* New York: Oxford University Press.

Morgan, R., Fischer, R., & Bulbulia, J. A. (2017). To be in synchrony or not? A meta-analysis of synchrony's effects on behavior, perception, cognition and affect. *Journal of Experimental Social Psychology, 72,* 13–20.

Norenzayan, A. (2013). *Big Gods: How religion transformed cooperation and conflict.* Princeton, NJ: Princeton University Press.

Norenzayan, A., Gervais, W. M., & Trzesniewski, K. H. (2012). Mentalizing deficits constrain belief in a personal god. *PLoS One, 7,* Article e36880.

Putnam, R. D. (2000). *Bowling alone: The collapse and revival of American community.* New York: Simon and Schuster.

Redman, R. R. (2001). Welcome to the worship awakening. *Theology Today, 58*(3), 369–383.

Routledge, C., Abeyta, A. A., & Roylance, C. (2017). We are not alone: The meaning motive, religiosity, and belief in extraterrestrial intelligence. *Motivation and Emotion, 41,* 135–146.

Rowatt, W. C., Shen, M. J., LaBouff, J. P., & Gonzalez, A. (2013). Religious fundamentalism, right-wing authoritarianism, and prejudice: Insights from meta-analysis, implicit social cognition, and social neuroscience. In R. F. Paloutzian, & C. L. Park (Eds.). *Handbook of the psychology of religion and spirituality,* pp. 457–475. New York: Guilford Press.

Slone, D. J. (2004). *Theological incorrectness: Why religious people believe what they shouldn't*. New York: Oxford University Press.

Sober, E. (2020). *Core Questions in Philosophy* (7th Ed.). New York: Routledge.

Sosis, R. (2019). Do religions promote cooperation? Testing signaling theories of religion. In D. Jason Slone & W. W. McCorkle Jr. (Eds), *The cognitive science of religion: A methodological introduction to key empirical studies*, pp. 155–162. London: Bloomsbury Academic Press.

Sosis, R., & Ruffle, B. J. (2003). Religious ritual and cooperation: Testing for a relationship on Israeli religious and secular kubbutzim. *Current Anthropology, 44*(5), 712–722.

Stanovich, K. E., & West, R. F. (2000). Individual differences in reasoning: Implications for the rationality debate. *Behavioral and Brain Sciences, 23*, 645–665.

Tarr, B., Launay, J., & Dunbar, R. I. M. (2016). Silent disco: Dancing in synchrony leads to elevated pain thresholds and social closeness. *Evolution and Human Behavior, 37*(5), 343–349.

Venema, D. R., & McKnight, S. (2017). *Adam and the genome*. Grand Rapids, MI: Brazos Press.

Watson-Jones, R. E., & Legare, C. H. (2016). The social functions of group rituals. *Current Directions in Psychological Science, 25*(1), 42–46.

Watson-Jones, R. E., Whitehouse, H., & Legare, C. H. (2016). In-group ostracism increases high-fidelity imitation in early childhood. *Psychological Science, 27*(1), 34–42.

Whitehouse, H. (2004). *Modes of religiosity: A cognitive theory of religious transmission*. Walnut Creek, CA: AltaMira Press.

Willard, A. K., & Norenzayan, A. (2013). Cognitive biases explain religious belief, paranormal belief, and belief in life's purpose. *Cognition, 129*, 379–391.

Wood, C. (2016). Ritual well-being: Toward a social signaling model of religion and mental health. *Religion, Brain & Behavior, 7*(3), 223–243.

Xygalatas, D. (2019). Do rituals promote social cohesion? In D. Jason Slone & W. W. McCorkle Jr. (Eds), *The cognitive science of religion: A methodological introduction to key empirical studies*, pp. 163–172. London: Bloomsbury Academic Press.

Xygalatas, D., Mitkidis, P., Fischer, R., Reddish, P., Skewes, J., Geertz, A. W., Roepstorff, A., &Bulbulia, J. (2013). Extreme rituals promote prosociality. *Psychological Science, 24*(8), 1602–1605.

INDEX

Due to the use of para id indexing, indexed terms that span two pages (e.g., 52–53) may, on occasion, appear on only one of those pages.

Tables, figures, and boxes are indicated by *t*, *f*, and *b* following the page number

A

Absolute Unitary Being, 328
afterlife, 3, 5–6, 7
  accounts, 262–63
  beliefs, 15–16, 22, 34, 39, 48, 67, 95–96, 97,
    100, 101–3, 146, 159, 192–93, 361–62,
    412–13
  experience, 4–5
agency, 23, 92–93, 193–95, 258. *See also*
    superhuman agents
  human agency, 416–17
  overattribution, 398
agency detection, 18, 114–15, 193–95, 229–30,
    258, 260–61, 353–54, 372, 412
agency-detection device (ADD), 114–15,
    193–95, 258, 357
agents. *See also* supernatural agents
  minimally counterintuitive, 261, 262
  properties of, 193–95
Ainu (Japan), 68*f*, 81–82
allocare, 356
Alston, W., 376–77
ancestors, 54. *See also* spirits
ancestor worship, 52–53
Andersen, M., 221–26, 341
animates, 111–12, 193–95, 195n.5, 197
anthropology
  anthropological approach, 418
  origin of, 215–16
anthropomorphism, 258, 259
  anthropomorphic biases, 399,
    403–4
  anthropomorphic ideas, 424

tendency, 378–79, 382–85
anti-secularization thesis, 314–15
antitheism, 303, 313–14
Anubis, 72
anxiety, 139. *See also* death anxiety
Archeology, 286
artificialism, 115
Asprem, E., 44
atheists, 121–22, 303, 314–15, 415–16
Atkinson, Q., 3, 285–86, 287
Atran, S., 33–34, 351–52
attachment, 71–72
authoritative-text hypothesis, 172
authority, 363
  "authoritative" view, 79*b*
  inconsistency, 79*b*
  scriptural authority, 179–81
Azande, 135

B

Bainbridge, W., 359
Balinese, 81–82
Barrett, J., 191, 358–59
  and hypersensitive agency-detection device
    (HADD) theory, 372–83
belief, 56–59
  defeater, 382, 382n.22, 384
  genealogy of, 372–73
  intuitive belief, 389, 390
  magical belief, 56–59
  prima facie belief, 382
  unreflective belief, 415–19
Bering, J., 5–6, 101, 259, 353, 354

INDEX

Bible, 174, 177, 178, 180, 183–85, 186, 188–89, 423–24. *See also* sacred texts
Bible interpretations, 179, 184*t*, 260
scriptural authority, 179–81
textual study of, 185–86
topical study of, 186
Big Gods theory, 288–89, 309–10, 311–12, 357, 360, 385n.30, 413n.1
Bjorklund, D. F., 101, 102, 259
Black Stone, 195, 201–2
body and identity, 90
Boyer, P., 28–29, 30, 31, 32, 33–34, 35–37, 40, 48, 261–63, 267, 351–52, 353, 358–59, 380, 419
brain, 99–101. *See also* neuroscience
conception of, 90
mind-brain distinction, 94
brain anatomy
and religion, 333–35, 336*b*
Buddhism, 49, 50
Buddha, 72
and death, 149
versus informal religious activity, 55
burial. *See* death practices
Burkert, W., 351
byproduct thesis, 28–30, 229–30, 307–10, 351–61, 374–75, 390
commitments of, 29

C

Calvinism, 56–57
canon, 177
Septuagint canon, 179
Catholicism, 314–17
and afterlife beliefs, 101–2
in the Republic of Ireland, 314–17
Centre for Science Communication, 3
childhood development, 393–97, 398–401. *See also* cognitive development
Chomsky, N., 16, 17, 364
Christianity. *See also* evangelical Christians
Christian theism, 310–14
Christian theology, 411–13, 414–19
concept of God, 414
versus informal religious activity, 55
rituals, 263–64
Clark, K., 382

cognition
automatic, 390–91
deep and shallow cognition, 70
effortful, 390–91
intuitive theories, 391
parental intuitive religious, 398–400
as result of religious teaching, 400–1
cognitive anthropology, 67
cognitive biases, 90, 310, 343, 416–17
and gods, 17–18
and intuition, 136–37, 260, 392
psychological essentialism, 97–98
and punishment, 266
cognitive development, 98, 391. *See also* childhood development; developmental niche theory
in infants, 91–92
cognitive mechanisms, 35–37, 43–44. *See also* agency-detection device
as a capacity, 38
and group-level tendencies, 38
language, 16
sensus divinitatis, 384
cognitive niche, 391–92
cognitive resource depletion, 222–24, 223n.6, 224n.9
cognitive science of religion (CSR)
commitments of, 30
concept of, 412–13
development of, 17
as epistemic friend, 382–85
and genealogy of belief, 372–73
history of, 13
limitations of, 24–25
and natural selection, 374–77
as neutral, 385–86
rationality, 373–82
standard model of, 21–22
cognitive science of religion (CSR), explanations, 34
belief-desire explanations, 36
casual models, 38
covering law model, 38, 43
evolutionary explanations of religion, 37–41
general laws, 38
mechanistic analysis of, 43
piecemeal approach, 7, 34, 35, 413

pluralism, 42–43
post-hoc rationalizations, 36
proximate and ultimate, 40–41
selective explanation, 39
comparative religion, 13–16
and interpretation of religious thought and behavior, 15–16
complexity drop, 220–21, 223–24, 224n.10
model of the supernatural, 220–21, 228
complexity-based reasoning, 217
conformity, 172, 173
consciousness
altered states of, 242–43
contagion
and special objects, 203–4
continuity theory, 226
costly signaling theory, 153–54, 246, 248, 279, 356, 419, 420–21
counterintuitive agents (CI agents). *See* counterintuitive concepts
counterintuitive concepts, 21–22, 59, 195–96, 195–96n.6, 199–200
counterintuitive agents (CI agents), 113–15, 124
maximally counterintuitive components, 308
minimally counterintuitive (MCI), 113–14, 124, 261–63, 307, 363–64, 412
religious, 112–13
counterschematic causal effects, 196, 199–200
creation accounts, 260, 262–63
Biblical, 260
Mongolian, 110
of objects and artifacts, 116–17
credibility-enhancing displays (CRED), 289–91, 291f, 312–13, 315–17
credibility-undermining displays (CRUD), 289–91
cults, 51
Cybele cult, 55
cultural evolution
in death practices, 156–58
cultural learning, 156–57
as form of social learning, 396
cultural selection, 38–39, 40
culture, 67
cultural cognition, 70–71

cultural construction of concepts, 393–95
cultural information, 69, 70–71
cultural niche hypothesis, 396
culturalness, 69
definition of, 69
Cummins, R., 38

D

D'Aquili, E., 328
danger
contamination, 151, 154
coping strategies, 139
Hazard Precaution System, 152, 157–58
responses, 138–40
and ritual, 151–52
Darwin, C., 40–41, 67, 77–78, 267–68, 350–52, 364
Darwinian evolution. *See* Darwinian evolution; evolution
de-automatization, 222–23
death, 145. *See also* death rituals
and disease, 151
and fear, 155
mortuary practices, 145
death anxiety, 71–72
death practices, 93, 103–4. *See also* death rituals; rituals
death rituals. *See also* death rituals; rituals
funerals, 152–53
deducing intentions, 229–30
deities. *See also* gods; superhuman agents
small-scale, 56
developmental niche theory, 396–97
child-care practices and customs, 397
parent ethnotheories, 397
physical and social settings, 397
religious, 398–404
developmental psychology, 90. *See also* cognitive development
dimensions of mental and physical states
nonembodied, 99
non-psychological body, 99
psychological body, 99
distinctiveness hypothesis, 178
Divergent Modes of Religiosity Theory (DMR Theory), 279–86, 288, 291–93, 308–9
divination, 51–52, 53–54

434 INDEX

divine, 413. *See also* gods; supernatural agents
  divine intervention, 380–81, 416–17
  divine sovereignty, 416–17
doctrine, 50
  doctrinal practices, 53, 308–9
domain
  definition of, 37
  specificity of, 37
dominance hierarchies, 71–72
dreams, 225–29
  definition of, 217
  dream fulfillment, 228–29
  dream repetition, 228–29
  good fortunes, 227
dual inheritance theory, 356–58
dual-process theory of cognition, 122. *See also*
  dual-system thinking
dual-system thinking, 412–13, 415–19
  and teleological thinking, 415–19
dualism, 72, 93–96, 262, 362
  Cartesian substance dualism, 93
  intuitive dualism, 93, 259, 307, 354, 412
  mind-body dualism, 413
  substance dualism, 93
Durkheim, É., 15, 278, 362
  sociological program, 32–33

E
ecology, 79–82, 352, 355–56
eisagesis
  and interpretive tradition, 183
electroencephalography (EEG), 327, 331–33
emergentists, 101
emulation
  and social learning, 395
Enga (tribe, Papua New Guinea), 81
epidemiology of beliefs, 167–68
eschatology, 50
essentialism, 97–99, 392, 398
  psychological, 97–98
  social essentialism, 98
ethics
  ethical intuition, 100
  ethical reasoning, 100
evangelical Christians
  and Biblical interpretations, 183–85, 184*t*,
    186

  and mega-churches, 422–23
  "seeker-sensitive" worship, 421, 421n.7
Evans-Pritchard, E., 53–54, 135
events, 219
  event cognition, 217, 219
  event models, 219
  event schemata, 219
evolution, 40, 121, 260
  cultural evolution, 37–41
  Darwinism, 40
  evolutionary explanations of religion, 37–41
  evolutionary psychology, 40
  Evolutionary Psychology of Religion (EPR),
    327, 353–54
  evolutionary study of religion, 350–58
  exaptations, 40–41
  naturalistic account, 374–77
  theistic accounts, 375
evolutionary theory of religion, 260
expectation sets, 111–12, 194
  and counterintuitive agents, 114
  transfer of, 113
explanatory coexistence, 135
extreme rituals, 238
  circumcision, 238
  description, 237
  fire-walking ceremonies, 419–20
  and gender dynamics, 248
  genital mutilation, 238
  and healing, 241–42
  and identity, 244
  individual participation, 239–43
  and meaning, 239–43
  self-flagellation, 237–38, 248
  self-mutilation, 237–38
  social cohesion, 243–44
extrovertive experience, 217–18, 222, 224–25

F
faith, 50
Fieser, J., 170–73
Finke, R., 359
folk theories, 35, 391
  folk anthropology, 97–105
  folk beliefs, 229–30
  folk biology, 91–92, 112
  folk dualism, 262

folk intuitions, 412
folk ontology, 261–62
folk physics, 91, 92
folk psychology, 92, 93–96, 112
force, 72. *See also* great spirit
Fortier, M., 220–21, 223–24
fractionation, 303–4
Functional Magnetic Resonance Imaging
    (fMRI). *See* Magnetic Resonance
    Imaging (MRI)
funerals, 152–53. *See also* death rituals

G

G/wi (Kalahari), 77–78
Gaia beliefs, 121–22, 123, 124
Ganesha, 80–81
Gantley, M., 286–87
Geertz, C., 31–32, 44
General genetic law of cultural development
    (Vygotsky), 393
ghosts. *See* spirits
goal competition, 58
god(s), 54, 55–56, 198–99. *See also* Big Gods
    theory
    Christian conception of, 414
    "Big Gods", 56
    cognitive foundations of, 258–61
    concepts, 373
    concepts of, anthropomorphically based,
        399–400
    features, 71–75
    interest, 75–77
    knowledge, 73–75, 74*f*
    local god, 73, 76–77
    minds, 72, 425
    moralistic gods, 73, 76–77, 81
    mysteriousness of, 77–78
    as perceived by children, 394, 398
    power, 77–79
    reverence/fear of, 77–78
    as systems, 80
Granth, A., 181 – –75
Gray, K., 377–82
Great Spirit
    dao (Chinese), 72
    karma (Indian), 72, 78, 260–61, 293–94
    mana (Polynesian), 72

manitou (Algonquian), 72
orenda (Iroqouian), 72
wakan tanka (Siouan), 72
grief, 147, 148–50
Griffiths, P., 374–77
group dynamics
    commitment to group, 152–54
    costly signaling, 153–54, 246, 248, 279, 356,
        419, 420–21
    and death practices, 154–56
    and extreme ritual, 243–48
    forming social bonds, 152–54, 421
    group cohesion, 103
    group identification, 152–54, 281–85
    identity fusion, 281–85
    in- and out-group categories, 104
    intergroup competition, 156–57
    prestige bias, 156–57
Guthrie, S., 29, 259, 351–52, 353–54, 372–80,
    381n.20

H

Hadza, 68*f*, 74*f*, 76*f*, 78*f*
Haitian earthquake, 2010
    and divine intervention, 416–17
Hardy, A., 350
hazard precaution system theory, 152,
    363–64
Heaven's Gate, 305, 305n.1
Hell, 3, 221, 262–63
Hierarchical Predictive Coding (HPC), 216,
    219–21, 229
Hinde, R., 351
Hinduism, 257
    religious rituals (puja), 263–64
    and the soul, 262
    and theological correctness, 56–57
homeostasis, 134, 139, 140
    psychological, 134
Hood, R., 217n.2
human
    conception of, 90–91
    human nature, 90
Human Behavioral Ecology of Religion,
    90–91
Human Relations Area Files, 51–52, 148–49,
    152–53, 155, 285–86, 287–88

INDEX

Hypersensitive Agency-Detection Device (HADD). *See* Agency-Detection Device (ADD)
hypnosis, 336–37

I

ideas
  transmission of, 39
identity
  group identification, 152–54, 281–85
  interlevel, 42
  religious, 423
illusion, 336–37
imagistic practices, 53, 239–40, 279–81, 285, 286–87, 289, 292, 293–94, 308–9
imitative learning
  as form of social learning, 395
impurity/contamination, 19, 22
ineffability, 224n.10
inspiration, 51–52, 180
interpretation, 182–87
  interpretive approach, 36
  interpretive process, 183–85
  interpretive traditions, 183
  interpretive-belief hypothesis, 172
introvertive experience, 218, 222–25
intuition, 56–57
  beliefs, 57
  ethical intuition, 100
  intuitive dualism, 93, 412
  intuitive ontologies, 37
  intuitive theism, 354
  materialist intuition, 93
  tripartite intuition, 93, 99–101
Islam, 172, 203, 262, 265–66, 267, 307–8, 310, 377–78, 383–84
  versus informal religious activity, 55
  and mate guarding, 57

J

James, W., 215–16
Jesus, 184, 414, 418–22
Jívaro, 72
Job, (Biblical text), 418–19
Johnson method, 100
Johnson, D., 40, 374–75
Jong, J., 383
Judaism, 201, 203, 384, 386

K

Kahneman, D., 17–18, 412
karma, 72, 78, 260–61, 293–94
Kavanagh, C., 383, 419–20
Kelemen, D., 5–6, 117–19, 123–24, 259–60, 354
Khaldun, I., 278
kibbutzim
  religious rituals and, 419–20
Kim, S., 220–21
knowledge
  attribution of, 74
Kung, H., 307–8
Kwak, C. H., 171

L

Lakota (Sioux), 72
Laudato si' (Praise Be to You), 81–82
laws of nature, 111
Lawson, E. T., 28, 30–31, 175–76, 358–59
Leech, D., 382
Legare, C., 419–21
Levering, M., 169–70
life history theory, 309–10, 311–12
linguistics
  generative linguistics, 16
living things, 111–12, 193–95, 195n.5, 197, 199–200
local enhancement
  as form of social learning, 395
Lord's Prayer, 175. *See also* prayer
Lovu (Pacific people group), 68f, 74f, 76f, 78f
Luhrmann, T., 418

M

M Scale, 217n.2
magic, 138–39, 168, 174, 204–5
  magical belief, 51, 56–59, 342, 401
Magnetic Resonance Imaging (MRI), 327, 331–35, 336–37, 338–40
magnetoencephalography (MEG), 327
Malinowski, B., 138–40, 151–52
Marajó (S. American people group), 68f, 74f, 76f, 78f, 270
Martu (Australia), 81–82
materialist intuition, 93
mating cognition, 268
mating strategies, 267–71
  mate guarding, 271–72
  and religiosity, 269

INDEX

Matsigenka (Peru), 73, 77–78
Mauritius, 68f, 73–74, 74f, 76f, 76–77, 78f
Mazu (goddess, Taiwan), 81
McCauley, R., 27–30, 33–34, 40, 41, 42–43, 175–76, 358–59, 361, 419, 420–23
meaning, 134, 136, 239–40, 363, 413
    effort justification, 240–41
    and memory, 239
medium
    complex, 51–53
memories
    episodic, 239–40, 280
    semantic, 280
methodological naturalism, 381
methodologically holistic, 32–33
mimicry
    as form of social learning, 395
mind, 99–101
    and identity, 96–97
    mind-body dualism (see dualism)
    mind-brain distinction, 94
minimally counterintuitive concepts. See counterintuitive concepts
miracles, 181, 197
misfortune, 51–52, 53–54
modularity, 59
    belief-adjudicating, 58
    modularity hypothesis, 36–37
monism. 93. See also dualism
moralistic gods, 81. See also god(s)
morality, 75n.7, 265, 363
    intuitive morality, 257, 265–67
    moral behavior, 76
    moral cognition, 75–77, 80
    moralizing religions, 267
    sexual morality, 267–71
mortuary practices, 145. See also rituals-death rituals
    acquisition and cultural transmission of, 154–56
    anthropology, 146, 148–49, 150–51
    and community effects, 152–54
    corpse interaction, 150–57
    cultural learning of, 156–57
    disgust, 151
    and evolution, 157–58

and fear, 156
    public ceremonies, 152–53
mortuary rituals. See also death rituals; rituals
    across cultures, 148–50
    corpse interaction, 148, 153–54
    Functions, 148–50
Mueller, F. M., 169
Müller-Lyer illusion, 71
mystical experience, 215, 376–77
    accounts of, 221–22
    definition, 217–18
myths, 82, 262–63, 363. See afterlife accounts; creation accounts

N

N!adima (Kalahari deity), 77–78
narrative themes, 21
natural
    explanations, 133–34
natural geographic areas (NGAs), 287–89
Natural Histories of Discourse, The, 175
naturalism, 37–41
    broad, nonreductionist, emergent, or soft, 42
    methodological naturalism, 41
    ontological naturalism, 41–42
    reductive naturalism, 41–42
    strict, hard, or reductive naturalism, 41–42, 43
    varieties of, 41–43
naturalistic approach, 30–34
naturalness
    maturationally natural, 361–63
naturalness of belief, 382–85, 391–93
naturalness of religion, 260, 303, 361–63, 412–13
nature-nurture debate, 69n.4
neural systems, 331–33
neuroenchantment, 329, 340–42
neurological development, 390–91
neuroscience, 327
    approaches to religion, 329
    versus neurotheology, 328
    and theoretical integration, 342–43
neuroscience of religion
    definition of, 327
    methodological problems, 329–30
Newberg, A. B., 328
non-natural consequence, 198–99, 402. See *also* divine intervention; miracle

438 INDEX

Norenzayan, A., 40, 311–12, 357
North American Association for the Study of Religion (NAASR), 17

O

objects
    and agents, 193–95
    properties of, 193–95
obligation, 363
obsessive-compulsive disorder, 137
Omaha (Ictinike), 80–81
omniscience, 73, 74–75, 79b
ontological categories, 111–14
organized religion. *See* religion
origin stories
    of scripture, 181
orthopraxy, 147

P

patterns
    of mental process, 32
persons, 193–95, 195n.5, 197–98, 200
philosophy, 414
    mechanical philosophy, 43–44
    philosophy of mind, 57
phylogeny, 360, 363, 392
physical and mental states, 102
physics, 41–42
Piaget, J., 115–22
piecemeal approach, 7, 34, 35, 413
Pope Francis, 69
possession, 51–52
power. *See* Great Spirit
Powers, J., 170–73
practice of scriptural authority, 185–86
    textual study, 185–86
    topical study, 186
    transitivity, 187
prayer, 425. *See also* Lord's Prayer
    as perceived by children, 394, 403–4
prediction error, 219, 221, 222, 223, 225, 227, 230
predictive processing framework, 342–43
prelife
    beliefs, 97, 101–3
Preus, S., 14
priest. *See also* religious specialists
    complex, 51–53

principle of superhuman immediacy, 207
propensities to form religious beliefs (PFRBs), 374–77, 381–82
psychedelics, 336
psychological processes
    body independent, 96
psychology
    beginnings, 215–16
    experimental psychology, 331–33, 333b
Psychology of Religion (PoR)
    afterlife experience and beliefs, 4–5
    in contrast to CSR, 3
puja (Hinduism), 263–64
punishment, 55–56, 72, 76, 288–89, 315–16, 354, 363–64
    by the dead, 156
    supernatural punishment theory, 374–75
pure consciousness, 222–23

Q

quintessence, 93, 97–101, 103–4
    and ritual change, 103–4
Qur'an, 177. *See also* sacred texts
    reading of, 176

R

randomness
    concept of, 220–21
Rappaport, R., 179–81, 362
rational choice theory, 373–74
recognition hypothesis, 177
reductionism, 41
reductive physicalism, 93
relational mobility, 291–93
religion
    bad religion, 425–26
    components of, 257
    concept of, 4–5, 48–50, 59–60, 304–6, 413
    hegemony of, 54–56
    historical study of, 55
    identity, 423
    issues in definition, 34
    naturalness of, 260
    organized religion, 59–60
    prehistoric, 50
religionist, 34, 171–72
religiosity, 7, 8, 306

and the brain, 333–35
divergent modes of, theory, 279–81
religious activity, 49–51
informal, 50–53, 55
informal, features of, 50–51
religious affiliation/community, 50
religious anthropology, 54–56
religious behavior
as maladaptive, 355
religious belief
and misattribution, 377–82
religious cognition
denial of, 34
religious explanation vs. interpretation, 30–34
religious features, 50
misleading, 50
religious leaders, 358. *See also* religious specialists
religious organization, 55
emergence, 52–53
religious phenomena and analogy, 336–37, 341
religious practice
and authenticity, 338–40, 340*b*
religious records, 55
religious representation
dark matter, 59–60
religious rituals, 19–20, 267. *See also* rituals
function of religious practices, 15
religious specialists, 50, 51–52, 79*b*
complexes, 51–53
features of, 51–52
lineage elders, 52
magic-religious, 51–53
religious teaching
in child development of religious
cognitions, 400–1
*Rethinking Religion: Connecting Cognition and
Culture* (Lawson & McCauley, 1990)., 263
Rif'at, M., 176
ritual, 136–38, 263, 362, 419–24. *See also*
extreme rituals
baptism, 103–4
causal opacity, 279, 283
child imitation of, 402–4
cognitive foundations of, 258–61
collective, 278–79
death practices, 103–4, 145
definition of, 402–4

doctrinal, 279–81
efficacy of, 402
as evolutionarily adaptive social function, 103
forms of, 264
goal demotion, 279
high-frequency/low-arousal, 280–81, 284–85,
288, 290*f*, 290–91, 291*f*
Hindu, 242, 243–44
imagistic, 279–81
kavadi, 33, 241, 243–44
low-frequency/high-arousal, 279–81, 283,
284, 284*f*, 290–91
in medical treatment, 139–40
membership/initiation rituals, 266
and memory, 239–40
and minimally counterintuitive concepts,
263–64
psychological mechanisms of, 152
and quintessence, 103–4
repetition of, 136–38
ritual form hypothesis, 202–3
sacrifice, 423–24
as shared religious activity, 402–4
and social bonds, 419–20, 423–24
special agent rituals (SARs), 202–3, 206,
209, 263–64, 422–23
and special instrument rituals (SIRs)., 202–3,
206, 209, 263–64
and special objects, 206
special patient rituals (SPRs), 202–3, 206,
263–64, 422–24
text-performance, 176
transmission of, 154–56
ritual action
and special objects, 202–3
ritual action representation system, 402
ritual behavior
apophatic, 222–24, 223nn.7–8, 224n.9
ritual form hypothesis (RFH), 202–3, 420,
422–23
ritual form theory, 363–64
ritualized behaviors, 19
Robertson-Smith, W., 278
Roman Catholic groups
Benedictines, 421–22
Franciscans, 421–22
Rozin, P., 57

440 INDEX

S
sacred, 363
sacred books of the East, 169
sacred objects, *See* special objects
sacred texts, 79*b*, 167, *See also* Bible; Qur'an
  Bible, 167, 174
  fixity of, 171
  Qur'an, 169–70, 175, 176, 177
  Torah, 167, 176
sacred ultimate sacred postulates, 179–80
sacrifice, 3, 423–24
science of religion
  study of, 30
ScienceTeller conference, 3
scriptural authority
  grounded, 179–81
  implications, 188
  principle of, 178–81
  and transitivity, 185–87
  and unification, 179
scriptural explanation, 172, 173
scriptural foundationalism, 172–73, 180
  and scripturalist communities, 172
scriptural uniqueness, 181–82
scripturalism, 167
  and authority, 167, 168, 170–73
  as a cultural tradition, 167–68
  community, 168
  definitional problem, 169–70
  and ritual, 168
  as set of named hypotheses, 168
  transmission, 168
scripture
  authority, 178–81
  compilation of, 171
  fixity of, 171
  hermeneutic prescription, 182–85
  interpretation of, 182
  interpretive process, 182–85
  intuitive notions of, 169–70
  origin stories, 181
  scriptural uniqueness, 181–82
  self-reference, 179
  traditional interpretation, 182–85
  traditions about, 178–82
  and unification, 179
scripture citation, 182–87

scripture interpretation, 182–87. *See also* interpretation
scripture-artifact, 175–76
scripture-concepts, 177–78
  distinctiveness, 178
  recognition, 177
  unification, 177
scripture-performances, 176
Scriptures of the World's Religions, 170–73
secularization, 303–4, 310–14
sense of control, 138–40, 241–42
  and death practices, 146
  illusion of control, 139
  and scripture-performance, 176
  and threat, 150–57
sensus divinitatis, 384
sexual activity, 267–71, 356
  and religiosity, 268–69
Shaman
  Shaman and healer complex, 51–52, 53
  Shamanism, 51
Shariff, A., 3
Silverstein, M., 175
Simplicity Principle, 197–98
sin, 315–16, 418–19, 423–24
  original sin, 414
Smith, W. C., 170
social cohesion, 67
social learning, 395–96
social synchrony, 278–79
social technology
  extreme ritual, 247
socially strategic information, 75
sociology
  social facts, 32–34
  sociological approaches, 32–33
solid objects, 193–95, 195n.5, 197–98, 199–200
Sørensen, J., 58–59, 136, 138, 195–96, 199–200, 204, 207
Sosis, R., 356
soul, 97, 99–101
  Christian concept of, 262
  and ethical reasoning, 100
  Hindu concept of, 262
  Muslim concept of, 262
special agents, 197–99, 263–64
special entities, 193–95, 195n.5, 197, 199–200

INDEX

special objects, 191
  agential, 199–200, 206
  altar, 191
  ark of the Covenant, 201
  definition, 192–200
  distinguishing, 195–97
  Eucharist (holy communion), 191, 206,
    206n.10
  holy water, 191, 195, 196, 202–3, 206, 208–9
  icon, 197
  interpretation concerns, 204–5
  invisible and intangible objects, 199n.9
  and magic, 204–5
  means of change, 208–9
  origin of, 201–5
  power or efficacy, 207–8
  relics, 203
  in rituals, 206
  types, 199–200
  vestments, 203
spells, 176
Sperber, D., 57, 180
spider god, 80–81
spirits, 51, 54, 425. *See also* supernatural agents
  fear of, 155
spiritualists, 101
Stace, W., 217–18
standard social science model, 33
Stark, R., 359
statements of scriptural authority, 172–73
Strassmann, B. I., 356
superhuman agents. *See* supernatural agents
superhuman effects, 175–76, 402. *See also* miracles
supernatural
  explanations, 133
  powers, 134
supernatural action
  and special objects, 201–2
supernatural agency
  "Big Gods", 288–89, 309
  belief in, 382–85
  and events, 416
  supernatural agents, 51, 54, 55–56, 59, 67, 134,
    196, 197, 198–99, 201–2, 206, 207–8, 221,
    223–24, 266, 267, 363, 399–400, 402, 403–4,
    411, 413, 423–24
  fear of, 155, 156

  high gods, 288–89
  moralizing gods, 289–91
supernatural monitoring theory, 360
supernatural phenomena, 135–40
Sword, G., 72

T

taboo, 363
Tamil Hindus
  religious rituals and, 419–20
Tanna (Pacific people group)
  Inland Tanna, 68*f*, 74*f*, 76*f*, 78*f*
  Coastal Tanna, 68*f*, 74*f*, 78*f*
Taves, A., 44
Taylor, C., 310–14
teaching
  as form of social learning, 395
teleological explanations, 259–61
teleological thinking, 412
teleology, 354, 398
  teleo-functioning reasoning, 115–22
  teleological reasoning, 117–18, 119–22, 124,
    415–19
  and theology, 415–19
text, 174–75, 174n.1, 262–63. *See also* sacred texts
  distinctions of, 174–75
  text-artifact, 175–76
  text-performance, 176
theodicy, 50
theological correctness, 56–57
  orthodoxy, 20
theology
  Christian theology, 411–13, 414–19
  concept of, 413
  corrective application of information, 416–18
  and CSR, 413
  generative application of information,
    418–24
  and other disciplines, 414
  and teleological reasoning, 415–19
theory of mind (ToM), 18, 74–75, 92–96, 104,
    112, 258, 259, 354, 362, 412, 425
  and MCI concepts, 113–14
  and agency-detection device (ADD), 114–15
  general-purpose learning machine vs
    collection of specialized systems, 35–37
  or "intentionality system", 72

442 INDEX

thick descriptions, 37–38
things
  ontological categories of, 194
Tillich, P., 307–8
Tinbergen, N., 360
top-down cognition, 241–42
Torah
  reading of, 176
tradition
  "great" and "little", 55
  wild tradition, 50–53, 55 (*see also* religious
    activity: informal)
trance, 51–52
transcranial direct-current stimulation
  (TDCS), 327
transcranial magnetic stimulation (TMS),
  80–81, 327
trickster, 80–81
tripartite intuition, 99–101. *See also* dualism
  tripartite concept, 93, 101
Tripitaka, 177
Tsembaga (Papua New Guinea), 81–82
Tylor, E.B., 215–16
Tyva Republic, 68*f*, 73, 74*f*, 76*f*, 76, 78*f*

U

ultimate sacred postulates, 179–81
  explicit transmission, 180
  generativity, 180
  symbolism, 180
unexpectedness
  concept of, 220–21
unification hypothesis, 177, 179
  in relation to canon, 177
universals, 71–79
Urban, G., 175

V

Vineyard congregations, 417–18
Visala, A., 382, 383
voodoo, 208–9, 341

W

Wakan Tanka (Siouan), 72, 377–82. *See also*
  great spirit
WEIRD (Western, educated, industrialized,
  rich, and democratic) societies, 312
What is Scripture? (Smith, 1993), 170
When God Talks Back (Luhrmann, 2012), 417–18
Whitehouse, H., 29, 53, 285–86, 287, 358–59,
  363–64, 419–20
Wicked Bible, The, 181
wild religion, 59–60. *See also* religious activity:
  informal
Wilkins, J.
  evolutionary debunking arguments (2013),
    374–77
Wilson, A., 171
Wilson, D.S., 351, 357, 359
Wilson, E.O., 351
Winkelman, M.J., 351, 357, 359
Winternitz, M., 169
Wishpoosh (American Pacific Northwest),
  80–81. *See also* gods
witchcraft, 53–54, 102–3, 341
*World Scripture: A Comparative Anthology of
  Sacred Texts*, 171

X

Xygalatas, D., 9, 237, 419–21

Y

Yasawa (Pacific), 68*f*, 73–74, 74*f*, 76*f*, 76–77, 78*f*